Nutritional Management and Outcomes in Malnourished Medical Inpatients

Nutritional Management and Outcomes in Malnourished Medical Inpatients

Special Issue Editors

Zeno Stanga
Philipp Schuetz

MDPI • Basel • Beijing • Wuhan • Barcelona • Belgrade • Manchester • Tokyo • Cluj • Tianjin

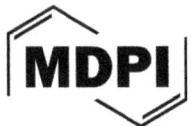

Special Issue Editors

Zeno Stanga
Bern University Hospital
Switzerland

Philipp Schuetz
Aarau and Medical Faculty of the University of Basel
Switzerland

Editorial Office
MDPI
St. Alban-Anlage 66
4052 Basel, Switzerland

This is a reprint of articles from the Special Issue published online in the open access journal *Journal of Clinical Medicine* (ISSN 2077-0383) (available at: https://www.mdpi.com/journal/jcm/special_issues/Nutritional_Malnourished_Medical).

For citation purposes, cite each article independently as indicated on the article page online and as indicated below:

LastName, A.A.; LastName, B.B.; LastName, C.C. Article Title. *Journal Name* **Year**, *Article Number*, Page Range.

ISBN 978-3-03936-491-6 (Hbk)
ISBN 978-3-03936-492-3 (PDF)

Cover image courtesy of Archive Nutritional Medicine, University Hospital Bern, Switzerland.

© 2020 by the authors. Articles in this book are Open Access and distributed under the Creative Commons Attribution (CC BY) license, which allows users to download, copy and build upon published articles, as long as the author and publisher are properly credited, which ensures maximum dissemination and a wider impact of our publications.

The book as a whole is distributed by MDPI under the terms and conditions of the Creative Commons license CC BY-NC-ND.

Contents

About the Special Issue Editors ix

Philipp Schuetz and Zeno Stanga
Nutritional Management and Outcomes in Malnourished Medical Inpatients in 2020: The Evidence Is Growing!
Reprinted from: *J. Clin. Med.* **2020**, *9*, 27, doi:10.3390/jcm9010027 1

Michael Hiesmayr, Silvia Tarantino, Sigrid Moick, Alessandro Laviano, Isabella Sulz, Mohamed Mouhieddine, Christian Schuh, Dorothee Volkert, Judit Simon and Karin Schindler
Hospital Malnutrition, a Call for Political Action: A Public Health and NutritionDay Perspective
Reprinted from: *J. Clin. Med.* **2019**, *8*, 2048, doi:10.3390/jcm8122048 5

Lena J. Storck, Reinhard Imoberdorf and Peter E. Ballmer
Nutrition in Gastrointestinal Disease: Liver, Pancreatic, and Inflammatory Bowel Disease
Reprinted from: *J. Clin. Med.* **2019**, *8*, 1098, doi:10.3390/jcm8081098 23

Emilie Reber, Kristina Norman, Olga Endrich, Philipp Schuetz, Andreas Frei and Zeno Stanga
Economic Challenges in Nutritional Management
Reprinted from: *J. Clin. Med.* **2019**, *8*, 1005, doi:10.3390/jcm8071005 37

Marina V. Viana, Olivier Pantet, Geraldine Bagnoud, Arianne Martinez, Eva Favre, Mélanie Charrière, Doris Favre, Philippe Eckert and Mette M. Berger
Metabolic and Nutritional Characteristics of Long-Stay Critically Ill Patients
Reprinted from: *J. Clin. Med.* **2019**, *8*, 985, doi:10.3390/jcm8070985 53

Peter J.M. Weijs, Kris M. Mogensen, James D. Rawn and Kenneth B. Christopher
Protein Intake, Nutritional Status and Outcomes in ICU Survivors: A Single Center Cohort Study
Reprinted from: *J. Clin. Med.* **2019**, *8*, 43, doi:10.3390/jcm8010043 71

Paweł Wiech, Dariusz Bazaliński, Izabela Sałacińska, Monika Binkowska-Bury, Bartosz Korczowski, Artur Mazur, Maria Kózka and Mariusz Dabrowski
Decreased Bioelectrical Impedance Phase Angle in Hospitalized Children and Adolescents with Newly Diagnosed Type 1 Diabetes: A Case-Control Study
Reprinted from: *J. Clin. Med.* **2018**, *7*, 516, doi:10.3390/jcm7120516 81

Emilie Reber, Natalie Friedli, Maria F. Vasiloglou, Philipp Schuetz and Zeno Stanga
Management of Refeeding Syndrome in Medical Inpatients
Reprinted from: *J. Clin. Med.* **2019**, *8*, 2202, doi:10.3390/jcm8122202 93

Emilie Reber, Markus Messerli, Zeno Stanga and Stefan Mühlebach
Pharmaceutical Aspects of Artificial Nutrition
Reprinted from: *J. Clin. Med.* **2019**, *8*, 2017, doi:10.3390/jcm8112017 111

Jessica Stirnimann and Guido Stirnimann
Nutritional Challenges in Patients with Advanced Liver Cirrhosis
Reprinted from: *J. Clin. Med.* **2019**, *8*, 1926, doi:10.3390/jcm8111926 133

Emilie Reber, Filomena Gomes, Ilka A. Dähn, Maria F. Vasiloglou and Zeno Stanga
Management of Dehydration in Patients Suffering Swallowing Difficulties
Reprinted from: *J. Clin. Med.* **2019**, *8*, 1923, doi:10.3390/jcm8111923 . . . . **145**

Maria F. Vasiloglou, Jane Fletcher and Kalliopi-Anna Poulia
Challenges and Perspectives in Nutritional Counselling and Nursing: A Narrative Review
Reprinted from: *J. Clin. Med.* **2019**, *8*, 1489, doi:10.3390/jcm8091489 . . . . **165**

Andrea Kopp Lugli, Aude de Watteville, Alexa Hollinger, Nicole Goetz and Claudia Heidegger
Medical Nutrition Therapy in Critically Ill Patients Treated on Intensive and Intermediate Care Units: A Literature Review
Reprinted from: *J. Clin. Med.* **2019**, *8*, 1395, doi:10.3390/jcm8091395 . . . . **175**

Marta Delsoglio, Najate Achamrah, Mette M. Berger and Claude Pichard
Indirect Calorimetry in Clinical Practice
Reprinted from: *J. Clin. Med.* **2019**, *8*, 1387, doi:10.3390/jcm8091387 . . . . **193**

Irene Hoyas and Miguel Leon-Sanz
Nutritional Challenges in Metabolic Syndrome
Reprinted from: *J. Clin. Med.* **2019**, *8*, 1301, doi:10.3390/jcm8091301 . . . . **213**

Emilie Reber, Rachel Strahm, Lia Bally, Philipp Schuetz and Zeno Stanga
Efficacy and Efficiency of Nutritional Support Teams
Reprinted from: *J. Clin. Med.* **2019**, *8*, 1281, doi:10.3390/jcm8091281 . . . . **225**

Paula Ravasco
Nutrition in Cancer Patients
Reprinted from: *J. Clin. Med.* **2019**, *8*, 1211, doi:10.3390/jcm8081211 . . . . **243**

Emilie Reber, Filomena Gomes, Lia Bally, Philipp Schuetz and Zeno Stanga
Nutritional Management of Medical Inpatients
Reprinted from: *J. Clin. Med.* **2019**, *8*, 1130, doi:10.3390/jcm8081130 . . . . **257**

Stephan R. Vavricka and Thomas Greuter
Gastroparesis and Dumping Syndrome: Current Concepts and Management
Reprinted from: *J. Clin. Med.* **2019**, *8*, 1127, doi:10.3390/jcm8081127 . . . . **269**

Emilie Reber, Filomena Gomes, Maria F. Vasiloglou, Philipp Schuetz and Zeno Stanga
Nutritional Risk Screening and Assessment
Reprinted from: *J. Clin. Med.* **2019**, *8*, 1065, doi:10.3390/jcm8071065 . . . . **283**

Cristina Cuerda, Maria F. Vasiloglou and Loredana Arhip
Nutritional Management and Outcomes in Malnourished Medical Inpatients:
Anorexia Nervosa
Reprinted from: *J. Clin. Med.* **2019**, *8*, 1042, doi:10.3390/jcm8071042 . . . . **303**

Julie Mareschal, Najate Achamrah, Kristina Norman and Laurence Genton
Clinical Value of Muscle Mass Assessment in Clinical Conditions Associated with Malnutrition
Reprinted from: *J. Clin. Med.* **2019**, *8*, 1040, doi:10.3390/jcm8071040 . . . . **321**

Dorothee Volkert, Anne Marie Beck, Tommy Cederholm, Emanuele Cereda, Alfonso Cruz-Jentoft, Sabine Goisser, Lisette de Groot, Franz Großhauser, Eva Kiesswetter, Kristina Norman, et al.
Management of Malnutrition in Older Patients—Current Approaches, Evidence and Open Questions
Reprinted from: *J. Clin. Med.* **2019**, *8*, 974, doi:10.3390/jcm8070974 . . . . **341**

Céline Isabelle Laesser, Paul Cumming, Emilie Reber, Zeno Stanga, Taulant Muka and Lia Bally
Management of Glucose Control in Noncritically Ill, Hospitalized Patients Receiving Parenteral and/or Enteral Nutrition: A Systematic Review
Reprinted from: *J. Clin. Med.* **2019**, *8*, 935, doi:10.3390/jcm8070935 . . . . **357**

Mette M Berger, Olivier Pantet, Antoine Schneider and Nawfel Ben-Hamouda
.Micronutrient Deficiencies in Medical and Surgical Inpatients
Reprinted from: *J. Clin. Med.* **2019**, *8*, 931, doi:10.3390/jcm8070931 . . . . **375**

An Jacobs, Ines Verlinden, Ilse Vanhorebeek and Greet Van den Berghe
Early Supplemental Parenteral Nutrition in Critically Ill Children: An Update
Reprinted from: *J. Clin. Med.* **2019**, *8*, 830, doi:10.3390/jcm8060830 . . . . **393**

Ulrich Keller
Nutritional Laboratory Markers in Malnutrition
Reprinted from: *J. Clin. Med.* **2019**, *8*, 775, doi:10.3390/jcm8060775 . . . . **405**

About the Special Issue Editors

Zeno Stanga studied medicine at the University of Bern and obtained board certification in internal and general medicine in 1995. He trained in general internal medicine, nutritional medicine and metabolism in several hospitals in Switzerland. After research fellowships in Nottingham (U.K.) and Charleston (USA), he founded a nutritional support team in 2001 and leads the nutritional medicine unit at the University Hospital of Bern. He is currently associate professor for internal and nutritional medicine at the Medical Faculty of the University of Bern. He is a member of the appointment commission and active in several working groups of the medical faculty. Professor Stanga was responsible for the Swiss Certificate of Advanced Studies in Clinical Nutrition and acted on the board of directors of the Swiss Society of Clinical Nutrition for 20 years. He has published over 150 scientific papers and is associate editor of the ESPEN Blue Book.

Philipp Schuetz was born in Switzerland and studied Medicine at the University of Basel, Switzerland, and the University Kremlin Bicetre in Paris, France. He is a board-certified internist and endocrinologist with special interest in clinical nutrition. He is the head of internal medicine and emergency medicine Kantonsspital Aarau and part of the faculty of medicine at the university in Basel, Switzerland. He has published more than 300 studies and research articles in high-impact journals including *Lancet, JAMA, Annals of Internal Medicine,* and many others. Prof. Schuetz obtained a research professorship from the Swiss National Science Foundation (SNF) and was principal investigator of the EFFORT trial, the largest-yet randomized controlled trial examining the clinical effects of clinical nutrition in medical ward patients.

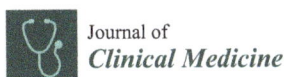

Editorial

Nutritional Management and Outcomes in Malnourished Medical Inpatients in 2020: The Evidence Is Growing!

Philipp Schuetz [1,2,*] and Zeno Stanga [3]

1 Department of Endocrinology, Diabetes and Clinical Nutrition, University Department of Internal Medicine, Kantonsspital, CH-5001 Aarau, Switzerland
2 Medical Faculty of the University of Basel, CH-4056 Basel, Switzerland
3 Department of Diabetes, Endocrinology, Nutritional Medicine and Metabolism, Inselspital, Bern University Hospital, and University of Bern, CH-3008 Bern, Switzerland; Zeno.Stanga@insel.ch
* Correspondence: Philipp.Schuetz@unibas.ch

Received: 16 December 2019; Accepted: 18 December 2019; Published: 20 December 2019

Access to adequate food is a fundamental human right. There is no doubt that nutrition is essential in maintaining health and preventing or treating disease. Particularly when patients are affected by disease-related malnutrition, their risk of adverse clinical outcomes increases significantly and optimizing nutritional support becomes mandatory [1,2].

There is ongoing debate about what constitutes an optimal nutritional care process in terms of screening, assessment, and use of nutritional support in different patient populations. Issues include dose and quality of proteins and total energy, route of delivery, and whether or how nutritional support needs to be adjusted for specific medical and metabolic conditions. As we move toward personalized medicine, which is based on patients' individual needs, an understanding of these different factors is important. Well-planned clinical studies of high methodological quality are needed to develop the best approach to providing individualized nutritional support [3].

Historically, much of the evidence regarding effects of nutritional support has come from small interventional trials and observational studies with cross-sectional or cohort-study designs, whereas there was an important lack of large-scale randomized interventional research, which is needed to establish causal effects rather than just statistical associations [4,5]. As a consequence, the medical community has struggled to design efficient, evidence-based approaches for the prevention and treatment of malnutrition [4].

Recently, however, the results of several high-quality trials have provided important new insights that advance nutritional science significantly and translate nutrition research into practice [6]. Regarding prevention of cardiovascular disease through nutrition, the PREDIMED (Prevención con Dieta Mediterránea) trial provided strong evidence that a Mediterranean diet supplemented with extra-virgin olive oil or with mixed nuts reduces the risk of cardiovascular and metabolic disease by about 30% over five years [7]. Regarding the use of clinical nutrition in patients at nutritional risk or with established malnutrition, two trials found nutritional support to be highly effective. First, the multicenter, randomized, placebo-controlled NOURISH trial (Nutrition effect On Unplanned ReadmIssions and Survival in Hospitalized patients) including 652 older adults affected by malnutrition found that a high-protein oral nutritional supplement containing beta-hydroxy-beta-methylbutyrate was associated with a significant reduction in 90 day mortality, with a number needed to treat (NNT) of 20 [8]. Second, the EFFORT (Effect of early nutritional support on Frailty, Functional Outcomes and Recovery of malnourished medical inpatients Trial) including 2028 medical inpatients at nutritional risk in eight Swiss hospitals showed that protocol-guided individualized nutritional support designed to achieve protein and energy targets results in significantly lower rates of severe complications (NNT = 25) and mortality (NNT = 37) compared to regular hospital food [9,10]. Moreover, functional decline was significantly lower, and quality of life as well as activities of daily living significantly improved. A recent meta-analysis including these two trials and several other trials also came to the conclusion that nutritional support in the malnourished medical inpatient population reduces the risk for both, mortality and hospital readmission by about 25% [6].

Evidence-based medicine is an approach used to optimize decision-making by emphasizing evidence from properly designed and well-conducted research, typically randomized trials and meta-analyses from such trials. With the growing number of high-quality trials such as the ones mentioned above, we are increasingly able to practice "evidence-based clinical nutrition" and to adapt nutrition to the individual patient's needs. This Special Issue of the *Journal of Clinical Medicine* (JCM) focuses on a topic that is critical for hospitals today: "Nutritional Management and Outcomes in Malnourished Medical Inpatients". This special edition presents a number of reviews and original research articles in the field of nutritional management and clinical outcomes in malnourished medical inpatients. Twenty-six important articles illustrate the different facets of this complex and timely topic.

The articles included cover the process of nutritional care, including screening tools to identify nutritional risk (Nutritional risk screening and assessment [11]), patient muscle mass assessment including bioimpedance analysis (Clinical value of muscle mass assessment in clinical conditions associated with malnutrition [12]; Decreased bioelectrical impedance phase angle in hospitalized children and adolescents with newly diagnosed type 1 diabetes: a case-control study [13]), nutritional biomarkers (Nutritional laboratory markers in malnutrition [14]), nutritional therapy planning (Indirect calorimetry in clinical practice [15]; Micronutrient deficiencies in medical and surgical inpatients [16]), use of nutritional support overall (Efficacy and efficiency of nutritional support teams [17]; Challenges and perspectives in nutritional counselling and nursing: a narrative review [18]) and in specific patient populations (e.g., medical patients, critical care patients, geriatric patients, oncologic patients, patients after allogenic stem cell transplantation, patients with dysphagia or eating disorders, as well as the nutritional challenges associated with metabolic disorders) (Nutritional management of medical inpatients [19]; Medical nutrition therapy in critically ill patients treated on intensive and intermediate care units: a literature review [20]; Metabolic and nutritional characteristics of long-stay critically ill patients [21]; Protein intake, nutritional status, and outcomes in intensive care unit survivors: a single-center cohort study [22]; Early supplemental parenteral nutrition in critically ill children: an update [23]; Management of malnutrition in older patients—current approaches, evidence, and open questions [24]; Nutrition in cancer patients [25]; Management of dehydration in patients suffering swallowing difficulties [26]; Nutrition in gastrointestinal diseases: liver, pancreatic, and inflammatory bowel diseases [27]; Nutritional management and outcomes in malnourished medical inpatients: anorexia nervosa [28]; Nutritional challenges in metabolic syndrome [29]; Nutritional challenges in patients with advanced liver cirrhosis [30]). Potential complications of nutritional interventions, such as refeeding syndrome (Management of refeeding syndrome in medical inpatients [31]), and treatment challenges posed by gastric motility disorders are discussed (Gastroparesis and dumping syndrome: current concepts and management [32]). Economic aspects of nutritional management (Economic challenges in nutritional management [33]) and specific considerations such as pharmaceutical/therapeutic aspects of artificial nutrition are additionally reviewed (Management of glucose control in non-critically ill, hospitalized patients receiving parenteral and/or enteral nutrition: a systematic review [34]; Pharmaceutical aspects of artificial nutrition [35]).

Last but not least, the call for political commitment in the treatment of malnutrition is of key importance. Health care institutions and associations must be mobilized to take action against malnutrition by expanding information and public-awareness-raising campaigns, adopting supportive policies, as well as allocating resources (Hospital malnutrition, a call for political action: a public health and nutritionDay perspective [36]). Stakeholders including political organizations, nutritional social networks, and researchers will be valuable promoters of this important political priority in the future.

Understanding the optimal use of nutritional therapy is highly complex. Timing, route of delivery, and the amount and type of nutrients all play important roles and potentially affect patient outcomes. Recent trials provide important information to strengthen the evidence regarding the use of nutritional therapy in specific patient populations, but there are still important questions to be addressed by robust clinical trials in the future. It is now important to incorporate these recent findings into clinical practice in order to ensure that our patients receive high-quality, safe, and optimal care.

Author Contributions: P.S. and Z.S. wrote this article and take full responsibility for its content. All authors have read and agreed to the published version of the manuscript.

Funding: The article processing charge was funded by the Research Fund of the Department of Diabetes, Endocrinology, Nutritional Medicine, and Metabolism and in part by Nestlé Health Science.

Conflicts of Interest: The authors declare no conflict of interest.

References

1. Felder, S.; Lechtenboehmer, C.; Bally, M.; Fehr, R.; Deiss, M.; Faessler, L.; Kutz, A.; Steiner, D.; Rast, A.C.; Laukemann, S.; et al. Association of nutritional risk and adverse medical outcomes across different medical inpatient populations. *Nutrition* **2015**, *31*, 1385–1393. [CrossRef] [PubMed]
2. Felder, S.; Braun, N.; Stanga, Z.; Kulkarni, P.; Faessler, L.; Kutz, A.; Steiner, D.; Laukemann, S.; Haubitz, S.; Huber, A.; et al. Unraveling the Link between Malnutrition and Adverse Clinical Outcomes: Association of Acute and Chronic Malnutrition Measures with Blood Biomarkers from Different Pathophysiological States. *Ann. Nutr. Metab.* **2016**, *68*, 164–172. [CrossRef] [PubMed]
3. Merker, M.; Gomes, F.; Stanga, Z.; Schuetz, P. Evidence-based nutrition for the malnourished, hospitalised patient: One bite at a time. *Swiss Med. Wkly.* **2019**, *149*, w20112. [CrossRef] [PubMed]
4. Schuetz, P. Food for thought: Why does the medical community struggle with research about nutritional therapy in the acute care setting? *BMC Med.* **2017**, *15*, 38. [CrossRef]
5. Ioannidis, J.P.A. The Challenge of Reforming Nutritional Epidemiologic Research. *JAMA* **2018**, *320*, 969–970. [CrossRef]
6. Gomes, F.; Baumgartner, A.; Bounoure, L.; Bally, M.; Deutz, N.E.; Greenwald, J.L.; Stanga, Z.; Mueller, B.; Schuetz, P. Association of nutritional support with clinical outcomes among hospitalized medical patients: an updated systematic review and meta-analysis. *JAMA Netw. Open* **2019**, *2*, e1915138. [CrossRef]
7. Estruch, R.; Ros, E.; Salas-Salvado, J.; Covas, M.I.; Corella, D.; Aros, F.; Gomez-Gracia, E.; Ruiz-Gutierrez, V.; Fiol, M.; Lapetra, J.; et al. Primary Prevention of Cardiovascular Disease with a Mediterranean Diet Supplemented with Extra-Virgin Olive Oil or Nuts. *N. Engl. J. Med.* **2018**, *378*, e34. [CrossRef]
8. Deutz, N.E.; Matheson, E.M.; Matarese, L.E.; Luo, M.; Baggs, G.E.; Nelson, J.L.; Hegazi, R.A.; Tappenden, K.A.; Ziegler, T.R. Readmission and mortality in malnourished, older, hospitalized adults treated with a specialized oral nutritional supplement: A randomized clinical trial. *Clin. Nutr.* **2016**, *35*, 18–26. [CrossRef]
9. Schuetz, P.; Fehr, R.; Baechli, V.; Geiser, M.; Gomes, F.; Kutz, A.; Tribolet, P.; Bregenzer, T.; Hoess, C.; Pavlicek, V.; et al. Individualized nutritional support in medical inpatients at nutritional risk: A randomized clinical trial. *Lancet* **2019**, *393*, 2312–2321. [CrossRef]
10. Schuetz, P.; Fehr, R.; Baechli, V.; Geiser, M.; Gomes, F.; Kutz, A.; Tribolet, P.; Bregenzer, T.; Hoess, C.; Pavlicek, V.; et al. Design and rationale of the effect of early nutritional therapy on frailty, functional outcomes and recovery of malnourished medical inpatients (EFFORT): A pragmatic, multicenter, randomized-controlled trial. *Int. J. Clin. Trials* **2018**, *5*, 142–150. [CrossRef]
11. Reber, E.; Gomes, F.; Vasiloglou, M.F.; Schuetz, P.; Stanga, Z. Nutritional Risk Screening and Assessment. *J. Clin. Med.* **2019**, *8*, 1065. [CrossRef] [PubMed]
12. Mareschal, J.; Achamrah, N.; Norman, K.; Genton, L. Clinical Value of Muscle Mass Assessment in Clinical Conditions Associated with Malnutrition. *J. Clin. Med.* **2019**, *8*, 1040. [CrossRef] [PubMed]
13. Wiech, P.; Bazalinski, D.; Salacinska, I.; Binkowska-Bury, M.; Korczowski, B.; Mazur, A.; Kozka, M.; Dabrowski, M. Decreased Bioelectrical Impedance Phase Angle in Hospitalized Children and Adolescents with Newly Diagnosed Type 1 Diabetes: A Case-Control Study. *J. Clin. Med.* **2018**, *7*, 516. [CrossRef] [PubMed]
14. Keller, U. Nutritional Laboratory Markers in Malnutrition. *J. Clin. Med.* **2019**, *8*, 775. [CrossRef]

15. Delsoglio, M.; Achamrah, N.; Berger, M.M.; Pichard, C. Indirect Calorimetry in Clinical Practice. *J. Clin. Med.* **2019**, *8*, 1387. [CrossRef]
16. Berger, M.M.; Pantet, O.; Schneider, A.; Ben-Hamouda, N. Micronutrient Deficiencies in Medical and Surgical Inpatients. *J. Clin. Med.* **2019**, *8*, 931. [CrossRef]
17. Reber, E.; Strahm, R.; Bally, L.; Schuetz, P.; Stanga, Z. Efficacy and Efficiency of Nutritional Support Teams. *J. Clin. Med.* **2019**, *8*, 1281. [CrossRef]
18. Vasiloglou, M.F.; Fletcher, J.; Poulia, K.A. Challenges and Perspectives in Nutritional Counselling and Nursing: A Narrative Review. *J. Clin. Med.* **2019**, *8*, 1489. [CrossRef]
19. Reber, E.; Gomes, F.; Bally, L.; Schuetz, P.; Stanga, Z. Nutritional Management of Medical Inpatients. *J. Clin. Med.* **2019**, *8*, 1130. [CrossRef]
20. Kopp Lugli, A.; de Watteville, A.; Hollinger, A.; Goetz, N.; Heidegger, C. Medical Nutrition Therapy in Critically Ill Patients Treated on Intensive and Intermediate Care Units: A Literature Review. *J. Clin. Med.* **2019**, *8*, 1395. [CrossRef]
21. Viana, M.V.; Pantet, O.; Bagnoud, G.; Martinez, A.; Favre, E.; Charriere, M.; Favre, D.; Eckert, P.; Berger, M.M. Metabolic and Nutritional Characteristics of Long-Stay Critically Ill Patients. *J. Clin. Med.* **2019**, *8*, 985. [CrossRef] [PubMed]
22. Weijs, P.J.M.; Mogensen, K.M.; Rawn, J.D.; Christopher, K.B. Protein Intake, Nutritional Status and Outcomes in ICU Survivors: A Single Center Cohort Study. *J. Clin. Med.* **2019**, *8*, 43. [CrossRef] [PubMed]
23. Jacobs, A.; Verlinden, I.; Vanhorebeek, I.; Van den Berghe, G. Early Supplemental Parenteral Nutrition in Critically Ill Children: An Update. *J. Clin. Med.* **2019**, *8*, 830. [CrossRef] [PubMed]
24. Volkert, D.; Beck, A.M.; Cederholm, T.; Cereda, E.; Cruz-Jentoft, A.; Goisser, S.; de Groot, L.; Grosshauser, F.; Kiesswetter, E.; Norman, K.; et al. Management of Malnutrition in Older Patients-Current Approaches, Evidence and Open Questions. *J. Clin. Med.* **2019**, *8*, 974. [CrossRef]
25. Ravasco, P. Nutrition in Cancer Patients. *J. Clin. Med.* **2019**, *8*, 1211. [CrossRef]
26. Reber, E.; Gomes, F.; Daehn, I.; Vasiloglou, M.F.; Stanga, Z. Management of Dehydration in Patients Suffering Swallowing Difficulties. *J. Clin. Med.* **2019**, *8*, 1923. [CrossRef]
27. Storck, L.J.; Imoberdorf, R.; Ballmer, P.E. Nutrition in Gastrointestinal Disease: Liver, Pancreatic, and Inflammatory Bowel Disease. *J. Clin. Med.* **2019**, *8*, 1098. [CrossRef]
28. Cuerda, C.; Vasiloglou, M.F.; Arhip, L. Nutritional Management and Outcomes in Malnourished Medical Inpatients: Anorexia Nervosa. *J. Clin. Med.* **2019**, *8*, 1042. [CrossRef]
29. Hoyas, I.; Leon-Sanz, M. Nutritional Challenges in Metabolic Syndrome. *J. Clin. Med.* **2019**, *8*, 1301. [CrossRef]
30. Stirnimann, J.; Stirnimann, G. Nutritional challenges in patients with advanced liver cirrhosis. *J. Clin. Med.* **2019**, *8*, 1926. [CrossRef]
31. Reber, E.; Friedli, N.; Vasiloglou, M.F.; Schuetz, P.; Stanga, Z. Management of refeeding syndrome in medical inpatients. *J. Clin. Med.* **2019**, *8*, 8614. [CrossRef] [PubMed]
32. Vavricka, S.R.; Greuter, T. Gastroparesis and Dumping Syndrome: Current Concepts and Management. *J. Clin. Med.* **2019**, *8*, 1127. [CrossRef] [PubMed]
33. Reber, E.; Norman, K.; Endrich, O.; Schuetz, P.; Frei, A.; Stanga, Z. Economic Challenges in Nutritional Management. *J. Clin. Med.* **2019**, *8*, 1005. [CrossRef] [PubMed]
34. Laesser, C.I.; Cumming, P.; Reber, E.; Stanga, Z.; Muka, T.; Bally, L. Management of Glucose Control in Noncritically Ill, Hospitalized Patients Receiving Parenteral and/or Enteral Nutrition: A Systematic Review. *J. Clin. Med.* **2019**, *8*, 935. [CrossRef]
35. Reber, E.; Messerli, M.; Stanga, Z.; Muehlebach, S. Pharmaceutical Aspects of Artificial Nutrition. *J. Clin. Med.* **2019**, *8*, 2017. [CrossRef]
36. Hiesmayr, M.; Tarantino, S.; Moick, S.; Laviano, A.; Sulz, I.; Mouhieddine, M.; Schuh, C.; Volkert, D.; Simon, J.; Schindler, K. Hospital malnutrition, a call for political action: A public health and nutritionDay perspective. *J. Clin. Med.* **2019**, *8*, 2048. [CrossRef]

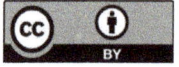

© 2019 by the authors. Licensee MDPI, Basel, Switzerland. This article is an open access article distributed under the terms and conditions of the Creative Commons Attribution (CC BY) license (http://creativecommons.org/licenses/by/4.0/).

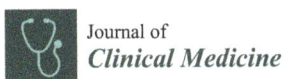 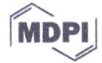

Article

Hospital Malnutrition, a Call for Political Action: A Public Health and NutritionDay Perspective

Michael Hiesmayr [1,*], Silvia Tarantino [1], Sigrid Moick [1], Alessandro Laviano [5], Isabella Sulz [2], Mohamed Mouhieddine [1], Christian Schuh [2], Dorothee Volkert [6], Judit Simon [3] and Karin Schindler [4]

- [1] Division Cardio-thoracic and Vascular Anesthesia and Intensive Care, Medical University Vienna, 1090 Vienna, Austria; silvia.tarantino@meduniwien.ac.at (S.T.); sigrid.moick@gmail.com (S.M.); mohamed.mouhieddine@meduniwien.ac.at (M.M.)
- [2] Center for Medical Statistics, Informatics and Intelligent Systems, Medical University Vienna, 1090 Vienna, Austria; isabella.sulz@meduniwien.ac.at (I.S.); christian.schuh@meduniwien.ac.at (C.S.)
- [3] Department of Health Economics, Center for Public Health, Medical University Vienna, 1090 Vienna, Austria; judit.simon@meduniwien.ac.at
- [4] Department of Internal Medicine III, Medical University Vienna, 1090 Vienna, Austria; karin.schindler@meduniwien.ac.at
- [5] Department of Translational and Precision Medicine, Università degli Studi di Roma "La Sapienza", 00185 Roma, Italy; alessandro.laviano@uniroma1.it
- [6] Institute for Biomedicine of Ageing, Friedrich-Alexander Universität Erlangen-Nürnberg, 90408 Nürnberg, Germany; dorothee.volkert@fau.de
- * Correspondence: michael.hiesmayr@meduniwien.ac.at; Tel.: +43-(0)1-40400-41080

Received: 29 September 2019; Accepted: 14 November 2019; Published: 22 November 2019

Abstract: Disease-related malnutrition (DRM) is prevalent in hospitals and is associated with increased care needs, prolonged hospital stay, delayed rehabilitation and death. Nutrition care process related activities such as screening, assessment and treatment has been advocated by scientific societies and patient organizations but implementation is variable. We analysed the cross-sectional nutritionDay database for prevalence of nutrition risk factors, care processes and outcome for medical, surgical, long-term care and other patients (n = 153,470). In 59,126 medical patients included between 2006 and 2015 the prevalence of recent weight loss (45%), history of decreased eating (48%) and low actual eating (53%) was more prevalent than low BMI (8%). Each of these risk factors was associated with a large increase in 30 days hospital mortality. A similar pattern is found in all four patient groups. Nutrition care processes increase slightly with the presence of risk factors but are never done in more than 50% of the patients. Only a third of patients not eating in hospital receive oral nutritional supplements or artificial nutrition. We suggest that political action should be taken to raise awareness and formal education on all aspects related to DRM for all stakeholders, to create and support responsibilities within hospitals, and to create adequate reimbursement schemes. Collection of routine and benchmarking data is crucial to tackle DRM.

Keywords: malnutrition; hospital; nutrition care; continuity of care; mortality; process indicators; benchmarking; disease related malnutrition

1. Introduction

Disease-related malnutrition (DRM) is highly prevalent in hospitalized patients and associated with complications and poor outcome [1–3]. Malnutrition in hospitals originates from imbalances, either deficiencies or excesses, in nutrients intake compared with body needs. Nutritional status and needs may be modified acutely or chronically by the disease process itself. Further deterioration may occur due to hospitalization, thus making the population of hospitalized patients very different from the general population. Prolonged nutrients imbalance is associated with change in body mass index (BMI). Association between body mass index (BMI) and mortality is U-shaped in the general population and J-shaped in patients, especially with chronic diseases, meaning that mortality is higher if BMI is low and lower in patients with increased lean body mass and even obesity [4,5]. This observation called "obesity paradox" underscores the importance of a "good" nutrition status for patients with illnesses for short and long-term outcomes.

Malnutrition in hospitalized patients often addresses an evident poor nutritional status (low BMI and low muscle mass) whereas being at risk of malnutrition is derived from a set of risk factors typically associated with a loss in lean body mass persisting over a certain period of time [6]. Nutrition care in hospitals is a treatment for patients with malnutrition and a preventive intervention for patients at risk of malnutrition. Nevertheless, nutrition care is still an underrated field when compared to medical diagnostics procedures, or pharmacological and technological interventions in hospitals.

There are several reasons why nutrition care has received so little attention in acute care hospitals. There is a common knowledge deficit reflected in a lack of proper education in university curricula for healthcare professionals (doctors, nurses, care assistants) combined with patients and relatives giving low value to nutrition as part of a successful therapy of the primary disease. Since no immediate effects of nutrition can be expected during a short hospital length of stay, the attention for nutrition related issues is often low. Standard nutrition care processes such as screening, assessment, planning and monitoring together with documentation and continuity of care are not regular parts of care on all hospital wards [7]. Moreover, food provision and related tasks are not considered part of healthcare responsibilities. Food provision is not part of the medical budget but usually of the administrative budget of a hospital where cost reduction is not considered to influence directly patient care. Inadequate management of food provision might affect food quality, presentation [8] and composition and, subsequently, patient care. Food costs are to be added to the overall malnutrition related costs. Patients with malnutrition usually stay longer in hospitals, are more often re-hospitalized or transferred to long-term care [9–12]. Each of these, together with the reimbursement schemes, do create additional costs for the healthcare system. Insights on improved hospital nutrition care processes and reduced healthcare costs come from the Swiss EFFORT study.

In patients with risk of malnutrition, nutrition intake was improved with enriched meals or oral nutritional supplements, food intake was monitored and was associated with better outcomes and reduced healthcare costs [11].

These multiple barriers and the lack of proper attention to DRM and nutrition care in hospitals has been formally addressed at a political level by a resolution of the European Council in 2003 but was not followed by national regulatory actions [3].This lack of action led to several independent initiatives. The European Society for Clinical Nutrition and Metabolism (ESPEN) (www.espen.org) together with the Medical University of Vienna developed a tailored action to tackle malnutrition in hospitals and healthcare institutions [4]. The resulting project "nutritionDay" aimed to generate more awareness on DRM with a yearly one-day data collection on patient's malnutrition risk factors, outcomes and quality indicators of nutrition care (www.nutritionday.org). In the nutritionDay analysis, several nutrition related risk factors, such as low BMI, recent weight loss and reduced food intake (in the week before nutritionDay or on nutritionDay itself), were found to be independently associated with death within 30 days in hospital [4]. In an another analysis that led to the development of the PANDORA score for prediction of death in hospital within 30 days after nutritionDay, decreased food intake was identified among the seven most important risk factors as it contributed 3–12 points out of a maximum of 75 points to the final score [5]. nutritionDay rapidly became a worldwide benchmarking tool for monitoring and improving nutrition care in hospital wards [13–15]. Patient related risk factors for decreased eating have a similar pattern in all world regions [16] and nutrition care processes implementation appears highly variable [7].

A multi-stakeholder initiative to promote screening for risk of disease-related malnutrition/undernutrition and implement nutritional care across Europe "Optimal Nutritional Care for All" has started an annual meeting with national nutrition societies and political representatives in 2008 [17]. The last meeting in Sintra, Portugal in 2018 involved representatives from 18 countries that had already joined the initiative and had the motto: "Optimal Nutrition Care across Europe: Fair Access and Shared Decision Making". The decision was taken together with the European Patient Forum [18] to translate relevant guidelines into a lay version to increase the possibility for patients to take informed responsibility [19].

The human right for proper nutrition care was acknowledged in the Cartagena declaration [20] and signed on 3rd May 2019 by all presidents of the Latin American Federation of Nutritional Therapy, Clinical Nutrition (FELANPE). The declaration includes 13 principles, such as patient empowerment, dignity, ethical principles, justice and equity and urges the United Nations and the Human Rights Council to recognize the Right to Nutrition Care as a human right in line with the "Sustainable Development Goals" [21].

The worldwide Global Leadership Initiative on Malnutrition (GLIM) composed by the major nutrition societies aims at defining universally accepted criteria for DRM [22]. This process is still ongoing with planned steps of validation and regular updating. Current recommendations from scientific societies emphasize that it is mandatory to identify the malnourished as well as those at risk early during hospitalization to trigger proper treatment or a set of preventive measures [19]. The recommended three step process consists of screening, assessing and developing a nutrition care plan. A further important and less appreciated step is that nutrition care needs to be monitored and adapted to the patient's changing condition. Finally, proper documentation and communication of a comprehensive care plan to the next sector, "extramural health care", and the patients themselves are essential to ensure continuity of care. To be efficient, responsibilities need to be cleared delineated and all relevant stakeholder (Table 1) involved.

Table 1. List and role of important stakeholders.

1. Within the hospital	
a. Patients and their relatives	
b. Care persons	
i. Nurses	Screening, diet ordering, documentation
ii. Physicians	Assessment, ordering, documentation, information
iii. Dieticians	Assessment, documentation
iv. Physiotherapists	Effect monitoring
v. Speech Therapists	Swallowing disorders
vi. Pharmacists	Clinical nutrition supply and counselling
c. Kitchen/Catering services	
i. Administrators	Budget
ii. Chefs	Standards, variety, quality control
iii. Kitchen aids	Presentation
iv. Delivering staff	Monitoring
d. Hospital administration	Budget, planning, controlling
2. Outside the hospital	
a. Patients and relatives	
b. Extramural medical services/family medicine/primary health care centres	
c. Extramural care services/mobile nursing	
d. Services for disabled and dependent persons	
e. Local food producers	
f. Medical food producing industries	

Table 1. *Cont.*

3. Scientific societies and stakeholder associations	
a. Medical	Guidelines, standards
b. Nursing	Guidelines, standards
c. Dietician	Guidelines, standards
d. Nutrition science	Research, standards
e. Patient organizations	Guidelines
4. Policy maker	
a. Health care system	Reimbursement
b. Social affairs	Equity
c. Agriculture	Local production integration
d. Environmental affairs	Sustainable planning, waste prevention
5. Payers	
a. Reimbursement of the nutrition care process in the whole health care system	
b. Public procurement of food supply and services	

This study aims to determine in the medical patients of the nutritionDay database 2006–2018, first, the prevalence of simple nutrition related risk factors and their association with outcome and, second, to determine the routine use of recommended nutrition care procedures such as screening, nutrition intake monitoring and documentation in patients with and without risk factors.

Based on the findings we will propose several options for political action to tackle malnutrition in hospitals.

2. Experimental Section

The nutritionDay audit is a cross-sectional international data collection in hospitalized patients with 30 days in hospital outcome assessment. The nutritionDay project was approved by the Ethical Committee of the Medical University of Vienna (EK407/2005) and it has been amended annually. In accordance with national regulations, the project was also submitted to national or local ethical committees in each participating country. This trial was registered at clinicaltrials.gov as NCT02820246. We analysed the complete nutritionDay database 2006–2015 for the association between nutrition related risk factors and 30 days hospital mortality. We assessed the 2016–2018 nutritionDay database for nutrition care process indicators newly introduced in 2016.

We included all adult patients with the exception of women before or after giving birth. Patients were divided into four groups: group surgical (patients admitted to a surgical unit or waiting for surgery or after surgery on any medical/other ward), group medical (all patients admitted to general medical, cardio, gastro, hepatology, nephrology, infectiology or oncology), group long-term (geriatric or long-term care wards) and others (all other specialties such as ear-nose-throat, gynecology, obstetrics, trauma, orthopedics, etc.). Risk factors were age, gender, BMI, weight change in the last three months, decreased eating during the previous week and on nutritionDay, fluid status (as intravascular or tissue fluid overload or depletion as observed by a clinician), reduced mobility and whether patients have been admitted to an intensive care unit at any time before nutritionDay during this index admission. In addition we included in the multivariate analysis the diagnostic categories derived from the 17 ICD 10 top categories (brain and nerves, eye and ear, nose and throat, heart and circulation, lung, liver, gastrointestinal tract, kidney/urinary tract/female genital tract, endocrine system, skeleton/bone/muscle, blood/bone marrow, skin, ischemia, cancer, infection, pregnancy, others) and six comorbidities (diabetes, stroke, COPD, myocardial infarction, cardiac failure and others), each one used as a unique variable as condition being present versus not present. All factors were used as categorical variables and included a missing category according to the STROBE guidelines [23]. Reference categories were either the "normal" category or the group including the median or the largest subgroup as appropriate. Age was divided into eight groups spanning 10 years with 60–70 years as reference; BMI was divided into 6 WHO groups with normal BMI 18.5–25 used as a reference [24].

Sensitivity analysis included only patients from units fulfilling quality criteria, such as >60% recruitment of admitted patients and outcome reporting for >80% of included patients. In addition a second sensitivity analysis was done for the multivariate modelling of the association between risk indicators and outcome after exclusion of all cases with missing values. The sensitivity study population includes 82,993 patients compared with 153,470 in the full study population.

Descriptive statistics report frequencies and median with interquartile range. Comparison of proportions were done with the χ^2 test and corrected for multiple testing. All associations between mortality and risk factors were done with logistic regression based on general linear models with units as clusters and weighting of patients to compensate for time-based bias from cross-sectional data acquisition [25]. In short, patients with a longer observed length of stay had less weight because they were more likely to be included in the study sample than short stay patients. We used univariate analysis for all risk factors and included all significant factors in the multivariate analysis. The effect of risk factors was also analysed within all four patient groups separately in the multivariate model (STATA 15.1, Statacorp, College Station, TX, USA). To show the extent of use of selected nutrition care processes, they are shown as percentages within different risk categories. Significant differences to each reference group were tested with a proportions test, comparisons were considered significant when $p < 0.005$ as we accounted for multiple tests for each reference category.

3. Results

Medical patients in the nutritionDay database ($n = 59,126/153,470$) (39%) represent the second largest group after surgical patients ($n = 63,289/153,470$) (41%). Patients were admitted in 61 countries and 19 countries recruited more than 1000 patients.

Medical patients were four years older than surgical patients (65.2 years SD 17.2 versus 61.2 years SD 18.0). The proportion of female was 48.3 in medical and 48.1 in surgical patients. Weight (71.3 kg SD 19.4 versus 71.9 kg SD 18.1) and height (166.1 cm SD 10.3 versus 166.5 cm SD 10.2) were similar in both groups. BMI was nearly identical (25.7 SD 6.3 versus 25.8 SD 5.8) ($p = 0.02$). Based on WHO categories (www.who.int) both groups have a similar proportion of obese with BMI > 30 (17.7% versus 17.4%) but the proportion with low BMI < 18.5 was significantly higher in medical than in surgical patients (7.5% versus 6%) ($p < 0.0001$).

3.1. Prevalence of Nutrition Risk Factors

Nutrition risk factors such as weight loss during the last three months (26,790, 45%), not eating normally in the previous week (28,950, 49%) and did not eat all food served on nutritionDay (30,965, 52%) were highly prevalent in the medical patients of the cohort 2006–2015 (Figure 1) and in the three other patient groups (Table 2).

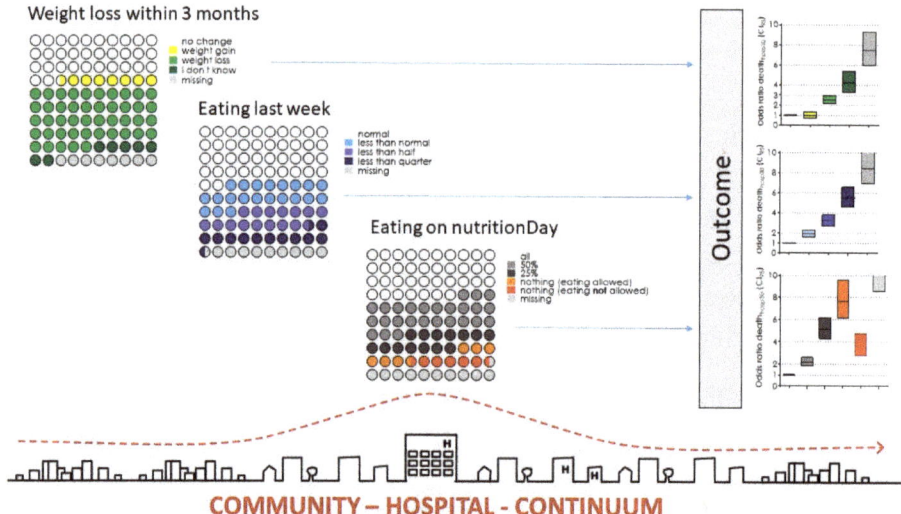

Figure 1. Prevalence of risk factors and association with odds ratio for death in hospital within 30 days after nutritionDay in medical patients. Prevalence is indicated by dots. Each dot represents 1% of the total population. All risk indicators are collected on one single day, the nutritionDay 2006–2015. Odds ratio are indicated with 95% confidence intervals and colours according to risk indicator categories Graph of Community–Hospital–Continuum from Magdalena Maierhofer's architectural diploma thesis: A Hospital is not a Tree (2016).

Table 2. Demographic characteristics and prevalence of nutrition risk factors of patients in the nutritionDay cohort 2006–2015, in the four studied groups.

	Medical		Surgical		Long-Term Care		Others	
Characteristics	n (%)	Mean ± SD	n (%)	Mean ± SD	n (%)	Mean ± SD	n (%)	Mean ± SD
Age (year)	59,046	65.1 ± 17.2		61.2 ± 18.0		80.7 ± 12.4		61.2 ± 18.8
Gender (female)	28,535 (49%)		30,445 (49%)		6937 (62%)		9992 (51%)	
Weight (kg)	52,735 (89%)	71.3 ± 19.4		71.9 ± 18.1		66.4 ± 16.9		71.8 ± 18.3
Height (cm)	52,735	166.1 ± 10.3		166.6 ± 10.2		163.0 ± 9.5		166.7 ± 10.4
BMI * (kg·cm^{-2})	52,735	25.7 ± 6.3		25.8 ± 5.8		24.9 ± 5.8		25.7 ± 5.9
Weight change within three months								
Unchanged *	19,139 (32%)		25,164 (40%)		3153 (28%)		7338 (37%)	
Increase	4335 (7.3%)		4997 (8%)		671 (6%)		1990 (10%)	
Loss	26,790 (45%)		24,928 (39%)		4989 (44%)		7356 (37%)	
Do not know	4020 (6.8%)		3679 (6%)		1339 (12%)		1205 (6%)	
Missing	4842 (8.2%)		4521 (7%)		1127 (10%)		1887 (10%)	
Eating last week								
Normal *	24,679 (42%)		29,898 (47%)		4731 (42%)		9973 (50%)	
Less than normal	12,613 (21%)		12,618 (20%)		2526 (22%)		4047 (20%)	
Less than a half	8979 (15%)		7894 (12%)		1628 (14%)		2262 (11%)	
Less than a quarter	7358 (12%)		7691 (12%)		1076 (9%)		1433 (7%)	
Missing	5497 (9.3%)		5188 (8%)		1318 (12%)		2061 (10%)	

Table 2. Cont.

	Medical	Surgical	Long-Term Care	Others
Eating on nutritionDay				
All *	22,046 (37%)	22,232 (35%)	4131 (37%)	8496 (43%)
Half	15,327 (26%)	15,141 (24%)	3363 (30%)	5054 (26%)
Quarter	8256 (14%)	7262 (11%)	1592 (14%)	2206 (11%)
Nothing (eating allowed)	3696 (6.3%)	3666 (6%)	698 (6%)	927 (5%)
Nothing (eating not allowed)	3686 (6.2%)	8717 (14%)	372 (3%)	875 (4%)
Missing	6115 (10%)	6271 (10%)	1123 (10%)	2218 (11%)
Mobility on nutritionDay				
Normal	35,846 (61%)	37,439 (59%)	3731 (33%)	12,227 (62%)
With help	12,299 (21%)	14,110 (22%)	4557 (40%)	3838 (19%)
Bedridden	5587 (9.4%)	6832 (11%)	1841 (16%)	1732 (9%)
Missing	5394 (9.1%)	4908 (8%)	1150 (10%)	1979 (10%)
Fluid status on nutritionDay				
Normal *	28,499 (48%)	3619 (6%)	1147 (10%)	1284 (6%)
Overload	6214 (11%)	33,636 (53%)	5836 (51%)	1142 (58%)
Deficit	3267 (6%)	2723 (4%)	985 (9%)	886 (4%)
Missing	21,146 (36%)	23,311 (37%)	3311 (29%)	6178 (31%)
Any Intensive Care Stay before nutritionDay	4143 (7.0%)	10,465 (17%)	564 (5%)	1464 (8%)
Medical specialty				
General internal medicine	29,173 (49%)	3958 (6%)		
Oncology	11,412 (19%)	1953 (3%)		
Gastroenterology/Hepatology	9744 (16%)	1350 (2%)		
Cardiology	5401 (9.1%)	1405 (2%)		
Nephrology	1785 (3.0%)	370 (1%)		
Infectiology	1611 (2.7%)	149 (0%)		
Neurology		592 (1%)		4442 (22%)
Psychiatry		17 (0%)		1409 (7%)
ENT		2195 (3%)		1272 (6%)
General surgery		28,310 (45%)		
Cardiothorcic surgery		2013 (3%)		
Characteristics	n (%)	Mean ± SD	n (%)	Mean ± SD	n (%)	Mean ± SD	n (%)	Mean ± SD
Orthopaedic surgery		7803 (12%)		
Trauma		2160 (3%)		
Neurosurgery		1717 (3%)		
Gynecology		1198 (2%)		1151 (6%)
Long-term care		526 (1%)	9885 (88%)	
Other		5955 (9%)		11,401 (58%)
Pediatrics		46 (0%)		101 (1%)
Geriatrics		1572 (2%)	1785 (12%)	

* indicates the reference categories.

There is some overlap between risk categories. Two third of patients (17,497/26,790) with weight loss reported not eating normal in the previous week and a similar proportion did not eat all served on nutritionDay (16,681/26,790).

Nearly 40% of patients (9551/24,679) that did eat normally in the previous week were eating less than all meal served on nutritionDay indicating a new nutrition risk associated with hospitalization.

In most patients (80%) all four nutrition risk factors, low BMI, weight loss, reduced eating during the previous week and on nutritionDay could be evaluated. 91% had no more than one risk factor missing. Only 32,216/140,418 (23%) of patients had no single nutrition related risk factor, 31% had one risk factor, 28% two risk factors and 16% had three risk factors.

3.2. Nutrition Care

3.2.1. Food provision

Oral diet, either normal hospital food or special diet, was mostly used in medical patients (Table 3). Two third of oral diets were given as hospital food and one third as special diet. Oral nutritional supplements were given to 9.3% of patients whereas enteral nutrition was used in 7.1% and parenteral nutrition in 3.5% (Table 3). Surprisingly, the use of enteral or parenteral nutrition only increased by a factor of three between patients who reported having eaten their full meal and those who had eaten nothing. Two-thirds of patients reporting eating nothing were on oral diet. The use of enteral and parenteral nutrition was not differentiating much in patients who have eaten nothing regardless of being allowed to eat or not.

Table 3. Nutrition care versus amount eaten on nutritionDay according to the patients in the four studied groups.

		Oral	ONS	EN	PN	Othercomb
Medical	all	19,484 (88.4%)	1651 (7.5%)	1154 (5.2%)	289 (1.3%)	794 (3.6%)
n = 59,126	half	13,657 (89.1%)	1560 (10.2%)	770 (5%)	311 (2%)	544 (3.5%)
	quarter	7176 (87%)	1132 (13.7%)	426 (5.2%)	354 (4.3%)	332 (4%)
	nothing_a	2760 (74.7%)	448 (12.1%)	428 (11.6%)	306 (8.3%)	278 (7.5%)
	nothing_na	2391 (65%)	226 (6.1%)	329 (8.9%)	417 (11.3%)	521 (14.1%)
	missing	3377 (55.2%)	462 (7.6%)	1083 (17.7%)	381 (6.2%)	323 (5.3%)
	Total	48,845 (82.6%)	5479 (9.3%)	4190 (7.1%)	2058 (3.5%)	2792 (4.7%)
Surgical	all	19,368 (87.1%)	1468 (6.6%)	1286 (5.8%)	429 (1.9%)	1184 (5.3%)
n = 63,289	half	13,106 (86.6%)	1294 (8.5%)	913 (6%)	506 (3.3%)	906 (6%)
	quarter	6066 (83.5%)	779 (10.7%)	472 (6.5%)	381 (5.2%)	536 (7.4%)
	nothing_a	2384 (65%)	324 (8.8%)	448 (12.2%)	415 (11.3%)	573 (15.6%)
	nothing_na	4611 (53%)	301 (3.5%)	810 (9.3%)	1535 (17.6%)	1906 (21.9%)
	missing	3596 (57.3%)	392 (6.3%)	819 (13.1%)	605 (9.6%)	689 (11%)
	Total	49,131 (77.6%)	4558 (7.2%)	4748 (7.5%)	3871 (6.1%)	5794 (9.2%)
Longterm	all	3480 (84.3%)	824 (19.9%)	370 (9%)	15 (0.4%)	135 (3.3%)
n = 11,279	half	2858 (85%)	790 (23.5%)	268 (8%)	29 (0.9%)	113 (3.4%)
	quarter	1312 (82.4%)	482 (30.3%)	130 (8.2%)	28 (1.8%)	70 (4.4%)
	nothing_a	473 (67.8%)	225 (32.2%)	111 (15.9%)	41 (5.9%)	53 (7.6%)
	nothing_na	200 (53.8%)	75 (20.2%)	85 (22.8%)	46 (12.4%)	43 (11.6%)
	missing	672 (59.8%)	177 (15.8%)	247 (22%)	36 (3.2%)	45 (4%)
	Total	8995 (79.7%)	2573 (22.8%)	1211 (10.7%)	195 (1.7%)	459 (4.1%)
Others	all	7435 (87.5%)	509 (6%)	672 (7.9%)	70 (0.8%)	392 (4.6%)
n = 19,776	half	4398 (87%)	380 (7.5%)	403 (8%)	84 (1.7%)	258 (5.1%)
	quarter	1885 (85.4%)	267 (12.1%)	147 (6.7%)	78 (3.5%)	118 (5.3%)
	nothing_a	628 (67.7%)	84 (9.1%)	160 (17.3%)	68 (7.3%)	90 (9.7%)
	nothing_na	544 (62.2%)	49 (5.6%)	100 (11.4%)	101 (11.5%)	131 (15%)
	missing	1214 (54.7%)	124 (5.6%)	355 (16%)	91 (4.1%)	128 (5.8%)
	Total	16,104 (81.4%)	1413 (7.1%)	1837 (9.3%)	492 (2.5%)	1117 (5.6%)

Percentages are indicated within each eating category. Multiple entries in the nutrition type for one patient are possible. Patients who ate nothing on nutritionDay were divided into those who did not eat even if they were allowed to (nothing_a) and those who did not eat because they were told not to eat by the doctor (nothing_na) as, for instance, before planned surgery or diagnostic tests. Combined enteral and parenteral nutrition was used in less than 2.5% of patients in any patient category and is not shown.

3.2.2. Process indicators

A total of 1415 units reported in 2016–2018 about the screening tool utilised (Figure 2). The majority, used a formal tool such as NRS-2002 (Nutrition Risk Screening 2002), MUST (Malnutrition Universal Screening Tool), MST (Malnutrition Screening Tool), or a local tool. Only 10% of the units did not have a routine screening nor fixed screening criteria. Patients identified as malnourished were overall 3340/28,100 (11.9%), with the highest proportion identified with an informal tool 722/4793 (15.1%) or NRS-2002 1169/8453 (13.8%) followed by MUST 134/1210 (11.1%), MST 269/2269 (11.9%) and visual experience 197/1666 (11.8%) whereas the proportion of identified malnourished patients was lower with no implemented routine 204/2154 (9.5%). The proportion of patients identified at nutritional risk was overall 4944/28,100 (17.6%). Of those, the highest proportion, 22.4% was identified with an unspecified tool while only 14–16% of patients were identified at risk when no routine, only visual appearance or MST was used. Only 28.9% of malnourished patients had a BMI below 18.5, 49.8% a normal BMI, 21.4% were overweight or obese. Being identified as malnourished was associated with unintentional weight loss within the last three months in 85% of patients, with reduced nutrient intake before admission in 57% of patients and with not eating a full lunch in hospital in 65% of patients. Not being identified as malnourished or at risk of malnutrition was associated with unintentional weight loss within the last three months in 47% of patients, with reduced nutrient intake before admission in 28% of patients and with not eating a full lunch in hospital in 48% of patients. The proportion of patients with two or more nutrition risk factors was 50% in the 2016–2018 cohort.

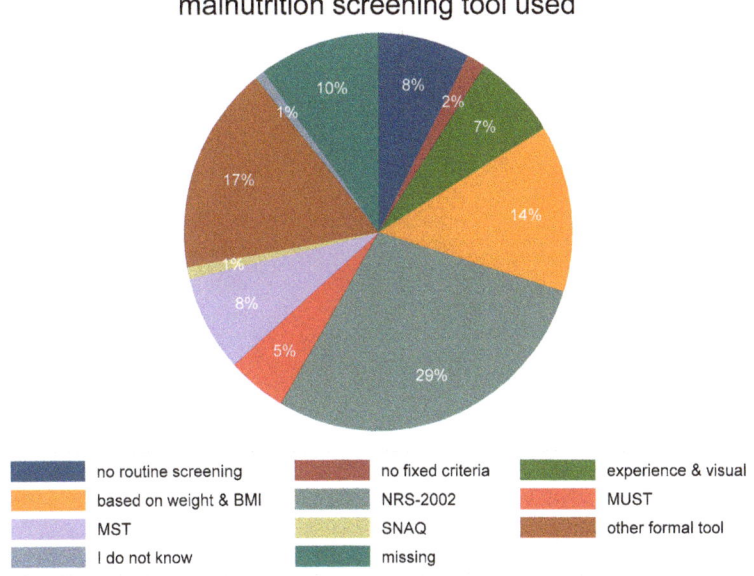

Figure 2. Proportion of different methods/approaches used for malnutrition screening in 1415 units from 46 countries in the nutritionDay cohort 2016–2018. NRS-2002 (nutrition risk screening 2002); MUST (Malnutrition Universal Screening Tool); MST (Malnutrition Screening Tool); SNAQ (Short Nutritional Assessment Questionnaire).

Nutrition intake monitoring was more frequent in patients with unintentional weight loss than in patients with stable weight (52% versus 41%) (Figure 3). Still, nearly 50% of patients with a history of weight loss did not have their nutrition intake monitored while in hospital. Similarly, history of poor nutrition intake before admission triggered more frequent monitoring compared with history of normal eating but intake was never monitored in more than 50% of patients with a history of poor nutritional intake. Actual poor food intake did not have any effect on monitoring of food intake.

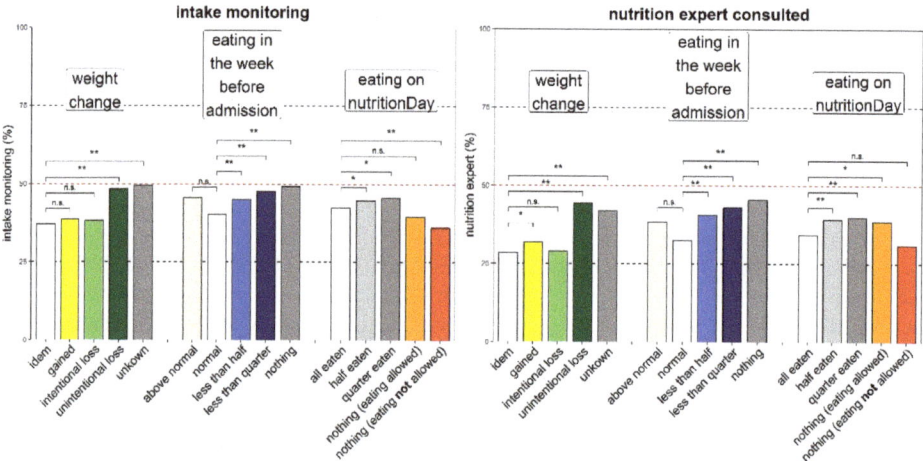

Figure 3. Nutrition care process indicators versus three nutrition associated risk factors. Daily nutrition intake monitoring (**left**) and nutrition expert consulted (**right**). Bars indicate percentage answering "yes", significant differences to each reference group are shown with * $p < 0.005$ and ** $p < 0.00001$, 'n.s.' indicates no significant difference. Missing values were <7.5% in all subcategories. Colour coding similar to Figure 1 (the empty bar is the reference).

A nutrition expert was consulted more frequently when an unintentional weight loss was reported by patients or when food intake was reported as reduced before hospital admission (Figure 3). A nutrition expert was never consulted in more than 46% of patients even when risk factors were reported. Documentation of malnutrition in patient's chart followed a similar pattern as consulting an expert and was always below 41%.

Low BMI was associated with a more frequent monitoring of intake (58% versus 47%) ($p < 0.0001$) and malnutrition reporting in patient record (52% versus 36%) ($p < 0.0001$) compared with normal BMI. In obese patients (BMI 30–35) we observed the lowest intake monitoring (40%) and malnutrition reporting (27%).

3.3. Outcome

Thirty days after nutritionDay we collected outcome data and found that 73% of the study patients had been discharged home, 11.8% had been transferred to another health care facility, hospital, long-term care or rehabilitation; 9.4% were still in the same hospital and 5.5% had died (Table 4). Similar results were observed in the sensitivity analysis. In medical patients, death was observed more than twice as frequently as in surgical patients (4.6% versus 1.7%, $p < 0.0001$) and was similar to the groups geriatrics and long-term care (4.6% versus 4.8%, $p < 0.0001$).

The group "other", which includes patients from neurology, psychiatry and non-operative patients in gynecology and ENT, has a lower mortality (2.6% versus 4.6%) ($p < 0.0001$) a lower proportion discharged home $p > 0.0001$) at day 30 after nutritionDay than medical patients (Table 4).

Table 4. Outcomes in hospital within 30 days after nutritionDay in the four patient groups.

Outcome	Surgery	Medical	Longterm	Other
in hospital	5740 (9.1%)	4639 (7.8%)	1560 (13.8%)	2303 (11.6%)
transfer other hospital	1500 (2.4%)	1343 (2.3%)	290 (2.6%)	390 (2%)
transfer longterm care	1424 (2.2%)	2109 (3.6%)	1471 (13%)	574 (2.9%)
transfer rehabilitation	1967 (3.1%)	1341 (2.3%)	441 (3.9%)	535 (2.7%)
discharge home	39,705 (62.7%)	36,439 (61.6%)	4710 (41.8%)	11,049 (55.9%)
death within 30 days	1053 (1.7%)	2721 (4.6%)	541 (4.8%)	512 (2.6%)
other destination	948 (1.5%)	1033 (1.7%)	322 (2.9%)	376 (1.9%)
missing	10,952 (17.3%)	9501 (16.1%)	1944 (17.2%)	4037 (20.4%)

Nutrition risk factors were associated with death in hospital within 30 days in a univariate analysis with odds ratios 2.6 CI 95 [2.2–3.0] for weight loss, 5.5 CI 95 [4.6–6.6] for eating less than a quarter of their meals in the previous week and 7.6 CI 95 [6.1–9.6] if eating nothing on nutritionDay despite being allowed to eat. The prevalence of individual risk categories for weight loss, decreased eating last week and on nutritionDay were associated with significantly worse outcomes (Figure 1), while increasing BMI was associated with decreasing odds ratios for death.

Other risk factors such as increasing age and male gender were also associated with poor outcome. The largest univariate association with hospital death was observed in patients with reduced mobility or those who were bedridden. Mortality within 30 days after nutritionDay increased with the number of nutrition risk factors present from 0.9% for no risk factor, 1.68% for one risk factor, 3.55% for two risk factors, 8.13% for three risk factors and 13% for four risk factors.

Multivariate Outcome Analysis

All risk factors that were significantly associated with 30 days hospital death in the univariate analysis were also significant in the multivariate analysis (Figures 4 and 5) including all affected organs and comorbidities that could be estimated. Most estimates indicated a reduced strength of the association of the individual risk factors compared with univariate analysis, which indicates confounding. In the multivariate analysis, history of decreased eating before hospital admission was associated with higher odds ratio for death in surgical patients than in medical patients, weight loss was associated with similar odds ratio. History of a stay in intensive care during the hospitalization before nutritionDay was found to be significantly associated with death only in medical patients. "Eating less than normal in the previous week" is associated with death 30 days after nDay in medical, surgical and long-term care patients but not in the "other" group. Weight loss is only associated with poor outcome in medical and surgical patients. Higher BMI was associated with better outcome in medical, surgical and "other" patients, an observation called "reverse epidemiology" and low BMI with worse outcome but not in long-term care patients. Higher age is in all groups associated with worse outcome. Abnormal fluid status, identified as either overloaded or dehydrated, based on clinical judgment, was a robust risk indicator in all patient groups. Decreased food intake on nutritionDay was always associated with worse outcome. A clear difference between eating nothing while not being allowed (nil by mouth) or being allowed is only found in the surgical patient group whereas in all three other groups there was no clear difference. A very robust risk indicator is "reduced mobility" in all patient groups (Figure 4). Having had an ICU stay before nutritionDay was only associated with worse outcome in medical patients.

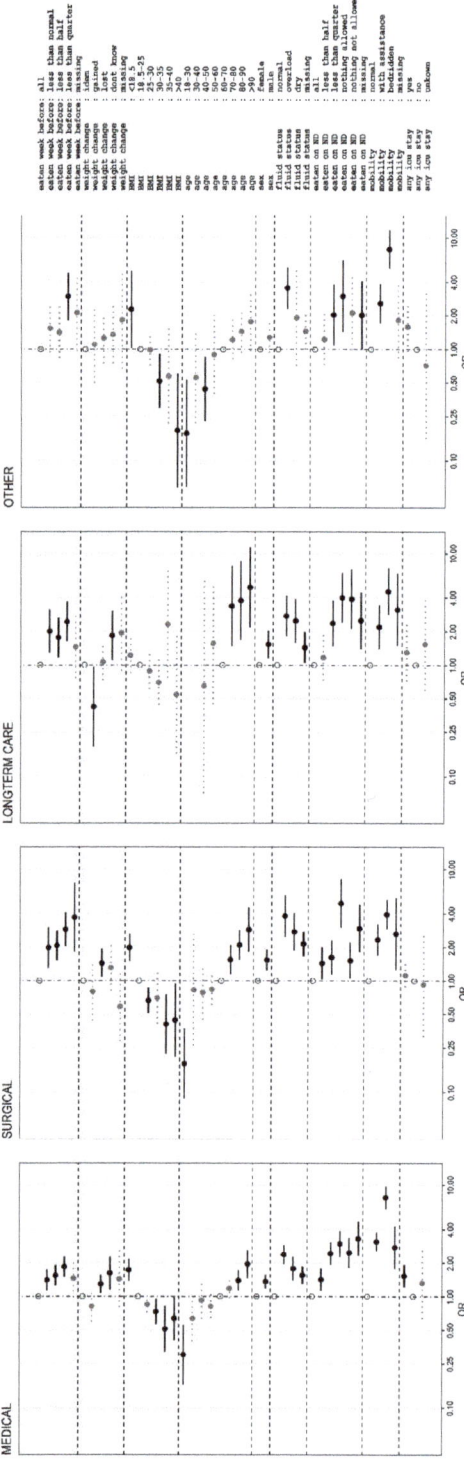

Figure 4. Multivariate analysis of association between demographic and nutrition related risk factors and death in hospital within 30 days after nutritionDay for medical, surgical, long-term care and other patient groups with the general linear model for logistic regression with wards as clusters and weighting of individual patients for sampling probability [25] and including all diagnostic categories and comorbidities (see Figure 5). Odds ratios (OR) with 95% confidence intervals indicated by horizontal line. Reference categories are indicated by an open symbol. Missing values are included in the model as individual categories.

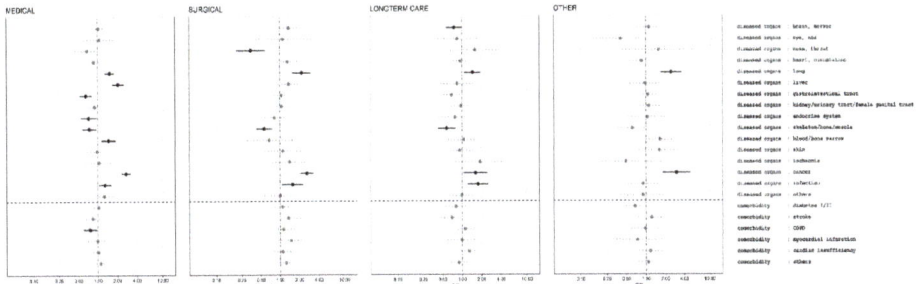

Figure 5. Multivariate analysis of association between organ related disease categories from ICD 10 as well as comorbidities and death in hospital within 30 days after nutritionDay for medical, surgical, long-term care and other patient groups with the general linear model for logistic regression with wards as clusters and weighting of individual patients for sampling probability [25] and including demographic and nutrition related risk factors (see Figure 4). Odds ratios (OR) with 95% confidence intervals indicated by horizontal line. Multiple entries are possible. Missing values are included in the model as individual categories.

The association between affected organs as derived from ICD 10 categories is very different for medical and surgical patients (Figure 5). No comorbidities had a negative prognostic effect in the multivariate analysis.

4. Discussion

This analysis of medical/surgical patients from the nutritionDay cohort 2006–2015 showed that individual nutrition risk indicators such as low BMI, weight loss in last three months, poor eating before admission and low nutrient intake in hospital are highly prevalent in hospitalized patients and are associated with poor hospital outcome within 30 days after nutritionDay. Each additional risk indicator observed was associated with a nearly two-times higher mortality in the overall population.

All four risk indicators were independently associated with death in the hospital within 30 days after nutritionDay in the multivariate analysis (Figure 4) in the two largest groups medical and surgical patients. There is no clear indication that a single risk indicator can be ignored because the presence of each risk indicator is associated with a higher rate of dying by nearly a factor of two for these two groups. Surprisingly recent weight-loss and lower BMI was not associated with worse prognosis in long-term care whereas only weight-loss was not associated with worse outcome for the group of non-medical and non-surgical patients including neurological and psychiatric disorders.

Three risk indicators emerge similarly for all four patient groups, poor eating in hospital, reduced mobility and altered fluid status. All three had also being found as individual risk indicators in the PANDORA risk scoring system whereas recent weight loss and history of poor eating were not included [5]. These robust factors may also serve as indicators that may trigger more consistent observation and initiation of treatments that have proven to efficacious [26].

In recent years (2016–2018) healthcare teams identified only half of the patients as having nutrition related risk factors such as being malnourished or at risk of malnutrition in comparison to the nutritionDay indicators 8701/28,013 (31%) versus 21,070/28,100 (75%) such as unintentional weight loss, low BMI or decreased food intake. Thus, it appears that a large group of patients with nutrition related risk factors is not identified in standard care practice. This observed gap may originate from the different type of data collected from patients during routine clinical practice and the targeted data collection of the nutritionDay audit.

The efficiency of interventions may depend on the size of risk of the individual patient. It has recently been demonstrated that patients identified at high risk of malnutrition by the Nutritional Risk Screening (NRS-2002) risk system benefit from an integrated intervention [26]. It is unknown, however, whether the large group of patients with moderate risk, which account for almost half of the hospitalized patients on any given day, would also benefit from some targeted interventions. Interventions effective for the moderate risk group may be less complex and costly, and potentially integrated in to routine care processes, and could lead to better outcomes and reduced hospital length of stay and better patient outcomes.

4.1. Nutrition Care

Nutrition care processes such as screening, prescribing nutrition treatment, monitoring daily nutrition intake and recording of malnutrition status are applied in less than 50% of patients. These observations may again arise from identification issues, from lack of a systematic screening processes which then lead to a weak targeting even in the presence of nutrition risk factors. Educational gaps of healthcare professionals in the field of nutrition, as well as the importance given to nutrition care might also be considered crucial to fight DRM. Recent results from a large randomized trial [26] from a Swiss team could demonstrate that a systematic approach to patients with nutrition risk factors is associated with a decreased short and long-term mortality.

Our data suggest that a systematic care for patients with nutrition related risk factors in hospitals is currently missing. Reception and dissemination of current recommendations from major clinical nutrition societies such as ESPEN and ASPEN requires further efforts to reach all the involved stakeholders, not only those directly involved in nutrition care but also those in management and decision making.

4.2. Political Action Derived from Observations

A structured approach to tackle the challenges of disease related malnutrition needs to include all involved stakeholders to implement universal screening for risk factors, apply systematically supportive nutrition care, monitor the effect in individual patients and take measures to promote continuity of care after discharge from acute care hospitals.

4.3. Limitations of the Study

A limitation of such a cross-sectional international data collection may be that clinical observations and their evaluation are not matching the same clinical pattern. Participants are provided with a document explaining all collected variables in English and with questionnaires which were translated and checked by clinicians in order to achieve as much as possible consistency between answers. Great care was taken to utilize a simple and self-explanatory wording. This was also essential because the patient questionnaires are intended to be answered by patients independently of their education level. For such factors as fluid status, overloaded or dehydrated, we had to accept the data as clinically evaluated.

Such large databases with participating centres from more than 60 countries carry also the risk of missing data and non-homogeneous data reporting. Over the years we found stable proportions of missing data in the individual risk indicators. Surprisingly, this missingness does not appear to be at random as missing data were often associated with a poor outcome and not with an intermediate outcome from the various strata of a variable. We have addressed this issue by including missing categories in all variables as recommended by the STROBE statement [23] and have performed in addition a sensitivity analysis with complete cases without missing data that yielded quite similar results.

In addition, large databases may identify risk indicators with a minimal clinical relevance despite a large univariate effect. We have, thus, selected to present multivariate analysis where spurious associations are less likely.

A further limitation is that cross-sectional observational data from a convenience sample are not appropriate to determine a causal association between risk indicators and outcome. Nevertheless only observational studies can identify risk indicators because risk indicators cannot be randomised (Table 5).

Table 5. Problem areas and suggested options for political action.

Problem Area	Political Action
Education of all healthcare professionals directly involved in patient care in disease related malnutrition and nutrition care insufficient.	Mandatory inclusion of disease related malnutrition and nutrition care processes in curriculum for nurses, doctors, dieticians, etc.
Limited awareness of the importance of nutrition in disease states in the public especially the population at risk.	National nutrition care campaigns targeting the general population, residents of nursing homes and also targeted nutrition campaigns run through general practitioners. Availability of an education platform for patients and families.
Nomination of responsible person or team for patient nutrition care missing. No monitoring of nutrition care processes part of hospital quality control.	Mandatory designation of a nutrition team/responsible person in each hospital with a threefold responsibility: coordination of expertise, definition of processes and regular benchmarking of applications of processes through initiatives like nutritionDay, the Dutch nutrition benchmarking program, the British malnutrition awareness week and the analysis of electronic patients records.
Inconsistent screening and collection of data. Missing documentation of nutrition risk factors and communication of nutrition status and care at discharge to the next sector.	Mandatory inclusion of data in a nutrition care benchmarking program. Definition and inclusion of mandatory harmonized fields for a systematic collection and documentation of nutrition risks factors and nutrition care processes in the electronic patient record. Inclusion of planned nutrition treatment recorded in patient's discharge letter/information to patients and relatives.
Missing patients and families empowerment due to insufficient communication of nutrition status and care to the patients and their families.	Mandatory monitoring of communication processes in quality assurance programs.
Lack of a harmonized reimbursement schemes for nutrition related processes such as screening, assessment and treatment such as oral nutritional supplements, enteral or parenteral nutrition.	Clear reimbursement schemes.
Missing a partnership for hospital food provision and of a positive image for hospital food.	Creation of a public best practice platform for food provision in hospitals. Supported use of local food in hospital kitchen for the creation of wealth not only for the community using the hospital but also for the local community.

5. Conclusions

In summary the analysis and dissemination of the nutritionDay data helps to increase awareness of nutrition related issues in hospitals and provides discussion for potential political actions. There are many options for political action. The key points appear to be the raised awareness about all the described aspects related to DRM to all stakeholders, as well as the proposal of easy and standardized nutrition care processes, defined responsibilities within hospitals, and the establishment of adequate reimbursement schemes. Collection of data is crucial to allow monitoring of DRM as well as food provision at all levels and to allow benchmarking and discussion within the teams. DRM is unlikely to disappear from hospitals because disease acts as a strong driver towards malnutrition. Appropriate nutrition care should be continued after discharge to prevent further deterioration in patient's autonomy, quality of life and poor outcome. A systematic approach to DRM in hospitals and an adequate continuity of care may lead to better outcomes [11,12,26]. nutritionDay in this regard has served and it will keep serving as a tool to monitor changes in clinical practice and associated outcome.

Author Contributions: Conceptualization: M.H., S.T., D.V., J.S. and K.S.; data curation: M.M. and C.S.; formal analysis: M.H. and I.S.; funding acquisition: M.H., S.T., D.V. and J.S.; investigation: S.M.; methodology: M.H., J.S. and K.S.; project administration: S.T., S.M. and D.V.; resources: M.H. and D.V.; software: M.M. and C.S.; supervision: A.L. and J.S.; validation: M.H. and I.S.; visualization: M.H., S.T. and I.S.; writing—original draft: M.H., S.T., D.V., J.S. and K.S.; writing—review and editing: M.H., S.T., A.L., I.S., D.V., J.S. and K.S.

Funding: This research was funded by The European Society for Clinical Nutrition and Metabolism (ESPEN) and supported by the Medical University of Vienna.

Acknowledgments: We acknowledge the nutritionDay national coordinators and the Austrian Society for Clinical Nutrition (AKE) for logistic support. We acknowledge all national coordinators contributing to nutritionDay: Jean-Charles Preiser and Brigitte Croix (Belgium), M. Cristina Gonzalez (Brazil), Luiza Kent-Smith (Canada), Angélica María Pérez Cano and Olga Lucía Pinzón Espitia (Colombia), Dina Ljubas (Croatia), Evelyn Frias Toral (Ecuador), Elina Ioannou (Cyprus), Frantisek Novak (Czech Republic), José Gutiérrez (El Salvador), Ulla Siljamäki-Ojansuu (Finland), Stéphane Schneider (France), Elke-Tatjana Schütz (Germany), Meropi Kontogianni and Kalliopi-Anna Poulia (Greece), Laszlo Harsányi (Hungary), Hartono (Indonesia), Pierre Singer (Israel), Marcello Maggio and Pietro Vecchiarelli (Italy), Hiroyoshi Takemoto (Japan), Laila Meija and Ilze Jagmane (Latvia), Gintautas Kekstas and Edita Gaveliene (Lithuania), Cora Jonkers-Schuitema (The Netherlands), Hugo Nilssen (Norway), Kinga Kupczyk (Poland), Paula Alves and Luis Matos (Portugal) Ioana Grintescu and Liliana Mirea (Romania), Vanessa Kotze (South Africa), Katja Kogovšek (Slovenia), Rosa Burgos (Spain), Barbara Hürlimann (Switzerland), Sonqsri Keawtanom (Thailand), Sadik Kilicturgay (Turkey), Sergii Dubrov and Olesia Gavrilenko (Ukraine), Kate Hall (United Kingdom) and Gail Gewirtz (USA).

Conflicts of Interest: The authors declare no conflict of interest. The funders had no role in the design of the study; in the collection, analyses, or interpretation of data; in the writing of the manuscript; or in the decision to publish the results.

References

1. Butterworth, C.E., Jr. Editorial: Malnutrition in the hospital. *JAMA* **1974**, *230*, 879. [CrossRef]
2. Bistrian, B.R.; Blackburn, G.L.; Vitale, J.; Cochran, D.; Naylor, J. Prevalence of malnutrition in general medical patients. *JAMA* **1976**, *235*, 1567–1570. [CrossRef]
3. Council of Europe Committee of Ministers. Resolution ResAP (2003) 3 on Food and Nutritional Care in Hospitals. Available online: https://search.coe.int/ (accessed on 18 November 2019).
4. Hiesmayr, M.; Schindler, K.; Pernicka, E.; Schuh, C.; Schoeniger-Hekele, A.; Bauer, P.; Laviano, A.; Lovell, A.D.; Mouhieddine, M.; Schuetz, T.; et al. Decreased food intake is a risk factor for mortality in hospitalised patients: The NutritionDay survey 2006. *Clin. Nutr.* **2009**, *28*, 484–491. [CrossRef]
5. Hiesmayr, M.; Frantal, S.; Schindler, K.; Themessl-Huber, M.; Mouhieddine, M.; Schuh, C.; Pernicka, E.; Schneider, S.; Singer, P.; Ljunqvist, O.; et al. The Patient- And Nutrition-Derived Outcome Risk Assessment Score (PANDORA): Development of a Simple Predictive Risk Score for 30-Day In-Hospital Mortality Based on Demographics, Clinical Observation, and Nutrition. *PLoS ONE* **2015**, *10*, e0127316. [CrossRef]
6. Kondrup, J.; Rasmussen, H.H.; Hamberg, O.; Stanga, Z. Nutritional risk screening (NRS 2002): A new method based on an analysis of controlled clinical trials. *Clin. Nutr.* **2003**, *22*, 321–336. [CrossRef]
7. Schindler, K.; Pernicka, E.; Laviano, A.; Howard, P.; Schutz, T.; Bauer, P.; Grecu, I.; Jonkers, C.; Kondrup, J.; Ljungqvist, O.; et al. How nutritional risk is assessed and managed in European hospitals: A survey of 21,007 patients findings from the 2007–2008 cross-sectional nutritionDay survey. *Clin. Nutr.* **2010**, *29*, 552–559. [CrossRef] [PubMed]
8. Navarro, D.A.; Boaz, M.; Krause, I.; Elis, A.; Chernov, K.; Giabra, M.; Levy, M.; Giboreau, A.; Kosak, S.; Mouhieddine, M.; et al. Improved meal presentation increases food intake and decreases readmission rate in hospitalizd patients. *Clin. Nutr.* **2016**, *35*, 1153–1158. [CrossRef]
9. Correia, M.I.; Waitzberg, D.L. The impact of malnutrition on morbidity, mortality, length of hospital stay and costs evaluated through a multivariate model analysis. *Clin. Nutr.* **2003**, *22*, 235–239. [CrossRef]
10. Lim, S.L.; Ong, K.C.; Chan, Y.H.; Loke, W.C.; Ferguson, M.; Daniels, L. Malnutrition and its impact on cost of hospitalization, length of stay, readmission and 3-year mortality. *Clin. Nutr.* **2012**, *31*, 345–350. [CrossRef] [PubMed]
11. Reber, E.; Norman, K.; Endrich, O.; Schuetz, P.; Frei, A.; Stanga, Z. Economic Challenges in Nutritional Management. *J. Clin. Med.* **2019**, *8*, 1005. [CrossRef]

12. Reber, E.; Strahm, R.; Bally, L.; Schuetz, P.; Stanga, Z. Efficacy and Efficiency of Nutritional Support Teams. *J. Clin. Med.* **2019**, *8*, 1281. [CrossRef] [PubMed]
13. Bendavid, I.; Singer, P.; Theilla, M.; Themessl-Huber, M.; Sulz, I.; Mouhieddine, M.; Schuh, C.; Mora, B.; Hiesmayr, M. NutritionDay ICU: A 7 year worldwide prevalence study of nutrition practice in intensive care. *Clin. Nutr.* **2017**, *36*, 1122–1129. [CrossRef] [PubMed]
14. Schindler, K.; Pichard, C.; Sulz, I.; Volkert, D.; Streicher, M.; Singer, P.; Ljungqvist, O.; Van Gossum, A.; Bauer, P.; Hiesmayr, M. nutritionDay: 10 years of growth. *Clin. Nutr.* **2017**, *36*, 1207–1214. [CrossRef] [PubMed]
15. Streicher, M.; Themessl-Huber, M.; Schindler, K.; Sieber, C.C.; Hiesmayr, M.; Volkert, D. nutritionDay in Nursing Homes-The Association of Nutritional Intake and Nutritional Interventions With 6-Month Mortality in Malnourished Residents. *J. Am. Med. Dir. Assoc.* **2017**, *18*, 162–168. [CrossRef]
16. Schindler, K.; Themessl-Huber, M.; Hiesmayr, M.; Kosak, S.; Lainscak, M.; Laviano, A.; Ljungqvist, O.; Mouhieddine, M.; Schneider, S.; de van der Schueren, M.; et al. To eat or not to eat? Indicators for reduced food intake in 91,245 patients hospitalized on nutritionDays 2006–2014 in 56 countries worldwide: A descriptive analysis. *Am. J. Clin. Nutr.* **2016**, *104*, 1393–1402. [CrossRef]
17. Man, F.D. Optimal Nutrition Care for All (ONCA). Available online: https://european-nutrition.org (accessed on 21 August 2019).
18. European Patient Forum. Available online: http://www.eu-patient.eu/ (accessed on 21 August 2019).
19. Kondrup, J.; Allison, S.P.; Elia, M.; Vellas, B.; Plauth, M. ESPEN guidelines for nutrition screening 2002. *Clin. Nutr.* **2003**, *22*, 415–421. [CrossRef]
20. Cardenas, D.; Bermudez, C.; Barazzoni, R. The Cartagena Declaration: A call for global commitment to fight for the right to nutritional care. *Clin. Nutr.* **2019**. [CrossRef]
21. United Nations. *Sustainable Development Goals*; United Nations: New York, NY, USA, 2015.
22. Cederholm, T.; Jensen, G.L.; Correia, M.; Gonzalez, M.C.; Fukushima, R.; Higashiguchi, T.; Baptista, G.; Barazzoni, R.; Blaauw, R.; Coats, A.; et al. GLIM criteria for the diagnosis of malnutrition—A consensus report from the global clinical nutrition community. *Clin. Nutr.* **2019**, *38*, 1–9. [CrossRef]
23. Von Elm, E.; Altman, D.G.; Egger, M.; Pocock, S.J.; Gotzsche, P.C.; Vandenbroucke, J.P.; Initiative, S. The Strengthening the Reporting of Observational Studies in Epidemiology (STROBE) statement: Guidelines for reporting observational studies. *Lancet* **2007**, *370*, 1453–1457. [CrossRef]
24. World Health Organisation. Body Mass Index. Available online: http://www.euro.who.int/en/health-topics/disease-prevention/nutrition/a-healthy-lifestyle/body-mass-index-bmi (accessed on 10 September 2019).
25. Frantal, S.; Pernicka, E.; Hiesmayr, M.; Schindler, K.; Bauer, P. Length bias correction in one-day cross-sectional assessments—The nutritionDay study. *Clin. Nutr.* **2016**, *35*, 522–527. [CrossRef]
26. Schuetz, P.; Fehr, R.; Baechli, V.; Geiser, M.; Deiss, M.; Gomes, F.; Kutz, A.; Tribolet, P.; Bregenzer, T.; Braun, N.; et al. Individualised nutritional support in medical inpatients at nutritional risk: A randomised clinical trial. *Lancet* **2019**, *393*, 2312–2321. [CrossRef]

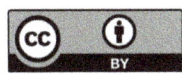

© 2019 by the authors. Licensee MDPI, Basel, Switzerland. This article is an open access article distributed under the terms and conditions of the Creative Commons Attribution (CC BY) license (http://creativecommons.org/licenses/by/4.0/).

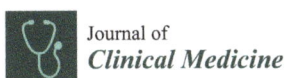

Article

Nutrition in Gastrointestinal Disease: Liver, Pancreatic, and Inflammatory Bowel Disease

Lena J. Storck [1,*], Reinhard Imoberdorf [1] and Peter E. Ballmer [1,2]

[1] Kantonsspital Winterthur, Department of Medicine, 8401 Winterthur, Switzerland
[2] Zürcher RehaZentrum Davos, 7272 Davos Clavadel, Switzerland
* Correspondence: lena.storck@ksw.ch; Tel.: +41-(0)52-266-23-27

Received: 13 June 2019; Accepted: 15 July 2019; Published: 25 July 2019

Abstract: Liver, pancreatic, and inflammatory bowel diseases are often associated with nutritional difficulties and necessitate an adequate nutritional therapy in order to support the medical treatment. As most patients with non-alcoholic fatty liver disease are overweight or obese, guidelines recommend weight loss and physical activity to improve liver enzymes and avoid liver cirrhosis. In contrast, patients with alcoholic steatohepatitis or liver cirrhosis have a substantial risk for protein depletion, trace elements deficiency, and thus malnutrition. Patients with chronic pancreatitis and patients with inflammatory bowel disease have a similar risk for malnutrition. Therefore, it clearly is important to screen these patients for malnutrition with established tools and initiate adequate nutritional therapy. If energy and protein intake are insufficient with regular meals, oral nutritional supplements or artificial nutrition, i.e., tube feeding or parenteral nutrition, should be used to avoid or treat malnutrition. However, the oral route should be preferred over enteral or parenteral nutrition. Acute liver failure and acute pancreatitis are emergencies, which require close monitoring for the treatment of metabolic disturbances. In most patients, energy and protein requirements are increased. In acute pancreatitis, the former recommendation of fasting is obsolete. Each disease is discussed in this manuscript and special recommendations are given according to the pathophysiology and clinical routine.

Keywords: monitoring; malnutrition; micronutrient deficiency; inflammation; oral nutritional supplements; artificial nutrition

1. Introduction

Gastrointestinal diseases are often associated with nutritional deficiencies. The complications range from digestive problems to nutrient absorption disorders and necessitate an adequate nutritional therapy in order to support the medical treatment. In this article, we focus on diseases of three important organs: Liver, pancreas, and intestine.

The liver is the main metabolic organ of the human organism because of its multiple functions; e.g., the liver controls the glucose homeostasis by regulation of glycogen synthesis, glycogenolysis, and gluconeogenesis. In addition, important body proteins and lipids are metabolized and synthesized in liver cells. Next to these metabolic pathways, the liver has an exocrine function by secretion of bile acids and detoxification of ammonia by urea production and glutamine synthesis. Taken these extensive functions into account, it is obvious that liver diseases and thus restrictions in liver functions have far-reaching consequences also for clinical nutrition. An important and by dietary habits increasing liver disease is non-alcoholic fatty liver disease (NAFLD), when the fat content of hepatocytes increases [1,2]. NAFLD aggregates benign hepatosteatosis, progressive and inflammatory non-alcoholic steatohepatitis (NASH) [3]. Insulin resistance, hyperinsulinemia, elevated plasma free fatty acids, fatty liver, hepatocyte injury, liver inflammation, oxidative stress, mitochondrial dysfunction, imbalanced pro-inflammatory cytokines, and fibrosis characterize NAFLD [4]. The other main cause for the development of steatosis is alcohol abuse. Chronic high alcohol consumption causes reduced fatty-acid oxidation as well as increased triglyceride synthesis and deposition, and thereby supports the development of alcoholic steatohepatitis (ASH). Usually, steatohepatitis can be reversible if the relevant noxious agent is eliminated. Inadequate or lack of treatment over many years increases the risk for the development of a liver cirrhosis. Thus, 15–20% of patients with NAFLD will develop liver cirrhosis [5]. Next to these liver diseases that develop over many years, acute liver failure may occur usually as a medical emergency.

Another important organ, which can develop inflammatory processes, is the pancreas. This organ plays a central role in digestion due to its exocrine and endocrine function. A total of 98% of pancreatic tissue is part of the exocrine function, whereby pancreatic enzymes are secreted for food digestion. The endocrine part is located in the Langerhans cells, secreting insulin and glucagon for regulation of glucose homeostasis. Acute pancreatitis is a severe disease, causing self-digestion of the pancreas due to prematurely activated digestive enzymes. Patients with chronic pancreatitis have recurrent inflammatory episodes that replace the pancreatic parenchyma by fibrous connective tissue resulting in a progressive loss of exocrine and endocrine function. Characteristic complications and symptoms are pain, pseudocysts, and pancreatic duct stenosis [6].

The largest digestive organ is the intestine, which regulates the absorption of nutrients. Two important diseases of the intestine are Crohn's disease (CD) and ulcerative colitis (UC) that are characterized by periods of remission and inflammatory flare-ups [7]. In CD, the small and large intestine as well as the mouth, esophagus, stomach, and the anus can be affected with typical ulcerations that occur discontinuously. In contrast, UC mostly affects the colon and rectum and usually shows a continuous pattern of the mucosa. Despite multiple differences, these two diseases share similar symptoms such as abdominal pain, diarrhea, and malnutrition. Hence, these diseases were grouped in the term inflammatory bowel disease (IBD) [7,8].

Nutritional care is clearly important in the treatment of patients with IBD, pancreas or liver disease. Nutritional management includes prevention and/or treatment of malnutrition and micronutrient deficiencies as well as specific recommendations for each condition.

2. Liver Diseases

2.1. Non-Alcoholic Fatty Liver Disease (NAFLD)

So far, there are no approved pharmacological therapies for NAFLD [3]. One reason is that the pathophysiology of NAFLD is not yet fully understood despite enormous advance in this field of research. Since overnutrition is the key problem of NAFLD and most of the patients are overweight or obese, weight loss is an obvious therapeutic possibility, hence, intensive lifestyle interventions are well studied [4,5]. The guideline on clinical nutrition in liver disease recommend a 7–10% weight loss to improve steatosis and liver enzymes [3,9]. To improve fibrosis, a weight loss of more than 10% is necessary [10]. Lifestyle interventions including diet and physical activity should be the first-line treatment and only if all efforts fail, bariatric surgery should be proposed [11,12].

In addition, the composition of the diet may also have an effect on liver fat. Low-carbohydrate diet may be helpful with weight loss, but over a long time, a low-carbohydrate diet stimulated NAFLD pathogenesis in an animal model [4]. It is speculated that the carbohydrate's composition is crucial [4]. For example, fructose can easily induce metabolic complications in the liver and in contrast, fiber might be helpful to maintain blood glucose and thus prevent NAFLD. Furthermore, a fat-rich diet induces hepatic steatosis, but only saturated fatty acids are detrimental for the liver metabolism. Monounsaturated fatty acids might be beneficial and polyunsaturated fatty acids might even be a treatment option for NAFLD [4].

The evidence suggest that increased oxidative stress and changes in several molecular factors like pro- and anti-inflammatory cytokines are mainly involved in the progression of NAFLD [13]. Therefore, antioxidants like vitamin C or polyphenols (e.g., resveratrol, curcumin, quercetin, anthocyanin, green tea polyphenols) might have beneficial effects to improve NAFLD [4]. Kitade et al. (2017) showed that the dietary administration of the carotenoids β-crypoxanthin and astaxanthin not only prevents but also reverses NASH progression in mice by regulating M1/M2 macrophage/Kupffer cell polarization [13]. NAFLD induced by diets high in sucrose/fructose or fat can be prevented or improved by soy protein (β-Conglycinin) by decreasing the expression and function of the two nuclear receptors SREBP-1c and PPAR γ2. Fish oil with ω-3 fatty acids inhibits SREBP-1c activity, but controversially increases PPAR γ2 expression [13,14]. In summary, research results for the effects of micronutrients on NAFLD showed positive effects on some factors in liver metabolism. However, it remains unclear whether the use of antioxidants and ω-3 fatty acids improve liver disease, thus, further investigations are needed and no recommendation can be given [4]. In contrast and only in non-diabetic adults, vitamin E (800 IU α-tocopherol daily) can improve liver enzymes and histologic pathology [11,15].

The Mediterranean Diet, which is characterized by a high content of antioxidants and fiber, a balanced lipid profile and a low content of simple sugar, seems to be the optimal diet for the management of NAFLD. This diet is a natural multi-ingredient supplement that may exert its related health benefits by the synergistic and/or complementary action of each food compound [16]. A Mediterranean diet low in carbohydrates mobilizes more liver fat compared to a low fat diet with a similar weight loss [17].

2.2. Alcoholic Steatohepatitis (ASH), Liver Cirrhosis, and Acute Liver Failure

The nutritional recommendations for patients with ASH and liver cirrhosis are fundamentally different compared to the recommendations for patients with NAFLD, because these patients have a high risk for protein depletion, trace elements deficiency, and malnutrition. Twenty percent of patients with a compensated and 60% of patients with a decompensated liver disease are malnourished [18–20].

Therefore, screening for malnutrition is highly recommended on a regular basis in patients with ASH and liver cirrhosis, but the nutritional assessment can be difficult in patients with cirrhosis especially if there is associated fluid retention and/or obesity. Patients with cirrhosis may have a combination of loss of skeletal muscle and gain of adipose tissue, culminating in the condition of "sarcopenic obesity". In addition, patients had a loss or deficiency of several other nutrients such as vitamin D and zinc [21]. The Nutritional Risk Screening-2002 and the Malnutrition Universal Screening Tool are validated and well-known tools to screen patients at risk for malnutrition [22]. Specifically in patients with liver disease, the Royal Free Hospital Nutrition Prioritizing Tool (RFH-NPT) was developed and when compared to Nutritional Risk Screening, it was more sensitive to identify malnourished liver patients. Next to the important variables unplanned weight loss and reduced dietary intake, the RFH-NPT has additional score points for complications like fluid overload and diuretics [23,24]. In addition, the presence or absence of sarcopenia may be assessed with radiological methods, because sarcopenia is a strong predictor of mortality and morbidity in patients with liver disease [25,26]. Next to radiological methods, handgrip strength is a simple, objective, and practical method to assess sarcopenia [21].

In case of malnutrition, patients need extensive nutritional counseling and therapy. The treatment is a challenge as the nutritional problems are multifactorial [11]. Usually, the resting energy expenditure is increased [27,28] and patients are required to consume 35–40 kcal/kg body weight [23]. Non-malnourished patients should eat 1.2 g protein/kg body weight per day to cover the protein needs, whereas the optimal intake of malnourished and/or sarcopenic patients is 1.5 g protein/kg body weight [11,23]. If energy and protein intake are not adequate with regular meals, oral nutritional supplements (ONS), or artificial nutrition (tube feeding or parenteral) should be used to avoid or treat malnutrition. However, the oral route should be preferred over enteral or parenteral nutrition. The standard formulas should be used, preferably formulas with high energy density (≥1.5 kcal/mL). In case of tube feeding, a percutaneous endoscopic gastrostomy placement is not recommended and can only be used in exceptional cases because of a higher risk of complications, e.g., infections, ascites, or oesophageal varices [22].

Patients with ASH or liver cirrhosis have poor hepatic glycogen stores due to the impaired synthetic capacity of hepatic cells, hence, an overnight fast in these patients is equivalent to a nearly 72 hours fast in healthy persons. As a result, metabolism shifts to fatty acids as a dominant substrate for oxidation. Some tissues dependent on glucose will need neoglucogenesis from amino acids as fatty acids cannot be used for this process. This leads to mobilization of amino acids from the skeletal muscles so that the adequate amount of glucose can be produced. Repeated and frequent fasting results in recurrent proteolysis resulting in muscle loss in human cirrhotic patients [21,29]. Therefore, fasting periods should be avoided and patients with severe liver disease, who have to fast for more than twelve hours, should receive intravenous glucose (2–3 g/kg body weight). When the fasting period lasts longer than 72 hours, total parenteral nutrition may be required [11]. At home, periods of starvation should also be kept short and, therefore, the consumption of three to five meals a day and a late evening snack are recommended [30]. One complication of severe liver disease is hepatic encephalopathy, a disorder of the central nervous system with a wide spectrum, ranging from psychomotor impairments to coma [31]. In case of hepatic encephalopathy, protein intake should no longer be restricted in cirrhotic patients as it increases protein catabolism and thus promotes malnutrition [32]. Advanced cirrhosis patients could benefit from branched-chain amino acids (0.25 g/kg body weight) in order to improve event-free survival and quality of life [33].

Acute liver failure may occur as a medical emergency. In multi-organ failure, a severe derangement of the whole metabolism can occur in these patients due to loss of hepatocellular functions. The metabolic condition is characterized by impaired hepatic glucose production and lactate clearance as well as protein catabolism associated with hyperaminoacidemia and hyperammonemia [11,34,35]. In general, patients with acute liver failure should be treated in the same way as other critically ill patients. Therefore, the patients need to be monitored regularly and if necessary, macronutrients, vitamins, and trace elements should be supplemented [11]. On the one hand, the energy requirement of patients with acute liver disease is increased [36], but on the other hand, a hypercaloric diet induces hyperglycemia and hyperlipidemia. Therefore, it is important to achieve an iso-energetic diet in order to avoid malnutrition and complications. For metabolic monitoring, the following target values should be aimed at: Blood glucose 8–10 mmol/L, serum lactate <5 mmol/L, triglycerides <3 mmol/L, and ammonia <100 mmol/L. The protein requirement is set at 0.8–1.2 g/kg body weight [11]. A summary of nutritional recommendations in liver disease are presented in Figure 1.

Non-alcoholic fatty liver disease
- Obese patients: 7-10% weight loss with intensive lifestyle interventions including physical activity
- Normal weight patients: Increasing physical activity

Alcoholic steatohepatitis and liver cirrhosis
- High risk for malnutrition: Regular screening and assessment using oral nutritional supplements or artificial nutrition
- 35-40 kcal/kg body weight and 1.2-1.5g protein/kg body weight
- Avoid periods of starvation
- Encephalopathy: Protein restriction obsolete
- 0.25g branched-chain amino acids/kg body weight

Acute liver failure
- Analog to other critically ill patients
- Iso-energetic nutrition intake
- Close monitoring and needs-based supplementation

Figure 1. Summary of nutritional recommendations in liver disease.

3. Pancreatic Diseases

3.1. Acute Pancreatitis

The degree of the inflammatory response of the pancreas plays an important role for the assessment of clinical nutrition. Normally, patients with a mild or moderately severe pancreatitis do not need a specific nutritional? intervention, but every patient with acute pancreatitis should be screened for malnutrition with the regular tools and in case of malnutrition, receive an adequate nutritional therapy [37]. The energy and protein requirements are usually not increased and the patients are allowed to eat normal food independently of lipase and amylase activity [37,38]. In contrast to former medical opinions, fasting after an inflammatory episode has no positive effect on the clinical course or prognosis of acute pancreatitis. During the course of pancreatitis, exocrine secretion is blocked and therefore a stimulation of the exocrine function by food intake or artificial nutrition is not expected [6,37]. For those patients who can tolerate an oral diet, an initial low-fat solid diet is preferred [39,40]. This early approach to oral feeding may reduce the length of hospital stay in these patients [41].

In contrast, patients with severe necrotizing pancreatitis need an adequate clinical nutritional? strategy. Initial short-time fasting could be beneficial for patients with ileus or nausea and vomiting, but within 24–48 hours, enteral nutrition should be started. Early enteral nutrition has a more preventive then a nutritive effect, because early enteral nutrition decreased mortality and complications [42–44]. Parenteral nutrition instead could result in an intestinal villous atrophy within a few days, which then facilitates bacterial translocation and may result in severe infections. The administration of enteral nutrition counteracts translocation, and therefore enteral nutrition should be administered whenever possible to prevent intestinal atrophy [6,45].

Due to inflammation and pain, patients with severe acute pancreatitis have an increased energy and protein requirement [46]. Energy requirement is set at 25–30 kcal/kg body weight, glucose intake at 2–4 g/kg body weight, and protein at 1.2–1.5 g/kg body weight. Infusion rate for lipids should be 0.8–1.5 g/kg body weight and the infusion should be monitored regularly since triglycerides in plasma should be <12 mmol/L. Trace elements are supplemented in normal concentrations and high-dose vitamin supplements are not required [37]. In addition, administration of pre- and probiotics as well as immunonutrition cannot be recommended since studies so far have not shown a clear beneficial effect [47,48]. To reach the nutritional goal, enteral nutrition can be completed with oral food intake or parenteral nutrition if necessary. In case of total parenteral nutrition over a long time period, administration of 0.2–0.5 g glutamine/kg body weight could protect against infections and reduce mortality [49]. In addition, monitoring of volume substitution is very important and can decrease mortality [6]. An early return to normal food intake should be pursued [6]. After an episode of acute pancreatitis, approximately 20% of the patients develop the common complications diabetes and exocrine pancreatic insufficiency [50]. Therefore, patients should be regularly screened for these complications in order to prevent nutritional status.

3.2. Chronic Pancreatitis

Patients with chronic pancreatitis have a high risk for malnutrition due to maldigestion from pancreatic exocrine insufficiency in combination with inflammation and increased energy metabolism. Pancreatic exocrine insufficiency is the main pancreatic cause of malnutrition in these patients [51]. In addition, due to diarrhea and steatorrhea, patients with chronic pancreatitis often have a deficiency of the fat-soluble vitamins A, D, E, and K. Malnutrition is associated with an increased complication rate and increased mortality [52]. Therefore, malnutrition should be avoided using nutritional counseling and if necessary artificial nutrition. Energy requirement is set at 25–30 kcal/kg body weight and protein requirement at 1.5 g protein/kg body weight. Since alcohol is an important cause for chronic pancreatitis, patients should avoid alcohol completely [6,37,53].

In the case of pancreatic exocrine insufficiency, patients should be supplemented with pancreas enzymes. The exocrine insufficiency is diagnosed if the patients have either steatorrhea (>15 g/day fecal fats) or suffer from manifest maldigestion, respective malabsorption. For a first indication, patients can be asked whether they see undigested food in their feces or if the feces are difficult to wash away. Further examination could be a pancreatic function test and the evaluation of maldigestion-related symptoms like diarrhea or flatulence, poor nutritional status, and fecal elastase-1 concentration [51,52]. In patients with an exocrine insufficiency, low levels of circulation fat-soluble vitamins, proteins like albumin, lipoproteins, apolipoproteins, and mineral trace elements like magnesium, zinc, or calcium, can occur [54–57]. Since most of these abnormalities are related to pancreatic exocrine insufficiency, a laboratory analysis might be helpful in order to diagnose the insufficiency. However, other factors like toxic habits or deficient food intake may play a relevant role, too [51]. Pancreas enzymes should be taken during the meals and the dosage is based on lipase activity. A range of 20.000 to 40.000 lipase units per main meal should be administered as an initial dose and 10.000 to 20.000 units for the digestion of smaller in-between snacks [6,58]. It is not necessary to avoid high fat intake if the exocrine pancreas function is compensated [37]. The replacement therapy should promote digestion, but a complete normalization of digestion is usually not achieved. However, there are several options for a failure of normalization. First, the pH value in the stomach inactivates the pancreatic enzymes. Therefore, the addition of a proton-pump inhibitor before breakfast and dinner is recommended in cases of an unsatisfactory clinical response to the standard dose of pancreatic enzymes [59]. Second, the enzyme dose should be increased if needed to normalize digestion and the nutritional status of the patients. If these two strategies fail, another cause for maldigestion like bacterial overgrowth should be evaluated [51]. A summary of nutritional recommendations in pancreatic disease is shown in Figure 2.

Acute pancreatitis
- Mild: Normal energy requirements and oral food intake
- Severe: Enteral nutrition should be started within 24-48 hours, energy and protein requirement are increased, combination with parenteral nutrition possible, early return to oral food intake should be pursued

Chronic pancreatitis
- High risk for malnutrition: Regular screening and assessment using oral nutritional supplements or artificial nutrition
- 25-30 kcal/kg body weight and 1.2-1.5g protein/kg body weight
- In case of steatorrhea or maldigestion: Supplementation of pancreas enzymes

Figure 2. Summary of nutritional recommendations in pancreatic disease.

4. Inflammatory Bowel Diseases (IBD)

IBD is a heterogeneous and multifactorial disorder resulting from a complex interplay between genetic variation, intestinal microbiota, the host immune system, and environmental factors such as diet, drugs, breastfeeding, and smoking [60–62]. The relationship between dietary nutrients and intestinal homeostasis is complex and influenced by several interactions between host immune system, the intestinal barrier, and the gut microbiota [60,63]. Patients with IBD have a high risk for malnutrition, which may be the result of reduced oral intake, increased nutrient requirement, increased gastrointestinal losses of nutrients, and occasionally from drug–nutrient interactions [7,64]. In pediatric patients, malnutrition is the main cause for growth retardation [65,66]. In CD, malnutrition is a great problem compared to UC because any part of the gastrointestinal tract can be affected. Therefore, the risk for malnutrition remains even when the disease is quiescent. UC is normally restricted to the colon and hence shows few malabsorptive problems except in active disease [64]. Due to the high risk, patients with IBD should be screened for malnutrition using the established tools at the time of diagnosis and thereafter on a regular basis [67,68]. Malnourished patients should receive an adequate nutritional therapy because otherwise it worsens the prognosis, complication rates, mortality, and quality of life [67,69,70]. The energy requirement of patients with IBD are normally not increased as well as the protein requirement in remission. In contrast, protein requirement is increased in active IBD and therefore, the protein intake should be 1.2–1.5 g/kg body weight [67,71,72].

In addition, patients with IBD have a high risk for micronutrient deficiencies due to losses from diarrhea and/or inadequate dietary intake. The most common micronutrient deficiencies are iron, calcium, selenium, zinc, and magnesium depletion. Vitamin deficiencies include all vitamins and in particular B_{12}, folic acid, and vitamins A, D, and K [73,74]. For example, selenium, zinc, and magnesium depletions are caused by an inadequate dietary intake and chronic loss because of diarrhea. Symptoms associated with deficiencies include bone health impairment, fatigue, poor wound healing, and cartilage degeneration [73,74]. An example for the influence of medication is cholestyramine that can interfere with absorption of fat-soluble vitamins, iron, and B_{12} vitamin. Main side effect is steatorrhea due to impair absorption of fats [75]. Therefore, laboratory values of patients should be checked on a regular basis and possible deficits should be appropriately corrected.

The most frequent extraintestinal manifestation of IBD is iron-deficiency and anemia, which occurs more frequently in CD and which should be supplemented with iron. Anemia is usually associated with other important symptoms like fatigue, sleeping disorders, restless legs syndrome, or attention deficit [75]. Patients with mild anemia can receive oral iron, when they are tolerant for oral iron and when the disease is inactive. Intravenous iron should be considered in patients with active IBD, with previous intolerance to oral iron, with hemoglobin below 100 g/L, and in patients who need erythropoiesis-stimulating agents [67,76,77]. Furthermore, patients may have deficiencies of calcium, vitamin D, folate, vitamin B_{12}, and zinc [64]. When more than 20 cm of the distal ileum is resected, vitamin B_{12} must be administered to patients [67].

Low levels of calcium and vitamin D are common in patients with IBD, especially in those with duodenal and jejunal disease [61,73,74]. Calcium deficiency is linked to vitamin D deficiency, which is related to inadequate daily intake, inflammation status, diarrhea, and glucocorticoid therapy. The prevalence among IBD patients is up to 70% in CD patients and up to 40% in UC patients. Nonetheless, it is not established if the vitamin D deficiency is a cause or a consequence of IBD. However, there are suggestions that in genetically predisposed individuals, vitamin D deficiency may be a contributing factor in the development of IBD [78]. Beneficial effects of vitamin D in IBD are supported by pre-clinical studies mainly in mouse models, where the active form of vitamin D has shown to regulate gastrointestinal microbiota function and promote anti-inflammatory response [61].

When oral nutritional intake is insufficient during active disease, ONS are the first step. If oral feeding is not sufficient, tube feeding is superior to parenteral feeding. Parenteral nutrition is indicated in IBD (i) when oral or tube feeding is not sufficiently possible, (ii) when there is an obstructed bowel, where there is no possibility of placement of a feeding tube beyond the obstruction or where this has failed, or (iii) when other complications occur such as an anastomotic leakage or a high-output intestinal fistula [67]. During active disease, specific formulations or substrates, e.g., glutamine, ω-3 fatty acids are not recommended, neither is the use of probiotics. Probiotic therapy using Escherichia coli Nissle 1917 or VSL#3 can be considered for use in patients with mild to moderate UC for the induction of remission [79].

Enteral exclusive nutrition has been extensively used for induction of remission in pediatric CD, in which avoidance of steroids is critical for childhood growth. Several recent pediatric studies have demonstrated and confirmed that enteral exclusive nutrition can induce remission in 60–86% of children [80–82] and is associated with higher remission rates, better growth, and longer steroids-free periods [60]. However, the benefit was lost when partial enteral nutrition was used with access to a free diet [83]. Nonetheless, a recent study has shown that partial enteral nutrition can be effective for induction of remission in children and young adults in combination with a diet, which is based on components hypothesized to affect the microbiome or intestinal permeability [84]. In remission, ONS or artificial nutrition are only recommended if malnutrition cannot be treated sufficiently by dietary counseling. In addition, specific diets or supplementations with ω-3 fatty acids are not recommended for maintenance of remission. A systematic review has not supported the hypothesis that supplementation of ω-3 fatty acids can induce and maintain remission in IBD [85]. However, several studies have demonstrated that different genotypes can be associated with the variable response to nutritional intervention with ω-3 fatty acids [86]. Probiotic therapy can be considered in UC but not CD for maintenance of remission [67]. In addition, clinical trials show that curcumin supplementation might be effective for the induction and maintenance of remission in UC patients [87,88]. Curcumin suppresses cytokine production by macrophages and intestinal epithelial cells via the inhibition of NF-kB activation [89,90] and thus mitigates induced colitis in mouse models [91,92]. A summary of nutritional recommendations in IBD is presented in Figure 3.

Inflammatory bowel disease
- Regular screening for malnutrition and micronutrient deficiency
- Energy and protein requirement are stable in remission, but increased in active disease
- Supplementation of iron in case of anemia
- If oral feeding is not sufficient then tube feeding is superior to parenteral feeding

Figure 3. Summary of nutritional recommendations in inflammatory bowel disease.

5. Future Perspectives

Clinical nutrition is clearly important in the treatment of patients with liver, pancreatic, and inflammatory bowel disease. However, there are many gaps of knowledge in the pathophysiology of these diseases despite an enormous research effort and thus the effects from clinical nutrition cannot be at a maximum so far.

A major gap in knowledge is associated with the evolution of NAFLD in children and adolescents. Weight loss is important for histological improvement and the benefits of weight loss will extend beyond those expected from drug treatment of high-risk NASH. It is postulated that only public health strategies will have the opportunity to improve the burden of obesity-related diseases in the future [93]. In addition, due to our aging population, it is expected that the burden of liver disease due to cirrhosis from NASH will increase over the next two decades unless effective preventive and therapeutic interventions are implemented as part of a public health strategy [93].

Furthermore, knowledge about the human microbiome constantly increases. Trillions of microbial cells, which form a symbiotic relationship with the host, play a crucial role in the development of diseases, when the balance of the microbiome becomes disrupted [94]. Increase intestinal permeability and dysbiosis are common characteristics linking the liver to a number of gastrointestinal diseases [95]. For example, alcohol consumption and endogenous alcohol production by gut bacteria in obese individuals can disrupt the tight junctions of the intestinal epithelial barrier, resulting in increased gut permeability. The bacterial endotoxin in the portal circulation leads to liver inflammation and fibrosis through activation of toll-like receptor 4 [95]. Although several mechanisms by which the microbiome might affect liver disease have been proposed, more work is needed to fully understand these relationship [93].

IBD is also associated with a dysbiotic microbiome. However, it is unclear if this dysbiosis plays a role in the pathophysiology or is a result of the disease. Due to the importance of the microbiome in IBD, therapies manipulating the microbiome have gained popularity. While there are some promising trials demonstrating the efficacy of antibiotic combinations in treating IBD, more controlled trials are required [94]. In addition, a more precise understanding of the complex interrelation between dietary nutrients, host immunity, and the microbiome is necessary to increase the effectiveness of dietary interventions used to treat IBD [63]. Moreover, an in-depth knowledge of the genetic background is important for personalized nutritional management, which might lead to a maximum efficacy in therapy [63].

New trials in acute pancreatitis showed that approximately one-third of patients will develop prediabetes or diabetes within five years of an index episode of acute pancreatitis and 24–40% of the patients develop an exocrine pancreatic insufficiency, but the mechanisms and risk factors remain to be specified [96–99]. Furthermore, further evidence is required to determine the optimal panel of laboratory markers for nutritional evaluation in chronic pancreatitis, and the utility, reliability, and accuracy of these markers in diagnosing pancreatic exocrine insufficiency [51].

Author Contributions: L.J.S., R.I. and P.E.B. contributed to the conceptualization of the manuscript. L.J.S. wrote the original draft. R.I. and P.E.B. reviewed and edited the original draft. All authors contributed to the final version of the manuscript.

Conflicts of Interest: There are no conflicts of interest to declare.

References

1. Mantovani, A.; Byrne, C.D.; Bonora, E.; Targher, G. Nonalcoholic fatty liver disease and risk of incident type 2 diabetes: A meta-analysis. *Diabetes Care* **2018**, *41*, 372–382. [CrossRef] [PubMed]
2. Loomba, R.; Abraham, M.; Unalp, A.; Wilson, L.; Lavine, J.; Doo, E.; Bass, N.M. Nonalcoholic steatohepatitis clinical research, N. association between diabetes, family history of diabetes, and risk of nonalcoholic steatohepatitis and fibrosis. *Hepatology* **2012**, *56*, 943–951. [CrossRef] [PubMed]
3. European association for the study of the liver, european association for the study of diabetes, european association for the study of obesity. EASL-EASD-EASO clinical practice guidelines for the management of non-alcoholic fatty liver disease. *Obes. Facts* **2016**, *9*, 65–90. [CrossRef] [PubMed]
4. Ullah, R.; Rauf, N.; Nabi, G.; Ullah, H.; Shen, Y.; Zhou, Y.D.; Fu, J. Role of nutrition in the pathogenesis and prevention of non-alcoholic fatty liver disease: Recent updates. *Int. J. Biol. Sci.* **2019**, *15*, 265–276. [CrossRef] [PubMed]
5. Vernon, G.; Baranova, A.; Younossi, Z.M. Systematic review: The epidemiology and natural history of non-alcoholic fatty liver disease and non-alcoholic steatohepatitis in adults. *Aliment. Pharm.* **2011**, *34*, 274–285. [CrossRef] [PubMed]
6. Hoffmeister, A.; Mayerle, J.; Beglinger, C.; Büchler, M.; Bufler, P.; Dathe, K.; Fölsch, U.; Friess, H.; Izbicki, J.; Kahl, S.; et al. S3-Leitlinie chronische pankreatitis: Definition, ätiologie, diagnostik, konservative, interventionell endoskopische und operative therapie der chronischen pankreatitis. leitlinie der Deutschen Gesellschaft für Verdauungs- und Stoffwechselkrankheiten (DGVS). *Zeitschrift für Gastroenterol.* **2012**, *50*, 1176–1224.
7. Hanauer, S.B. Inflammatory Bowel Disease: Epidemiology, Pathogenesis, and Therapeutic Opportunities. *Inflamm. Bowel Dis.* **2006**, *12*, S3–S9. [CrossRef]
8. Wedrychowicz, A.; Zajac, A.; Tomasik, P. Advances in nutritional therapy in inflammatory bowel diseases: Review. *World J. Gastroenterol.* **2016**, *22*, 1045–1066. [CrossRef]
9. Promrat, K.; Kleiner, D.E.; Niemeier, H.M.; Jackvony, E.; Kearns, M.; Wands, J.R.; Fava, J.L.; Wing, R.R. Randomized controlled trial testing the effects of weight loss on nonalcoholic steatohepatitis. *Hepatology* **2010**, *51*, 121–129. [CrossRef]
10. Vilar-Gomez, E.; Martinez-Perez, Y.; Calzadilla-Bertot, L.; Torres-Gonzalez, A.; Gra-Oramas, B.; Gonzalez-Fabian, L.; Friedman, S.L.; Diago, M.; Romero-Gomez, M. Weight loss through lifestyle modification significantly reduces features of nonalcoholic steatohepatitis. *Gastroenterology* **2015**, *149*, 367–378. [CrossRef]
11. Plauth, M.; Bernal, W.; Dasarathy, S.; Merli, M.; Plank, L.D.; Schutz, T.; Bischoff, S.C. ESPEN guideline on clinical nutrition in liver disease. *Clin. Nutr.* **2019**, *38*, 485–521. [CrossRef] [PubMed]
12. Mummadi, R.R.; Kasturi, K.S.; Chennareddygari, S.; Sood, G.K. Effect of bariatric surgery on nonalcoholic fatty liver disease: Systematic review and meta-analysis. *Clin. Gastroenterol. Hepatol.* **2008**, *6*, 1396–1402. [CrossRef] [PubMed]
13. Kitade, H.; Chen, G.; Ni, Y.; Ota, T. Nonalcoholic fatty liver disease and insulin resistance: New insights and potential new treatments. *Nutrients* **2017**, *9*, 387. [CrossRef] [PubMed]
14. Yamazaki, T.; Li, D.; Ikaga, R. Effective food ingredients for fatty liver: Soy protein beta-conglycinin and fish oil. *Int. J. Mol. Sci.* **2018**, *19*, 4107. [CrossRef] [PubMed]

15. Del Ben, M.; Polimeni, L.; Baratta, F.; Pastori, D.; Angelico, F. The role of nutraceuticals for the treatment of non-alcoholic fatty liver disease. *Br. J. Clin. Pharm.* **2017**, *83*, 88–95. [CrossRef] [PubMed]
16. Suarez, M.; Boque, N.; Del Bas, J.M.; Mayneris-Perxachs, J.; Arola, L.; Caimari, A. Mediterranean diet and multi-ingredient-based interventions for the management of non-alcoholic fatty liver disease. *Nutrients* **2017**, *9*, 1052. [CrossRef]
17. Gepner, Y.; Shelef, I.; Schwarzfuchs, D.; Zelicha, H.; Tene, L.; Yaskolka Meir, A.; Tsaban, G.; Cohen, N.; Bril, N.; Rein, M.; et al. Effect of distinct lifestyle Interventions on mobilization of fat storage pools: Central magnetic resonance imaging randomized controlled trial. *Circulation* **2018**, *137*, 1143–1157. [CrossRef]
18. Mendenhall, C.L.; Anderson, S.; Weesner, R.E.; Goldberg, S.J.; Crolic, K.A. Protein-calorie malnutrition associated with alcoholic hepatitis. *Am. J. Med.* **1984**, *76*, 211–222. [CrossRef]
19. Merli, M.; Riggio, O.; Dally, L. Italian Multicenter Cooperative Project on nutrition in liver cirrhosis. Nutritional status in cirrhosis. *J. Hepatol.* **1994**, *21*, 317–325.
20. Lautz, H.U.; Selberg, O.; Körber, J.; Bürger, M.; Müller, M.J. Protein-calorie malnutrition in liver cirrhosis. *Clin. Investig.* **1992**, *70*, 478–486. [CrossRef]
21. Anand, A.C. Nutrition and muscle in cirrhosis. *J. Clin. Exp. Hepatol.* **2017**, *7*, 340–357. [CrossRef] [PubMed]
22. Kondrup, J.; Allison, S.P.; Elia, M.; Vellas, B.; Plauth, M. ESPEN guidelines for nutrition screening 2002. *Clin. Nutr.* **2003**, *22*, 415–421. [CrossRef]
23. Amodio, P.; Bemeur, C.; Butterworth, R.; Cordoba, J.; Kato, A.; Montagnese, S.; Uribe, M.; Vilstrup, H.; Morgan, M.Y. The nutritional management of hepatic encephalopathy in patients with cirrhosis: International society for hepatic encephalopathy and nitrogen metabolism consensus. *Hepatology* **2013**, *58*, 325–336. [CrossRef] [PubMed]
24. Borhofen, S.M.; Gerner, C.; Lehmann, J.; Fimmers, R.; Gortzen, J.; Hey, B.; Geiser, F.; Strassburg, C.P.; Trebicka, J. The royal free hospital-nutritional prioritizing tool is an independent predictor of deterioration of liver function and survival in cirrhosis. *Dig. Dis. Sci.* **2016**, *61*, 1735–1743. [CrossRef] [PubMed]
25. Carey, E.J.; Lai, J.C.; Wang, C.W.; Dasarathy, S.; Lobach, I.; Montano-Loza, A.J.; Dunn, M.A.; Fitness, L.E. Exercise in liver transplantation, C. A multicenter study to define sarcopenia in patients with end-stage liver disease. *Liver Transpl.* **2017**, *23*, 625–633. [CrossRef] [PubMed]
26. Montano-Loza, A.J.; Meza-Junco, J.; Prado, C.M.; Lieffers, J.R.; Baracos, V.E.; Bain, V.G.; Sawyer, M.B. Muscle wasting is associated with mortality in patients with cirrhosis. *Clin. Gastroenterol. Hepatol.* **2012**, *10*, 166–173. [CrossRef] [PubMed]
27. Jhangiani, S.S.; Agarwal, N.; Holmes, R.; Cayten, C.G.; Pitchumoni, C.S. Energy expenditure in chronic alcoholics with and without liver disease. *Am. J. Clin. Nutr.* **1986**, *44*, 323–329. [CrossRef]
28. Schneeweiss, B.; Pammer, J.; Ratheiser, K.; Schneider, B.; Maldl, C.; Kramer, L.; Kranz, A.; Ferenci, P.; Druml, W.; Grimm, G.; et al. Energy metabolism in acute hepatic failure. *Gastroenterology* **1993**, *105*, 1515–1521. [CrossRef]
29. Tsien, C.D.; McCullough, A.J.; Dasarathy, S. Late evening snack: Exploiting a period of anabolic opportunity in cirrhosis. *J. Gastroenterol. Hepatol.* **2012**, *27*, 430–441. [CrossRef]
30. Plank, L.D.; Gane, E.J.; Peng, S.; Muthu, C.; Mathur, S.; Gillanders, L.; McIlroy, K.; Donaghy, A.J.; McCall, J.L. Nocturnal nutritional supplementation improves total body protein status of patients with liver cirrhosis: A randomized 12-month trial. *Hepatology* **2008**, *48*, 557–566. [CrossRef]
31. Ferenci, P.; Lockwood, A.; Mullen, K.; Tarter, R.; Weissenborn, K.; Blei, A.T. Hepatic encephalopathy–definition, nomenclature, diagnosis, and quantification: Final report of the working party at the 11th World Congresses of Gastroenterology, Vienna, 1998. *Hepatology* **2002**, *35*, 716–721. [CrossRef] [PubMed]
32. Cordoba, J.; Lopez-Hellin, J.; Planas, M.; Sabin, P.; Sanpedro, F.; Castro, F.; Esteban, R.; Guardia, J. Normal protein diet for episodic hepatic encephalopathy: Results of a randomized study. *J. Hepatol.* **2004**, *41*, 38–43. [CrossRef] [PubMed]
33. Ney, M.; Vandermeer, B.; van Zanten, S.J.; Ma, M.M.; Gramlich, L.; Tandon, P. Meta-analysis: Oral or enteral nutritional supplementation in cirrhosis. *Aliment. Pharm.* **2013**, *37*, 672–679. [CrossRef] [PubMed]
34. Clemmesen, J.O.; Kondrup, J.; Ott, P. Splanchnic and leg exchange of amino acids and ammonia in acute liver failure. *Gastroenterology* **2000**, *118*, 1131–1139. [CrossRef]
35. Rosen, H.M.; Yoshimura, N.; Hodgman, J.M.; Fischer, J.E. Plasma amino acid patterns in hepatic encepathalopathy of differing etiology. *Gastroenterology* **1977**, *72*, 483–487. [PubMed]

36. Walsh, T.S.; Wigmore, S.J.; Hopton, P.; Richardson, R.; Lee, A. Energy expenditure in acetaminophen-induced fulminant hepatic failure. *Crit. Care. Med.* **2000**, *28*, 649–654. [CrossRef] [PubMed]
37. Ockenga, J.; Löser, C.; Kraft, M.; Madl, C. S3-Leitlinie der Deutschen Gesellschaft für Ernährungsmedizin (DGEM) in Zusammenarbeit mit der GESKES, der AKE und der DGVS. *Aktuelle Ernährungsmedizin* **2014**, *39*, e43–e56. [CrossRef]
38. Meier, R.; Ockenga, J.; Pertkiewicz, M.; Pap, A.; Milinic, N.; Macfie, J.; Dgem; Loser, C.; Keim, V. ESPEN guidelines on enteral nutrition: Pancreas. *Clin. Nutr.* **2006**, *25*, 275–284. [CrossRef]
39. Larino-Noia, J.; Lindkvist, B.; Iglesias-Garcia, J.; Seijo-Rios, S.; Iglesias-Canle, J.; Dominguez-Munoz, J.E. Early and/or immediately full caloric diet versus standard refeeding in mild acute pancreatitis: A randomized open-label trial. *Pancreatology* **2014**, *14*, 167–173. [CrossRef]
40. Vaughn, V.M.; Shuster, D.; Rogers, M.A.M.; Mann, J.; Conte, M.L.; Saint, S.; Chopra, V. Early versus delayed feeding in patients with acute pancreatitis: A systematic review. *Ann. Intern. Med.* **2017**, *166*, 883–892. [CrossRef]
41. Aaronson, N.K.; Ahmedzai, S.; Bergman, B.; Bullinger, M.; Cull, A.; Duez, N.J.; Filiberti, A.; Flechtner, H.; Fleishman, S.B.; de Haes, J.C.J.M. The european organization for research and treatment of cancer qlq-c30: A quality-of-life instrument for use in international clinical trials in oncology. *J. Natl. Cancer Inst.* **1993**, *85*, 365–376. [CrossRef] [PubMed]
42. Marik, P.E.; Zaloga, G.P. Meta-analysis of parenteral nutrition versus enteral nutrition in patients with acute pancreatitis. *BMJ* **2004**, *328*, 1407. [CrossRef] [PubMed]
43. McClave, S.A.; Chang, W.K.; Dhaliwal, R.; Heyland, D.K. Nutrition support in acute pancreatitis: A systematic review of the literature. *J. Parenter. Enter. Nutr.* **2006**, *30*, 143–156. [CrossRef] [PubMed]
44. Al-Omran, M.; Albalawi, Z.H.; Tashkandi, M.F.; Al-Ansary, L.A. Enteral versus parenteral nutrition for acute pancreatitis. *Cochrane Database Syst. Rev.* **2010**, CD002837. [CrossRef] [PubMed]
45. Imrie, C.W.; Carter, C.R.; McKay, C.J. Enteral and parenteral nutrition in acute pancreatitis. *Best Pract. Res. Clin. Gastroenterol.* **2002**, *16*, 391–397. [CrossRef] [PubMed]
46. Shaw, J.H.F.; Wolfe, R.R. Glucose, fatty acid, and urea kinetics in patients with severe pancreatitis—The response to substrate infusion and total parenteral nutrition. *Ann. Surg.* **1986**, *204*, 665–672. [CrossRef] [PubMed]
47. Sun, S.; Yang, K.; He, X.; Tian, J.; Ma, B.; Jiang, L. Probiotics in patients with severe acute pancreatitis: A meta-analysis. *Langenbecks Arch. Surg.* **2009**, *394*, 171–177. [CrossRef]
48. Petrov, M.S.; Atduev, V.A.; Zagainov, V.E. Advanced enteral therapy in acute pancreatitis: Is there a room for immunonutrition? A meta-analysis. *Int. J. Surg.* **2008**, *6*, 119–124.
49. Asrani, V.; Chang, W.K.; Dong, Z.; Hardy, G.; Windsor, J.A.; Petrov, M.S. Glutamine supplementation in acute pancreatitis: A meta-analysis of randomized controlled trials. *Pancreatology* **2013**, *13*, 468–474. [CrossRef]
50. Lee, P.J.; Papachristou, G.I. New insights into acute pancreatitis. *Nat. Rev. Gastroenterol. Hepatol.* **2019**. [Epub ahead of print]. [CrossRef]
51. Dominguez-Munoz, J.E.; Phillips, M. Nutritional therapy in chronic pancreatitis. *Gastroenterol. Clin. North. Am.* **2018**, *47*, 95–106. [CrossRef] [PubMed]
52. Ockenga, J. Importance of nutritional management in diseases with exocrine pancreatic insufficiency. *HPB* **2009**, *11* (Suppl. S3), 11–15. [CrossRef] [PubMed]
53. Lévy, P.; Mathurin, P.; Roqueplo, A.; Rueff, B.; Bernades, P. A Multidimensional case-control study of dietary, alcohol, and tobacco habits in alcoholic men with chronic pancreatitis. *Pancreas* **1995**, *10*, 231–238. [CrossRef] [PubMed]
54. Duggan, S.N.; Smyth, N.D.; O'Sullivan, M.; Feehan, S.; Ridgway, P.F.; Conlon, K.C. The prevalence of malnutrition and fat-soluble vitamin deficiencies in chronic pancreatitis. *Nutr. Clin. Pr.* **2014**, *29*, 348–354. [CrossRef] [PubMed]
55. Lindkvist, B.; Dominguez-Munoz, J.E.; Luaces-Regueira, M.; Castineiras-Alvarino, M.; Nieto-Garcia, L.; Iglesias-Garcia, J. Serum nutritional markers for prediction of pancreatic exocrine insufficiency in chronic pancreatitis. *Pancreatology* **2012**, *12*, 305–310. [CrossRef] [PubMed]
56. Lindkvist, B.; Phillips, M.E.; Dominguez-Munoz, J.E. Clinical, anthropometric and laboratory nutritional markers of pancreatic exocrine insufficiency: Prevalence and diagnostic use. *Pancreatology* **2015**, *15*, 589–597. [CrossRef] [PubMed]

57. Montalto, G.; Soresi, M.; Carroccio, A.; Scafidi, E.; Barbagallo, C.M.; Ippolito, S.; Notarbartolo, A. Lipoproteins and chronic pancreatitis. *Pancreas* **1994**, *9*, 137–138. [CrossRef]
58. Dominguez-Munoz, J.E. Pancreatic exocrine insufficiency: Diagnosis and treatment. *J. Gastroenterol. Hepatol.* **2011**, *26* (Suppl. S2), 12–16. [CrossRef]
59. Lohr, J.M.; Dominguez-Munoz, E.; Rosendahl, J.; Besselink, M.; Mayerle, J.; Lerch, M.M.; Haas, S.; Akisik, F.; Kartalis, N.; Iglesias-Garcia, J.; et al. United european gastroenterology evidence-based guidelines for the diagnosis and therapy of chronic pancreatitis (HaPanEU). *United Eur. Gastroenterol. J.* **2017**, *5*, 153–199. [CrossRef]
60. Saez-Gonzalez, E.; Mateos, B.; Lopez-Munoz, P.; Iborra, M.; Moret, I.; Nos, P.; Beltran, B. Bases for the adequate development of nutritional recommendations for patients with inflammatory bowel disease. *Nutrients* **2019**, *11*, 1062. [CrossRef]
61. Fletcher, J.; Cooper, S.C.; Ghosh, S.; Hewison, M. The role of vitamin D in inflammatory bowel disease: Mechanism to management. *Nutrients* **2019**, *11*, 1019. [CrossRef] [PubMed]
62. De Souza, H.S.; Fiocchi, C. Immunopathogenesis of IBD: Current state of the art. *Nat. Rev. Gastroenterol. Hepatol.* **2016**, *13*, 13–27. [CrossRef] [PubMed]
63. Sugihara, K.; Morhardt, T.L.; Kamada, N. The role of dietary nutrients in inflammatory bowel disease. *Front. Immunol.* **2018**, *9*, 3183. [CrossRef] [PubMed]
64. Goh, J.; O'Morain, C.A. Review article: Nutrition and adult inflammatory bowel disease. *Aliment. Pharm.* **2003**, *17*, 307–320.
65. Hill, R.J.; Cleghorn, G.J.; Withers, G.D.; Lewindon, P.J.; Ee, L.C.; Connor, F.; Davies, P.S. Resting energy expenditure in children with inflammatory bowel disease. *J. Pediatr. Gastroenterol. Nutr.* **2007**, *45*, 342–346. [CrossRef] [PubMed]
66. Wiskin, A.E.; Wootton, S.A.; Culliford, D.J.; Afzal, N.A.; Jackson, A.A.; Beattie, R.M. Impact of disease activity on resting energy expenditure in children with inflammatory bowel disease. *Clin. Nutr.* **2009**, *28*, 652–656. [CrossRef]
67. Forbes, A.; Escher, J.; Hebuterne, X.; Klek, S.; Krznaric, Z.; Schneider, S.; Shamir, R.; Stardelova, K.; Wierdsma, N.; Wiskin, A.E.; et al. ESPEN guideline: Clinical nutrition in inflammatory bowel disease. *Clin. Nutr.* **2017**, *36*, 321–347. [CrossRef]
68. Sandhu, A.; Mosli, M.; Yan, B.; Wu, T.; Gregor, J.; Chande, N.; Ponich, T.; Beaton, M.; Rahman, A. Self-screening for malnutrition risk in outpatient inflammatory bowel disease patients using the malnutrition universal screening tool (MUST). *J. Parenter. Enter. Nutr.* **2016**, *40*, 507–510. [CrossRef]
69. Gajendran, M.; Umapathy, C.; Loganathan, P.; Hashash, J.G.; Koutroubakis, I.E.; Binion, D.G. Analysis of hospital-based emergency department visits for inflammatory bowel disease in the USA. *Dig. Dis. Sci.* **2016**, *61*, 389–399. [CrossRef]
70. Ananthakrishnan, A.N.; McGinley, E.L. Infection-related hospitalizations are associated with increased mortality in patients with inflammatory bowel diseases. *J. Crohns. Colitis.* **2013**, *7*, 107–112. [CrossRef]
71. O'Keefe, S.J.D.; Ogden, J.; Rund, J.; Potter, P. Steroids and bowel rest versus elemental diet in the treatment of patients with Crohn's disease: The effects on protein metabolism and immune function. *J. Parenter. Enter. Nutr.* **1989**, *13*, 455–460. [CrossRef] [PubMed]
72. Royall, D.; Greenberg, G.R.; Allard, J.P.; Baker, J.P.; Jeejeebhoy, K.N. Total enteral nutrition support improves body composition of patients with active Crohn's disease. *J. Parenter. Enter. Nutr.* **1995**, *19*, 95–99. [CrossRef] [PubMed]
73. Weisshof, R.; Chermesh, I. Micronutrient deficiencies in inflammatory bowel disease. *Curr. Opin. Clin. Nutr. Metab. Care.* **2015**, *18*, 576–581. [CrossRef] [PubMed]
74. Hwang, C.; Ross, V.; Mahadevan, U. Micronutrient deficiencies in inflammatory bowel disease: From A to zinc. *Inflamm. Bowel Dis.* **2012**, *18*, 1961–1981. [CrossRef] [PubMed]
75. Scaldaferri, F.; Pizzoferrato, M.; Lopetuso, L.R.; Musca, T.; Ingravalle, F.; Sicignano, L.L.; Mentella, M.; Miggiano, G.; Mele, M.C.; Gaetani, E.; et al. Nutrition and IBD: Malnutrition and/or sarcopenia? A practical guide. *Gastroenterol. Res. Pr.* **2017**, *2017*, 1–11. [CrossRef]
76. Bergamaschi, G.; Di Sabatino, A.; Albertini, R.; Ardizzone, S.; Biancheri, P.; Bonetti, E.; Cassinotti, A.; Cazzola, P.; Markoupoulos, K.; Massari, A.; et al. Prevalence and pathogenesis of anemia in inflammatory bowel disease. Influence of anti-tumor necrosis factor-alpha treatment. *Haematologica* **2010**, *95*, 199–205. [CrossRef] [PubMed]

77. Reinisch, W.; Staun, M.; Bhandari, S.; Munoz, M. State of the iron: How to diagnose and efficiently treat iron deficiency anemia in inflammatory bowel disease. *J. Crohns Colitis* **2013**, *7*, 429–440. [CrossRef]
78. Cantorna, M.T. Vitamin D and its role in immunology: Multiple sclerosis, and inflammatory bowel disease. *Prog. Biophys. Mol. Biol.* **2006**, *92*, 60–64. [CrossRef]
79. Fujiya, M.; Ueno, N.; Kohgo, Y. Probiotic treatments for induction and maintenance of remission in inflammatory bowel diseases: A meta-analysis of randomized controlled trials. *Clin. J. Gastroenterol.* **2014**, *7*, 1–13. [CrossRef]
80. Connors, J.; Basseri, S.; Grant, A.; Giffin, N.; Mahdi, G.; Noble, A.; Rashid, M.; Otley, A.; van Limbergen, J. Exclusive enteral nutrition therapy in paediatric Crohn's disease results in long-term avoidance of corticosteroids: results of a propensity-score matched cohort analysis. *J. Crohns Colitis* **2017**, *11*, 1063–1070. [CrossRef]
81. Levine, A.; Turner, D.; Pfeffer Gik, T.; Amil Dias, J.; Veres, G.; Shaoul, R.; Staiano, A.; Escher, J.; Kolho, K.L.; Paerregaard, A.; et al. Comparison of outcomes parameters for induction of remission in new onset pediatric Crohn's disease: Evaluation of the porto IBD group "growth relapse and outcomes with therapy" (GROWTH CD) study. *Inflamm. Bowel Dis.* **2014**, *20*, 278–285. [CrossRef] [PubMed]
82. Cohen-Dolev, N.; Sladek, M.; Hussey, S.; Turner, D.; Veres, G.; Koletzko, S.; Martin de Carpi, J.; Staiano, A.; Shaoul, R.; Lionetti, P.; et al. Differences in outcomes over time with exclusive enteral nutrition compared with steroids in children with mild to moderate Crohn's disease: Results from the GROWTH CD study. *J. Crohns Colitis* **2018**, *12*, 306–312. [CrossRef] [PubMed]
83. Levine, A.; Wine, E. Effects of enteral nutrition on Crohn's disease: Clues to the impact of diet on disease pathogenesis. *Inflamm. Bowel Dis.* **2013**, *19*, 1322–1329. [CrossRef] [PubMed]
84. Sigall-Boneh, R.; Pfeffer-Gik, T.; Segal, I.; Zangen, T.; Boaz, M.; Levine, A. Partial enteral nutrition with a Crohn's disease exclusion diet is effective for induction of remission in children and young adults with Crohn's disease. *Inflamm. Bowel Dis.* **2014**, *20*, 1353–1360. [CrossRef] [PubMed]
85. Turner, D.; Shah, P.S.; Steinhart, A.H.; Zlotkin, S.; Griffiths, A.M. Maintenance of remission in inflammatory bowel disease using omega-3 fatty acids (fish oil): A systematic review and meta-analyses. *Inflamm. Bowel Dis.* **2011**, *17*, 336–345. [CrossRef] [PubMed]
86. Paradis, A.M.; Fontaine-Bisson, B.; Bosse, Y.; Robitaille, J.; Lemieux, S.; Jacques, H.; Lamarche, B.; Tchernof, A.; Couture, P.; Vohl, M.C. The peroxisome proliferator-activated receptor alpha Leu162Val polymorphism influences the metabolic response to a dietary intervention altering fatty acid proportions in healthy men. *Am. J. Clin. Nutr.* **2005**, *81*, 523–530. [CrossRef] [PubMed]
87. Hanai, H.; Iida, T.; Takeuchi, K.; Watanabe, F.; Maruyama, Y.; Andoh, A.; Tsujikawa, T.; Fujiyama, Y.; Mitsuyama, K.; Sata, M.; et al. Curcumin maintenance therapy for ulcerative colitis: Randomized, multicenter, double-blind, placebo-controlled trial. *Clin. Gastroenterol. Hepatol.* **2006**, *4*, 1502–1506. [CrossRef] [PubMed]
88. Lang, A.; Salomon, N.; Wu, J.C.; Kopylov, U.; Lahat, A.; Har-Noy, O.; Ching, J.Y.; Cheong, P.K.; Avidan, B.; Gamus, D.; et al. Curcumin in combination with mesalamine induces remission in patients with mild-to-moderate ulcerative colitis in a randomized controlled trial. *Clin. Gastroenterol. Hepatol.* **2015**, *13*, 1444–1449.e1441. [CrossRef]
89. Wang, J.; Ghosh, S.S.; Ghosh, S. Curcumin improves intestinal barrier function: Modulation of intracellular signaling, and organization of tight junctions. *Am. J. Physiol. Cell Physiol.* **2017**, *312*, C438–C445. [CrossRef]
90. Pan, M.H.; Lin-Shiau, S.Y.; Lin, J.K. Comparative studies on the suppression of nitric oxide synthase by curcumin and its hydrogenated metabolites through down-regulation of IkappaB kinase and NFkappaB activation in macrophages. *Biochem. Pharm.* **2000**, *60*, 1665–1676. [CrossRef]
91. Yang, J.Y.; Zhong, X.; Kim, S.J.; Kim, D.H.; Kim, H.S.; Lee, J.S.; Yum, H.W.; Lee, J.; Na, H.K.; Surh, Y.J. Comparative effects of curcumin and tetrahydrocurcumin on dextran sulfate sodium-induced colitis and inflammatory signaling in mice. *J. Cancer Prev.* **2018**, *23*, 18–24. [CrossRef] [PubMed]
92. Sugimoto, K.; Hanai, H.; Tozawa, K.; Aoshi, T.; Uchijima, M.; Nagata, T.; Koide, Y. Curcumin prevents and ameliorates trinitrobenzene sulfonic acid-induced colitis in mice. *Gastroenterology* **2002**, *123*, 1912–1922. [CrossRef] [PubMed]
93. Sanyal, A.J. Past, present and future perspectives in nonalcoholic fatty liver disease. *Nat. Rev. Gastroenterol. Hepatol.* **2019**, *16*, 377–386. [CrossRef] [PubMed]
94. Ihekweazu, F.D.; Versalovic, J. Development of the pediatric gut microbiome: Impact on health and disease. *Am. J. Med. Sci.* **2018**, *356*, 413–423. [CrossRef] [PubMed]

95. Mandato, C.; Di Nuzzi, A.; Vajro, P. Nutrition and liver disease. *Nutrients* **2017**, *10*, 9. [CrossRef] [PubMed]
96. Nikkola, J.; Laukkarinen, J.; Lahtela, J.; Seppanen, H.; Jarvinen, S.; Nordback, I.; Sand, J. The long-term prospective follow-up of pancreatic function after the first episode of acute alcoholic pancreatitis: Recurrence predisposes one to pancreatic dysfunction and pancreatogenic diabetes. *J. Clin. Gastroenterol.* **2017**, *51*, 183–190. [CrossRef] [PubMed]
97. Das, S.L.; Kennedy, J.I.; Murphy, R.; Phillips, A.R.; Windsor, J.A.; Petrov, M.S. Relationship between the exocrine and endocrine pancreas after acute pancreatitis. *World J. Gastroenterol.* **2014**, *20*, 17196–17205. [CrossRef] [PubMed]
98. Hollemans, R.A.; Hallensleben, N.D.L.; Mager, D.J.; Kelder, J.C.; Besselink, M.G.; Bruno, M.J.; Verdonk, R.C.; van Santvoort, H.C. Pancreatic exocrine insufficiency following acute pancreatitis: Systematic review and study level meta-analysis. *Pancreatology* **2018**, *18*, 253–262. [CrossRef] [PubMed]
99. Das, S.L.; Singh, P.P.; Phillips, A.R.; Murphy, R.; Windsor, J.A.; Petrov, M.S. Newly diagnosed diabetes mellitus after acute pancreatitis: A systematic review and meta-analysis. *Gut* **2014**, *63*, 818–831. [CrossRef]

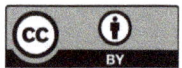

© 2019 by the authors. Licensee MDPI, Basel, Switzerland. This article is an open access article distributed under the terms and conditions of the Creative Commons Attribution (CC BY) license (http://creativecommons.org/licenses/by/4.0/).

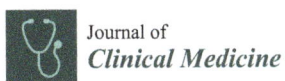

Article

Economic Challenges in Nutritional Management

Emilie Reber [1,*,†], Kristina Norman [2,3,†], Olga Endrich [4], Philipp Schuetz [5], Andreas Frei [6] and Zeno Stanga [1]

1. Department for Diabetes, Endocrinology, Nutritional Medicine and Metabolism, Bern University Hospital, and University of Bern, 3010 Bern, Switzerland
2. Department of Nutrition and Gerontology, German Institute for Human Nutrition Potsdam-Rehbrücke, 14558 Nuthetal, Germany
3. Research Group on Geriatrics, Charité Universitätsmedizin Berlin, Corporate Member of Freie Universität Berlin, Humboldt-Universität zu Berlin, and Berlin Institute of Health, 13347 Berlin, Germany
4. Health Data Management and Health Economics, Medical Directorate, Bern University Hospital, and University of Bern, 3010 Bern, Switzerland
5. Medical University Department, Division of General Internal and Emergency Medicine, Kantonsspital Aarau, 5001 Aarau, Switzerland
6. Freelance Health Economist, 4133 Pratteln, Switzerland
* Correspondence: emilie.reber@insel.ch
† Equally contributing first authors.

Received: 31 May 2019; Accepted: 4 July 2019; Published: 10 July 2019

Abstract: Disease-related malnutrition (DRM) is a highly prevalent independent risk and cost factor with significant influence on mortality, morbidity, length of hospital stay (LOS), functional impairment and quality of life. The aim of our research was to estimate the economic impact of the introduction of routinely performed nutritional screening (NS) in a tertiary hospital, with subsequent nutritional interventions (NI) in patients with potential or manifest DRM. Economic impact analysis of natural detection of inpatients at risk and estimation of the change in economic activity after the implementation of a systematic NS were performed. The reference population for natural detection of DRM is about 20,000 inpatients per year. Based on current data, DRM prevalence is estimated at 20%, so 4000 patients with potential and manifest DRM should be detected. The NI costs were estimated at CHF 0.693 million, with savings of CHF 1.582 million (LOS reduction) and CHF 0.806 million in additional revenue (SwissDRG system). Thus, the introduction of routine NS generates additional costs of CHF 1.181 million that are compensated by additional savings of CHF 2.043 million and an excess in additional revenue of CHF 2.071 million. NS with subsequent adequate nutritional intervention shows an economic potential for hospitals.

Keywords: economic challenges; nutritional management; malnutrition

1. Introduction

Disease-related malnutrition (DRM) is a debilitating, important and frequently occurring problem with an estimated prevalence of 20–50% on hospital admission [1–5]. The consequences of DRM are well known: Increases in morbidity, complication and mortality rates, resource use for inpatient treatment, prolonged hospital length of stay (LOS), decreased quality of life (QoL) and decreased body function. Many studies have shown the positive effects of nutritional interventions (NI), mainly in the reduction of complication rates, LOS, or rates of non-elective re-hospitalizations [3,6–10]. The recently published study by Schuetz et al.—a multicenter study with 2088 medical patients at nutritional risk, from eight Swiss hospitals—showed a significant reduction in serious complications and mortality as well as an improvement in physical function and quality of life after 30 days [11]. The study by Deutz et al. also showed a significant reduction in mortality after 90 days [12]. Available studies on cost-effectiveness clearly show that NI can save money and that the costs of NI are more than offset by the savings [7,9,13].

Since 2012, hospitals in Switzerland are remunerated using per-case rates for inpatients through the Swiss Diagnosis Related Groups (SwissDRG) system. In the SwissDRG it is possible to take DRM into account by coding it as a principal or secondary diagnosis. This requires optimal nutritional management from the hospitals, with an initial screening and adequate therapy in the course of treatment. Coding DRM may have the effect that a certain percentage of the patients will be assigned to a DRG with a higher cost-weight, generating additional revenue for the hospital (like a bonus system). Aeberhard et al. investigated the financial effects of coding DRM in the SwissDRG system, including all inpatients from the years 2013 to 2016 in our university hospital. During the observation period, 3.2% of the patients were coded with DRM. In 8.3% of these cases, the coding led to the attribution of a DRG with an increased cost-weight. This resulted in total additional revenue of circa CHF 3.5 million, which was offset by costs of CHF 2.8 million for assessment and treatment of DRM [1]. Thus, the costs of screening and treatment of DRM were already overcompensated for as a result of the DRM coding and changes in SwissDRG attribution. These results have been confirmed in similar studies [14,15].

As regularly performed nutritional risk screening is not established at the Bern University Hospital, these results reflect the natural detection (ND) of DRM. If nutritional screening (NS) is performed routinely on all patients, the detection rate of DRM will likely increase, leading to earlier detection and treatment. Performing routine screening will generate further costs. Besides that, the same costs for each patient at nutritional risk occurs when the NS is performed, as in the natural detection of DRM. However, due to an increased detection rate, the number of patients with treated and coded DRM will rise, with NI costs increasing as a consequence, but with additional revenues generated [16,17]. If DRM is detected and adequately treated, three types of consequences will occur:

- There will be costs for the detection of DRM and consequently for nutritional treatment,
- Treatment of DRM will lead to improvements in clinical outcomes that transfer to savings in the costs of basic treatment, and
- Patients may be attributed to DRGs with increased cost-weights, causing additional revenues for the hospital.

Previous economic analyses have always compared either the costs of NI with savings in the costs of basic nutritional treatments [3,7,13] or with the additional revenues due to DRG changes [14,16,17]. No study is known to have compared costs with a combination of both savings and additional revenue.

The objective of this study was to estimate the economic impact of the introduction of a systematically performed NS on all patients in our hospital, with subsequent NI in all patients at nutritional risk.

2. Materials and Methods

The data for this economic impact analysis were collected from the electronic patient record system of the Bern University Hospital in Bern, Switzerland, between 1 January and 31 December 2018. This is a cost-minimization analysis of the short-term economic consequences of inpatient hospitalization for the year 2018. Included were direct medical costs for NS and NI, cost savings due to NI, and additional revenues due to DRM coding and DRG changes. Using a population-based approach, the economic effects of a systematically performed NS were projected and compared with the existing situation reflecting the natural detection of DRM and routine nutritional management. To this end, a flow chart was created, and the patient flows and resource use were assessed. The costs of ND were subtracted from those of a systematic NS. Furthermore, the number of additional staff needed to perform routine NS was estimated. Data were obtained through analyses of the literature, the use of secondary statistics, and data collection at the Bern University Hospital. In cases of unclear or controversial data, assumptions were made. The flow chart is presented in Figure 1.

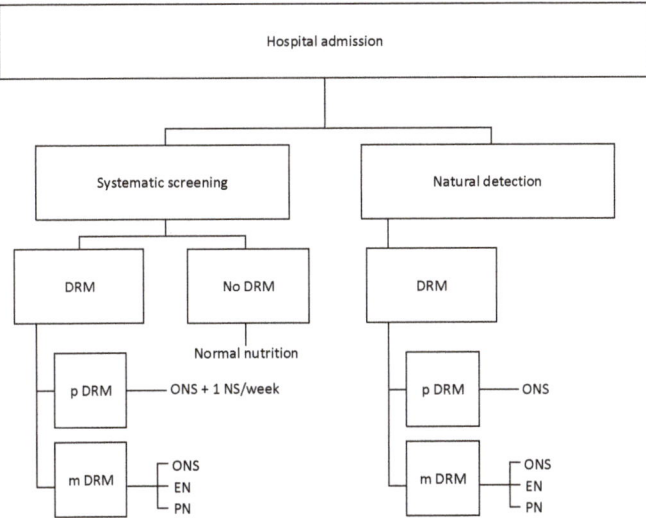

Figure 1. Nutritional screening (NS) and natural detection (ND). DRM: Disease-related malnutrition; p DRM: potential DRM; m DRM: manifest DRM; ONS: oral nutritional supplements; EN: enteral nutrition; PN: parenteral nutrition.

In a systematic NS, all patients are screened on admission to the hospital using a validated tool—in our case, the Nutritional Risk Screening 2002 (NRS 2002) [18]. Patients with an NRS score of 2 points or less are likely to be unaffected. Patients with an NRS score of 3 are considered at risk of DRM, and those with a score >3 points are considered to have manifest DRM. Patients with potential DRM undergo NS once per week. Patients with potential DRM will receive oral nutritional supplements (ONS) in addition to the customary nutrition and will also undergo NS once per week. Patients with manifest DRM will receive specific NI such as ONS, enteral nutrition (EN), or parenteral nutrition (PN) as needed and indicated in addition to the customary hospital nutrition. Their nutritional status will be regularly observed so that in these patients no additional NS will be needed [19].

3. Input Data

In Table 1 the input data are summarized.

Table 1. Overview of the input data.

Item	Both	Natural Detection	Nutritional Screening
Target population		Variable	20,000
Detection rate DRM		6.4%	20.0%
Proportions p DRM:m DRM		25% vs. 75%	45% vs. 55%
Number of nutritional screenings			No DRM, m DRM: 1; p DRM: 2
Nutritional interventions			
p DRM: ONS	100%	25%	45%
m DRM: ONS	45%	34%	25%
m DRM: EN	39%	29%	21%
m DRM: PN	16%	12%	9%
Reduction LOS in mDRM, days	1.2		
SwissDRG attribution change		8.3%	15.0%
Average increase cw		0.694	0.44

DRM: disease-related malnutrition; p DRM: potential DRM; m DRM: manifest DRM; ONS: oral nutritional supplements; EN: enteral nutrition; PN: parenteral nutrition; LOS: length of hospital stay; SwissDRG: Swiss diagnosis-related group, cw: cost-weight.

3.1. Target Population

For a systematic NS with subsequent NI, patients with an expected LOS of >3 days were considered eligible. In 2018, this amounted to 21,819 patients (information from Bern University Hospital). The average LOS of these patients was 10.01 days. This number also included healthy newborns. Therefore, it was assumed that the target population for a systematic NS at the Bern University Hospital would amount to approximately 20,000 patients yearly. Even though Aeberhard et al. [1] included all inpatients, it is unlikely that DRM was detected in patients with a LOS ≤3. Therefore, the reference population for ND patients with DRM was also assumed to be about 20,000 patients per year.

3.2. Detection Rate

Detection rates of 19% and 25.6% were obtained from two German studies [16,17]. The latter, however, also included patients with NRS ≥2, and the rate of patients with NRS >3 was computed at 20.7%. A Dutch study found that NS could increase the detection rate of DRM from 50% to 80% given a DRM prevalence of 32% [20]. Based on these data, the detection rate was estimated at 20%. For natural detection, we doubled the rate of 3.2% from Aeberhard et al. [1], using 6.4%.

3.3. Proportions with Potential and Manifest DRM

In patients with NS, the proportion of potential versus manifest DRM was estimated at 45%:55% based on [17]. In the naturally detected patients, these proportions were assumed to be 25%:75% as in [1].

3.4. Number of Screenings

Patients potentially having DRM are screened on admission and then once weekly. Patients with manifest DRM are only screened once on admission [19].

The number of screenings therefore depends on the proportions of patients with potential and manifest DRM and their expected LOS. Two studies showed that LOS in patients with DRM is longer than in well-nourished patients (11 vs. 7 days [16], 14 vs. 7.6 days [17]). Thus, it was assumed that LOS in patients without DRM was one week or less, and that LOS detected in DRM patients detected by NS was 12–14 days (1–2 weeks). Therefore, it was assumed that patients without DRM receive one NS, patients with potential DRM receive two NS, and patients with manifest DRM receive one.

3.5. Types and Proportions of NI

We distinguish between three types of NI: ONS, EN, and PN. In the study by Aeberhard et al., 59% of ND patients received ONS, 29% received EN, and 12% received PN [1]. All patients with potential DRM received ONS. Of the 59% of patients prescribed ONS, 25% were patients with potential DRM and 34% were patients with manifest DRM. The proportions of potential and manifest DRM differ in patients with NS. This implies that 45% with potential DRM will be prescribed ONS. In addition, of the 55% with manifest DRM, 25% will receive ONS, 21% will receive EN, and 9% will receive PN.

3.6. Reduction of LOS

Available data suggest that hospital LOS can be reduced by NI. However, it is difficult to quantify the amount. It seems that this effect is more likely to occur in patients with manifest DRM than with potential DRM and that it is more pronounced in connection with severe DRM [5,20–22]. Based on the findings of Elia et al. (−13.8% in relation to 22.5 hospital days) [3], Sriram et al. (−10% in relation to 6 days) [5] and Bally et al. (0%, calculated −3.2% of 13 days, not significant) [6], it was assumed here that NS will reduce LOS in patients with manifest DRM by 10%. This results in a reduction in LOS of 1.2 days. The same assumption is also made for ND patients.

3.7. DRG Changes

In ND, coding of a case of DRM led to a DRG change in 8.3% of all coded cases [1]. In patients with NS this proportion was substantially higher, amounting to 27% [16] and 15% [17]. Therefore, it was conservatively estimated to be 15%.

3.8. Increase in Cost-Weight

The average amount of additional revenue per case with a DRG change amounted to CHF 7564 [1]. Given a base rate of CHF 10,900, this corresponds to an average increase in the cost-weight of 0.694. However, in patients with NS, the average increase was clearly smaller (0.44) [16,17].

3.9. Ethics

This study was conducted in accordance with the ethical guidelines of the 1957 Declaration of Helsinki and approved by the Bernese Cantonal Ethics committee (BASEC ID 2017-00480), Bern, Switzerland.

4. Cost and Savings

4.1. Cost of NS

The costs of NS were calculated based on the time needed in minutes multiplied by the cost per minute of nursing staff. According to Wenger et al., the time needed to administer NS is about 5 min [19]. The costs per minute were calculated from an hourly rate (gross wage including employers' contributions to social insurance, information University Hospital Bern) and amounted to CHF 3.93.

4.2. Costs per Patient with NI

Therapy costs per patient for NI patients with DRM included daily personnel and materials costs multiplied by the duration of NI in days. In the case of EN and PN, one-time costs per therapy were added (Table 2). These values were based on Aeberhard et al. [1] and updated for 2019.

For ONS, the time expended by staff members was 10 min for a nutritional therapist, 10 min for nursing staff, and 2 min for a physician; for EN it was 10 min for a nutritional therapist, 40 min for nursing staff, and 2 min for a physician; and for PN it was 12 min for a nutritional therapist, 70 min for nursing staff, and 2.4 min for physicians. The costs were CHF 41.40 per hour for a nutritional therapist, CHF 47.11 per hour for nursing staff, and CHF 78.24 per hour for physicians (information provided by the Bern University Hospital). Data on materials costs, duration of NI and one-time costs were obtained from Aeberhard et al. [1]. Thus, the costs per patient for NI were calculated as CHF 187.57 for ONS, CHF 842.96 for EN, and CHF 1557.84 for PN.

Table 2. Costs of nutritional interventions (NI) per patient and intervention.

	ONS	EN	PN
Per day			
Personnel costs, CHF	17.36	40.91	66.37
Materials costs, CHF	4.97	40.09	75.02
Personnel and materials costs, CHF	22.33	81.00	141.39
Per therapy			
Duration of therapy, days	8.4	10.3	9.6
Personnel and material costs, CHF	187.57	834.35	1357.36
One-time costs, CHF		8.61	200.48
Total therapy costs, CHF	187.57	842.96	1557.84

ONS: oral nutritional supplements; EN: enteral nutrition; PN: parenteral nutrition.

4.3. Savings per Prevented Inpatient Day

It was assumed that the reduction of LOS occurred at the end of the hospitalization period. The costs then were mainly related to accommodation, food, medical care, follow-up visits, hospital buildings and the like. Such LOS-dependent costs are also used for the remuneration of hospital services in DRG outliers. In such cases, in addition to the per-case rate, the hospital is reimbursed a daily rate for each day exceeding the upper trim point delimiting inlier LOS. These daily rates are based on cost-weights per day. The cost-weight per day was calculated at 0.126 as a weighted average across the SwissDRGs based on Aeberhard et al. [1]. This was multiplied by the base rate of the Bern University Hospital (CHF 10,900). Thus, the cost per prevented hospital day was estimated at CHF 1373.

4.4. Additional Revenue due to SwissDRG Change

The number of patients with SwissDRG changes were multiplied by the average increases in the cost-weights and the CHF 10,900 base rate of the Bern University Hospital.

5. Results

5.1. Effect of a Systematic NS

The patient flow and performance of systematic NS are summarized in Table 3.

Table 3. Patient flow and resource use in connection with a systematic nutritional screening (NS).

Patients Flow and Performance	Proportion/Rate	Number
Target population		20,000
Detection rate, of which:	20%	4000
- proportion p DRM	0.45	1800
- proportion m DRM	0.55	2200
Number of systematic nutritional screenings		
- On hospital admission	1	20,000
- Weekly in cases with p DRM	1	1800
Total screenings		21,800
Nutritional interventions		
p DRM		
- ONS	45.0%	1800
m DRM		
- ONS	24.9%	997
- EN	21.3%	851
- PN	8.8%	352
Total nutritional interventions	100.0%	4000
Saved hospital days	Per Patient	Total
expected LOS	12	
reduction %	10%	
Reduction LOS, days	1.2	2640
Swiss DRG changes	Detected Cases	
Changes in DRG attribution	0.15	600

DRM: disease-related malnutrition; p DRM: potential DRM; m DRM: manifest DRM; ONS: oral nutritional supplements; EN: enteral nutrition; PN: parenteral nutrition; LOS: length of hospital stay; DRG: diagnosis-related groups.

For a systematic NS, 20,000 patients per year would have to be screened on hospital admission. Assuming a detection rate of 20%, 4000 patients (including potential and manifest DRM) would be detected. Of these, 45% (1800) will have potential DRM and 55% (2200) will have manifest DRM. Patients with potential DRM and a projected LOS of 12 days will experience a second instance of NS in the second week of their hospital stay. So, in total, 21,800 NS will be performed. The 1800 patients with potential DRM and an absolute 24.9% of the 2200 patients with manifest DRM (=997 patients) will receive ONS. Furthermore, 21.3% (=851 patients) will receive EN, and 8.8% (=352 patients) will receive PN. These NI will effect a reduction of LOS of 1.2 days per case in patients with manifest DRM. This will result in global savings of 2640 hospital days in 2200 patients.

In all 4000 DRM patients, DRM will be coded as a complication or comorbidity in the DRG system. This coding will cause a DRG change in 15% of all DRM coded cases (i.e., 600 patients). The resulting costs are summarized in Table 4.

A total of 21,800 NS will be performed per year at a cost of CHF 3.93 per unit of NS. Thus, the costs of NS will amount to CHF 85,583. The costs of NI are calculated in a similar way using the number of patients multiplied by the NI costs per patient. The costs for all 2797 patients with ONS (1800 with potential, 997 with manifest DRM) were calculated as CHF 524,694, the costs of the 851 patients with EN as CHF 717,076, and those of the 352 patients with PN as CHF 548,358. Overall, the costs of NI amount to CHF 1,790,128. Combined with the costs of NS, global costs amount to 1,875,711. These costs are balanced by savings of CHF 3,625,930 due to the reduction of LOS. Furthermore, additional revenue of CHF 2,877,600 results from DRG changes. So, after deduction of the costs, there is a net monetary gain of CHF 4,627,818 for the hospital.

Table 4. Costs resulting from a systematic NS.

	Number	Value	Costs
Costs			
Systematic nutritional screening	21,800	3.93	85,583
Nutritional interventions			
ONS	2797	187.57	524,694
EN	851	842.96	717,076
PN	352	1557.84	548,358
Total nutritional interventions	4000		1,790,128
Total costs			1,875,711
Savings (LOS reduction) (−)	2640	1373.46	−3,625,930
Additional revenue (SwissDRG) (−)	600	4796.00	−2,877,600
Net effect			−4,627,818

Costs are indicated with positive (+), savings and additional revenue with negative (−) prefix. DRM: disease-related malnutrition; p DRM: potential DRM; m DRM: manifest DRM; ONS: oral nutritional supplements; EN: enteral nutrition; PN: parenteral nutrition.

5.2. Effects of ND, Treatment and Coding of DRM

Table A1 (Appendix A) shows the patient flow in the case of natural detection of DRM. In relation to the target population of 20,000 patients, the detection rate is 6.4%, which results in 1280 patients per year with DRM detected, treated and coded. Of these, 25% (320 patients) will be patients with potential DRM and 75% (960 patients) will be with manifest DRM. ONS will be provided to 755 patients (59%), EN to 371 patients (29%), and PN to 154 patients (12%).

It can be assumed that the average LOS in patients with naturally detected DRM would have been longer if they had not been treated for DRM and if NI had not reduced this LOS in the 960 patients with manifest DRM by 1.2 days. This amounts to a savings of 1152 hospital days. In 8.33% of the patients, i.e., in 107 cases, there is a DRG change.

Table A2 (Appendix A) shows the costs related to natural detection of DRM. The costs of NI amounts to CHF 141,652 for the treatment of 755 patients with ONS, CHF 312,906 for the 371 patients with EN, and CHF 239,284 for the 154 patients with PN. Total costs amount to CHF 693,842 per year. The savings due to a reduction of LOS amounted to CHF 1,582,224. The additional revenue resulting from SwissDRG changes amounts to CHF 806,579. The costs are overcompensated for by the savings and the additional revenue, resulting in an overall net savings of CHF 1,694,961.

5.3. Costs, Savings, and Additional Revenue Attributable to NS

As compared with the actual state of a natural detection, a systematic NS would generate additional costs of CHF 85,583 for screening and CHF 1,096,286 for NI, totaling CHF 1,181,869. These would be compensated for by savings of CHF 2,043,706 due to a reduction in LOS and by additional revenue of CHF 2,071,021 arising from coding and DRG changes (Table 5).

Table 5. Net monetary effects of the introduction of a systematic NS.

	Nutritional Screening	Natural Detection	Extra Costs/ Savings NS
Costs			
Systematic screening	85,583		85,583
Nutritional interventions	1,790,128	693,842	1,096,286
Total costs	1,875,711	693,842	1,181,869
Savings (reduction LOS) (−)	−3,625,930	−1,582,224	−2,043,706
Additional revenue (SwissDRG) (−)	−2,877,600	−806,579	−2,071,021
Net effect	−4,627,818	−1,694,961	−2,932,858

5.4. Staff Needed

Table A3 shows (Appendix A) the calculation of the staff needed, broken down by professional group. The total number of working hours and days was based on the time needed per day and the duration of the therapy in days (see Table 1) and on the number of patients undergoing therapy. Details are given in Table A4 (Appendix A). The number of positions was calculated using an average working day of 8.4 h, 220 working days per year and a fulltime position, and a productivity of 80%.

For a systematic NS, 4.09 positions for nutritional therapists, 9.27 positions for nursing staff, and 0.82 positions for physicians is needed. The treatment of naturally detected patients with DRM presently requires 1.35 positions for nutritional therapists, 3.6 positions for nursing staff, and 0.27 positions for physicians. Thus, the additional staff needed amounts to 2.75 positions for nutritional therapists, 5.66 positions for nursing staff and 0.55 positions for physicians.

5.5. Scenario Analyses

The results show that the savings and the additional revenue are each separately greater than the costs. Scenario analyses were performed based on few important assumptions to determine the minimum savings or additional revenues needed in order to cover only the costs. To find a best estimate for the reduction of LOS, the value of a saved hospital day, the proportion of DRG changes, and the average increases in the cost-weights, the following scenario analyses were performed:

Analysis 1, cost consequences in case the savings = 0, shows that even if no savings could be realized, NS could still achieve a net benefit through the additional revenue of CHF 1,001,889.

Analysis 2, cost consequences if additional revenue = 0, reveals that, even if no additional revenue were realized, NS would still lead to net savings of CHF 1,750,218.

Analysis 3, minimal additional revenue needed if savings = 0, shows that, in order to compensate for the costs, additional revenue of CHF 1,875,711 is needed. This could be achieved (1) by reducing the proportion of cases with changes in DRG attribution to 9.8% while keeping the increase in the cost-weight constant, or (2) by leaving the percentage of cases with changes in DRG attribution unchanged while increasing the average cost-weight by only 0.29.

Analysis 4 shows that a 5% reduction in LOS with a constant value per day would be sufficient to achieve the minimum required savings of CHF 1,875,711. On the other hand, if the reduction of LOS were left unchanged, a valuation of CHF 710 per saved hospital day would be sufficient.

6. Discussion

The introduction of a systematic NS would be accompanied by yearly costs of CHF 1.875 million. These costs would be compensated for by savings of CHF 3.635 million from a reduction in LOS and by additional revenue of CHF 2.877 million due to changes in documentation and coding of DRM. These numbers include the costs, savings and additional revenue produced by natural detection of DRM. These were estimated at CHF 0.693 million for the costs, CHF 1.582 million for the savings, and CHF 0.806 million for the additional revenue. Thus, the introduction of a systematic NS would generate additional costs of CHF 1.181 million that would be compensated for by additional savings of CHF 2.043 million and additional revenue of CHF 2.071 million.

These figures are based on projections using data from literature analyses, use of secondary statistics and data collected from the Bern University Hospital. It is notable that the savings per se are almost twice the costs, and the additional revenue alone is about 1.5 times the costs. These results are based on a few central assumptions about the data collected. The most important of these are discussed here.

The detection rate of NS was estimated to be 20%. Compared with data from the literature showing prevalence rates of 20–50% and even greater, this is a cautious assumption. The assumption regarding the size of the target population seems well justified, as only patients with an expected LOS of >3 days were considered. In estimating the expected LOS of patients with DRM, neither the average LOS (barely 6 days) of all patients from the Bern University Hospital nor the LOS (20 days) of the naturally detected patients in the study by Aeberhard et al. [1] can be considered representative. The expected LOS in patients with DRM (12 days) is plausible given that the average LOS of the target population is 10 days.

The costs of NS are very low compared with those of NI. The costs as well as the savings and the additional revenue are determined by the detection rate and the number of patients with DRM. Varying the assumptions relating to the detection rate will therefore result in a corresponding almost proportional variation in the difference between the costs and the savings and the additional revenue. This difference depends strongly on the assumptions regarding the savings and the additional revenue.

The projected savings are based on assumptions about the reduction of LOS due to NI. These are based on the results of meta-analyses, reviews and single studies. The literature is not consistent, but it shows evidence of or tendencies toward reduction of LOS, complication rates or rates of non-elective rehospitalizations [5,6,10–13]. However, for an economic assessment, available data on types and frequencies of avoided complications are not specific enough. Reductions in rehospitalizations are also difficult to evaluate because of varying follow-up periods. Therefore, it seems justified to use the reduction in LOS as a proxy for the many and various effects, with evidence of an improvement in clinical and economic outcomes due to NI.

For each one-day reduction in LOS, CHF 1371 was saved. This reflects the high costs associated with medical care in Switzerland and at university hospitals. A Danish study found the costs of outliers to be \$224 per day in 2006. A Dutch study from the year 2005 estimated these costs at 476 €, and a US study reported costs of \$1770 in 2018. The global average costs per hospital day at the Bern University Hospital amounted to CHF 2848 (information provided by the Federal Office of Public Health). So, valuing the LOS-dependent cost with per diem additional rates for DRG outliers seems justified.

The amount of additional revenues received is determined by the proportion of cases with DRG changes and the resulting increase in the average cost-weight in these cases. In the study by Aeberhard et al. [1], the proportion with changes in DRG attribution amounted to 8.3%. Compared with other studies in patients without NS, this is quite low. The average increase in the cost-weight was 0.694, a figure confirmed by other studies as well. In patients with NS, these numbers are not valid. The proportion of cases with changes in DRG attributions was assumed to be 15%. This is a conservative estimate and corresponds with the lower of two values from studies with NS (15% and 27%). The average increase in the cost-weight in these patients was lower, amounting to circa 0.44 in both studies, a figure, which was therefore applied in the current study.

7. Cost Effectiveness of Nutritional Therapy in the Post-Hospital or Community Setting: A Brief Statement

Prevalence of malnutrition has been studied less often in the community setting due to the lack of systematic or standardized screening programs, for example at healthcare institutions or in the offices of general practitioners. It is well established, however, that between 20% and 40% of patients admitted from the community setting to a hospital are already malnourished. Also, nutritional status frequently worsens during a hospital stay, which means that a large proportion of patients, particularly those older than 60 years, are discharged to a community setting or to other institutions with malnutrition. It is estimated that only around 10% of malnourished patients are in fact hospital patients, with the rest dwelling in a community or nursing home setting [23].

Few studies have addressed the costs of malnutrition and the economic impact of nutritional support in these settings [24]. Due to feasibility, the majority of studies investigating cost effectiveness of nutritional therapy are in-hospital analyses, but these only reflect a short period in terms of the patients' needs for nutritional therapy. Malnourished patients, particularly those who are old, frequently need continued nutritional support. This is a challenge for the analysis of cost effectiveness, as the costs of management in one setting may be offset by greater cost savings in another setting, such as when patients are moving from one care setting to another and a more comprehensive perspective is needed. Not surprisingly, nutritional therapy is frequently discontinued after a hospital stay. Most studies that have assessed cost effectiveness of NI in the community-dwelling population are initiated at hospital discharge [25–28]. These frequently use oral nutritional supplements and are carried out for 3–6 months after a hospital stay. Studies of community-dwelling or nursing home residents more frequently address further types of nutritional support, such as dietary counseling, snacks between meals, or multi-component nutritional support.

Table A5 (Appendix A) gives an overview of the type and design of studies investigating the cost effectiveness of nutritional support following hospital discharge in the community-dwelling elderly or in nursing home residents. Despite the different methodologies used, nutritional therapy was generally found to be cost effective, with the higher costs incurred by nutritional support being ultimately associated with decreased use of health care resources and improved quality of life.

8. Conclusions

This is the first study to compare the costs of a systematic NS and subsequent adequate NI, with the combined effects of savings due to reduced LOS and additional revenue resulting from SwissDRG changes. The costs of the intervention could be separately compensated for by savings in the costs of basic treatment and by the additional revenue generated. NS with subsequent adequate NI is thus associated with high economic potential for the hospital. Moreover, the EFFORT trial was able to demonstrate an impressive effect of NI, with a significant reduction in mortality and severe complications as well as improvement of physical function and quality of life in medical inpatients [11]. These clinical benefits, in terms of savings in supplemental hospital costs, were not included in the current economic impact analysis. If they had been, this would have greatly increased the financial efficacy.

Author Contributions: Conceptualization, E.R. and Z.S.; data analysis and curation, O.E. and A.F.; writing—original draft preparation, E.R. and K.N.; writing—review and editing, A.F. and O.E. and P.S. and Z.S.; supervision, Z.S.

Funding: The APC was funded by the Research Fund of the Department of Diabetes, Endocrinology, Nutritional Medicine and Metabolism and in part by Nestlé Health Science (grant to the institution).

Conflicts of Interest: The authors declare no conflicts of interest.

Appendix A

Table A1. Patient flow and resource use in connection with ND.

Patients Flow and Performance	Proportion/Rate	Number
Target population	20,000	
	Proportion/Rate	n
Detection rate, of which:	6.4%	1280
proportion p DRM	0.25	320
proportion m DRM	0.75	960
Nutritional interventions		
	Proportion	n
ONS	59%	755
EN	29%	371
PN	12%	154
Saved hospital days	Per Patient	total
Reduction in LOS, days	1.2	1152
SwissDRG changes	Detected Cases	
	Proportion	n
Changes in DRG attribution	0.0833	107

DRM: disease-related malnutrition; p DRM: potential DRM; m DRM: manifest DRM; ONS: oral nutritional supplements; EN: enteral nutrition; PN: parenteral nutrition; LOS: length of hospital stay; DRG: diagnosis-related groups.

Table A2. Consequences of the costs of ND.

	Number	Value	Costs
Costs nutritional Interventions			
ONS	755	187.57	141,652
EN	371	842.96	312,906
PN	154	1557.84	239,284
Total costs	1280		693,842
Savings (reduction LOS) (−)	1152	1373.46	−1582,224
Additional revenue (SwissDRG) (−)	107	7564.70	−806,579
Net effect			−1,694,961

Costs are indicated with positive (+), savings and additional revenue with negative (−) prefix. DRM: disease-related malnutrition; p DRM: potential DRM; m DRM: manifest DRM; ONS: oral nutritional supplements; EN: enteral nutrition; PN: parenteral nutrition.

Table A3. Hours, workdays and positions needed for NI in the case of systematic NS, ND and additional needs for systematic NS.

	Nutritional Therapy	Nursing	Physician
Systematic nutritional screening			
Hours total	6052	13,700	1210
Days total	721	1631	144
Positions needed	4.09	9.27	0.82
Natural Detection			
Hours total	1989	5327	398
Days total	237	634	47
Positions needed	1.35	3.60	0.27
Additional needs for systematic nutritional screening			
Hours total	4063	8373	813
Days total	484	997	97
Positions needed	2.75	5.66	0.55

Table A4. Staff time per nutritional intervention and professional group.

		Dietician	Nursing Staff	Physician
ONS				
Duration of therapy, days	8.4			
Minutes/patient/day		10	10	2
Minutes/patient		84	84	16.8
N patients NS	2797			
Minutes for NS		234,976	234,976	46,995
N patients ND	755			
Minutes for ND		63,437	63,437	12,687
EN				
Duration of therapy, days	10.3			
Minutes/patient/day		10	40	2
Minutes/patient		103	412	20.6
N patients NS	851			
Minutes for NS		87,619	350,475	17,524
N patients ND	371			
Minutes for ND		38,234	152,934	7647
PN				
Duration of therapy, days	9.6			
Minutes/patient/day		12	70	2.4
Minutes/patient		115.2	672	23.04
N patients NS	352			
Minutes for NS		40,550	236,544	8110
N patients ND	154			
Minutes for ND		17,695	103,219	3539

DRM: disease-related malnutrition; p DRM: potential DRM; m DRM: manifest DRM; ONS: oral nutritional supplements; EN: enteral nutrition; PN: parenteral nutrition.

Table A5. Studies addressing the economic impact of nutritional support after hospital discharge in the community or nursing home setting.

Nutritional Support After Hospital Discharge

Author	Population	Type of Study	Cost Analysis	Results
Edington et al., 2004 [29] United Kingdom	mixed malnourished ≥ 65 y; (n = 100)	RCT intervention ONS for 8 weeks, 24 weeks follow-up	Cost-effectiveness analysis, direct and indirect costs	No difference regarding quality of life, post-hospital health care resource use or cost
Norman et al., 2011 [25] Germany	gastrointestinal disease, malnourished (n = 114)	RCT intervention Dietary counseling at discharge and high-protein ONS for months vs. dietary counseling at discharge	Cost-effectiveness analysis, direct costs of nutritional support	Intervention patients: increase in quality of life after 3 months ICER: EUR9497–12099/QALY
Neelemaat et al., 2012 [26] The Nederlands	mixed, malnourished ≥ 60 y (n = 210)	RCT: ONS, dietary counseling, vitamin D for 3 months after hospital discharge vs. usual care	Cost-effectiveness analysis, direct and indirect costs	No significant difference in QALYs at 3 months follow-up, intervention group: improvement in functional limitations, EUR618/functional limitation improvement (0.95 probability the intervention is cost effective)
Zhong et al., 2016 [27] United States of America	Mixed, malnourished ≥ 65 y (n = 622)	RCT: high-protein ONS, enriched b-hydroxy-b-methylbutyrate for 3 months after hospital discharge compared to placebo	Cost-effectiveness analysis, direct and indirect costs	Intervention group: increase in quality of life ICER: USD 33,818/QALY lifetime ICER: USD 524/LY

Nutritional support in the community or nursing home setting

Author	Population	Type of study	Cost analysis	Results
Arnaud-Battandier et al., 2004 [30] France	Malnourished ≥ 70 y community or nursing home residents (n = 287)	prospective, cohort study of patients from 2 groups of physicians (high vs. low ONS prescription rate), 12-month follow-up	Comparison of direct costs	Higher costs of ONS in intervention group (EUR M, but lower costs of medical care: hospital admissions (EUR1631 vs. EUR 2203) and medical visits (EUR 299 vs. EUR 462)
Lorefält et al., 2011 [31] Sweden	nursing home residents, ≥ 65 y (n = 109)	Prospective cohort study of nutrition education and care (individualized meals) for 3 months	Comparison of direct costs	Higher costs in intervention group (EUR 830 vs. EUR 760 for nutritional support, EUR 652 vs. EUR 402 for education program)
Freijer et al., 2013 [32] The Nederlands	malnourished ≥ 65 y; community or nursing home residents (n = 720,223)	Health economic evaluation of published studies	Budget impact analysis	Annual cost savings of EUR 11.62 million due to intervention with ONS
Schilp et al., 2014 [28] The Nederlands	malnourished ≥ 65 y; community-dwelling old (n = 146)	RCT, dietary counseling vs. usual care	Cost-effectiveness analysis	No differences regarding gain in weight, QALY or costs
Simmons et al., 2015 [33] United States of America	Malnourished/at risk ≥ 65 y; nursing home residents (n = 154)	3-arm RCT: ONS vs. in-between snacks vs. usual care for 6 months	Cost-effectiveness analysis	No change in body weight, intervention costs per person per day; ONS group 2.54 and snack group 3.85; ICER: 103 kcal/USD in ONS group vs. 79 kcal/USD in snack group
van der Pols-Vijlbrief et al., 2017 [34] The Nederlands	community-dwelling older adults receiving home care with or at risk of malnutrition ≥65 y (n = 155)	RCT, multifactorial personalized intervention for 6 months	Cost-effectiveness analysis	No differences regarding gain in weight, functional status, QALY or costs
Elia et al., 2018 [35] United Kingdom	Malnourished, nursing home residents ≥65 y (n = 104)	RCT, comparing ONS versus dietary advice for 3 months	Cost effectiveness analysis with direct and indirect costs	Intervention group improved quality of life: ICER: GBP 10,961/QALY

ONS: oral nutritional supplements; QALY: quality of life adjusted life year; ICER: incremental cost-effectiveness ratio.

References

1. Aeberhard, C.; Abt, M.; Endrich, O.; Aubry, E.; Leuenberger, M.S.; Schütz, P.; Sterchi, A.B.; Stanga, Z. Auswirkung, der Kodierung der Mangelernährung im SwissDRGSystem. *Aktuell. Ernährungsmed.* **2018**, *43*, 92–100.
2. Aeberhard, C.; Birrenbach, T.; Joray, M.; Muhlebach, S.; Perrig, M.; Stanga, Z. Simple training tool is insufficient for appropriate diagnosis and treatment of malnutrition: A pre-post intervention study in a tertiary center. *Nutrition* **2016**, *32*, 355–361. [CrossRef] [PubMed]
3. Elia, M. The Cost of Malnutrition in England and Potential Cost Savings from Nutritional Interventions (short version). BAPEN. 2015. Available online: www.bapen.org.uk/pdfs/economic-report-short.pdf (accessed on 8 July 2019).
4. Imoberdorf, R.; Meier, R.; Krebs, P.; Hangartner, P.J.; Hess, B.; Staubli, M.; Wegmann, D.; Rühlin, M.; Ballmer, P.E. Prevalence of undernutrition on admission to Swiss hospitals. *Clin. Nutr.* **2010**, *29*, 38–41. [CrossRef] [PubMed]
5. Sriram, K.; Sulo, S.; VanDerBosch, G.; Partridge, J.; Feldstein, J.; Hegazi, R.A.; Summerfelt, W.T. A Comprehensive Nutrition-Focused Quality Improvement Program Reduces 30-Day Readmissions and Length of Stay in Hospitalized Patients. *JPEN J. Parenter. Enteral Nutr.* **2017**, *41*, 384–391. [CrossRef] [PubMed]
6. Bally, M.R.; Blaser Yildirim, P.Z.; Bounoure, L.; Gloy, V.L.; Mueller, B.; Briel, M.; Schuetz, P. Nutritional Support and Outcomes in Malnourished Medical Inpatients: A Systematic Review and Meta-analysis. *JAMA Int. Med.* **2016**, *176*, 43–53. [CrossRef] [PubMed]
7. Elia, M.; Normand, C.; Laviano, A.; Norman, K. A systematic review of the cost and cost effectiveness of using standard oral nutritional supplements in community and care home settings. *Clin. Nutr.* **2016**, *35*, 125–137. [CrossRef] [PubMed]
8. National Institute for Health and Care Excellence (NICE). Nutritional support for adults: oral nutrition support, enteral tube feeding and parenteral nutrition. Clinical Guideline 32, published February 2006m last modified August 2017. Available online: https://www.nice.org.uk/Guidance/CG32 (accessed on 8 July 2019).
9. Stratton, R.J.; Green, C.J.; Elia, M. *Disease-Related Malnutrition: An Evidence-Based Approach to Treatment*; CABI: Wallingford, UK, 2003; pp. 1128–1129.
10. Stratton, R.J.; Hebuterne, X.; Elia, M. A systematic review and meta-analysis of the impact of oral nutritional supplements on hospital readmissions. *Ageing Res. Rev.* **2013**, *12*, 884–897. [CrossRef]
11. Schuetz, P.; Fehr, R.; Baechli, V.; Geiser, M.; Deiss, M.; Gomes, F.; Bilz, S.; Sigrist, S.; Brändle, M.; Benz, C.; et al. Individualised nutritional support in medical inpatients at nutritional risk: A randomised clinical trial. *Lancet* **2019**, *393*, 8–14. [CrossRef]
12. Deutz, N.E.; Matheson, E.M.; Matarese, L.E.; Luo, M.; Baggs, G.E.; Nelson, J.L.; Hegazi, R.A.; Tappenden, K.A.; Ziegler, T.R. NOURISH Study Group. Readmission and mortality in malnourished, older, hospitalized adults treated with a specialized oral nutritional supplement: A randomized clinical trial. *Clin. Nutr.* **2016**, *35*, 18–26. [CrossRef]
13. Muscaritoli, M.; Krznaric, Z.; Singer, P.; Barazzoni, R.; Cederholm, T.; Golay, A.; Van Gossum, A.; Kennedy, N.; Kreymann, G.; Laviano, A.; et al. Effectiveness and efficacy of nutritional therapy: A systematic review following Cochrane methodology. *Clin. Nutr.* **2017**, *36*, 939–957. [CrossRef]
14. Voltz, C.; Seegler, S.; Keil, J.-P.; Fleßa, S. Malnutrition in Hospital Care – Potential Revenues of Nutrition. *Aktuelle Ernährungsmedizin.* **2016**, *41*, 187–189.
15. Vonzun, N.; Sterchi, A.-B.; Imoberdorf, R.; Rühlin, M. Malnutrition and DRG—The Swiss Solution. *Aktuell. Ernährungsmed.* **2014**, *39*, 392–396.
16. Ockenga, J.; Freudenreich, M.; Zakonsky, R.; Norman, K.; Pirlich, M.; Lochs, H. Nutritional assessment and management in hospitalised patients: Implication for DRG-based reimbursement and health care quality. *Clin. Nutr.* **2005**, *24*, 913–919. [CrossRef]
17. Reinbold, T.; Broß, I.; Lenfers, B. Malnutrition in the G-DRG-System—Effects of a Structured Nutritional Management on Codification and Revenues. *Aktuell. Ernährungsmed.* **2013**, *38*, 24–29.
18. Kondrup, J.; Rasmussen, H.H.; Hamberg, O.; Stanga, Z. Nutritional risk screening (NRS 2002): A new method based on an analysis of controlled clinical trials. *Clin. Nutr.* **2003**, *22*, 321–336. [CrossRef]

19. Wenger, C.; Hischier, T.; Rhyner, A.; Iff, S.; Sterchi, A.-B.; Stanga, Z. Introduction of Malnutrition Management on two Specialized University Clinics. *Aktuell. Ernährungsmed.* **2008**, *33*, 296–301. [CrossRef]
20. Kruizenga, H.M.; Van Tulder, M.W.; Seidell, J.C.; Thijs, A.; Ader, H.J.; Van Bokhorst-de van der Schueren, M.A. Effectiveness and cost-effectiveness of early screening and treatment of malnourished patients. *Am. J. Clin. Nutr.* **2005**, *82*, 1082–1089. [CrossRef]
21. Holyday, M.; Daniells, S.; Bare, M.; Caplan, G.A.; Petocz, P.; Bolin, T. Malnutrition screening and early nutrition intervention in hospitalised patients in acute aged care: A randomised controlled trial. *J. Nutr. Health Aging* **2012**, *16*, 562–568. [CrossRef] [PubMed]
22. Somanchi, M.; Tao, X.; Mullin, G.E. The facilitated early enteral and dietary management effectiveness trial in hospitalized patients with malnutrition. *JPEN J. Parenter. Enteral Nutr.* **2011**, *35*, 209–216. [CrossRef] [PubMed]
23. Elia, M.; Russell, C. *Combating Malnutrition: Recommendations for Action*; Nutrition Advisory Group on Malnutrition Led by BAPEN 2009; BAPEN: Redditch, UK, 2009.
24. Abizanda, P.; Sinclair, A.; Barcons, N.; Lizan, L.; Rodriguez-Manas, L. Costs of Malnutrition in Institutionalized and Community-Dwelling Older Adults: A Systematic Review. *J. Am. Med. Dir. Assoc.* **2016**, *17*, 17–23. [CrossRef] [PubMed]
25. Norman, K.; Pirlich, M.; Smoliner, C.; Kilbert, A.; Schulzke, J.D.; Ockenga, J.; Lochs, H.; Reinhold, T. Cost-effectiveness of a 3-month intervention with oral nutritional supplements in disease-related malnutrition: A randomised controlled pilot study. *Eur. J. Clin. Nutr.* **2011**, *65*, 735–742. [CrossRef] [PubMed]
26. Neelemaat, F.; Bosmans, J.E.; Thijs, A.; Seidell, J.C.; van Bokhorst-de van der Schueren, M.A. Oral nutritional support in malnourished elderly decreases functional limitations with no extra costs. *Clin. Nutr.* **2012**, *31*, 183–190. [CrossRef] [PubMed]
27. Zhong, Y.; Cohen, J.T.; Goates, S.; Luo, M.; Nelson, J.; Neumann, P.J. The Cost-Effectiveness of Oral Nutrition Supplementation for Malnourished Older Hospital Patients. *Appl. Health Econ. Health Policy.* **2017**, *15*, 75–83. [CrossRef] [PubMed]
28. Schilp, J.; Bosmans, J.E.; Kruizenga, H.M.; Wijnhoven, H.A.H.; Visser, M. Is dietetic treatment for undernutrition in older individuals in primary care cost-effective? *J. Am. Med. Dir. Assoc.* **2014**, *15*, 226.e7–226.e13. [CrossRef] [PubMed]
29. Edington, J.; Barnes, R.; Bryan, F.; Dupree, E.; Frost, G.; Hickson, M.; Lancaster, J.; Mongia, S.; Smith, J.; Torrance, A.; et al. A prospective randomised controlled trial of nutritional supplementation in malnourished elderly in the community: Clinical and health economic outcomes. *Clin. Nutr.* **2004**, *23*, 195–204. [CrossRef]
30. Arnaud-Battandier, F.; Malvy, D.; Jeandel, C.; Schmitt, C.; Aussage, P.; Beaufrere, B.; Cynober, L. Use of oral supplements in malnourished elderly patients living in the community: A pharmaco-economic study. *Clin. Nutr.* **2004**, *23*, 1096–1103. [CrossRef] [PubMed]
31. Lorefalt, B.; Andersson, A.; Wirehn, A.B.; Wilhelmsson, S. Nutritional status and health care costs for the elderly living in municipal residential homes–an intervention study. *J. Nutr. Health Aging* **2011**, *15*, 92–97. [CrossRef] [PubMed]
32. Freijer, K.; Nuijten, M.J.; Schols, J.M. The budget impact of oral nutritional supplements for disease related malnutrition in elderly in the community setting. *Front. Pharmacol.* **2012**, *3*, F78. [CrossRef] [PubMed]
33. Simmons, S.F.; Keeler, E.; An, R.; Liu, X.; Shotwell, M.S.; Kuertz, B.; Silver, H.J.; Schnelle, J.F. Cost-Effectiveness of Nutrition Intervention in Long-Term Care. *J. Am. Geriatr. Soc.* **2015**, *63*, 2308–2316. [CrossRef] [PubMed]
34. van der Pols-Vijlbrief, R.; Wijnhoven, H.A.H.; Bosmans, J.E.; Twisk, J.W.R.; Visser, M. Targeting the underlying causes of undernutrition. Cost-effectiveness of a multifactorial personalized intervention in community-dwelling older adults: A randomized controlled trial. *Clin. Nutr.* **2017**, *36*, 1498–1508. [CrossRef] [PubMed]
35. Elia, M.; Parsons, E.L.; Cawood, A.L.; Smith, T.R.; Stratton, R.J. Cost-effectiveness of oral nutritional supplements in older malnourished care home residents. *Clin. Nutr.* **2018**, *37*, 651–658. [CrossRef] [PubMed]

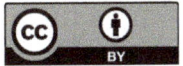

© 2019 by the authors. Licensee MDPI, Basel, Switzerland. This article is an open access article distributed under the terms and conditions of the Creative Commons Attribution (CC BY) license (http://creativecommons.org/licenses/by/4.0/).

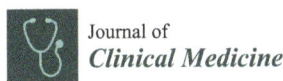

Article

Metabolic and Nutritional Characteristics of Long-Stay Critically Ill Patients

Marina V. Viana [1], Olivier Pantet [1], Geraldine Bagnoud [1,2], Arianne Martinez [1], Eva Favre [1], Mélanie Charrière [1,2], Doris Favre [1,2], Philippe Eckert [1,†] and Mette M. Berger [1,*,†]

[1] Service of Adult Intensive Care Medicine and Burns, Lausanne University Hospital (CHUV), 1011 Lausanne, Switzerland
[2] Service of Endocrinology, Diabetes and Metabolism, Lausanne University Hospital, 1011 Lausanne, Switzerland
* Correspondence: Mette.Berger@chuv.ch
† These authors contributed equally as co-seniors to this paper.

Received: 30 May 2019; Accepted: 4 July 2019; Published: 7 July 2019

Abstract: Background: insufficient feeding is frequent in the intensive care unit (ICU), which results in poor outcomes. Little is known about the nutrition pattern of patients requiring prolonged ICU stays. The aims of our study are to describe the demographic, metabolic, and nutritional specificities of chronically critically ill (CCI) patients defined by an ICU stay >2 weeks, and to identify an early risk factor. Methods: analysis of consecutive patients prospectively admitted to the CCI program, with the following variables: demographic characteristics, Nutrition Risk Screening (NRS-2002) score, total daily energy from nutritional and non-nutritional sources, protein and glucose intakes, all arterial blood glucose values, length of ICU and hospital stay, and outcome (ICU and 90-day survival). Two phases were considered for the analysis: the first 10 days, and the next 20 days of the ICU stay. Statistics: parametric and non-parametric tests. Results: 150 patients, aged 60 ± 15 years were prospectively included. Median (Q1, Q3) length of ICU stay was 31 (26, 46) days. The mortality was 18% at ICU discharge and 35.3% at 90 days. Non-survivors were older ($p = 0.024$), tended to have a higher SAPSII score ($p = 0.072$), with a significantly higher NRS score ($p = 0.033$). Enteral nutrition predominated, while combined feeding was minimally used. All patients received energy and protein below the ICU's protocol recommendation. The proportion of days with fasting was 10.8%, being significantly higher in non-survivors (2 versus 3 days; $p = 0.038$). Higher protein delivery was associated with an increase in prealbumin over time ($r^2 = 0.19$, $p = 0.027$). Conclusions: High NRS scores may identify patients at highest risk of poor outcome when exposed to underfeeding. Further studies are required to evaluate a nutrition strategy for patients with high NRS, addressing combined parenteral nutrition and protein delivery.

Keywords: chronic critical illness; protein; Nutrition Risk Screening (NRS-2002); age; nutrition; vasopressors; shock; glucose; diabetes; underfeeding

1. Introduction

The intensive care unit (ICU) patient population has evolved over the last two decades with the appearance of an increasing number of patients requiring very long ICU stays, lasting up to several months after surviving the initial acute insult [1]. A long stay is usually defined as the requirement of more than one week of mechanical ventilation (MV) and of ICU therapy, but different definitions have been used [2]. Chronic critical illness (CCI) is the most frequent designation for these patients, which is characterized by lengthy hospital stays, intense suffering, high mortality rates, and substantial resource consumption [3]. Genetic influence has also been shown to be increasingly present, particularly in pediatric ICUs [4]. Preexisting chronic comorbidities are strong, independent predictors of this condition [5]. In the ICU, mechanical ventilation, sepsis, Glasgow score < 15, inadequate calorie intake, and higher body mass index (BMI) have been identified as independent predictors of this condition [6].

Recently, a study including 185 chronic, critically ill patients showed that the preadmission nutritional status reflected by the Nutrition Risk Screening (NRS-2002) (hereafter NRS) [7] might be a good predictor of the outcome: a score ≥ 5 points seemed to be a cutoff predictor of mortality [8]. Entering the acute disease with deficits such as weight loss, being older, or malnourished, seems to constitute a metabolic handicap that threatens the patient's response capacity and survival. In 2013, the same group observed that inadequate nutrition (defined as the provision of less than 60% of needs) and organ failure (defined by the sequential organ failure assessment (SOFA) score) are mortality risk factors [6].

The optimal timing and amount of feeding has been much debated. Indeed, the intestine of the sickest patients is not always available to accommodate full feeding as shown by the French randomized controlled, multicenter, parallel group trial called NUTRIREA-2 including 2410 patients with septic shock [9]. Furthermore, many patients are at risk of the refeeding syndrome [10]. A recent Brazilian study showed in a cohort of 100 critically ill patients with a mean ICU stay of 19 days, that those 45 patients receiving a caloric intake ≥70% during the first 72 h of hospitalization did not present better outcomes in the short term (mechanical ventilation, length of ICU stay) or after 1 year (functional capacity, mortality) [11]. For both above reasons, i.e., risk of stressing the intestine and of relative overfeeding [12], the early full feeding strategy seems unable to promote a good outcome. In this context, the most recent European Society for Clinical Nutrition and Metabolism (ESPEN) guidelines propose increasing progressively (ramping up) the energy delivery whatever the feeding route over 3–4 days [13]. Furthermore, prescribed energy goals should be covered somewhere between day 4 and 7, and preferentially be determined by indirect calorimetry.

To better coordinate the treatment of the long stay patients admitted to our ICU, and to identify procedures that could be improved, the service initiated a dedicated program enrolling patients requiring more than 2 weeks of ICU treatment. The present study aims to describe the metabolic and nutritional specificities of these patients, to analyze those associated with poor outcome, and to identify a factor that might enable early detection of CCI risk.

2. Methods

With the approval of the Commission Cantonale d'Ethique sur la Recherche humaine (CER 2018-02018), consecutive patients admitted to the 35 bed multidisciplinary ICU of the Lausanne University Hospital were analyzed. The patients had been prospectively enrolled in the long-stay program of the ICU, a plan of action called PLS (Patients Long Séjour) created in January 2017 to improve the care of patients requiring more than 2 weeks of ICU therapy (clinical trial identifier: NCT03938961). The PLS program consisted of weekly interdisciplinary meetings addressing ventilation, nutrition, cognitive and functional issues, symptom management, psychological support, and complication prevention. The meetings ended with detailed evaluation and a plan of action.

2.1. Patients

The inclusion criteria were age >18 years, and inclusion in the PLS program with an ICU stay >2 weeks. The exclusion criteria were admission for major burns >20% body surface, traumatic brain injury, and patients who refused participation.

2.2. Study Variables

Data were extracted from the computerized information system (Metavision® iMDsoft, Tel Aviv, Israel, version 5.46.44) and included age, admission (dry weight) and discharge body weight, body mass index (BMI), NRS-2002 score [7], severity of disease (SAPSII), Sequential Organ Failure Assessment (SOFA) score on days 1, 2, 5, 10, 30, and discharge [14]), requirement of continuous renal replacement therapy (CRRT), admission for sepsis, presence of diabetes, daily intakes (energy, protein, glucose: raw data and per kg), all arterial blood glucose values, 24 h insulin dose, arterial blood lactate (maximal value), daily feeding route, pressure ulcers occurring during the ICU stay, discharge Medical Research Council force score (MRC), length of mechanical ventilation, ICU and hospital length of stay, ICU and 90-days mortality. Laboratory: blood prealbumin (determined weekly), C-reactive protein (CRP), and procalcitonin (mean of the ICU stay).

2.3. Nutrition Protocol

The ICU's protocol called NUTSIA (NUTrition aux Soins Intensifs Adultes) is based on the ESPEN guidelines [13]. Enteral nutrition is recommended as the first option when nutritional therapy is indicated (i.e., for patients for whom oral intake is not possible), and should be initiated within the first 3 days after hemodynamic stabilization. Parenteral nutrition (PN) may be used as combined feeding, or total PN from day 4 and earlier in selected malnutrition situations. Energy goals are 20 kcal/kg/day during the first week, to be increased or adapted thereafter—indirect calorimetry is recommended from day 7. The initial energy goal should be reached by day 4–5. Energy intakes include the energy from feeding products and oral intakes, and the energy resulting from glucose (drug dilution) and fat (sedative propofol), which are administered for non-nutritional purposes.

Feeding products were: Peptamen Intense (Nestlé, Switzerland), Promote Fiber plus (Abbott, Switzerland), Isosource Energy Fiber (Nestlé, Switzerland), Nutriflex Omega special (BBraun, Switzerland), and Pharmacy compounded PN in individual cases.

Energy balances were calculated as the daily difference between the total substrate intakes (nutritional and non-nutritional sources) and the prescribed value. The mean daily and the cumulated values were calculated for the first 10 days, and a cutoff of cumulated deficit −70 kcal/kg was considered critical [15,16]. For proteins, the daily delivery was compared to the recommended target of 1.2 g/kg/day. The cumulated deficit was calculated for the first 10 days and a cutoff of −300 g was considered critical.

Glucose control is handled by nurses, with a blood glucose (BG) goal of 6–8 mmol/L (6–10 mmol/L in diabetic patients) maintained using continuous insulin infusion. Blood glucose is presented as the daily mean value, and is measured on a point of care blood gas analyzer. Its variability is indicated as the daily standard error of the daily BG values. Daily total insulin was recorded.

The 2 dieticians (one full time position present on working days) attended to patients requiring >3 ICU days. These individuals are in charge of checking route of feeding, energy needs (indirect calorimetry), proteins delivery, and adapting the feeding solutions [17]. They attend the weekly PLS meetings.

2.4. Other Variables

Muscle strength upon discharge was assessed using the MRC score [18], where the patient's effort is graded on a *scale* of 0–5. Six muscle groups were bilaterally measured (abduction of the arm, flexion of the forearm, extension of the wrist, flexion of the hip, extension of the knee, and dorsal flexion of the foot). All muscle groups were scored between 0 and 5 (0, no visible/palpable contraction; 1, visible/palpable contraction without movement of the limb; 2, movements of the limb but not against gravity; 3, movements against gravity (almost full passive range of motion) but not against resistance; 4, movement against gravity and resistance, arbitrarily judged to be sub-maximal for gender and age; 5, normal). Therefore, the maximal score is 60 points.

2.5. Statistical Analysis

Data of the entire stay were extracted, but analysis was limited to the first 30 days. The data are presented as means ± standard deviation (SD), or median (interquartile Q1, Q3) depending on normal distribution, which was assessed through histograms and calculation of skewness and kurtosis. For non-parametric variables, the Kruskal-Wallis test was used. Two phases were considered for the analysis of the nutritional related variables: the first days (D1–D10), and the next 20 days of the ICU stay (D11–D30). The continuous variables in survivors versus non-survivors were compared using the one-way and two-way ANOVA, while the categorical variables were compared using Chi^2 tests. For non-parametric variables, Kruskal–Wallis rank sum test was used. Kaplan–Meier analysis and Cox regression were used to compare mortality. For the Kaplan–Meier analysis, the log rank test was used to compare the curves of each NRS group (3–4 and 5–6–7 points). The generalized linear model (GLM) was used to analyze response variables that were not normally distributed such as substrate administration or blood glucose over the 30 days. Statistical programs were JMP version 14.2 for Windows, (SAS Institute GMH, Böblingen, Germany), and R Version 3.5.3, 2019 (R Foundation for Statistical Computing, Vienna, Austria). Significance level was set at $p < 0.05$.

3. Results

3.1. Patients

The current study included prospectively 150 patients admitted between 1 February 2017 and 31 December 2018. During the same period, 589 patients were admitted who required ICU for >7 days, but the majority were discharged before entering the PLS program. Table 1 summarizes patient demographics and clinical outcomes, with the details of survivors/non-survivors at ICU discharge. Most patients (60.7%) were admitted for medical causes (17/91 with a surgical background), followed by emergency surgery, and elective surgery (52% were admitted for sepsis, and 48% needed continuous renal replacement during their stay).

Table 1. Demographics, severity of illness, laboratory and outcome variables according to ICU vital status.

	Overall	Non-Survivors	Survivors	p
N (%)	150	27 (18%)	123 (82%)	
Age (mean (SD))	60.2 (14.6)	66.0 (10.9)	59.0 (15.0)	0.024
Sex (Males, %)	116 (77.3)	24 (88.9)	92 (74.8)	0.184
Body weight admission (kg, mean (SD)) discharge	78.3 (18.4) 75.7 (17.8)	77.4 (18.8) 81.5 (18.5)	78.4 (18.4) 74.3 (17.5)	0.785 0.054
BMI (mean (SD))	26.47 (6.09)	26.15 (6.42)	26.54 (6.05)	0.761
SAPS2 (mean (SD))	52.9 (18.3)	58.7 (15.8)	51.7 (18.6)	0.072
SOFA on Day1 (median (Q1, Q3))	8 (5, 11)	11 (9, 14)	9 (6, 12)	0.134
NRS (median (Q1, Q3))	5 (3, 6)	5 (4, 6)	4 (3, 6)	0.033
Medical/Emergency surgery/elective surgery	91/40/19	20/6/1	71/34/18	0.141
Diabetes (%)	26 (17.3)	7 (25.9)	19 (15.4)	0.307
Renal failure requiring CRRT (n, % of n)	72 (48.0%)	22 (81.5%)	50 (40.5%)	<0.001
Sepsis on admission (n, % of n)	78 (52.0)	15 (55.6)	63 (51.2)	0.845
CRP (median (Q1, Q3)) mean of stay	125 (81,170)	153 (97, 183)	116(77, 166)	0.096
Procalcitonin (median (Q1, Q3)) mean of stay	1.4 (0.4, 4.6)	3.2 (1.6, 7.7)	1.0 (0.3, 3.7)	0.008
Glucose (daily means (median (Q1, Q3))	7.7 (7.2, 8.4)	7.8 (7.4, 8.2)	7.6 (7.1, 8.4)	0.408
Lactate (daily max (median (Q1, Q3))	1.7 (1.4, 2.1)	2.0 (1.7, 2.7)	1.6 (1.4, 2.1)	0.004
Pressure ulcers (n patients with)	72 (48%)	12	60	0.835
MRC on discharge (median (Q1, Q3) (n = 91))	34 (24,42)	31 (25, 43)	35 (25,42)	0.825
Length of Mech.Ventilation (days) (median (Q1, Q3))	16.1 (10.0, 21.6)	17.8 (13.2, 26.8)	15.7 (9.8, 20.3)	0.152
Total length of ICU stay (median (Q1, Q3))	31 (23, 46)	29 (18, 44)	31 (24, 46)	0.268
Hospital length of stay (median (Q1, Q3))	57 (39, 82)	30 (24, 47)	63 (44, 91)	<0.001

Abbreviations: SOFA = Sequential Organ Failure Assessment, SAPS = Simplified Acute Physiology Score, BMI = Body Mass Index, NRS = Nutrition risk screening, CRP = C-reactive protein, Q1 and Q3 = q quartiles 25, 75.

Gender was equally distributed, but the non-survivors were older ($p = 0.024$) and tended to have a higher SAPSII score ($p = 0.072$). The admission SOFA score did not differ significantly but its evolution was different over time, decreasing significantly in survivors ($p < 0.0001$) (Figure A1). The cardiac component of the score remained elevated for a longer period of time (i.e., at 3–4 points) in the non-survivors. A significantly higher NRS score ($p = 0.033$) was observed in non-survivors. The Kaplan–Meier analysis showed that the scores NRS 5–6–7 are associated with a higher 90-days mortality of 43.8% versus 25.7% with NRS scores 3 and 4, respectively (Figure 1). Admission weight (mean 78.3 kg) and BMI were similar, but the weight change over time differed significantly ($p < 0.0001$) depending on the outcome. By the end of the stay, survivors had lost weight, while non-survivors had gained weight due to a persistent positive fluid balance. While 28 patients (18%) died in the ICU, further 26 patients died within 90 days, resulting in a total of 56 (35.3%) deaths—age and NRS differences became even more pronounced by day 90 (age $p < 0.001$; NRS $p = 0.005$; Table A1). A Cox regression model with 90-days mortality as an outcome showed an increased risk of death in patients with NRS ≥ 5 (HR 2.2 (1.18–4.2), $p = 0.013$), but not for the SAPS2 score (HR 1.0 (0.99–1.0), $p = 0.235$). Diabetes mellitus was present in 17.3% of patients, but was not associated with any mortality difference.

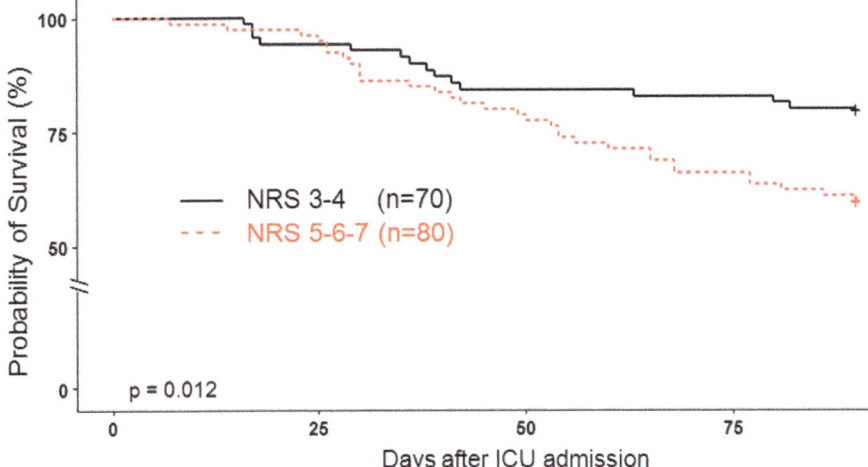

Figure 1. Kaplan–Meier analysis comparing elevated and low NRS scores. NRS: Nutrition Risk Screening and ICU: intensive care unit.

3.2. Nutrition

The proportion of days with intentional absence of feeding (fasting) was 10.8% of total days (Table 2 and Figure 2), being significantly higher in non-survivors ($p = 0.038$), with fasting contributing to the high day-to-day variability of intakes (Figure 3)—except for the number of fasting days (3 versus 2, $p = 0.043$). Table 2 shows that there was no difference between survivors and non-survivors. Fasting days were mostly observed during the first 5 days, but did occur throughout the 30 days. The feeding route was predominantly enteral, representing 55.7% of total days; combined enteral (EN) and parenteral (PN) feeding represented 8.1% and 14.1% of total days, respectively, and variable route combinations was used in 1% of total days.

Table 2. Nutrition characteristics according to ICU outcome (D = day).

	Overall	Non-Survivors	Survivors	p
N (%)	150	27 (18%)	123 (82%)	
Days of fasting: N per patient (median (Q1, Q3))	2.0 (1.0, 3.0)	3.0 (1.0, 4.0)	2.0 (1.0, 3.0)	0.043
Percentage of days (median (Q1, Q3))	5.4 (2.4, 10.0)	7.8 (4.3, 10.9)	4.9 (2.0, 9.3)	0.031
Prealbumin (delta of stay) (median (Q1, Q3)) g/L	0.07 (0.04, 0.12)	0.06 (0.02, 0.10)	0.07 (0.04, 0.13)	<0.001
Energy delivery D1–10 (median (Q1, Q3)) kcal/day	1161 (957, 1370)	1121 (936, 1385)	1161 (983, 1368)	0.719
(median (Q1, Q3)) kcal/kg/day	15.8 (11.8, 18.9)	16.4 (12.1, 17.9)	15.7 (11.8, 19.1)	0.838
Energy delivery D11–30 (median (Q1, Q3)) kcal/day	1559 (1368, 1762)	1504 (1284, 1645)	1581 (1387, 1772)	0.104
(median (Q1, Q3)) Kcal/kg/day	20.8 (17.9, 23.9)	20.2 (15.5, 21.9)	20.9 (18.1, 24.1)	0.151
Cumulated Energy balance D1–10 (median (Q1, Q3)) kcal/day	−5266 (−8365, −2697)	−5365 (−9208, −2852)	−5234 (−8043, −2651)	0.519
(median (Q1, Q3)) kcal/kg/day	−70 (−102, −37)	−74 (−125, −38)	−69 (−101, −36)	0.345
Cumulated Energy balance D1–30 (median (Q1, Q3)) kcal /day	−7700 (−11,607, −4702)	−7710 (−12,197, −5097)	−7677 (−11,350, −4554)	0.532
(median (Q1, Q3)) kcal /kg/day	−96.8 (−148.2, −59.7)	−92.4 (−151.1, −67.1)	−97.5 (−146.9, −58.4)	0.801
Protein delivery D1–10 (median (Q1, Q3)) g/day	53.7 (40.7, 64.3)	54.0 (40.2, 61.9)	53.4 (41.7, 65.7)	0.673
(median (Q1, Q3)) g/kg/day	0.69 (0.52, 0.86)	0.73 (0.57, 0.86)	0.68 (0.50, 0.87)	0.768
Protein delivery D11–30 (median (Q1, Q3)) g/day	75.4 (62.0, 90.3)	70.0 (49.4, 83.7)	76.4 (63.3, 90.4)	0.051
(median (Q1, Q3)) g/kg/day	1.0 (0.6, 1.4)	0.95 (0.68, 1.1)	1.0 (0.8, 1.2)	0.104
Cumulate protein balance D1–10 (median (Q1, Q3)) g/day	−374 (−595, −223)	−352 (−538, −244)	−379 (−608, 216)	0.803
(median (Q1, Q3)) g/kg/day	−4.86 (−6.82, −3.36)	−4.63 (−6.18, −3.49)	−4.98 (−7.07, −3.34)	0.938
Cumulate protein balance D1–30 g/day	−603 (−1070, −304)	−531 (−1006, −355)	−611 (−1069, −299)	0.912
(median (Q1, Q3)) g/kg/day	−7.91 (−12.47, −4.13)	−7.89 (−13.62, 4.74)	−8.43 (−12.34, −4.11)	0.816

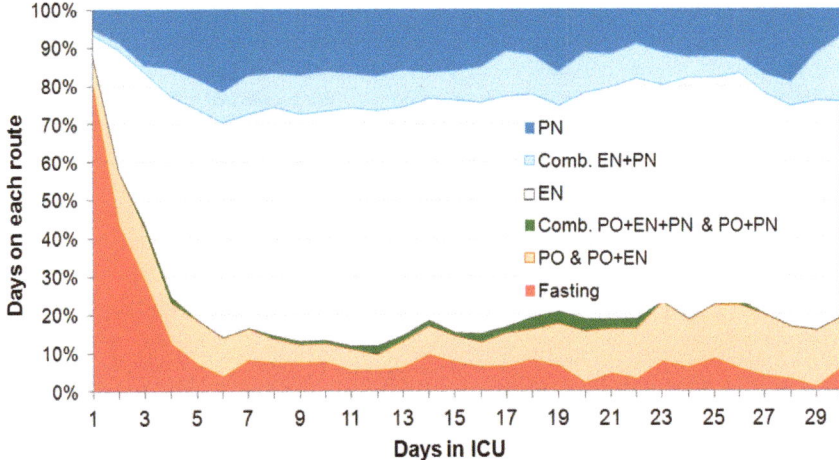

Figure 2. Evolution of the route of feeding over time presented as percentage of all patients over the first 30 days—there is a variable time of fasting during the first week. Enteral feeding was predominant, with a stable proportion of combined enteral–parenteral feeding (Comb EN + PN), or total parenteral nutrition (PN), and a variable proportion of the combinations oral–enteral, or oral–parenteral. Abbreviations: EN = enteral nutrition, PN = parenteral nutrition, Comb = combined, PO = oral.

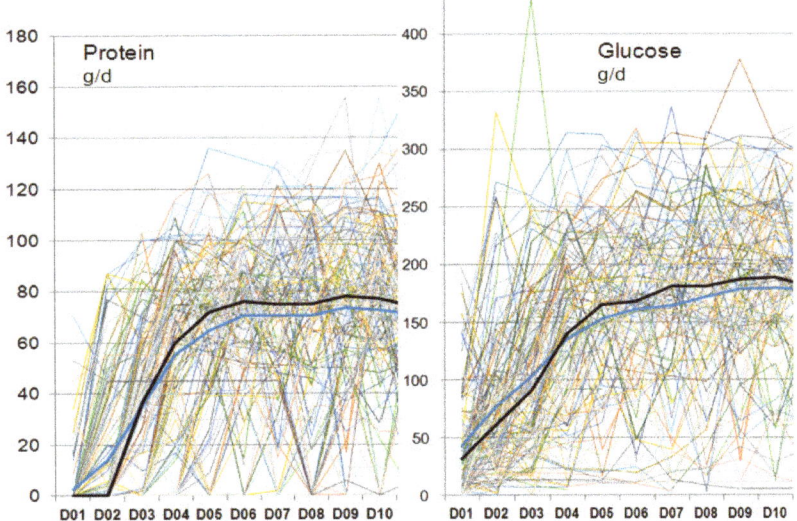

Figure 3. Individual delivery of protein and glucose by day during the first 10 days. Each line represents individual patient values. The erratic aspect aims at showing a phenomenon which is the extreme day to day variability and multiple interruptions that characterize the nutrition in the early phase. The thick dark lines show median (blue) and mean (black) values.

3.2.1. Energy

The mean prescribed energy during the first 10 days was 21.7 kcal/kg/day, and 23.4 kcal/kg/day thereafter (1750 kcal/day). The individual patients were characterized by a high variability of feeding, and total protein and glucose intakes (Figure 3). The progression of feeding occurred over the first 10 days (and not over 5 days as per protocol), i.e., before inclusion in the dedicated program (no difference between the two categories). Figure 4 shows the mean values for protein and energy, which were below the service's recommendations and below the prescribed values. Both groups were underfed, resulting in a median cumulated negative balance of −5266 kcal by day 10 (−70 kcal/kg). Nutrition delivery improved over time, but stagnated below the prescribed value.

Indirect calorimetry was available in 95 patients. The prescription was −236 kcal (range: −1391 to +483 kcal) below the measured energy expenditure. When this deficit is added to the daily energy deficit (difference between prescribed and delivered), the median deficit becomes −741 kcal/day (range: −2971 to −123 kcal per day) for the first 10 days.

3.2.2. Proteins

The delivery was lowest during the first 10 days (Figure 4), with a median of 64.3 g/day (0.70 g/kg/day), which is below the 1.2 g/kg/day service NUTSIA recommendation. By day 10, 80 patients (53.3%) exceeded −300 g of cumulated deficit. Protein intake thereafter increased to 1 g/kg/day remaining below recommendation, with a tendency to be lower in non-survivors.

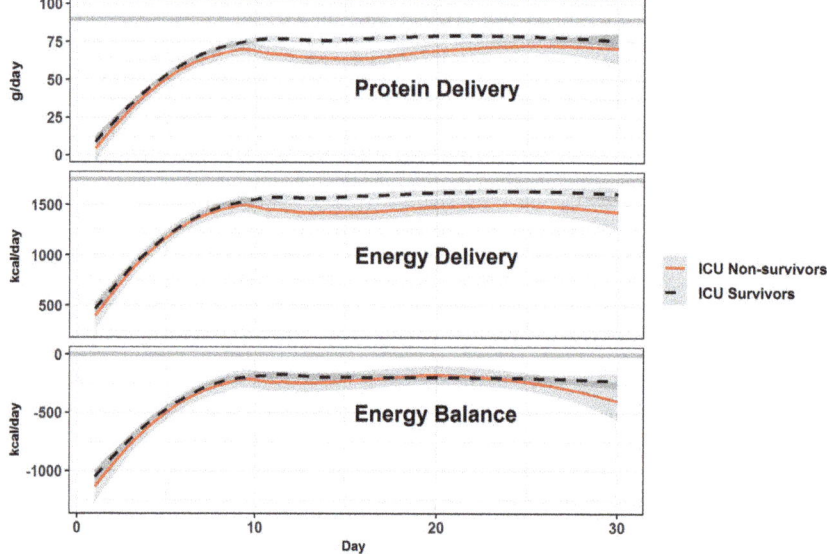

Figure 4. Mean protein and energy delivery with the resulting energy balance over the first 30 days according to ICU vital status (mean ± SD). The thick gray lines show protein target (1.2 g/kg/day), energy goal (prescribed value), and neutral energy balance. The differences in protein and energy delivery between survivors and non-survivors were significant after day 10 ($p < 0.001$). Energy balances were similarly negative.

Prealbumin, the lowest values were observed in patients with high NRS scores ($p = 0.067$). Prealbumin increased over time in the majority of patients in association with higher protein delivery ($r^2 = 0.19$; $p = 0.027$), and the increase (difference between first and last value of the ICU stay) was lower in non-survivors ($p < 0.001$).

3.2.3. Blood glucose

Altogether, 30,769 arterial blood glucose values were available for analysis (4–10 blood samples per day). Blood glucose and related variables differed between survivors and non-survivors (Figure 5), and over time. While glucose intakes were identical and low, non-survivors had higher BG values during the first 10 days, but not thereafter. Variability was higher, but not significant. Insulin needs were significantly higher and became again higher after day 20, while survivors' insulin needs declined, reaching below 30 u/day. Blood maximal lactate was also significantly higher during the first days in non-survivors.

The BG pattern differed in diabetic patients, being higher throughout the stay as per protocol, with higher variability and higher 24 h insulin requirements (Figure A2). This was particularly marked in surviving diabetic patients (Figure A3). Diabetic non-survivors were characterized by lower BG values and higher insulin needs during the first 5 days. Arterial lactate was elevated during the first 5 days in the majority of patients, being significantly higher in diabetic non-survivors.

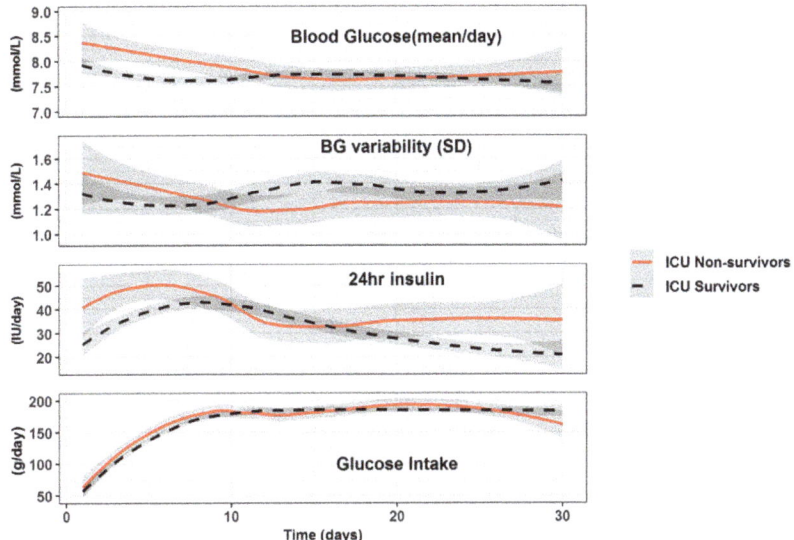

Figure 5. Evolution of mean blood glucose (mmol/L), Blood Glucose (BG) variability (standard error = SD of the individual daily values), 24 h insulin (total dose/24 h), and glucose intake (total in g/day). The figure shows that the 24 h Insulin delivery is not related to the glucose intake, which was similar in both groups (data are represented as mean ± SD).

3.3. MRC Discharge Score

MRC discharge score was available in 91 patients. The median value on discharge was low with 34 points. In those patients who did not suffer significant persistent renal failure on discharge (which results in elevated creatinine values), the median serum creatinine was 52 µmol/L (a low value in adult patients, and a surrogate for muscle mass).

4. Discussion

The main finding in our study is that CCI patients are not equal upon admission. Many patients begin their ICU journey without metabolic reserves reflected by a high NRS score. However, the impact is not immediate. During the first 10 days, the patients were exposed to very low and highly variable energy and protein intakes, and many were exposed to prolonged and repeated fasting. The acute underfeeding generated important energy and protein deficits, resulting in an additional malnutrition diagnosis in these critically ill patients. Combined EN and PN feeding was minimally used, despite being included in the service's protocol based on randomized trials [19,20]. In patients at risk of malnutrition upon admission, the underfeeding further erodes a previously altered metabolic status, resulting in a poor outcome. These results confirm recent observational data [16], where patients at low risk are likely to have a reasonable outcome despite several days of inadequate nutrition, while those at higher risk do not. The 2019 ESPEN recommendations [13] emphasize that no patient should be left longer than 72 h without initiating a balanced feeding. The majority of nutrition-related studies focus on the first days after admission, and have often included moderately sick or young patients that did not really benefit from artificial nutrition. By extracting the data of the entire stay, we observed that there was an early phase, and a later phase with a turning point around day 10. Thereafter, the patients were better fed, but the majority did not reach their prescribed goals.

The patient cohort was critically ill, as reflected by an elevated admission SAPSII score and an 18% ICU mortality, which was significantly higher than the general ICU patient's mortality (14.4%). The non-survivors were older, which belongs to the risk factors of CCI [1]. At the 90 days time point, a further 26 patients had died, increasing the total mortality to 35.3%. The initial SOFA score did not differ, but the score's evolution differed in survivors and non-survivors, remaining higher in the latter. The inclusion of the evolution of organ failure over time assessed by the SOFA score is an important strength of this study. Our data do not confirm those of a Brazilian cohort of 453 CCI patients, in which the initial SOFA score was a predictor of mortality [6]. One of the aims of the study was to find a variable facilitating the early detection of patients at critical illness risk. The total SOFA score did not predict the outcome, while the NRS score was able to detect them, confirming other Brazilian results [8]. A NRS score ≥ 5 should raise an alert, especially when associated with hemodynamic instability and high lactate values.

Timing and route of feeding in the critically ill has long been debated, and particularly the timing of PN initiation. The pragmatic CALORIES trial in 2400 mechanically ventilated patients randomized to EN or PN from day 1 showed no difference between the two routes [21]. The NUTRIREA-2 study included 2410 patients with septic shock, and showed that full early EN from day 1 was associated with more intestinal complications ($p < 0.001$) compared to the same dose of PN [9], with no benefit of EN on infectious complications. Providing early full feeding does not seem to prevent patients from becoming CCI, as shown by a Brazilian study including 100 critically ill patients. The study further shows that providing a caloric intake $\geq 70\%$ in the first 72 h of admission did not improve short term or 1-year outcomes [11]. Among the possible explanations of these disappointing results, the early endogenous glucose production [20,22] in response to acute illness should be considered. This production covers approximately two thirds of energy expenditure during the first days of disease. In addition, enteral full feeding is not always tolerated, as shown by NUTRIREA-2 [9], and the risk of refeeding syndrome is a reality [10]. The dose of both feeding and vasopressors might be the explanation as shown by the secondary analysis of a large septic cohort which showed that EN providing close to recommended intakes of energy and proteins over the stay was associated with a better outcome [23]. A propensity-matched analysis, including 52,563 ventilated adult patients stratified by dose of noradrenalin [24], suggests that in patients on low- or medium-dose noradrenalin, early EN seems associated with a reduction in mortality but not in the patients requiring high-dose noradrenalin. The recommendation to provide early, but progressive feeding starting ideally during the first 48 h, while discouraging early full feeding whatever the route, formulated in the latest ESICM [25] and ESPEN [13] guidelines was built on such data.

The ICU's internal protocol recommends progressing to the goal by day 4–5 based on ESPEN recommendations, which was not achieved without any difference between survivors and non-survivors. The latter were characterized by a higher percentage of fasting days during the first days after admission (associated with hemodynamic instability), but also occurring at random thereafter. The reasons for the feeding interruptions are multiple in an ICU, and have not changed much over the last decades [26]. The elevated mean cardiovascular SOFA scores reflect a persistent hemodynamic instability, which is probably one of the reasons for withholding feeding, and for difficult EN progression. These poor results may need a change in our ICU feeding procedure. Volume based feeding needs consideration as recent studies show that it is safe, and effectively improves energy and protein delivery compared to traditional rate-based feeding [27].

An American study analyzed the discharge destinations of critically ill surgical patients according to the magnitude of their energy and protein deficit. The authors showed that nutrition was a major outcome determinant [16]. Yeh et al. used a cumulated deficit cutoff of −6000 kcal and of −300 g protein. The patients who remained below those cutoffs were three times more likely to be discharged home. The authors also observed a longer ICU stay and higher mortality in those patients exceeding these values. In the present cohort, the patients entered the PLS program only after 2 weeks. Large energy and protein deficits had built up, but did not differ between survivors and non-survivors, both being similarly underfed by day 10: 80 patients (53.3%) exceeded the −300 g protein deficit and 50 patients (33%) exceeded the −6000 kcal cutoff. Knowing that the indirect calorimetry values for energy expenditure were higher than prescription in the majority of patients, the real deficit is even greater. Malnutrition causes loss of lean body mass, which is a determinant of the outcome [28,29], with the early protein deficit being an important contributor to the loss. The positive response of prealbumin to higher protein delivery shows that increasing proteins delivery is a treatment option. Critical illness is characterized by a high degree of stress with an accelerated protein degradation that results in malnutrition, systemic inflammation, and organ dysfunction [30]. Supporting this hypothesis, Briassoulis et al. showed that in critically ill children, only 22.7% of patients without protein deficiencies versus 37% of those at risk or already deficient, developed multiple-organ system failure [31]. Further transferrin and prealbumin levels increased already after 5 days of early EN, and the patients with positive nitrogen balance had higher prealbumin levels [32]. In critically ill patients, this muscle loss occurs very rapidly as shown in the landmark study by Puthucheary et al. [33]. In patients with two or more organ failures, the mean loss of muscle measured by ultrasound of the thigh was 22% in 10 days. The present patients were in multiple organ failure as reflected by their high SOFA score. However, there is currently no standardized procedure to assess sarcopenia in long-stay catabolic patients [34], and only surrogates are available: low (33 points) muscle strength at discharge (MRC score) and the discharge creatinine values below those recorded at admission reflect the loss of muscle mass. These results highlight the importance of an early multidisciplinary awareness for metabolic and nutritional issues, i.e., waiting 2 weeks to address them is too long. The timing, dose, and route of feeding must be addressed more stringently and earlier, and the recommendations of the dieticians applied more diligently in the high risk patients already by day 3–4.

Among the factors associated with ICU weakness, hyperglycemia has been considered important, as insulin therapy might be an attenuating factor of muscle loss through its anabolic properties [35]. Hyperglycemia is associated with increased mortality in critically ill patients [36], an issue that appears to improve by tight glycemic control [37]. The debate regarding optimal glycemic control continues as diabetic patients are frequent and exhibit a different response to tight glucose control [38]. However, there is little data in patients with prolonged ICU stay. One study reported that tighter glycemic control was associated with improved outcomes in CCI patients with stress hyperglycemia, but not in CCI patients with diabetes [39]. In the present study, the initial BG values were elevated, independently of low glucose intake. BG normalized around day 10, and remained stable thereafter, being higher in the non-survivors despite similar glucose intakes. The observed changes in BG and insulin needs over time may be related to the decrease in lean body mass. The future non-survivors also required more insulin during the 2nd phase, possibly reflecting a metabolic derangement. Diabetic patients exhibited a different pattern compared to non-diabetics corresponding to the application of the internal protocol.

Limitations of the study: our current study is observational, including only 150 patients, but the patients were enrolled prospectively to the PLS program and the study was aimed at identifying early risk criteria. The strength of the data comes from the quality of data extraction from the computer system, resulting in longitudinal continuous daily data. Regarding fasting, the study was not designed to record the reasons for the feeding interruptions, so exact causes are missing but are unlikely to differ from other observations [26]. Furthermore, our study lacks a measure for the loss of lean body mass. Except for ultrasound, which was not available in our clinical setting, there is currently no standardized procedure to assess sarcopenia in CCI patients [34]. Whole body multi-frequency bioimpedance, phase angle, and ultrasound assessment of the cross-sectional area of the thigh might become clinically useful tools, as they are non-invasive and little costly. We therefore consider integrating them into the nutrition protocol.

In randomized trials, our group showed that, in case of insufficient enteral feeding during the first 3 days (i.e., <60% of 25 kcal/kg/day which is <15 kcal/kg/day), supplemental PN (SPN) guided by indirect calorimetry to cover the measured value from day 4, reduced nosocomial infections [19] and related costs [40]. Furthermore, our group recently showed that this reduction was explained by modifications of the immune response and attenuation of the inflammatory response [20], with a trend to less loss of muscle mass ($p = 0.07$). This combined strategy should probably be applied more frequently, especially in patients with NRS ≥ 5 who obviously are not covering their needs, and who have persistent high cardiac SOFA scores. The two above Swiss SPN studies also show that a two-phase approach may be the most respectful of physiological mechanisms. Critically ill patients are generally unstable during the first days, and their endogenous energy production is elevated [22], providing 200–300 g glucose per day. This endogenous glucose production has an elevated protein cost, and 120 g/day were shown to be catabolized for neoglucogenesis. Full feeding during this period is therefore associated with a risk of overfeeding [12]. The present study shows that the very simple NRS score is probably able to identify patients who will not tolerate a prolonged underfeeding. This two-step, more physiological approach and the absence of difference between the enteral and parenteral feeding was recently summarized [41]. It is also important to integrate that "nutrition is more than the sum of its parts" as described by Briassoulis et al. [42], who emphasized that focusing only and separately on proteins or energy is not sufficient. An integrated, individualized approach, including all substrates and micronutrients is needed [43].

5. Conclusions

The present study shows that high NRS scores upon admission may identify patients at higher risk of a poor outcome, and those who require individualized nutrition therapy [43]. Exposing these high-risk patients to underfeeding further deteriorates their response capacity, including immune defenses [40], possibly favoring the development of chronic critical illness. The NRS score is not a malnutrition score, but identifies those patients who are at risk of high mortality at an early stage, this risk increasing further with underfeeding. Having no reserves, these patients will cope worse, and continue eroding their lean body mass, contributing to the poor prognosis [28,29]. Our study also shows that the most unstable patients, who become chronic, are exposed to discontinuous feeding, partly explained by persistent shock and high blood lactate values which question the clinicians about intestinal integrity, and the feasibility of EN [25]. In our previous studies [15], and in others [16], the cutoff of −70 kcal/kg of cumulated energy deficit was associated with increasing complications. Preventing such a deficit to build up requires identifying the patients at risk by their elevated NRS and hemodynamic instability. This would enable the introduction of combined feeding by day 4–5, while checking the real needs by indirect calorimetry. This strategy should be tested prospectively.

Author Contributions: Conceptualization P.E., E.F., O.P., and M.M.B.; methodology M.M.B., M.V.V., and P.E.; validation, M.V.V., O.P., G.B., A.M., E.F., M.C., D.F., P.E., and M.M.B.; formal analysis, M.M.B. and M.V.V.; methodology, M.V.V., E.V., A.M., and M.M.B.; supervision, M.M.B.; validation, M.V.V., G.B., M.C., and D.F.; investigation, M.V.V., O.P., A.M., E.F., M.C., D.F., and G.B.; resources, P.E. and M.M.B.; data curation, G.B., M.V.V., M.M.B., M.C., and D.F.; writing—original draft preparation, M.M.B. and M.V.V.; writing—review and editing, M.V.V., O.P., G.B., A.M., E.F., M.C., D.F., P.E., and M.M.B.; project administration, M.M.B., P.E., and O.P.

Conflicts of Interest: The authors declare no conflict of interest for the present research.

Appendix A

Table A1. Demographics, severity of illness, laboratory, and outcome variables according to the 90-day outcome.

	Overall	Non-Survivors	Survivors	p
N (%)	150	53 (35.3%)	97 (64.7%)	
Age (mean (SD))	60.2 (14.6)	66.1 (12.3)	57.0 (14.9)	<0.001
Sex (Males, %)	116 (77.3)	45 (84.9)	71 (73.2)	0.093
BMI (mean (SD))	26.47 (6.09)	26.56 (5.9)	26.42 (6.23)	0.899
SAPS2 (mean (SD))	52.9 (18.3)	55.5 (16.9)	51.6 (18.9)	0.211
SOFA on Day1 (median (Q1, Q3))	8 (5,11)	11 (8, 13)	9 (6, 12)	0.056
NRS (median (Q1, Q3))	5 (3, 6)	5 (4, 6)	4 (3, 6)	0.005

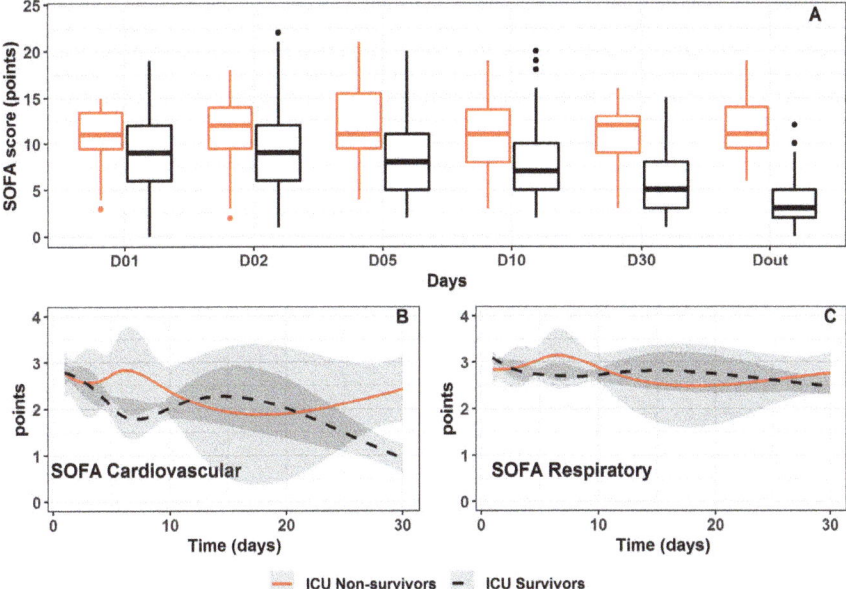

Figure A1. Evolution of the total SOFA score (**A**), and of its cardiac (**B**) and respiratory (**C**) components over time. The total SOFA score is shown as box plots (median is the line within the box, whiskers are 10th and 90th percentiles, the points above and below indicate outliers; "Dout" on time axis is the day of discharge). The boxes B and C show smooth curve uniting the days of available SOFA. The gray bands represent the 95% confidence intervals. Total SOFA changes over time were significantly different ($p < 0.0001$) between survivors and non-survivors, driven by the cardiovascular component of the score. The respiratory score did not differ between groups, remaining around three points for a long period: respiratory insufficiency was a frequent reason for prolonged ICU stay.

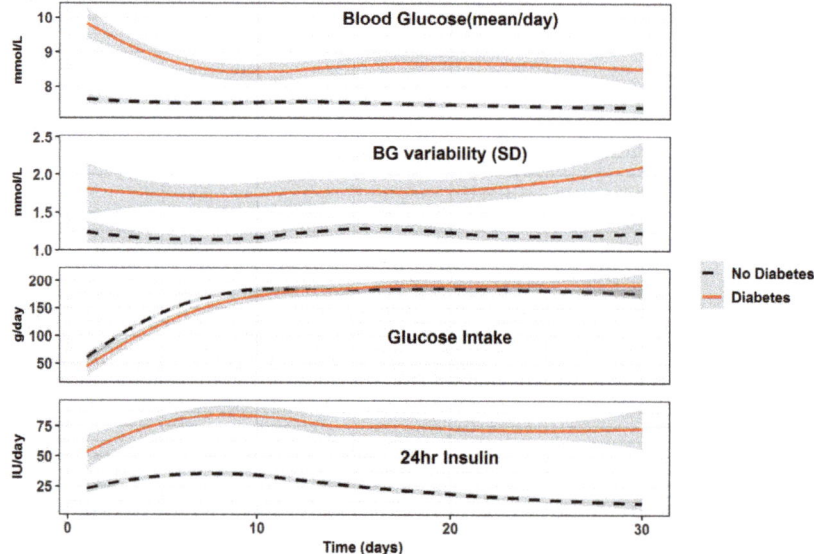

Figure A2. Evolution of glucose variables in the patients with diabetes ($n = 26$) versus those without diabetes ($n = 124$). Blood glucose (BG) and insulin needs were significantly higher in diabetic patients ($p < 0.0001$), as was the BG variability ($p < 0.001$) through the stay, with similar glucose intakes.

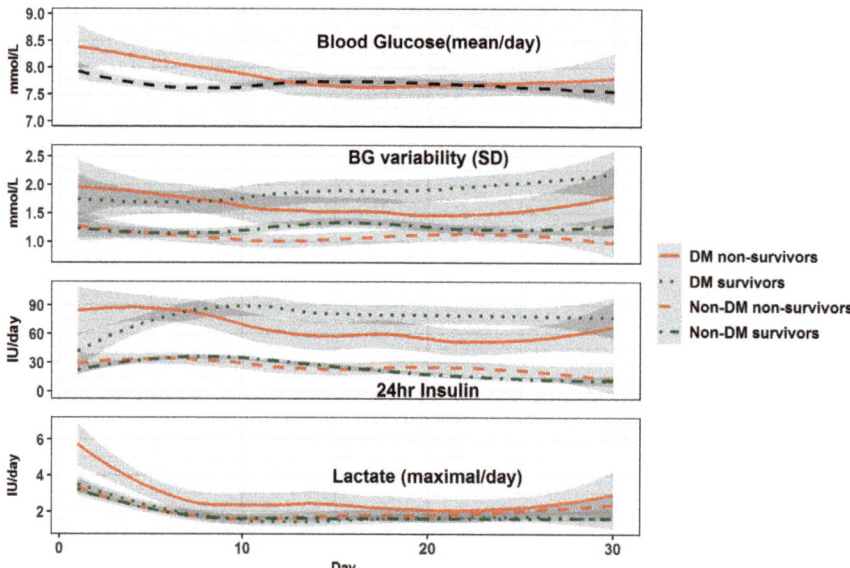

Figure A3. Glucose variables according to ICU outcome in patients with diabetes (DM) versus those without diabetes. Blood glucose (BG) was highest ($p < 0.001$) in DM-survivors compared to all, While the insulin needs did not differ in non-diabetic patients between survivors and non-survivors, the DM-non-survivors were characterized by significantly higher insulin needs during the first 6 days ($p < 0.001$), and lower needs than DM-survivors thereafter. Arterial lactate was elevated in all patients groups, and significantly higher in DM-non-survivors during the first 7 days ($p < 0.001$).

References

1. Nelson, J.E.; Cox, C.E.; Hope, A.A.; Carson, S.S. Chronic critical illness. *Am. J. Respir. Crit. Care Med.* **2010**, *182*, 446–454. [CrossRef] [PubMed]
2. Kahn, J.M.; Le, T.; Angus, D.C.; Cox, C.E.; Hough, C.L.; White, D.B.; Yende, S.; Carson, S.S.; ProVent Study Group Investigators. The epidemiology of chronic critical illness in the United States. *Crit. Care Med.* **2015**, *43*, 282–287. [CrossRef] [PubMed]
3. Loss, S.H.; Nunes, D.S.L.; Franzosi, O.S.; Salazar, G.S.; Teixeira, C.; Vieira, S.R.R. Chronic critical illness: Are we saving patients or creating victims? *Rev. Bras. Ter. Intensiva* **2017**, *29*, 87–95. [CrossRef] [PubMed]
4. Briassoulis, G.; Filippou, O.; Mavrikiou, M.; Natsi, L.; Ktistaki, M.; Hatzis, T. Current trends of clinical and genetic characteristics influencing the resource use and the nurse-patient balance in an intensive care setting. *J. Crit. Care* **2005**, *20*, 139–146. [CrossRef] [PubMed]
5. Frengley, J.D.; Sansone, G.R.; Kaner, R.J. Chronic Comorbid Illnesses Predict the Clinical Course of 866 Patients Requiring Prolonged Mechanical Ventilation in a Long-Term, Acute-Care Hospital. *J. Intensive Care Med.* **2018**, 0885066618783175. [CrossRef] [PubMed]
6. Loss, S.H.; Marchese, C.B.; Boniatti, M.M.; Wawrzeniak, I.C.; Oliveira, R.P.; Nunes, L.N.; Victorino, J.A. Prediction of chronic critical illness in a general intensive care unit. *Rev. Assoc. Med. Bras.* **2013**, *59*, 241–247. [CrossRef] [PubMed]
7. Kondrup, J.; Rasmussen, H.H.; Hamberg, O.; Stanga, Z. Nutritional risk screening (NRS 2002): A new method based on an analysis of controlled clinical trials. *Clin. Nutr.* **2003**, *22*, 321–336. [CrossRef]
8. Maciel, L.R.M.D.A.; Franzosi, O.S.; Nunes, D.S.L.; Loss, S.H.; Dos Reis, A.M.; Rubin, B.A.; Vieira, S.R.R. Nutritional Risk Screening 2002 Cut-Off to Identify High-Risk Is a Good Predictor of ICU Mortality in Critically Ill Patients. *Nutr. Clin. Pract.* **2019**, *34*, 137–141. [CrossRef]
9. Reignier, J.; Boisrame-Helms, J.; Brisard, L.; Lascarrou, J.B.; Ait Hssain, A.; Anguel, N.; Argaud, L.; Asehnoune, K.; Asfar, P.; Bellec, F.; et al. Enteral versus parenteral early nutrition in ventilated adults with shock: A randomised, controlled, multicentre, open-label, parallel-group study (NUTRIREA-2). *Lancet* **2018**, *391*, 133–143. [CrossRef]
10. Doig, G.S.; Simpson, F.; Heighes, P.T.; Bellomo, R.; Chesher, D.; Caterson, I.D.; Reade, M.C.; Harrigan, P.W.; Refeeding Syndrome Trial Investigators Group. Restricted versus continued standard caloric intake during the management of refeeding syndrome in critically ill adults: A randomised, parallel-group, multicentre, single-blind controlled trial. *Lancet Respir. Med.* **2015**, *3*, 943–952. [CrossRef]
11. Couto, C.F.L.; Dariano, A.; Texeira, C.; Silva, C.H.D.; Torbes, A.B.; Friedman, G. Adequacy of enteral nutritional support in intensive care units does not affect the short- and long-term prognosis of mechanically ventilated patients: A pilot study. *Rev. Bras. Ter. Intensiva* **2019**, *31*, 34–38. [CrossRef] [PubMed]
12. Oshima, T.; Berger, M.M.; De Waele, E.; Guttormsen, A.B.; Heidegger, C.P.; Hiesmayr, M.; Singer, P.; Wernerman, J.; Pichard, C. Indirect calorimetry in nutritional therapy. A position paper by the ICALIC study group. *Clin. Nutr.* **2017**, *36*, 651–662. [CrossRef] [PubMed]
13. Singer, P.; Reintam-Blaser, A.; Berger, M.M.; Alhazzani, W.; Calder, P.C.; Casaer, M.; Hiesmayr, M.J.; Mayer, K.; Montejo, J.M.; Pichard, C.; et al. ESPEN Guidelines: Nutrition in the ICU. *Clin. Nutr.* **2019**, *38*, 48–79. [CrossRef] [PubMed]
14. Vincent, J.L.; de Mendonca, A.; Cantraine, F.; Moreno, R.; Takala, J.; Suter, P.M.; Sprung, C.L.; Colardyn, F.; Blecher, S. Use of the SOFA score to assess the incidence of organ dysfunction/failure in intensive care units: Results of a multicenter, prospective study. Working group on "sepsis-related problems" of the European Society of Intensive Care Medicine. *Crit. Care Med.* **1998**, *26*, 1793–1800. [CrossRef] [PubMed]
15. Berger, M.M.; Pichard, C. Parenteral nutrition in the ICU: Lessons learned over the past few years. *Nutrition* **2019**, *59*, 188–194. [CrossRef]
16. Yeh, D.D.; Fuentes, E.; Quraishi, S.A.; Cropano, C.; Kaafarani, H.; Lee, J.; King, D.R.; DeMoya, M.; Fagenholz, P.; Butler, K.; et al. Adequate Nutrition May Get You Home: Effect of Caloric/Protein Deficits on the Discharge Destination of Critically Ill Surgical Patients. *J. Parenter. Enter. Nutr.* **2016**, *40*, 37–44. [CrossRef] [PubMed]
17. Soguel, L.; Revelly, J.P.; Schaller, M.D.; Longchamp, C.; Berger, M.M. Energy deficit and length of hospital stay can be reduced by a two-step quality improvement of nutrition therapy: The intensive care unit dietitian can make the difference. *Crit. Care Med.* **2012**, *40*, 412–419. [CrossRef]

18. Paternostro-Sluga, T.; Grim-Stieger, M.; Posch, M.; Schuhfried, O.; Vacariu, G.; Mittermaier, C.; Bittner, C.; Fialka-Moser, V. Reliability and validity of the Medical Research Council (MRC) scale and a modified scale for testing muscle strength in patients with radial palsy. *J. Rehabil. Med.* **2008**, *40*, 665–671. [CrossRef]
19. Heidegger, C.P.; Berger, M.M.; Graf, S.; Zingg, W.; Darmon, P.; Costanza, M.C.; Thibault, R.; Pichard, C. Optimisation of energy provision with supplemental parenteral nutrition in critically ill patients: A randomised controlled clinical trial. *Lancet* **2013**, *381*, 385–393. [CrossRef]
20. Berger, M.M.; Pantet, O.; Jacquelin-Ravel, N.; Charriere, M.; Schmidt, S.; Becce, F.; Audran, R.; Spertini, F.; Tappy, L.; Pichard, C. Supplemental parenteral nutrition improves immunity with unchanged carbohydrate and protein metabolism in critically ill patients: The SPN2 randomized tracer study. *Clin. Nutr.* **2018**. [CrossRef]
21. Harvey, S.E.; Parrott, F.; Harrison, D.A.; Bear, D.E.; Segaran, E.; Beale, R.; Bellingan, G.; Leonard, R.; Mythen, M.G.; Rowan, K.M.; et al. Trial of the route of early nutritional support in critically ill adults—Calories Trial. *N. Engl. J. Med.* **2014**, *371*, 1673–1684. [CrossRef] [PubMed]
22. Tappy, L.; Schwarz, J.M.; Schneiter, P.; Cayeux, C.; Revelly, J.P.; Fagerquist, C.K.; Jéquier, E.; Chioléro, R. Effects of isoenergetic glucose-based or lipid-based parenteral nutrition on glucose metabolism, de novo lipogenesis, and respiratory gas exchanges in critically ill patients. *Crit. Care Med.* **1998**, *26*, 860–867. [CrossRef] [PubMed]
23. Elke, G.; Wang, M.; Weiler, N.; Day, A.G.; Heyland, D.K. Close to recommended caloric and protein intake by enteral nutrition is associated with better clinical outcome of critically ill septic patients: Secondary analysis of a large international nutrition database. *Crit. Care* **2014**, *18*, R29. [CrossRef] [PubMed]
24. Ohbe, H.; Jo, T.; Matsui, H.; Fushimi, K.; Yasunaga, H. Differences in effect of early enteral nutrition on mortality among ventilated adults with shock requiring low-, medium-, and high-dose noradrenaline: A propensity-matched analysis. *Clin. Nutr.* **2019**. [CrossRef] [PubMed]
25. Reintam Blaser, A.; Starkopf, J.; Alhazzani, W.; Berger, M.M.; Casaer, M.P.; Deane, A.M.; Fruhwald, S.; Hiesmayr, M.; Ichai, C.; Jakob, S.M.; et al. Early enteral nutrition in critically ill patients: ESICM clinical practice guidelines. *Intensive Care Med.* **2017**, *43*, 380–398. [CrossRef] [PubMed]
26. Heyland, D.K.; Cook, D.J.; Winder, B.; Brylowski, L.; Van de Mark, H.; Guyatt, G.H. Enteral nutrition in the critically ill patient: A prospective survey. *Crit. Care Med.* **1995**, *23*, 1055–1060. [CrossRef] [PubMed]
27. Brierley-Hobson, S.; Clarke, G.; O'Keeffe, V. Safety and efficacy of volume-based feeding in critically ill, mechanically ventilated adults using the 'Protein & Energy Requirements Fed for Every Critically ill patient every Time' (PERFECT) protocol: A before-and-after study. *Crit. Care* **2019**, *23*, 105. [CrossRef]
28. Friedman, J.; Lussiez, A.; Sullivan, J.; Wang, S.; Englesbe, M. Implications of sarcopenia in major surgery. *Nutr. Clin. Pract.* **2015**, *30*, 175–179. [CrossRef]
29. Moisey, L.L.; Mourtzakis, M.; Cotton, B.A.; Premji, T.; Heyland, D.K.; Wade, C.E.; Bulger, E.; Kozar, R.A.; Nutrition and Rehabilitation Investigators Consortium (NUTRIC). Skeletal muscle predicts ventilator-free days, ICU-free days, and mortality in elderly ICU patients. *Crit. Care* **2013**, *17*, R206. [CrossRef] [PubMed]
30. Bouharras El Idrissi, H.; Molina Lopez, J.; Perez Moreno, I.; Florea, D.I.; Lobo Tamer, G.; Herrera-Quintana, L.; Perez De La Cruz, A.; Rodriguez Elvira, M.; Planells Del Pozo, E.M. Imbalances in protein metabolism in critical care patient with systemic inflammatory response syndrome at admission in intensive care unit. *Nutr. Hosp.* **2015**, *32*, 2848–2854. [CrossRef]
31. Briassoulis, G.; Zavras, N.; Hatzis, T. Malnutrition, nutritional indices, and early enteral feeding in critically ill children. *Nutrition* **2001**, *17*, 548–557. [PubMed]
32. Briassoulis, G.; Tsorva, A.; Zavras, N.; Hatzis, T. Influence of an aggressive early enteral nutrition protocol on nitrogen balance in critically ill children. *J. Nutr. Biochem.* **2002**, *13*, 560. [PubMed]
33. Puthucheary, Z.A.; Rawal, J.; McPhail, M.; Connolly, B.; Ratnayake, G.; Chan, P.; Hopkinson, N.S.; Padhke, R.; Dew, T.; Sidhu, P.S.; et al. Acute skeletal muscle wasting in critical illness. *JAMA* **2013**, *310*, 1591–1600. [CrossRef] [PubMed]
34. Hernandez-Socorro, C.R.; Saavedra, P.; Lopez-Fernandez, J.C.; Ruiz-Santana, S. Assessment of Muscle Wasting in Long-Stay ICU Patients Using a New Ultrasound Protocol. *Nutrients* **2018**, *10*, 1849. [CrossRef]
35. Hermans, G.; De Jonghe, B.; Bruyninckx, F.; Van den Berghe, G. Interventions for preventing critical illness polyneuropathy and critical illness myopathy. *Cochrane Database Syst. Rev.* **2014**. [CrossRef] [PubMed]

36. Krinsley, J.S.; Chase, J.G.; Gunst, J.; Martensson, J.; Schultz, M.J.; Taccone, F.S.; Wernerman, J.; Bohe, J.; De Block, C.; Desaive, T.; et al. Continuous glucose monitoring in the ICU: Clinical considerations and consensus. *Crit. Care* **2017**, *21*, 197. [CrossRef] [PubMed]
37. Mesotten, D.; Preiser, J.C.; Kosiborod, M. Glucose management in critically ill adults and children. *Lancet Diabetes Endocrinol.* **2015**, *3*, 723–733. [CrossRef]
38. Krinsley, J.S.; Maurer, P.; Holewinski, S.; Hayes, R.; McComsey, D.; Umpierrez, G.E.; Nasraway, S.A. Glucose Control, Diabetes Status, and Mortality in Critically Ill Patients: The Continuum From Intensive Care Unit Admission to Hospital Discharge. *Mayo Clin. Proc.* **2017**, *92*, 1019–1029. [CrossRef]
39. Schulman, R.C.; Moshier, E.L.; Rho, L.; Casey, M.F.; Godbold, J.H.; Mechanick, J.I. Association of glycemic control parameters with clinical outcomes in chronic critical illness. *Endocr. Pract.* **2014**, *20*, 884–893. [CrossRef]
40. Pradelli, L.; Graf, S.; Pichard, C.; Berger, M.M. Supplemental parenteral nutrition in intensive care patients: A cost saving strategy. *Clin. Nutr.* **2018**, *37*, 573–579. [CrossRef]
41. Arabi, Y.M.; Al-Dorzi, H.M. Trophic or full nutritional support? *Curr. Opin. Crit. Care* **2018**, *24*, 262–268. [CrossRef]
42. Briassoulis, G.; Briassoulis, P.; Ilia, I. Nutrition Is More Than the Sum of Its Parts. *Pediatr. Crit. Care Med.* **2018**, *19*, 1087–1089. [CrossRef]
43. Berger, M.M.; Pichard, C. Feeding should be individualized in the critically ill patients. *Curr. Opin. Crit. Care* **2019**, *25*, 307–313. [CrossRef]

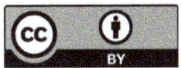

© 2019 by the authors. Licensee MDPI, Basel, Switzerland. This article is an open access article distributed under the terms and conditions of the Creative Commons Attribution (CC BY) license (http://creativecommons.org/licenses/by/4.0/).

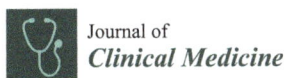

Article

Protein Intake, Nutritional Status and Outcomes in ICU Survivors: A Single Center Cohort Study

Peter J.M. Weijs [1,2], Kris M. Mogensen [3], James D. Rawn [4] and Kenneth B. Christopher [5,*]

1. Department of Nutrition and Dietetics, Amsterdam University Medical Centers, VU University, 1081 HV Amsterdam, The Netherlands; p.weijs@vumc.nl
2. Faculty of Sports and Nutrition, Amsterdam University of Applied Sciences, 1067 SM Amsterdam, The Netherlands
3. Department of Nutrition, Brigham and Women's Hospital, Boston, MA 02115, USA; kmogensen@bwh.harvard.edu
4. Department of Surgery, Brigham and Women's Hospital, Boston, MA 02115, USA; jrawn@bwh.harvard.edu
5. The Nathan E. Hellman Memorial Laboratory, Division of Renal Medicine, Brigham and Women's Hospital, Boston, MA 02115, USA
* Correspondence: kbchristopher@bwh.harvard.edu; Tel.: +1-617-272-0535

Received: 16 December 2018; Accepted: 31 December 2018; Published: 4 January 2019

Abstract: Background: We hypothesized that protein delivery during hospitalization in patients who survived critical care would be associated with outcomes following hospital discharge. Methods: We studied 801 patients, age $\geq$ 18 years, who received critical care between 2004 and 2012 and survived hospitalization. All patients underwent a registered dietitian formal assessment within 48 h of ICU admission. The exposure of interest, grams of protein per kilogram body weight delivered per day, was determined from all oral, enteral and parenteral sources for up to 28 days. Adjusted odds ratios for all cause 90-day post-discharge mortality were estimated by mixed-effects logistic regression models. Results: The 90-day post-discharge mortality was 13.9%. The mean nutrition delivery days recorded was 15. In a mixed-effect logistic regression model adjusted for age, gender, race, Deyo-Charlson comorbidity index, acute organ failures, sepsis and percent energy needs met, the 90-day post-discharge mortality rate was 17% (95% CI: 6–26) lower for each 1 g/kg increase in daily protein delivery (OR = 0.83 (95% CI 0.74–0.94; $p = 0.002$)). Conclusions: Adult medical ICU patients with improvements in daily protein intake during hospitalization who survive hospitalization have decreased odds of mortality in the 3 months following hospital discharge.

Keywords: protein; malnutrition; critical care; mortality; outcomes; hospital readmission; ICU Survivors

1. Introduction

A hallmark of critical illness is muscle wasting related to a dramatic increase in muscle protein catabolism in the setting of inflammation [1]. Catabolic critical illness results in a protracted and dramatic loss of nitrogen and reduces exogenous amino acid deposition into endogenous proteins [2]. Nutritionally compromised hospitalized patients commonly present with sarcopenia [3]. Inflammation related endogenous skeletal muscle protein catabolism that can quickly progress to severe muscle atrophy [4]. In the critically ill, muscle mass loss and decreased strength are common complications [5].

Protein intake recommended for healthy adults is 0.8 g/kg per day. While the most common recommended protein intake in the critically ill is 1.5 g/kg per day [6,7], up to 1.5–2.5 g protein/kg per day may be most advantageous [7,8]. ICU patients commonly receive less than even the lowest guideline recommendation regarding adequate protein intake [7,9–11]. Recent trials [12–15] demonstrate that "calorie-supplemented, protein-deficient nutrition" [4] does not improve clinical outcomes. Early energy provision of 70–80% of measured energy expenditure appears to be associated with improved outcome [16,17]. Although the correct amount of protein to provide critically ill patients is unknown, higher than 1.2 g/kg is associated with reduced mortality in non-septic non-energy overfed ICU patients [16]. A recent large observational study suggests achieving ≥80% of prescribed protein intake in the ICU is associated with decreased mortality [18].

Although short term survival is studied in the critically ill regarding protein delivery [18], post-hospital discharge outcomes in such ICU survivors relative to protein intake and nutrition status is not known. In patients who survive critical illness, pre-existing malnutrition may be a risk factor for adverse events following hospital discharge [19]. As ICU patients with low protein delivery [18] and with malnutrition [20] have elevated in-hospital mortality, we studied the association between increases in daily protein delivery in malnourished critically ill patients would be associated with lower 90-day mortality following hospital discharge. We hypothesized that in hospital survivors who received critical care, those with higher daily protein delivery would have a lower risk of post discharge mortality and this effect would be magnified in patients with pre-existing malnutrition.

2. Materials and Methods

2.1. Data Sources

We obtained administrative and laboratory data from critically ill medical patients admitted to the Brigham and Women's Hospital (BWH), an academic medical center in Boston with 777 beds. Patient data was collected by the Research Patient Data Registry (RPDR) a clinical data warehouse for patient records at BWH that has been utilized and validated in other studies [20]. The Partners Human Research Committee Institutional Review Board granted approval for the study. Between 2004 and 2012 there were 801 unique patients ≥18 years, assigned the CPT code 99291 (critical care, first 30–74 min) [21] who had nutrition risk assessed, protein intake measured, and survived to hospital discharge.

2.2. Exposure of Interest and Comorbidities

All medical ICU patients at BWH are screened by a registered dietitian (RD). Patients at risk for malnutrition are then evaluated by an RD with a structured objective assessment. The exposure of interest, grams of protein per kilogram body weight delivered per day, was determined by an RD from all oral, enteral and parenteral sources for up to 28 days. We included all nutrition data collected by an RD in the ten days prior to ICU admission to two days following an ICU discharge. The determination of nutrition status is described in detail previously [20,22]. The RD determines the diagnosis of malnutrition based on literature [23,24], clinical judgment, and on data related to inadequate nutrient intake, muscle wasting, subcutaneous fat wasting and unintended weight loss [22]. As in our prior study, we categorized nutrition diagnoses a priori into four groups of increasing severity: malnutrition absent, at risk for malnutrition, non-specific malnutrition, or any protein-energy malnutrition [22]. Patients that meet criteria for non-specific malnutrition have risk factors for malnutrition (insufficient intake of energy, protein, and micronutrients) in addition to metabolic stress and/or obvious signs of malnutrition (muscle and/or subcutaneous fat wasting) without supporting biochemical or anthropometric data. Patients that meet criteria for protein-energy malnutrition have a combination of disease-related weight loss, obvious muscle wasting, peripheral edema, inadequate energy or protein intake and are considered underweight by percent ideal body weight [25]. Patients with absence of malnutrition are diagnosed by an RD as well-nourished and not at risk for malnutrition.Race was self-determined or determined by the patient's family or healthcare proxy. The Deyo-Charlson comorbidity index was determined using validated ICD-9 coding algorithms [26]. To define sepsis we used the presence of the ICD-9 codes 038, 785.52, 995.91, or 995.92 in the three days before ICU admission to the 7 days after ICU admission [27]. The vasopressors/inotropes covariate is the prescription of any vasopressor or inotrope in the three days prior to ICU admission to the seven days after ICU admission [20].

The number of acute organ failures was a combination of ICD-9-CM and CPT codes relating to acute organ dysfunction assigned from three days prior to ICU admission day to the 30 days after [28,29]. Intubation was defined as the presence of ICD-9 codes mechanical ventilation (96.7×) following hospital admission [30]. Acute kidney injury is the RIFLE class Injury or Failure taking place in the three days prior to ICU admission and the seven days after ICU admission [31]. Chronic kidney disease is <60 mL/min glomerular filtration rate calculated from the Modification of Diet in Renal Disease (MDRD) equation using pre-hospital or hospital admission creatinine as baseline [32]. Changes from the expected hospital length of stay (LOS) are determined by subtracting the actual LOS from the geometric mean LOS for each Diagnostic Related Grouping (DRG) a classification system for hospital cases [33]. The geometric mean LOS is the United States national mean LOS for each DRG per the Centers for Medicare & Medicaid Services [34].

2.3. End Points

Our primary outcome was all cause 90-day post-discharge mortality. Mortality status for the study cohort was obtained from the United States Social Security Administration Death Master File. Mortality determination via the Death Master File is validated in our administrative database [21]. The entire cohort had mortality status present for the year following hospital discharge. The censoring date was 15 March 2012. All patients in the cohort had at least 90-day follow-up after hospital discharge or expired before the 90-days post-hospitalization.

2.4. Power Calculations and Statistical Analysis

90-day post-discharge mortality rate was 9.6% in our prior study nutrition in critical illness [35]. From these data, we assumed that 90-day post-discharge mortality would be 6.0% greater in patients with <1.0 g/kg/day protein delivery compared to those with >1.0 g/kg/day protein delivery. With a power of 80% and an alpha error level of 5%, the sample size required for the 90-day post-discharge mortality outcome was 393 patients with >1.0 g/kg/day protein delivery and 393 patients with <1.0 g/kg/day protein delivery.

We described categorical covariates via frequency distribution, and compared variables in outcome groups with chi-square testing. We compared continuous variables across outcome groups using one-way analysis of variance (ANOVA) or the Kruskal–Wallis test. We utilized mixed-effect logistic regression models [36,37] which contain both fixed and random-effects for analysis of the association between g/kg/day protein delivery and 90-day post-discharge mortality by use of the command xtmelogit [38] in STATA 14.1 MP (College Station, TX, USA). The dates of protein delivery of individual patients were used as the random effect. We assessed the following covariates for confounding: age, gender, race, Deyo-Charlson comorbidity index, energy delivery, nutrition status, acute organ failure, sepsis, metastatic malignancy, acute kidney injury and chronic kidney disease. We selected the final model confounders by analyzing the maximum model and then conducting backward elimination of covariates with a $p > 0.10$. The final model had an independent covariance structure of the random effects; a fixed effect for age, gender, race, Deyo-Charlson comorbidity index, energy delivery, nutrition status, acute organ failure and sepsis; and gaussian-distributed random intercepts and slopes. We then used mixed-effect linear regression to analyze the association between the change in daily protein delivery and hospital LOS where random effects accounted for the dates of protein delivery within individual patients. Data visualization was performed utilizing the DistillerSR Forest Plot Generator (Evidence Partners, Ottawa, ON, Canada). p-values presented are two-tailed with $p < 0.05$ considered to be significant. We utilized STATA 14.1MP (College Station, TX, USA) for all analyses.

3. Results

Patient characteristics were stratified according to 90-day post-discharge mortality (Table 1). In our cohort the mean (SD) age was 62.3 (16.6) years, 55.3% were male and 78.9% were white. The majority of patients were assessed by an RD within 24 hours of ICU admission (median [IQR] time between ICU admission and RD assessment was 0 [1, 1] days). The mean number of recorded nutrition delivery days was 15. A total of 8735 days with protein intake were determined. The mean peak protein daily delivery was 0.32 g protein/kg. Figure 1 shows protein delivery over time in the cohort.

The mean (SD) length of hospital stay was 22.1 (15.2) days. The 30-, 90- and 365-day post-discharge mortality rates were 7.1%, 13.9%, and 24.5%, respectively. Age, race, Deyo-Charlson comorbidity index, malnutrition, the acute organ failure score and chronic kidney disease are significantly associated with 90-day post-discharge mortality (Table 1).

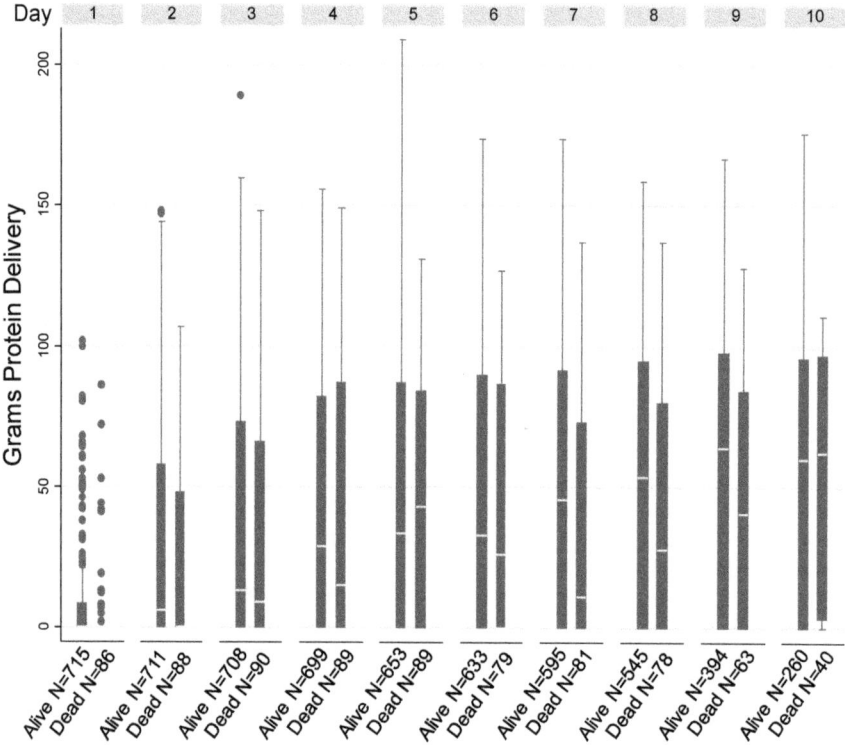

Figure 1. Box plots of daily protein delivery up to 10 days in patients who did and did not survive to 90-day post-discharge mortality, showing the median (white line), the third quartile (Q3) and first quartile (Q1) range of the data and data outliers (observations outside the 9–91 percentile range).

Table 1. Clinical and demographic characteristics of the study cohort ($n = 801$).

Characteristics	Alive at 90-Days Post-Discharge	Expired by 90-Days Post-Discharge	Total	p-Value	Unadjusted OR (95%CI) for 90-Day Post-Discharge Mortality
	690	111	801		
Age-Mean ± SD	61.1 ± 16.7	69.8 ± 14	62.3 ± 16.6	<0.001 *	1.04 (1.02, 1.05)
Male Gender-No. (%)	384 (56)	58 (52)	442 (55)	0.50	0.87 (0.58, 1.30)
Non-White Race-No. (%)	154 (22)	15 (14)	169 (21)	0.035	0.54 (0.31, 0.96)
Deyo-Charlson Index-No. (%)				0.003	
0	182 (26.38)	15 (13.39)	197 (24.56)		1.00 (Referent)
1–2	440 (63.77)	75 (66.96)	515 (64.21)		2.07 (1.16, 3.70)
≥3	68 (9.86)	22 (19.64)	90 (11.22)		3.93 (1.92, 8.01)
Acute Organ Failures-No. (%)				0.030	
0	86 (12)	16 (14)	102 (13)		1.00 (Referent)
1	217 (31)	29 (26)	246 (31)		0.72 (0.37, 1.39)
2	192 (28)	26 (23)	218 (27)		0.73 (0.37, 1.43)
3	136 (20)	20 (18)	156 (19)		0.79 (0.39, 1.61)
≥4	59 (9)	20 (18)	79 (10)		1.82 (0.87, 3.80)
Sepsis-No. (%)	138 (20)	28 (25)	166 (21)	0.21	1.35 (0.85, 2.15)
Intubation-No. (%)	400 (58)	60 (54)	460 (57)	0.44	0.85 (0.57, 1.28)
Acute Organ Failure Score-Mean ± SD	10.2 ± 4.4	11.4 ± 4.6	10.4 ± 4.5	0.0082 *	1.06 (1.02, 1.11)
Vasopressors/Inotropes-No. (%)	264 (38)	51 (46)	315 (39)	0.12	1.37 (0.92, 2.05)
Metastatic Malignancy-No. (%)	296 (43)	58 (52)	354 (44)	0.066	1.46 (0.97, 2.18)
Acute Kidney Injury-No. (%) †	55 (10)	6 (7)	61 (10)	0.381	0.68 (0.28, 1.63)
Chronic Kidney Disease-No. (%) ††	169 (31)	42 (49)	211 (33)	0.001	1.23 (1.06, 1.41)
Malnutrition-No. (%)				0.035	
At Risk for Malnutrition	291 (43)	33 (30)	324 (41)		1.00 (Referent)
Non-Specific Malnutrition	343 (51)	65 (60)	408 (52)		1.67 (1.07, 2.61)
Protein-Energy Malnutrition	45 (7)	11 (10)	56 (7)		2.16 (1.02, 4.57)

Data presented as n (%) unless otherwise indicated. p values determined by chi-square unless designated by (*) then p value determined by ANOVA. † Data available to determine Acute Kidney Injury in 638 patients. †† Data available to determine Chronic Kidney Disease was present in 638 patients.

Primary Outcome

Higher protein delivery in ICU survivors was associated with lower 90-day post-discharge mortality. In our mixed-effect logistic regression model adjusted for age, gender, race, Deyo-Charlson comorbidity index, energy delivery, nutrition status, acute organ failure, sepsis and the random-effects structure, the 90-day post-discharge mortality rate decreased by 18% for each 1 g/kg/day elevation in protein delivery following ICU admission (OR 0.82, 95% CI 0.73–0.92). Following stratification for nutrition status, the same multivariable mixed-effect logistic regression model shows the 90-day post-discharge mortality rate significantly decreased for each 1 g/kg elevation in daily protein delivery. Specifically, in patients diagnosed with malnutrition ($n = 473$), 90-day post-discharge mortality rate was 30% (95% CI: 6–26) less for each 1 g/kg elevation in daily protein delivery following ICU admission (OR = 0.70 (95% CI 0.61–0.81; $p < 0.001$)).

We next determined if protein delivery was associated with longer term mortality outcomes. When patients were evaluated using a multivariable mixed-effect logistic regression model with the same covariates and structure as the primary outcome model, 180-day post-discharge mortality was significantly reduced for each 1 g/kg elevation in daily protein delivery (OR 0.74, 95% CI 0.67–0.83; $p < 0.001$). When patients were evaluated using the multivariable mixed-effect logistic regression model with the same covariates and structure as the primary outcome model, the 365- and 720-day post-discharge mortality rate was significantly reduced for each 1 g/kg elevation in daily protein delivery (OR 0.76, 95% CI 0.69–0.83; $p < 0.001$), (OR 0.77, 95% CI 0.71–0.84; $p < 0.001$) respectively (Table 2, Figure 2). All estimates are for each 1 g/kg/day increase in protein delivery.

Table 2. Associations between Protein Delivery and post-hospital mortality outcomes.

Outcome	OR	95% CI	p-Value	Association for Each 1 g/kg/Day Increase in Protein Delivery
90-day post-discharge Mortality				
Full Cohort (n = 801)	0.83	0.74–0.94	0.002	17% decrease odds of death
Malnutrition (n = 473)	0.70	0.61–0.81	<0.001	30% decrease odds of death
180-day post-discharge Mortality				
Full Cohort (n = 801)	0.74	0.67–0.83	<0.001	26% decrease odds of death
365-day post-discharge Mortality				
Full Cohort (n = 801)	0.76	0.69–0.83	<0.001	24% decrease odds of death
720-day post-discharge Mortality				
Full Cohort (n = 801)	0.77	0.71–0.84	<0.001	23% decrease odds of death

All estimates were produced via a mixed-effect logistic regression model adjusted for age, gender, race, Deyo-Charlson comorbidity index, energy delivery, nutrition status, acute organ failure, sepsis and the random-effects structure.

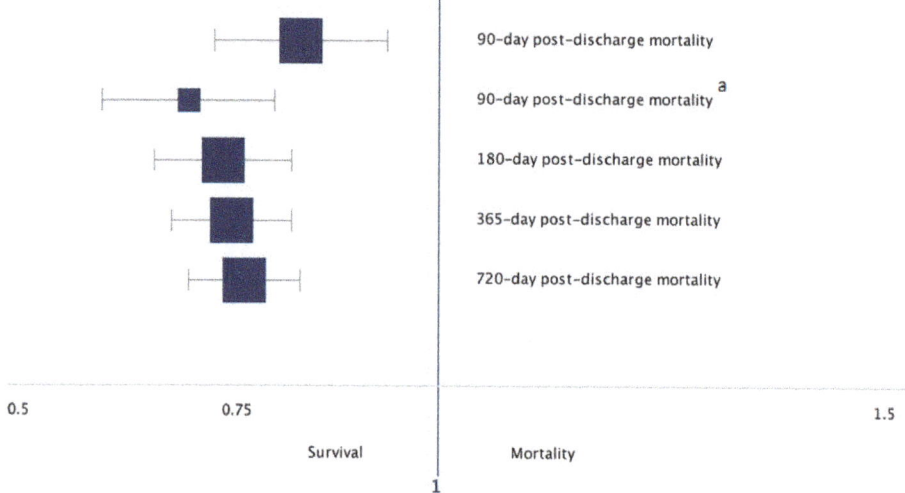

Figure 2. Forest plot of post-discharge mortality associated for each 1 g/kg/day increase in protein delivery in our study cohort. Odds ratios with corresponding 95% CIs shown of the individual outcomes under study. [a] Restricted to patients diagnosed with Malnutrition.

Finally we examined the association between protein delivery and hospital length of stay. In a mixed-effect linear regression model adjusted for age, gender, race, Deyo-Charlson comorbidity index, energy delivery, nutrition status, acute organ failure, sepsis and the random-effects structure, the actual hospital length of stay (LOS) was reduced by 0.87 days (95% CI −1.7 to −0.10) compared with the average LOS for the DRG for each 1 g/kg/day increase in protein delivery ($p = 0.028$).

4. Discussion

In our study, we examined the association between protein delivery in critical illness survivors and post-hospital discharge outcomes. We demonstrate that improvement in daily protein delivery is associated with a significant decrease in the odds of post-discharge hospital mortality. We also show that patients with improved daily protein delivery have decreased hospital length of stay.

Long-term morbidity and mortality are substantial problems in ICU survivors [39]. Adverse events following discharge from an ICU admission are known to include comorbidity, illness severity and organ failures [40]. In critical illness survivors, the risk factors for outside hospital adverse events are not well known. Our results show an association between higher daily protein delivery during hospitalization and improved post-discharge mortality in critical illness survivors. While our observational study cannot be interpreted as causal, the protein delivery-post-discharge outcome association has biologic plausibility.

Our study may have limitations due to its observational design. Causality is limited and as such our observations should be considered hypothesis generating. As protein intake in our cohort is only collected in patients considered to be at least at risk for malnutrition, ascertainment bias may be present. Unmeasured variables may influence outcomes following hospitalization independent of protein delivery, which can result in bias. We are unable to adjust for gut failure which associated with lower nutrition tolerance, lower protein intake and contributes to adverse outcomes [41]. Though ICD-9 code assignment data is collected from individual provider encounters, determination of covariates via ICD-9 codes may not completely capture the true incidence or prevalence. Finally, residual confounding may remain despite multivariable adjustment which may contribute to observed estimates.

Our study has several strengths. We utilize mixed-effects models to incorporate multiple measures and sources of protein intake over a total of 8735 days which allow for more complete information to be captured in parameter estimations. Mixed-effects models are ideal for such longitudinal data because each patient may have an unequal number of repeated measures. Additionally, a highly trained RD utilized weight loss history, clinical assessment, anthropometric metrics and protein intake to make an in person assessment of nutritional risk and daily protein delivery. Finally, the Master Death File is shown to capture post discharge mortality in our cohort accurately [21].

5. Conclusions

Our data show that in critically ill patients who survive hospitalization, higher daily protein delivery during hospitalization is associated with decreased mortality following hospital discharge. Increasing protein delivery following the acute phase of illness may be a strategy to assist with critical illness recovery and longer term outcomes.

Author Contributions: Conceptualization, P.J.M.W. and K.B.C.; Methodology, P.J.M.W. and K.B.C.; Software, K.B.C.; Validation, K.B.C.; Formal Analysis, K.B.C.; Investigation, P.J.M.W., K.M.M., and K.B.C.; Resources, K.M.M., J.D.R., and K.B.C.; Data Curation, J.D.R., and K.B.C.; Writing—Original Draft Preparation, P.J.M.W., K.M.M., and K.B.C.; Writing—Review & Editing, P.J.M.W., K.M.M., J.D.R., and K.B.C.; Supervision, K.B.C.; Project Administration, K.B.C.; Funding Acquisition, K.B.C.

Funding: This manuscript was funded by NIH R01GM115774.

Acknowledgments: This manuscript is dedicated to the memory of our dear friend and colleague Nathan Edward Hellman. The authors thank Shawn Murphy and Henry Chueh and the Partners Health Care Research Patient Data Registry group for facilitating use of their database.

Conflicts of Interest: The authors declare no conflict of interest.

References

1. Gabay, C.; Kushner, I. Acute-phase proteins and other systemic responses to inflammation. *N. Engl. J. Med.* **1999**, *340*, 448–454. [CrossRef] [PubMed]
2. Hoffer, L.J.; Bistrian, B.R. Nutrition in critical illness: A current conundrum. *F1000Research* **2016**, *5*, 2531. [CrossRef] [PubMed]
3. Cerri, A.P.; Bellelli, G.; Mazzone, A.; Pittella, F.; Landi, F.; Zambon, A.; Annoni, G. Sarcopenia and malnutrition in acutely ill hospitalized elderly: Prevalence and outcomes. *Clin. Nutr.* **2015**, *34*, 745–751. [CrossRef] [PubMed]
4. Hoffer, L.J. Protein requirement in critical illness. *Appl. Physiol. Nutr. Metab.* **2016**, *41*, 573–576. [CrossRef] [PubMed]

5. Batt, J.; dos Santos, C.C.; Cameron, J.I.; Herridge, M.S. Intensive care unit-acquired weakness: Clinical phenotypes and molecular mechanisms. *Am. J. Respir. Crit. Care Med.* **2013**, *187*, 238–246. [CrossRef] [PubMed]
6. Ziegler, T.R. Parenteral nutrition in the critically ill patient. *N. Engl. J. Med.* **2009**, *361*, 1088–1097. [CrossRef] [PubMed]
7. Hoffer, L.J.; Bistrian, B.R. Why critically ill patients are protein deprived. *JPEN J. Parenter. Enter. Nutr.* **2013**, *37*, 300–309. [CrossRef]
8. Hoffer, L.J.; Bistrian, B.R. What is the best nutritional support for critically ill patients? *Hepatobiliary Surg. Nutr.* **2014**, *3*, 172–174. [CrossRef]
9. Heyland, D.K. Should We PERMIT Systematic Underfeeding in All Intensive Care Unit Patients? Integrating the Results of the PERMIT Study in Our Clinical Practice Guidelines. *JPEN J. Parenter. Enter. Nutr.* **2016**, *40*, 156–158. [CrossRef]
10. Alberda, C.; Gramlich, L.; Jones, N.; Jeejeebhoy, K.; Day, A.G.; Dhaliwal, R.; Heyland, D.K. The relationship between nutritional intake and clinical outcomes in critically ill patients: Results of an international multicenter observational study. *Intensive Care Med* **2009**, *35*, 1728–1737. [CrossRef]
11. Heyland, D.K.; Dhaliwal, R.; Wang, M.; Day, A.G. The prevalence of iatrogenic underfeeding in the nutritionally 'at-risk' critically ill patient: Results of an international, multicenter, prospective study. *Clin. Nutr.* **2015**, *34*, 659–666. [CrossRef] [PubMed]
12. Doig, G.S.; Simpson, F.; Sweetman, E.A.; Finfer, S.R.; Cooper, D.J.; Heighes, P.T.; Davies, A.R.; O'Leary, M.; Solano, T.; Peake, S.; et al. Early parenteral nutrition in critically ill patients with short-term relative contraindications to early enteral nutrition: A randomized controlled trial. *JAMA* **2013**, *309*, 2130–2138. [CrossRef] [PubMed]
13. Casaer, M.P.; Mesotten, D.; Hermans, G.; Wouters, P.J.; Schetz, M.; Meyfroidt, G.; Van Cromphaut, S.; Ingels, C.; Meersseman, P.; Muller, J.; et al. Early versus late parenteral nutrition in critically ill adults. *N. Engl. J. Med.* **2011**, *365*, 506–517. [CrossRef] [PubMed]
14. Heidegger, C.P.; Berger, M.M.; Graf, S.; Zingg, W.; Darmon, P.; Costanza, M.C.; Thibault, R.; Pichard, C. Optimisation of energy provision with supplemental parenteral nutrition in critically ill patients: A randomised controlled clinical trial. *Lancet* **2013**, *381*, 385–393. [CrossRef]
15. Singer, P.; Anbar, R.; Cohen, J.; Shapiro, H.; Shalita-Chesner, M.; Lev, S.; Grozovski, E.; Theilla, M.; Frishman, S.; Madar, Z. The tight calorie control study (TICACOS): A prospective, randomized, controlled pilot study of nutritional support in critically ill patients. *Intensive Care Med.* **2011**, *37*, 601–609. [CrossRef] [PubMed]
16. Weijs, P.J.; Looijaard, W.G.; Beishuizen, A.; Girbes, A.R.; Oudemans-van Straaten, H.M. Early high protein intake is associated with low mortality and energy overfeeding with high mortality in non-septic mechanically ventilated critically ill patients. *Crit. Care* **2014**, *18*, 701. [CrossRef]
17. Zusman, O.; Theilla, M.; Cohen, J.; Kagan, I.; Bendavid, I.; Singer, P. Resting energy expenditure, calorie and protein consumption in critically ill patients: A retrospective cohort study. *Crit. Care* **2016**, *20*, 367. [CrossRef]
18. Nicolo, M.; Heyland, D.K.; Chittams, J.; Sammarco, T.; Compher, C. Clinical Outcomes Related to Protein Delivery in a Critically Ill Population: A Multicenter, Multinational Observation Study. *JPEN J. Parenter. Enter. Nutr.* **2016**, *40*, 45–51. [CrossRef]
19. Weijs, P.J.; Looijaard, W.G.; Dekker, I.M.; Stapel, S.N.; Girbes, A.R.; Oudemans-van Straaten, H.M.; Beishuizen, A. Low skeletal muscle area is a risk factor for mortality in mechanically ventilated critically ill patients. *Crit. Care* **2014**, *18*, R12. [CrossRef]
20. Mogensen, K.M.; Robinson, M.K.; Casey, J.D.; Gunasekera, N.S.; Moromizato, T.; Rawn, J.D.; Christopher, K.B. Nutritional Status and Mortality in the Critically Ill. *Crit. Care Med.* **2015**, *43*, 2605–2615. [CrossRef]
21. Zager, S.; Mendu, M.L.; Chang, D.; Bazick, H.S.; Braun, A.B.; Gibbons, F.K.; Christopher, K.B. Neighborhood poverty rate and mortality in patients receiving critical care in the academic medical center setting. *Chest* **2011**, *139*, 1368–1379. [CrossRef] [PubMed]
22. Robinson, M.K.; Mogensen, K.M.; Casey, J.D.; McKane, C.K.; Moromizato, T.; Rawn, J.D.; Christopher, K.B. The relationship among obesity, nutritional status, and mortality in the critically ill*. *Crit. Care Med.* **2015**, *43*, 87–100. [CrossRef] [PubMed]
23. Swails, W.S.; Samour, P.Q.; Babineau, T.J.; Bistrian, B.R. A proposed revision of current ICD-9-CM malnutrition code definitions. *J. Am. Diet. Assoc.* **1996**, *96*, 370–373. [CrossRef]

24. Blackburn, G.L.; Bistrian, B.R.; Maini, B.S.; Schlamm, H.T.; Smith, M.F. Nutritional and metabolic assessment of the hospitalized patient. *JPEN J. Parenter. Enter. Nutr.* **1977**, *1*, 11–22. [CrossRef] [PubMed]
25. Simopoulos, A.P. Obesity and body weight standards. *Annu. Rev. Public Health* **1986**, *7*, 481–492. [CrossRef] [PubMed]
26. Quan, H.; Sundararajan, V.; Halfon, P.; Fong, A.; Burnand, B.; Luthi, J.C.; Saunders, L.D.; Beck, C.A.; Feasby, T.E.; Ghali, W.A. Coding algorithms for defining comorbidities in ICD-9-CM and ICD-10 administrative data. *Med. Care* **2005**, *43*, 1130–1139. [CrossRef]
27. Liu, V.; Escobar, G.J.; Greene, J.D.; Soule, J.; Whippy, A.; Angus, D.C.; Iwashyna, T.J. Hospital deaths in patients with sepsis from 2 independent cohorts. *JAMA* **2014**, *312*, 90–92. [CrossRef]
28. Martin, G.S.; Mannino, D.M.; Eaton, S.; Moss, M. The epidemiology of sepsis in the United States from 1979 through 2000. *N. Engl. J. Med.* **2003**, *348*, 1546–1554. [CrossRef]
29. McMahon, G.M.; Mendu, M.L.; Gibbons, F.K.; Christopher, K.B. Association between hyperkalemia at critical care initiation and mortality. *Intensive Care Med.* **2012**, *38*, 1834–1842. [CrossRef]
30. Thickett, D.R.; Moromizato, T.; Litonjua, A.A.; Amrein, K.; Quraishi, S.A.; Lee-Sarwar, K.A.; Mogensen, K.M.; Purtle, S.W.; Gibbons, F.K.; Camargo, C.A., Jr.; et al. Association between prehospital vitamin D status and incident acute respiratory failure in critically ill patients: A retrospective cohort study. *BMJ Open Respir. Res.* **2015**, *2*, e000074. [CrossRef]
31. Braun, A.B.; Litonjua, A.A.; Moromizato, T.; Gibbons, F.K.; Giovannucci, E.; Christopher, K.B. Association of low serum 25-hydroxyvitamin D levels and acute kidney injury in the critically ill*. *Crit. Care Med.* **2012**, *40*, 3170–3179. [CrossRef] [PubMed]
32. Levey, A.S.; Bosch, J.P.; Lewis, J.B.; Greene, T.; Rogers, N.; Roth, D. A more accurate method to estimate glomerular filtration rate from serum creatinine: A new prediction equation. Modification of Diet in Renal Disease Study Group. *Ann. Intern. Med.* **1999**, *130*, 461–470. [CrossRef] [PubMed]
33. Rapoport, J.; Gehlbach, S.; Lemeshow, S.; Teres, D. Resource utilization among intensive care patients. Managed care vs traditional insurance. *Arch. Intern. Med.* **1992**, *152*, 2207–2212. [CrossRef] [PubMed]
34. Amrein, K.; Litonjua, A.A.; Moromizato, T.; Quraishi, S.A.; Gibbons, F.K.; Pieber, T.R.; Camargo, C.A., Jr.; Giovannucci, E.; Christopher, K.B. Increases in pre-hospitalization serum 25(OH)D concentrations are associated with improved 30-day mortality after hospital admission: A cohort study. *Clin. Nutr.* **2016**, *35*, 514–521. [CrossRef] [PubMed]
35. Mogensen, K.M.; Horkan, C.M.; Purtle, S.W.; Moromizato, T.; Rawn, J.D.; Robinson, M.K.; Christopher, K.B. Malnutrition, Critical Illness Survivors, and Postdischarge Outcomes: A Cohort Study. *JPEN J. Parenter. Enter. Nutr.* **2017**, *42*, 557–565. [CrossRef] [PubMed]
36. Hedeker, D. A mixed-effects multinomial logistic regression model. *Stat. Med.* **2003**, *22*, 1433–1446. [CrossRef]
37. Hartzel, J.; Agresti, A.; Caffo, B. Multinomial logit random effects models. *Stat. Model.* **2001**, *1*, 81–102. [CrossRef]
38. Nicholson, B.D.; Shinkins, B.; Pathiraja, I.; Roberts, N.W.; James, T.J.; Mallett, S.; Perera, R.; Primrose, J.N.; Mant, D. Blood CEA levels for detecting recurrent colorectal cancer. *Cochrane Database Syst. Rev.* **2015**, CD011134. [CrossRef]
39. Desai, S.V.; Law, T.J.; Needham, D.M. Long-term complications of critical care. *Crit. Care Med.* **2011**, *39*, 371–379. [CrossRef]
40. Horkan, C.M.; Purtle, S.W.; Mendu, M.L.; Moromizato, T.; Gibbons, F.K.; Christopher, K.B. The association of acute kidney injury in the critically ill and postdischarge outcomes: A cohort study. *Crit. Care Med.* **2015**, *43*, 354–364. [CrossRef]
41. Puleo, F.; Arvanitakis, M.; Van Gossum, A.; Preiser, J.C. Gut failure in the ICU. *Semin. Respir. Crit. Care Med.* **2011**, *32*, 626–638. [CrossRef] [PubMed]

© 2019 by the authors. Licensee MDPI, Basel, Switzerland. This article is an open access article distributed under the terms and conditions of the Creative Commons Attribution (CC BY) license (http://creativecommons.org/licenses/by/4.0/).

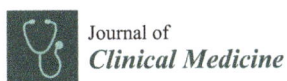

Article

Decreased Bioelectrical Impedance Phase Angle in Hospitalized Children and Adolescents with Newly Diagnosed Type 1 Diabetes: A Case-Control Study

Paweł Więch [1,*], Dariusz Bazaliński [1], Izabela Sałacińska [1], Monika Binkowska-Bury [1], Bartosz Korczowski [2], Artur Mazur [2], Maria Kózka [3] and Mariusz Dąbrowski [1,4]

1. Institute of Nursing and Health Sciences, Faculty of Medicine, University of Rzeszów, 35-959 Rzeszów, Poland; darek.bazalinski@wp.pl (D.B.); izabela.salacinska@wp.pl (I.S.); monika.binkowska@yahoo.com (M.B.-B.); mariusz.dabrowski58@gmail.com (M.D.)
2. Pediatric Department, Clinical Provincial Hospital No. 2 in Rzeszów, Faculty of Medicine, University of Rzeszów, 35-301 Rzeszów, Poland; korczowski@op.pl (B.K.); drmazur@poczta.onet.pl (A.M.)
3. Department of Clinical Nursing, Faculty of Health Sciences, Collegium Medicum, Jagiellonian University, 31-501 Kraków, Poland; makozka@cm-uj.krakow.pl
4. Diabetic Outpatient Clinic, Medical Center "Beta-Med", 35-073 Rzeszów, Poland; mariusz.dabrowski58@gmail.com
* Correspondence: p.k.wiech@gmail.com; Tel.: +48-667-192-696

Received: 25 October 2018; Accepted: 3 December 2018; Published: 4 December 2018

Abstract: The aim of this study was to assess the body composition and nutritional status of hospitalized pediatric patients with newly diagnosed type 1 diabetes by using bioelectrical impedance analysis (BIA) with phase angle (PA) calculation. PA is considered to be a useful and very sensitive indicator of the nutritional and functional status, and it has not yet been evaluated in such a population. Sixty-three pediatric patients aged 4 to 18 years, with newly diagnosed type 1 diabetes, were included in the study. The control group consisted of 63 healthy children and adolescents strictly matched by gender and age in a 1:1 case: control manner. In both groups, BIA with PA calculation was performed. Diabetic patients, in comparison to control subjects, had a highly significantly lower PA of 4.85 ± 0.86 vs. 5.62 ± 0.81, $p < 0.001$. They also demonstrated a lower percentage of body cell mass (BCM%), $46.89 \pm 5.67\%$ vs. $51.40 \pm 4.19\%$, $p < 0.001$; a lower body cell mass index (BCMI), 6.57 ± 1.80 vs. 7.37 ± 1.72, $p = 0.004$; and a lower percentage of muscle mass (MM%), $44.61 \pm 6.58\%$ vs. $49.40 \pm 7.59\%$, $p < 0.001$, compared to non-diabetic controls. The significantly lower PA value in diabetic patients indicate their worse nutritional and functional status compared to healthy subjects. To assess the predictive and prognostic value of this finding in this population, further prospective studies involving larger sample of patients are required.

Keywords: type 1 diabetes mellitus; bioelectrical impedance analysis; phase angle; children; adolescents

1. Introduction

Application of bioelectrical impedance analysis (BIA) to assess the body composition dates back to late 1980s [1]. Although differences between results obtained by BIA and Dual-Energy X-Ray Absorptiometry (DXA) are observed both in adult and in pediatric populations, BIA is considered as an easy to use, reliable, safe, non-invasive, and non-expensive method of the assessment of body composition, and it has been widely used in a number of epidemiological studies [2–5].

Bioelectrical impedance phase angle (PA) is considered to be a more sensitive and more accurate indicator of the nutritional and functional status than BIA alone, because PA better reflects the degree of cellular health and indicates early water shift from intracellular to extracellular compartment in subjects with malnutrition [6–8].

The reference values of PA in healthy subjects differ depending on age, sex, and body mass index (BMI) [9–11]. The PA values in adults are different compared with children and adolescents. Growing up is associated with increasing phase angles, a situation that is probably due to an increase in cell mass with age, especially in periods of childhood and adolescence [9]. This trend was observed by Redondo-Del-Río et al. for both genders (4–5 years: 5.2 vs. 12–13 years: 5.7–5.8 vs. 15–16 years: 6.1–6.5) [10].

Norman et al. summarized in their review the prognostic value of PA in dialysis subjects, patients with cancer, liver cirrhosis, heart failure, systemic sclerosis, human immunodeficiency virus (HIV) positive, geriatric, and surgical patients. In all cases lower PA values were associated with increased mortality and lower survival rates [12]. PA also correlates with function, disease severity, and prognosis in people with stable chronic obstructive pulmonary disease (COPD) [13]. Low PA at hospital admission appeared also to be associated with malnutrition and nutritional risk [14]. In the study by Zhang et al., patients with a better nutrition state demonstrated relatively higher PA than the patients with severe malnutrition, which suggests that PA has the potential to be a quantitative index in assessing nutrition state, while current assessing methods such as the Subjective Global Assessment (SGA) contain many subjective factors [7]. Thus, PA can be considered not only as an indicator of nutritional status but also as an important prognostic factor of malnutrition risk and clinical outcome, especially in chronic diseases leading to malnutrition and cachexia. The European Society for Clinical Nutrition and Metabolism (ESPEN) strongly recommends PA as a reliable prognostic nutritional measure [15]. Currently, it is expected that nutrition state assessment based on PA will be established and implemented in clinical trials [7].

The primary objective of our study was to assess the PA value in hospitalized children and adolescents with newly diagnosed type 1 diabetes compared to healthy controls. To our knowledge, it is the first study in such a group, as through searching Embase, Web of Science, PubMed, and Scopus databases by use of the terms "type 1 diabetes mellitus" and "children"; combined with "body composition" or/and "phase angle"; "bioelectrical impedance analysis", "type 1 diabetes mellitus", and "children"; and combined with "nutritional status" and "phase angle", we found only two full-text papers assessing the PA in diabetic patients, but both of them were conducted in adult populations [16,17].The search was limited to articles published in English from 1990 to 30 July 2018. The secondary objective was to analyze body composition in this group of patients.

2. Experimental Section

2.1. Ethics

The study was approved by the institutional Bioethics Committee at the University of Rzeszów (Resolution No. 5/02/2012) and by all appropriate administrative bodies. The study was conducted in accordance with ethical standards laid down in an appropriate version of the Declaration of Helsinki and in Polish national regulations.

2.2. Subjects

This pair-matched, case control study was carried out between March 2012 and August 2014. Sixty-three children and adolescents (28 girls, 44.4%) with type 1 diabetes hospitalized in the Clinical Department of Pediatrics with the Pediatric Neurology Unit at the Clinical Regional Hospital No. 2 in Rzeszow comprised the study group. The flow chart demonstrating the selection of the study and control groups is presented in Figure 1, while characteristics of both groups are presented in Table 1.

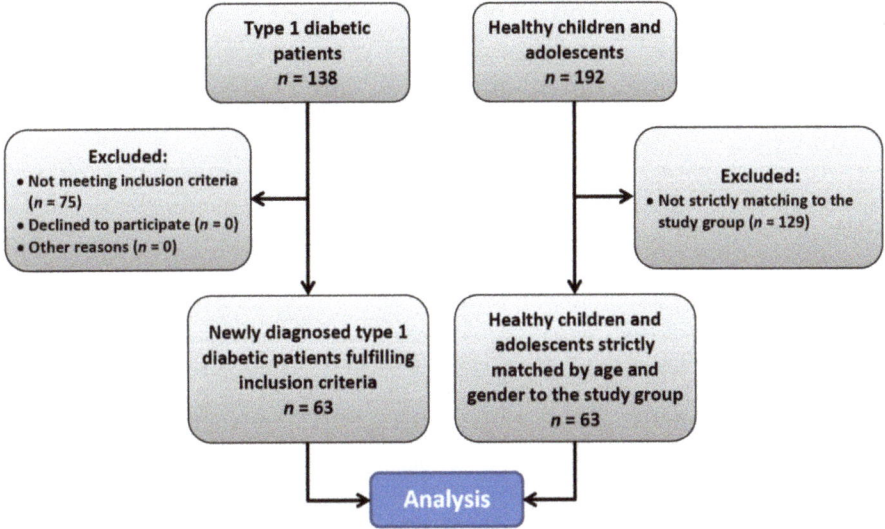

Figure 1. Flow chart of the selection of study participants.

Table 1. Demographic and anthropometric parameters of the study participants.

Parameter	Type 1 Diabetes Group	Control Group	p-Value
Age (years)	10.78 ± 3.72	10.80 ± 3.73	0.967
Girls	10.93 ± 3.55	10.96 ± 3.56	0.947
Boys	10.66 ± 3.90	10.66 ± 3.90	1.000
Body weight (kg)	42.15 ± 21.08	39.93 ± 14.97	0.907
Girls	38.71 ± 16.69	38.53 ± 11.92	0.962
Percentile * (n):			
<3	2	1	0.613
3–10	4	1	
10–90	20	23	
90–97	1	1	
>97	1	2	
Boys	44.89 ± 23.91	41.05 ± 17.11	0.720
Percentile * (n):			
<3	0	1	0.400
3–10	4	2	
10–90	24	26	
90–97	3	5	
>97	4	1	
Height (cm)	145.80 ± 22.16	144.12 ± 19.63	0.653
Girls	143.93 ± 19.64	143.66 ± 18.60	0.958
Low-to-age *	1	1	0.354
Normal *	27	25	
High-to-age *	0	2	
Boys	147.30 ± 24.17	144.49 ± 20.68	0.602
Low-to-age *	0	0	0.673
Normal *	31	33	
High-to-age *	4	2	

Table 1. Cont.

Parameter	Type 1 Diabetes Group	Control Group	p-Value
BMI (kg/m^2)	18.56 ± 4.57	18.52 ± 3.30	0.460
Girls	17.76 ± 3.40	18.26 ± 3.08	0.244
Underweight *	10	5	0.371
Normal weight *	15	19	
Overweight *	3	3	
Obesity *	0	1	
Boys	19.21 ± 4.94	18.72 ± 3.49	0.939
Underweight *	1	1	0.573
Normal weight *	27	24	
Overweight *	6	10	
Obesity *	1	0	

SD—standard deviation; BMI—body mass index. Values are presented as mean ± SD. * According to Polish normative values [18].

The inclusion criteria were as follows: newly diagnosed type 1 diabetes; age 4 to 18 years; no other autoimmune or chronic diseases having impact on height, weight, or nutritional status; and written informed consent signed by parents or legal guardians and also by adolescents aged over 16 years. The control group consisted of the same number of children and adolescents taken from primary, junior high, and high schools from urban and rural areas. The inclusion criteria for this group were the same, with the exception of having type 1 diabetes. The diabetic and healthy subjects were strictly matched by gender and age (to the nearest possible date of birth) in a 1:1 case:control manner.

2.3. Assessments

Body height was measured to the nearest 0.1 cm using a portable stadiometer (Seca 213). The measurements were performed under standard conditions in an upright position and barefoot. Body mass was assessed with an accuracy of 0.1 kg using a personal scale (Seca 799). Body mass index (BMI) was calculated as weight (kg)/height (m)^2. To avoid bias associated with dehydration at the time of diabetes diagnosis, in the first step, acid–base and water–electrolyte balance in the study group were normalized. In the treatment of hyperglycemia, a continuous intravenous insulin infusion was used in the first several hours after admission. After glucose metabolism control was achieved, children and adolescents were switched to subcutaneous multiple daily injections of insulin using the basal/bolus method. The assessment of body composition and nutritional status in diabetic subjects was performed between the 5th and 7th days after admission after when stable metabolic state was achieved. BIA was performed using an AKERN BIA 101 analyzer (Akern SRL, Pontassieve, Florence, Italy). PA was calculated from the following equation:

$$PA = \left(\frac{X_C}{R}\right) \times \left(\frac{180°}{\pi}\right) \tag{1}$$

(Xc—reactance, R—resistance)

The equations used by the software to assess the specific parameters are restricted property of the company, but to a significant degree, they are based on computed algorithms developed by Sun S. et al. [19] and Horlick et al. [20]. According to widely accepted and available methodologies [21], participants were in a fasting state and, before measurement (24 h), they did not practice physical exercises. Before the BIA measurement, they were asked to empty the bladder completely and to remove all clothing and metal elements. The measurements were carried out between 07:00 and 12:00 in a fasting state, in the supine position, with abducted upper (30°) and lower (45°) extremities, and after at least 5 min of rest. A tetrapolar system with a contralateral mode was used (amplitude of measured current: 800 uA; sinusoidal; 50 kHz). To ensure reliability and repeatability of the results obtained, two measurements, one after another, were performed. All the measurements were performed by the same person. The accuracy of the equipment was checked before the measurements with a 500 ohm resistor supplied by the manufacturer. The disposable electrodes (Biatrodes, Pontassieve, FI, Italy; the individual impedance of a single electrode: 25–30 Ω; compliance with the Medical Directive 93/42/EEC; accordance with ISO 10993-1:2003) were placed on the dorsal surface of the right upper limb (over the wrist) and the right lower limb (on the ankle) while the minimum distance between the two electrodes was 5 cm. The results were transferred and analyzed by specialized software (Bodygram1_31 by AKERN).

In all children and adolescents, weight and height was measured and BMI was calculated. The obtained results were compared to Polish normative values charts according to age and gender [18]. Weight was divided into five categories according to percentiles: <3 low-to-age weight, 3–10 alert level, 10–90 normal weight, 90–97 alert level, and >97 high-to-age weight. Height was divided into three percentile categories: >97 high-to-age height, 3–97 normal range, and <3 low-to-age height. BMI was divided into four categories: underweight, normal weight, overweight, and obese, according to normative charts for age and gender. BIA analysis included: fat mass (FM), fat free mass (FFM) muscle mass (MM) (kg and %), total body water (TBW), intra- and extracellular water (ICW and ECW; liters and %), body cell mass (BCM; kg and %), and body cell mass index (BCMI). Upon resistance and reactance results, phase angle was calculated. In addition, fat mass index (FMI) and fat free mass index (FFMI) were calculated.

Phase angle results were compared between diabetic and control groups as a whole and separately for each gender. In addition, we analyzed PA values in relation to the reference values for age, gender, and BMI obtained by Bosy-Westphal et al. in the study conducted in Germany, the neighboring country, which can be considered applicable for our population [9].

2.4. Statistical Analysis

Statistical analysis of the data was performed using SigmaPlot for Windows, version 12.5 (Systat Software Inc., San Jose, CA, USA). The continuous data are presented as mean ± SD (standard deviation). Differences between study and control groups were analyzed using a two-tailed Student's t-test for independent samples after performing a Shapiro-Wilk normality test and a constant variance test. In the case of normality and constant variance test failure, the Mann-Whitney rank sum test was performed. The categorical data were compared using the χ^2 test. The linear correlation between PA and HbA1c was assessed using the Pearson product moment correlation test after checking the normality of distribution by the Shapiro-Wilk test. A p-value of <0.05 was considered statistically significant.

3. Results

The phase angle value in diabetic patients was highly significantly lower compared to healthy subjects. Among components of the PA equation, only reactance appeared to be significantly different between the study and control groups (Table 2) regardless of gender (Table 3). Resistance, although higher in diabetic subjects, did not reach statistical significance. Although the muscle mass and body cell mass measured in kg were not significantly different between the diabetic and control groups, MM%, BCM%, and BCMI were also significantly lower in diabetic subjects (Table 2). The differences remained significant when these variables were also analyzed separately for each gender (Table 3).

Table 2. Bioelectrical Impedance Analysis results in study participants.

Parameter	Type 1 Diabetes Group (N = 63) Mean ± SD	Control group (N = 63) Mean ± SD	p-Value
Fat mass (kg)	10.84 ± 8.33	9.07 ± 5.20	0.481
Fat mass (% of body mass)	23.96 ± 9.50	22.49 ± 9.44	0.386
Fat mass index (kg/m^2)	4.66 ± 2.78	4.24 ± 2.33	0.364
Fat free mass (kg)	31.31 ± 14.49	30.86 ± 12.26	0.840
Fat free mass (% of body mass)	76.04 ± 9.50	77.51 ± 9.44	0.386
Fat free mass index (kg/m^2)	13.81 ± 2.74	14.20 ± 2.26	0.218
Muscle mass (kg)	18.87 ± 10.01	20.03 ± 9.17	0.341
Muscle mass (% of body mass)	44.61 ± 6.58	49.40 ± 7.59	**<0.001**
Total body water (L)	24.48 ± 10.61	24.28 ± 9.10	0.903
Total body water (% of body mass)	59.95 ± 8.62	61.36 ± 8.56	0.359
Extracellular water (L)	11.10 ± 4.44	10.57 ± 3.85	0.707
Extracellular water (% of body mass)	46.89 ± 7.34	44.05 ± 3.67	0.064
Intracellular water (L)	13.70 ± 6.49	13.76 ± 5.44	0.946
Intracellular water (% of body mass)	53.11 ± 7.34	55.95 ± 3.67	0.064
Body cell mass (kg)	15.14 ± 8.27	16.23 ± 7.57	0.308
Body cell mass (% of body mass)	46.89 ± 5.67	51.40 ± 4.19	**<0.001**
Body cell mass index (kg/m^2)	6.57 ± 1.80	7.37 ± 1.72	**0.004**
Resistance (ohm)	684.92 ± 99.29	659.98 ± 94.10	0.150
Reactance (ohm)	57.62 ± 10.41	63.83 ± 6.93	**<0.001**
Phase angle (—)	4.85 ± 0.86	5.62 ± 0.81	**<0.001**

A tetrapolar system with a contralateral mode; amplitude of a measured current of 800 uA, sinusoidal, 50kHz. Significant differences are in bold and indicate significant values ($p < 0.05$). Values are presented as mean ± SD.

Table 3. BIA results in study participants according to gender.

Parameter	Girls			Boys		
	Diabetes (N = 28)	Control (N = 28)	p-Value	Diabetes (N = 35)	Control (N = 35)	p-Value
Fat mass (kg)	9.98 ± 6.53	9.77 ± 4.53	0.891	11.53 ± 9.57	8.50 ± 5.67	0.215
Fat mass (% of body mass)	23.65 ± 9.72	25.12 ± 8.56	0.555	24.21 ± 9.46	20.38 ± 9.47	0.072
Fat mass index (kg/m^2)	4.37 ± 2.40	4.71 ± 2.39	0.611	4.90 ± 3.06	3.86 ± 2.25	0.079
Fat free mass (kg)	28.74 ± 11.00	28.76 ± 9.52	0.994	33.37 ± 16.63	32.55 ± 13.98	0.930
Fat free mass (% of body mass)	76.35 ± 9.72	74.88 ± 8.86	0.555	75.79 ± 9.46	79.62 ± 9.47	0.072
Fat free mass index (kg/m^2)	13.18 ± 2.52	13.46 ± 1.78	0.628	14.32 ± 2.84	14.78 ± 2.45	0.247
Muscle mass (kg)	16.79 ± 7.25	18.29 ± 6.59	0.421	20.53 ± 11.60	21.42 ± 10.70	0.597
Muscle mass (% of body mass)	43.62 ± 5.70	47.20 ± 6.17	0.028	45.41 ± 7.19	51.15 ± 8.23	**0.003**
Total body water (L)	22.25 ± 7.82	22.35 ± 6.92	0.958	26.25 ± 12.23	25.81 ± 10.37	0.893
Total body water (% of body mass)	59.75 ± 9.02	58.55 ± 7.54	0.590	60.11 ± 8.42	63.61 ± 8.77	0.093
Extracellular water (L)	10.48 ± 3.64	9.85 ± 3.12	0.629	11.59 ± 4.98	11.15 ± 4.30	0.930
Extracellular water (% of body mass)	48.31 ± 8.70	44.25 ± 3.08	0.119	45.76 ± 5.92	43.89 ± 4.12	0.131
Intracellular water (L)	12.13 ± 4.99	12.65 ± 4.05	0.793	14.95 ± 7.31	14.65 ± 6.25	0.995
Intracellular water (% of body mass)	51.69 ± 8.70	55.75 ± 3.08	0.119	54.24 ± 5.92	56.11 ± 4.12	0.131
Body cell mass (kg)	13.39 ± 5.99	14.79 ± 5.38	0.362	16.55 ± 9.57	17.37 ± 8.86	0.565
Body cell mass (% of body mass)	45.60 ± 6.30	50.90 ± 3.05	**<0.001**	47.91 ± 4.96	51.79 ± 4.93	**0.002**
Body cell mass index (kg/m^2)	6.11 ± 1.50	6.91 ± 1.27	**0.037**	6.93 ± 1.95	7.73 ± 1.96	**0.039**
Resistance (ohm)	712.75 ± 102.10	700.57 ± 79.01	0.620	662.66 ± 92.47	627.51 ± 93.53	0.119
Reactance (ohm)	58.07 ± 12.66	66.71 ± 5.14	**0.003**	57.26 ± 8.38	61.51 ± 7.36	**0.027**
Phase angle (−)	4.66 ± 0.84	5.49 ± 0.56	**<0.001**	5.00 ± 0.85	5.72 ± 0.97	**0.001**

A tetrapolar system with a contralateral mode; amplitude of a measured current of 800 uA, sinusoidal, 50kHz. Significant differences ($p < 0.05$) indicated in bold. Values are presented as mean ± SD.

We also found significant differences between the study and control group for both genders in the analysis of PA values in relation to the reference values for a healthy population obtained by Bosy-Westphal et al. in the study conducted in Germany, the neighboring country [9]. In our study, among girls with diabetes, only 14 (50.0%) had a PA value equal or higher than the 10th percentile expected for gender, age and BMI, while among healthy girls such number was 27 (96.4%), $p < 0.001$ for the difference. Among boys these numbers were 20 (57.1%) and 30 (85.7%) respectively and this difference was also statistically significant, $p = 0.017$. The more detailed results are presented in the Table 4.

Table 4. Number of subjects with PA value according to age, gender and BMI in relation to reference values.

Age Range (years)	Phase Angle Percentiles	Girls		Boys	
		Diabetes	Control	Diabetes	Control
All (n)		28	28	35	35
	≥10th percentile	14	27	20	30
	<10th percentile	14	1	15	5
	<5th percentile	13	1	11	1
4–9 (n)		10	10	13	13
	≥10th percentile	3	10	7	10
	<10th percentile	7	0	6	3
	<5th percentile	7	0	5	0
10–13 (n)		13	13	16	16
	≥10th percentile	9	13	10	14
	<10th percentile	4	0	6	2
	<5th percentile	3	0	5	1
14–18 (n)		5	5	6	6
	≥10th percentile	2	4	3	6
	<10th percentile	3	1	3	0
	<5th percentile	3	1	1	0

Phase angle (PA) value ≥10th percentile, <10th percentile and <5th percentile according to age, gender and body mass index (BMI) in relation to reference values from Bosy-Westphal et al. [9].

The mean HbA1c value in children and adolescents with newly diagnosed type 1 diabetes was 11.37% ± 2.26% (100.7 ± 24.7 mmol/mol). Girls had a mean HbA1c value significantly higher compared to boys, 12.22% ± 1.89% (110.1 ± 20.7 mmol/mol) vs. 10.71% ± 2.32% (93.4 ± 25.3 mmol/mol), respectively, $p = 0.012$. A trend towards negative linear correlation between the PA value and the HbA1c value in diabetic patients was observe; however, it did not attain a statistical significance ($r = -0.220$, $p = 0.085$).

In a subgroup of patients (four with newly diagnosed diabetes and nine with longer-lasting diabetes), we performed a follow-up after 13 to 21 (mean of 15.5) months of treatment. We found a significant improvement in the mean PA value and BCMI (from 5.52 ± 0.77 to 5.84 ± 0.67, $p = 0.003$, and from 6.85 ± 1.99 to 8.04 ± 2.15, $p < 0.001$, respectively). However, at baseline, six patients had a PA value above the mean value expected for age, gender, and BMI, while at follow-up, this number decreased to five. The percentage of FM, FFM, TBW, ECW, ICW, and MM did not change significantly compared to baseline.

No significant differences between the study and control groups regarding mean weight, height, and BMI were found, nor when individual results were analyzed in relation to Polish normative values.

4. Discussion

The primary objective of our study was to assess PA values in children and adolescents with newly diagnosed type 1 diabetes in comparison to healthy subjects, which has not yet been studied. The PA value is calculated from resistance (R) and reactance (Xc) values and reflects the nutritional and functional status. In the human body, resistance is related to tissue hydration while reactance occurs due to the cell membrane capacitance (i.e., the ability of the non-conducting object to save electrical charges) [8]. Data regarding PA assessment in the diabetic population are scarce. In the study by Buscemi et al. conducted in both type 1 and type 2 diabetic subjects, PA values appeared to be significantly lower in young adult type 1 diabetic male patients compared to control subjects, while in women, this difference was insignificant [16]. Dittmar et al. revealed significantly lower PA among men and women with type 2 diabetes compared to control subjects. They also found inverse relationships between the PA value and HbA1c levels and concluded that lower PA values at 50 and 100 kHz might indicate catabolism and long duration of the disease in type 2 diabetic patients [17]. No other studies assessing PA values in patients with diabetes were found in the PubMed, Scopus, or EMBASE databases.

Obviously, body composition of children and adolescents with type 1 diabetes significantly changes over the course of the disease, and, in many of them, an excess of fat mass develops, which was observed in different studies. Davis et al. observed a significantly lower FM% and similar lean mass in children with type 1 diabetes at the time of diagnosis compared to the non-diabetic group. After insulin introduction, sharp increases in fat mass and an insignificant loss of lean body mass during the first six weeks of treatment in diabetic group was revealed. The authors explained this phenomenon as a consequence of severe insulin deficiency and a catabolic state at the time of type 1 diabetes diagnosis [22]. In contrast to this study, in our observations, neither fat mass nor percentage of body fat in children and adolescents with newly diagnosed type 1 diabetes were significantly different compared to the control group, though we found a significantly lower percentage of muscle mass. We did not observe significant changes in body composition during the follow-up in the study group; however, the follow-up period was not long enough to find more pronounced changes. Interestingly, in the Greek study in children and adolescents with short-lasting type 1 diabetes (3.7 ± 2.0 years), FFMI was significantly higher compared to non-diabetic subjects, while FM% and FMI were not significantly different between the groups [23]. Patients with type 1 diabetes gain more weight than their peers, mainly due to the increase in fat mass, which was documented in the study by Szadkowska et al. In their observation, the prevalence of overweight and obesity among young adults (up to 40 years) with type 1 diabetes and an age at diabetes onset <20 years was significantly higher compared to the control group, and diabetic patients were characterized by higher fat mass [24]. Such unfavorable changes in body composition might have a negative impact on health in the future. Excessive weight gain in diabetic patients was associated with elevated waist circumference and blood pressure, lower insulin sensitivity, dyslipidemia, and with more extensive atherosclerosis in further observations [25,26].

It is well known that type 1 diabetes is associated with an elevated risk of complications, and poor metabolic control correlates with microangiopathy, macroangiopathy, and diabetic neuropathy [26,27]. Uncontrolled type 1 diabetes also has an impact on bone and muscle, i.e., lean body mass; moreover, it also impairs their function [28,29]. Coleman et al. indicate that decreased muscle mass and impaired muscle function has a significant impact on insulin sensitivity, glucose and lipids disposal, and on basal metabolic rate, which makes it difficult to achieve a stable metabolic control of type 1 diabetes. Thus, physical activity, which leads to an improvement in muscle mass and function, can also be helpful in the improvement of metabolic control and in delaying or even preventing the development of diabetic complications [30].

Poor metabolic control in childhood and adolescence and bad glycemic legacy (metabolic memory) is associated with an elevated risk of future complications in adulthood and can also lead to premature death, mainly due to cardiovascular disease. Thus, good diabetes care in early years can improve this prognosis [26,31].

Phase angle has not yet been analyzed prospectively in type 1 diabetic patients. The significant increases in PA values during the follow-up observed in our study can be simply explained by the growth of children and adolescents, because number of subjects with PA exceeding mean for age, gender, and BMI did not increase; on the contrary, it even decreased during observation. This may indicate the persistence of worse nutritional and functional status in this population.

The main limitation of our study was the relatively small number of participants, which did not allow us to find other differences between diabetic and control groups. Furthermore, only thirteen patients with diabetes were followed-up. Nevertheless, our study presents some new data and interesting findings which may indicate the directions of future research.

5. Conclusions

Low values of phase angle and altered body composition in newly diagnosed type 1 diabetic patients indicate their worse nutritional and functional status. However, although phase angle is a predictor of unfavorable clinical outcome in people with a number of chronic diseases, the predictive and prognostic value of our findings in patients with type 1 diabetes needs to be determined in further long-term prospective studies to establish its role in this population.

Author Contributions: Study concept and design: P.W., B.K., M.D.; funding acquisition: P.W., D.B., M.B.-B., A.M.; data acquisition: P.W., D.B., I.S.; statistical analysis: M.D.; analysis and interpretation of data: M.D., P.W.; supervision: B.K., A.M., M.B.-B; M.K.; manuscript drafting: M.D., P.W.; critical revision of the work for important intellectual content: P.W., D.B., I.S., M.B.-B., B.K., M.K., A.M., M.D.

Funding: The study was conducted under the grant for statutory activity (Research Potential) of the Institute of Nursing and Health Sciences, Faculty of Medicine, University of Rzeszów for 2018 and 2019 years (Resolution No. WM/21/2018/P-M). Also the study co-financed by the University of Rzeszów as the project of the Natural and Medical Center for Innovative Research, and by the Regional Operational Program for the Podkarpackie Province for the years 2007–2013, contract number UDA-RPPK.01.03.00-18-004/12-00.

Acknowledgments: The abstract based on these data was accepted for the American Diabetes Association 78th Scientific Sessions held in Orlando, FL in June 2018. The raw data used in this paper are deposited in the University of Rzeszów Repository: https://repozytorium.ur.edu.pl/ under the title of the manuscript or under the name of any of the authors.

Conflicts of Interest: The authors declare no conflict of interest.

References

1. Baumgartner, R.N.; Chumlea, W.C.; Roche, A.F. Estimation of body composition from bioelectric impedance of body segments. *Am. J. Clin. Nutr.* **1989**, *50*, 221–226. [CrossRef] [PubMed]
2. Shafer, K.J.; Siders, W.A.; Johnson, L.K.; Lukaski, H.C. Validity of segmental multiple-frequency bioelectrical impedance analysis to estimate body composition of adults across a range of body mass indexes. *Nutrition* **2009**, *25*, 25–32. [CrossRef]
3. Stoklossa, C.A.J.; Forhan, M.; Padwal, R.S.; Gonzalez, M.C.; Prado, C.M. Practical considerations for body composition assessment of adults with class II/III obesity using Bioelectrical Impedance Analysis or Dual-Energy, X.-Ray Absorptiometry. *Curr. Obes. Rep.* **2016**, *5*, 389–396. [CrossRef] [PubMed]
4. Wan, C.S.; Ward, L.C.; Halim, J.; Gow, M.L.; Ho, M.; Briody, J.N.; Leung, K.; Cowell, C.T.; Garnett, S.P. Bioelectrical impedance analysis to estimate body composition, and change in adiposity, in overweight and obese adolescents: Comparison with dual-energy x-ray absorptiometry. *BMC Pediatr.* **2014**, *14*, 249. [CrossRef] [PubMed]
5. Böhm, A.; Heitmann, B.L. The use of bioelectrical impedance analysis for body composition in epidemiological studies. *Eur. J. Clin. Nutr.* **2013**, *67*, S79. [CrossRef] [PubMed]
6. Selberg, O.; Selberg, D. Norms and correlates of bioimpedance phase angle in healthy human subjects, hospitalized patients, and patients with liver cirrhosis. *Eur. J. Appl. Physiol.* **2002**, *86*, 509–516. [CrossRef] [PubMed]
7. Zhang, G.; Huo, X.; Wu, C.; Zhang, C.; Duan, Z. A bioelectrical impedance phase angle measuring system for assessment of nutritional status. *Biomed. Mater. Eng.* **2014**, *24*, 3657–3664. [CrossRef] [PubMed]
8. Khalil, S.F.; Mohktar, M.S.; Ibrahim, F. The theory and fundamentals of bioimpedance analysis in clinical status monitoring and diagnosis of diseases. *Sensors* **2014**, *14*, 10895–10928. [CrossRef] [PubMed]

9. Bosy-Westphal, A.; Danielzik, S.; Dörhöfer, R.P.; Later, W.; Wiese, S.; Müller, M.J. Phase angle from bioelectrical impedance analysis: Population reference values by age, sex, and body mass index. *JPEN J. Parenter. Enteral. Nutr.* **2006**, *30*, 309–316. [CrossRef]
10. Redondo-del-Río, M.P.; Camina-Martín, M.A.; Marugan-de-Miguelsanz, J.M.; de-Mateo-Silleras, B. Bioelectrical impedance vector reference values for assessing body composition in a Spanish child and adolescent population. *Am. J. Hum. Biol.* **2017**, *29*, e22978. [CrossRef] [PubMed]
11. Kuchnia, A.J.; Teigen, L.M.; Cole, A.J.; Mulasi, U.; Gonzalez, M.C.; Heymsfield, S.B.; Vock, D.M.; Earthman, C.P. Phase angle and impedance ratio: Reference cut-points from the United States National Health and Nutrition Examination Survey 1999-2004 from bioimpedance spectroscopy data. *JPEN J. Parenter. Enteral. Nutr.* **2017**, *41*, 1310–1315. [CrossRef] [PubMed]
12. Norman, K.; Stobäus, N.; Pirlich, M.; Bosy-Westphal, A. Bioelectrical phase angle and impedance vector analysis–clinical relevance and applicability of impedance parameters. *Clin. Nutr.* **2012**, *31*, 854–861. [CrossRef] [PubMed]
13. Maddocks, M.; Kon, S.S.; Jones, S.E.; Canavan, J.L.; Nolan, C.M.; Higginson, I.J.; Gao, W.; Polkey, M.I.; Man, W.D. Bioelectrical impedance phase angle relates to function, disease severity and prognosis in stable chronic obstructive pulmonary disease. *Clin. Nutr.* **2015**, *34*, 1245–1250. [CrossRef] [PubMed]
14. Kyle, U.G.; Genton, L.; Pichard, C. Low phase angle determined by bioelectrical impedance analysis is associated with malnutrition and nutritional risk at hospital admission. *Clin. Nutr.* **2013**, *32*, 294–299. [CrossRef] [PubMed]
15. Cederholm, T.; Barazzoni, R.; Austin, P.; Ballmer, P.; Biolo, G.; Bischoff, S.C.; Compher, C.; Correia, I.; Higashiguchi, T.; Holst, M.; et al. ESPEN guidelines on definitions and terminology of clinical nutrition. *Clin. Nutr.* **2017**, *36*, 49–64. [CrossRef] [PubMed]
16. Buscemi, S.; Blunda, G.; Maneri, R.; Verga, S. Bioelectrical characteristics of type 1 and type 2 diabetic subjects with reference to body water compartments. *Acta. Diabetol.* **1998**, *35*, 220–223. [CrossRef]
17. Dittmar, M.; Reber, H.; Kahaly, G.J. Bioimpedance phase angle indicates catabolism in Type 2 diabetes. *Diabet. Med.* **2015**, *32*, 1177–1185. [CrossRef]
18. Kułaga, Z.; Różdżyńska-Świątkowska, A.; Grajda, A.; Gurzkowska, B.; Wojtyło, M.; Góźdź, M.; Świąder-Leśniak, A.; Litwin, M. Percentile charts for growth and nutritional status assessment in Polish children and adolescents from birth to 18 year of age. *Standard. Med. Ped.* **2015**, *12*, 119–135.
19. Sun, S.S.; Chumlea, W.C.; Heymsfield, S.B.; Lukaski, H.C.; Schoeller, D.; Friedl, K.; Kuczmarski, R.J.; Flegal, K.M.; Johnson, C.L.; Hubbard, V.S. Development of bioelectrical impedance analysis prediction equations for body composition with the use of a multicomponent model for use in epidemiologic surveys. *Am. J. Clin. Nutr.* **2003**, *77*, 331–340. [CrossRef]
20. Horlick, M.; Arpadi, S.M.; Bethel, J.; Wang, J.; Moye, J. Jr.; Cuff, P.; Pierson, R.N.Jr.; Kotler, D. Bioelectrical impedance analysis models for prediction of total body water and fat-free mass in healthy and HIV-infected children and adolescents. *Am. J. Clin. Nutr.* **2002**, *76*, 991–999. [CrossRef]
21. Kyle, U.G.; Bosaeus, I.; De Lorenzo, A.D.; Deurenberg, P.; Elia, M.; Gómez, J.M.; Heitmann, B.L.; Kent-Smith, L.; Melchior, J.C.; Pirlich, M.; et al. Bioelectrical impedance analysis—part I: Review of principles and methods. *Clin. Nutr.* **2004**, *23*, 1226–1243. [CrossRef] [PubMed]
22. Davis, N.L.; Bursell, J.D.; Evans, W.D.; Warner, J.T.; Gregory, J.W. Body composition in children with type 1 diabetes in the first year after diagnosis: Relationship to glycaemic control and cardiovascular risk. *Arch. Dis. Child.* **2012**, *97*, 312–315. [CrossRef] [PubMed]
23. Galli-Tsinopoulou, A.; Grammatikopoulou, M.G.; Stylianou, C.; Kokka, P.; Emmanouilidou, E. A preliminary case-control study on nutritional status, body composition, and glycemic control of Greek children and adolescents with type 1 diabetes. *J. Diabetes.* **2009**, *1*, 36–42. [CrossRef] [PubMed]
24. Szadkowska, A.; Madej, A.; Ziółkowska, K.; Szymańska, M.; Jeziorny, K.; Mianowska, B.; Pietrzak, I. Gender and Age—Dependent effect of type 1 diabetes on obesity and altered body composition in young adults. *Ann. Agric. Environ. Med.* **2015**, *22*, 124–128. [CrossRef] [PubMed]
25. DCCT Research Group. Weight gain associated with intensive therapy in the Diabetes Control and Complications Trial. *Diabetes Care* **1988**, *11*, 567–573. [CrossRef]
26. Purnell, J.Q.; Zinman, B.; Brunzell, J.D.; DCCT/EDIC Research Group. The effect of excess weight gain with intensive diabetes mellitus treatment on cardiovascular disease risk factors and atherosclerosis in type 1 diabetes mellitus: Results from the Diabetes Control and Complications Trial/Epidemiology of Diabetes

Interventions and Complications Study (DCCT/EDIC) study. *Circulation.* **2013**, *127*, 180–187. [CrossRef] [PubMed]
27. Gubitosi-Klug, R.A.; DCCT/EDIC Research Group. The Diabetes Control and Complications Trial/Epidemiology of Diabetes Interventions and Complications Study at 30 years: Summary and future directions. *Diabetes Care.* **2014**, *37*, 44–49. [CrossRef]
28. Wierzbicka, E.; Swiercz, A.; Pludowski, P.; Jaworski, M.; Szalecki, M. Skeletal Status, Body Composition, and Glycaemic Control in Adolescents with Type 1 Diabetes Mellitus. *J. Diabetes Res.* **2018**, *2018*, 8121634. [CrossRef]
29. Maratova, K.; Soucek, O.; Matyskova, J.; Hlavka, Z.; Petruzelkova, L.; Obermannova, B.; Pruhova, S.; Kolouskova, S.; Sumnik, Z. Muscle functions and bone strength are impaired in adolescents with type 1 diabetes. *Bone* **2018**, *106*, 22–27. [CrossRef]
30. Coleman, S.K.; Rebalka, I.A.; D'Souza, D.M.; Hawke, T.J. Skeletal muscle as a therapeutic target for delaying type 1 diabetic complications. *World J. Diabetes* **2015**, *6*, 1323–1336. [CrossRef]
31. Mameli, C.; Mazzantini, S.; Nasr, M.B.; Fiorina, P.; Scaramuzza, A.E.; Zuccotti, G.V. Explaining the increased mortality in type 1 diabetes. *World J. Diabetes* **2015**, *6*, 889–895. [CrossRef] [PubMed]

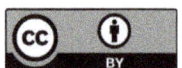

© 2018 by the authors. Licensee MDPI, Basel, Switzerland. This article is an open access article distributed under the terms and conditions of the Creative Commons Attribution (CC BY) license (http://creativecommons.org/licenses/by/4.0/).

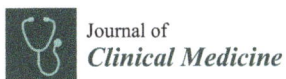

Review

Management of Refeeding Syndrome in Medical Inpatients

Emilie Reber [1,*], Natalie Friedli [2], Maria F. Vasiloglou [3], Philipp Schuetz [2,4] and Zeno Stanga [1]

1. Department of Diabetes, Endocrinology, Nutritional Medicine and Metabolism, Inselspital, Bern University Hospital, and University of Bern, 3010 Bern, Switzerland; zeno.stanga@insel.ch
2. Medical University Department, Division of General Internal and Emergency Medicine, Kantonsspital Aarau, 5001 Aarau, Switzerland; natalie.friedli@gmx.ch (N.F.); schuetzph@gmail.com (P.S.)
3. AI in Health and Nutrition Laboratory, ARTORG Center for Biomedical Engineering Research, University of Bern, 3008 Bern, Switzerland; maria.vasiloglou@artorg.unibe.ch
4. Medical Faculty of the University of Basel, 4056 Basel, Switzerland
* Correspondence: emilie.reber@insel.ch

Received: 14 October 2019; Accepted: 11 December 2019; Published: 13 December 2019

Abstract: Refeeding syndrome (RFS) is the metabolic response to the switch from starvation to a fed state in the initial phase of nutritional therapy in patients who are severely malnourished or metabolically stressed due to severe illness. It is characterized by increased serum glucose, electrolyte disturbances (particularly hypophosphatemia, hypokalemia, and hypomagnesemia), vitamin depletion (especially vitamin B1 thiamine), fluid imbalance, and salt retention, with resulting impaired organ function and cardiac arrhythmias. The awareness of the medical and nursing staff is often too low in clinical practice, leading to under-diagnosis of this complication, which often has an unspecific clinical presentation. This review provides important insights into the RFS, practical recommendations for the management of RFS in the medical inpatient population (excluding eating disorders) based on consensus opinion and on current evidence from clinical studies, including risk stratification, prevention, diagnosis, and management and monitoring of nutritional and fluid therapy.

Keywords: refeeding syndrome; diagnosis; management; malnutrition; hypophosphatemia; nutritional support; nutritional therapy

---

1. Introduction

During World War II, many people suffered from hunger and starvation. Under these circumstances, Ancel Keys investigated the physical and mental effects of prolonged dietary restriction and the subsequent refeeding of 36 conscientious objectors in the Minnesota Starvation Experiment [1]. Most of the subjects experienced periods of severe emotional distress, depression, social withdrawal, isolation, decline in concentration, and decreases in metabolic rate, respiration, and heart rate. Several of the participants developed edema in their extremities. Later, at the end of World War II, further observations were made by Schnitker and Burger [2,3]. Numerous starving detainees developed severe symptoms such as heart failure, peripheral edema, and neurological disorders after a normal diet was reintroduced, and one of five died within the next few days [2,3]. Those observations led to the first description of the refeeding syndrome (RFS), almost 75 years ago.

To date, there is still no commonly accepted definition of RFS, and its detailed pathophysiology remains largely unclear. This is primarily due to the fact that the clinical manifestations of RFS are nonspecific, leading to RFS frequently being overlooked, underdiagnosed, and subsequently untreated. In the study of Hernandez-Aranda et al., up to 48% of malnourished inpatients developed RFS [4]. A sub-analysis of the just-published study of Schuetz et al. demonstrates that medical patients with confirmed RFS have significant mortality rates and increased non-elective hospital readmission, thus confirming the negative effect of RFS on clinical outcome [5,6].

Nutritional treatment is a central aspect of modern multimodal inpatient therapy. It aims to reduce complications and mortality rates, and to improve patients' quality of life and autonomy [5,7]. Even though well tolerated, nutritional treatment has a potential risk of complications, including RFS, which is an exacerbated response to the metabolic change from a starvation to a fed state as a consequence of large amount of food in the replenishment phase. RFS is characterized by an imbalance of electrolytes (mainly phosphate, potassium, and magnesium), vitamin disturbances (e.g., vitamin B1 thiamine deficiency), and fluid imbalances, as well as limited organ functions, in some cases leading to mortality [8–12]. This article highlights, discusses, and reviews RFS in medical inpatients (excluding patients with eating disorders) in terms of pathophysiological aspects, preventive measures, clinical manifestations, risk evaluation, diagnostic procedures, and treatment methods.

2. Pathophysiology and Clinical Manifestations

RFS is an exaggerated physiological response to glucose reintroduction (refeeding) after a prolonged phase of starvation or scarce food intake [13]. The precise pathophysiological mechanisms remain unclear, but recent assumptions are based on the processes described below (Figure 1).

In a catabolic state (due to reduced food intake or even starvation), insulin production is decreased, whereas glucagon and catecholamine are slightly stimulated [14]. During a fasting period, glucose oxidation is reduced and only takes place in the glucose-dependent tissues, such as the brain, renal medulla and red blood cells. The glycogen stores are reduced, leading to activation of gluconeogenesis and the production of glucose from endogenous amino acids, which are released by increased proteolysis. This process causes a reduction in muscle mass, thus inducing functional weakness and weight loss. Vitamin and electrolyte levels are decreased and stores are depleted [15]. After a few days, lipolysis increases, subsequently leading to raised levels of free fatty acids in the circulation. These free fatty acids stimulate ketogenesis in the liver, leading to high production of ketone bodies (in particular acetoacetate and beta-hydroxybuturate), which become the main suppliers of energy for the body [16]. During the catabolic state, metabolic processes are reduced to 30–50% of normal (adaptation phase) [13].

If balanced nutritional support with carbohydrates (refeeding) is introduced, glucose becomes the main energy supplier again, causing hyperglycemia and consequently an increase in insulin secretion. Anabolic processes are stimulated, leading to intracellular shifts of glucose, water, and electrolytes, and resulting in a potentially severe drop in serum micronutrient levels. The resulting electrolyte imbalances can cause life-threatening complications such as arrhythmia, spasms, or tetany [8,11,15,17,18]. Acid-base balance can cause significant electrolyte shifts and this needs to be considered as a differential diagnosis/contributing cause when suspecting refeeding syndrome (e.g., respiratory acidosis). A significant drop in phosphate, potassium, or magnesium levels may occur when the patient has been acidotic, and this is starting to resolve. As the intracellular shift of glucose is thiamine dependent, a deficiency in thiamine, as observed during catabolism, can lead to symptoms of beriberi. The more compromised the nutritional state, the higher the risk of RFS and the greater the severity of its manifestations [8,12]. There are many non-specific symptoms that potentially occur during RFS; the most commonly observed clinical symptoms in daily practice are tachycardia, tachypnea, and peripheral edema [8,15,19,20].

Clinical consequences due to electrolyte changes following increases in insulin include:

- Phosphate is an important electrolyte in the metabolism of macronutrients for both the energy production and transport processes. Phosphate is especially important in the refeeding phase, since glycolysis requires only phosphorylated glucose. Hypophosphatemia may cause several clinical manifestations, such as rhabdomyolysis, hemolysis, respiratory failure, and musculoskeletal disorders. Severe hypophosphatemia (<0.32 mmol/L) is considered a typical hallmark of RFS and in several studies is a central defining criterion [15,18].

- Potassium and magnesium are also important intercellular cations. Severe hypokalemia (<2.5 mmol/L) and/or hypomagnesemia (<0.50 mmol/L) may trigger potentially lethal arrhythmia, neuromuscular dysfunctions such as paresis, rhabdomyolysis, confusion, and respiratory insufficiency [15].
- Thiamine is an essential coenzyme in the metabolism of carbohydrates, allowing the conversion from glucose to adenosine triphosphate (ATP) via the Krebs cycle. When thiamine is lacking (human body stores last for approximately 14 days), glucose is converted to lactate, leading to metabolic acidosis. Thiamine deficiency may also lead to neurologic (Wernicke's encephalopathy: dry beriberi) or cardiovascular disorders (wet beriberi) [15,16].
- Sodium: The major influence on the serum sodium level during the refeeding phase is the shift of sodium out of the cell as the potassium is pumped back into the cell (sodium-potassium-ATPase pump). In addition, the increased insulin level in the early phase of refeeding leads to sodium retention in the kidneys. Sodium concentration subsequently increases, thus inducing water retention. Noradrenaline and angiotensin II are stimulated and lead to augmented peripheral resistance and vasoconstriction [21]. This may cause peripheral edema and heart failure.

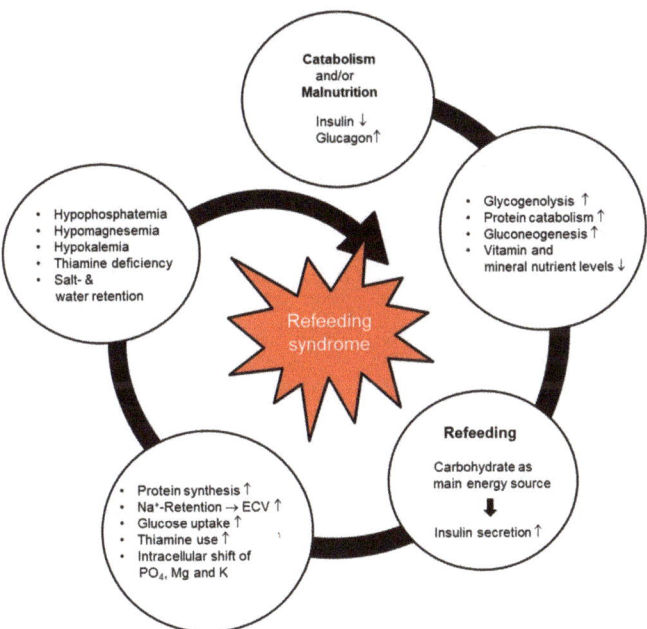

Figure 1. Pathophysiology of refeeding syndrome [22]. Used by permission of the Division of Diabetes, Endocrinology, Nutritional Medicine and Metabolism, Prof. Dr. med. Zeno Stanga (2019).

3. Current Level of Evidence

The current state of evidence for RFS was recently summarized in a systematic review by Friedli et al. [20]. It is mainly based on case series and retrospective, cohort, and case-control studies. To date, very few randomized controlled trials have been published. A recent experts' consensus defined risk factors, occurrence, incidence rate, preventive measures, and treatment recommendations in medical inpatients [19]. A literature search for newly published studies was performed according to the criteria of Friedli et al. for the systematic literature review, excluding anorexia nervosa [20]. Due to the scarce evidence, the National Institute for Health and Care Excellence (NICE) guidelines on nutritional support in adults, containing recommendations on identification and treatment of malnutrition as well as management of nutritional therapy, are often used as the standard of care [23]. Consistent data on the management of RFS and adverse clinical outcome are largely lacking, and justify further research on specific preventive, screening, and treatment measures in patients at risk.

A secondary analysis of a large randomized controlled trial (EFFORT trial [5]) showing the beneficial effects of nutritional support in hospitalized patients provides evidence that, due to the consequences of RFS (higher mortality and non-elective readmission rates), patients at risk may benefit from a specific treatment [5,6]. This secondary analysis relying on the risk stratification and definition from the above-mentioned experts' consensus [19] largely confirms the proposed risk factors and occurrence of RFS [6,8,12,19].

4. Prevention

4.1. Nutritional Support Teams

RFS is most likely to occur within the first 72 h after the start of nutritional therapy (replenishment phase), and to progress rapidly [20]. Quick recognition is crucial and requires well-trained medical staff [24]. In most hospitals, multidisciplinary nutritional support teams are available and assist the attending medical staff in the management of malnutrition. Such teams—consisting of physicians, dieticians, nurses, and pharmacists—contribute to improved quality and safety and optimal clinical outcomes [25–27].

4.2. Individual Risk Assessment

Although RFS is associated with severe and potentially lethal complications, it is a preventable condition [4,28,29]. It can occur with any kind of nutritional intervention (oral, enteral, or parenteral) [28]. RFS risk predictors have been investigated in many studies, but sensitivity and specificity are low [29–31]. Starvation remains the most reliable predictor of RFS [28]. Nutritional risk screening 2002 ≥ 3 points, polymorbidity, older age, and low serum magnesium (<0.7 mmol/L) were found to be risk factors for RFS in many studies [19,20,28,32–38]. According to the literature and to our long-lasting daily clinical experience, there are many clinical conditions at particular risk of developing RFS (see Table 1). Oncological and geriatric patients are very likely to develop RFS [4,39]. Underlying diseases and conditions affecting nutrient absorption (e.g., short bowel syndrome, bariatric surgery, eating disorders) may be risk factors as well [35]. Moreover, chronic gastrointestinal symptoms (e.g., diarrhea, vomiting) and polypharmacy may increase the risk of RFS [19,20,40]. Additionally, medical therapeutic interventions like hemodialysis or chemotherapy are associated with a high risk of RFS [14,23,26]. Before starting nutritional therapy, it is therefore recommended by the experts' consensus of Friedli et al. (Figure 2) to assess the patient's individual risk of RFS and to adapt the nutritional care plan accordingly [19,20,23].

Table 1. Clinical conditions at particular risk of developing RFS.

Clinical Conditions	
- Malnourished, catabolic patients	- Chronic wasting disease
- Geriatric patients	- Chronic pancreatitis
- Oncologic patients	- Chronic infectious disease
- Trauma patients	- Inflammatory bowel syndrome
- Critically ill patients	- Liver cirrhosis
- Hunger strikers or prolonged fasting	- Patients with dysphagia
- Short -bowel syndrome	- Patients with hemodialysis
- Bariatric surgery	- Patients with chemotherapy
- Anorexia nervosa	- Patients with chronic alcoholism
- Cystic fibrosis	- Drug dependent patients

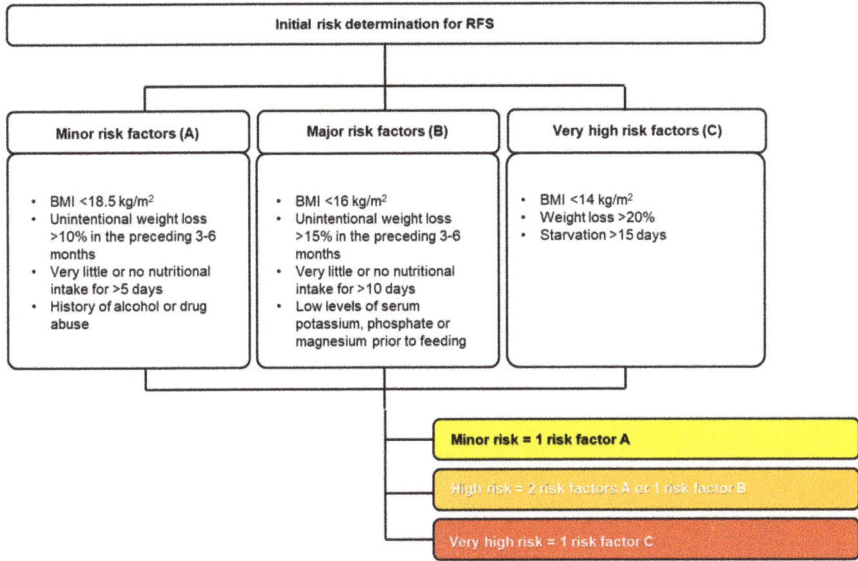

Figure 2. Risk stratification for RFS, according to [19,23]. This stratification has not been validated in a clinical trial [22]. Used by permission of the Division of Diabetes, Endocrinology, Nutritional Medicine and Metabolism, Prof. Dr. med. Zeno Stanga (2019).

5. Diagnostic Procedure

Even though RFS was identified more than 75 years ago, no common definition exists. Therefore, the diagnosis is often delayed or can even be overlooked. Electrolyte imbalance, mainly hypophosphatemia, was used to define RFS in several studies [8,15,41]. Clinical manifestations such as edemas, respiratory failure, or heart failure may occur as a consequence of the electrolyte imbalances, vitamin deficiencies, and fluid overload. The diagnostic procedure proposed by Friedli et al. consists of pathophysiological and clinical characteristics (Figure 3). RFS is probable if the phosphate level in the blood drops >30% under the lower normal value or under 0.6 mmol/L, or if two of the three electrolytes (phosphate, magnesium, and potassium) drop under the normal values within the first 72 h after the start of the replenishment phase in the absence of other possible causes [19,20]. RFS manifests as soon as clinical symptoms occur in addition to electrolyte imbalance [19,20].

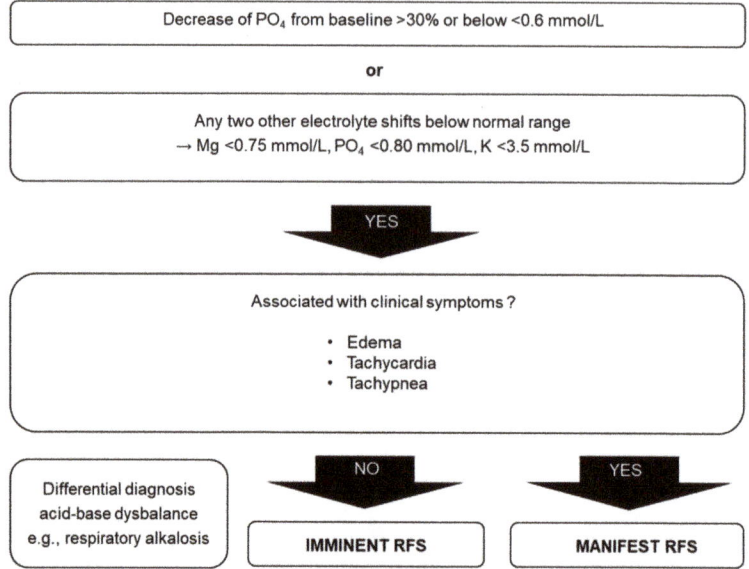

Figure 3. Diagnosis of RFS according to [19], and adapted from Rio et al. [28]. These diagnostic criteria have not been validated in a clinical trial [22]. Used by permission of the Division of Diabetes, Endocrinology, Nutritional Medicine and Metabolism, Prof. Dr. med. Zeno Stanga (2019).

6. Clinical Management

Each malnourished, catabolic patient should receive the best nutritional support according to the highest quality standards in a timely fashion. A recent randomized controlled trial demonstrated the efficacy of adequate nutritional management [5]. Patients at risk of developing RFS need replenishment of electrolytes and vitamins (especially thiamine) serum levels to help prevent/treat symptoms. In this study, the data from 967 malnourished patients were analyzed for RFS; 141 (14.6%) had confirmed RFS, indicating the high incidence of this metabolic state in medical patients receiving nutritional support [6]. The clinical manifestation can vary from mild forms with limited clinical signs and symptoms to severe forms with potentially lethal complications.

Diverse trials evaluated preventive approaches for RFS, such as substitution of electrolytes, thiamine administration, and hypocaloric feeding. Most studies used for the proposed nutritional management were observational and not interventional, pointing to the overall low level of evidence (see Table 2 for guidelines and Table 3 for trials). From the 45 studies included in the systematic review of Friedli et al. [20], only a few reported on therapeutic strategies to treat RFS; some of them reported phosphate supplementation to be effective. Several studies demonstrated a preventive effect of hypocaloric feeding and a reduced risk of RFS when replacing electrolytes. Moreover, close monitoring of serum electrolytes is a further measure for the reduction of risk of RFS.

Based on a previously published systematic review, international experts in the field of starvation metabolism and refeeding published a consensus paper [20]. There was a moderate agreement concerning the initial treatment of high-risk patients and prophylactic measures to prevent RFS. For the proposed treatment of imminent or manifest RFS, there was a strong agreement. In this regard, it is advantageous to manage nutritional and fluid intake as proposed in Figure 4.

Table 2. Relevant guidelines and reviews regarding the management of RFS.

Reference	Type of Study	Level of Evidence	Initial Energy/day	Proteins/day	Fluids/day	Vitamins (Before/During)
Solomon et al. 1990 [11]	Review	4	20 kcal/kg	1.2–1.5 g	NR	NR
Dewar et al. 2000 [42]	Review, guidelines	4	20 kcal/kg	NR	NR	Thiamine IV or PO for 2 days
Crook et al. 2001 [8]	Review	4	10 kcal/kg high risk: 5 kcal/kg 50–60% CHO, 15–25% fat	20–30% 1.2–1.5 g	20–30 mL/kg, 0 fluid balance	Thiamine 300 mg IV, than 100 mg daily during refeeding. In addition, Vit B12, Vit B6 and folate
Stroud et al. 2003 [43]	Review	4	10–20 kcal/kg	NR	NR	Thiamine and B vitamins IV for 3 days
Kraft et al. 2005 [44]	Review, guidelines	4	7.5 kcal/kg	NR	<1000 mL/day	Thiamine 50–100 mg IV or 100 mg PO for 5–7 days and multivitamin
NICE 2006 [23]	Review, guidelines	4	10 kcal/kg high risk: 5 kcal/kg	NR	0 fluid balance	Thiamine 200–300 mg PO for 10 days and multivitamin for 10 days
Stanga et al. 2008 [12]	Case series	4	10–15 kcal/kg high risk: 5 kcal/kg 50–60% CHO, 30–40% fat	15–20%	20–30 mL/kg, 0 fluid balance	Thiamine 200–300 mg IV or PO for 3 days and multivitamin for 10 days
Mehanna et al. 2008 [16]	Review	4	10 kcal/kg high risk: 5 kcal/kg	NR	carefully fluid repletion	Thiamine 200–300 mg PO for 10 days and multivitamin for 10 days
Boateng et al. 2010 [15]	Case series	4	10 kcal/kg high risk: 5 kcal/kg 50–60% CHO, 15–25% fat	20–30% 1.2–1.5 g	20–30 mL/kg, 0 fluid balance	Thiamine 300 mg IV, then 100 mg daily during refeeding. In addition, Vit B12, Vit B6 and folate
ESPEN 2019 [45]	Review, guidelines	4	10–15 kcal/kg high risk: 5 kcal/kg 50–60% CHO, 30–40% fat	15–20%	20–30 mL/kg, 0 fluid balance	Thiamine 200–300 mg IV or PO for 3 days and multivitamin for 10 days
Crook et al. 2014 [46]	Review	4	10 kcal/kg high risk: 5 kcal/kg 50–60% CHO, 15–25% fat	20–30% 1.2–1.5 g	20–30 mL/kg, 0 fluid balance	Thiamine 300 mg IV, then 100 mg daily during refeeding. In addition, Vit B12, Vit B6 and folate
Friedli et al. 2017 [20]	Systematic review	3a	10–15 kcal/kg high risk: 5 kcal/kg 50–60% CHO, 30–40% fat	15–20%	20–30 mL/kg, 0 fluid balance	Thiamine 200–300 mg IV or PO for 3 days and multivitamin for 10 days
Friedli et al. 2018 [19]	Systematic review, consensus paper	3a	10–15 kcal/kg high risk: 5 kcal/kg 50–60% CHO, 30–40% fat	15–20%	20–30 mL/kg, 0 fluid balance	Thiamine 200–300 mg IV or PO for 3 days and multivitamin for 10 days

CHO: carbohydrates, IV: intravenous, NR: not reported, PO: per os. Level of evidence after level of evidence for clinical studies from the Oxford centre for evidence-based medicine, http://www.cebm.net; 4 case series (and poor-quality cohort and case-control studies); 3a systematic review (with homogeneity) of case-control studies; 3b individual case-control study.

Table 3. Relevant studies regarding the management of RFS.

Reference	Type of Study	Level of Evidence	N	Preventive Medication	Therapeutic Medication	Effectivity
Hofer et al. 2014 [25]	Retrospective study	3b	86	Hypocaloric feeding, restricted fluid administration (0 fluid balance), thiamine 200–300 mg IV or PO for 3 days and multivitamin for 10 days, electrolyte supplementation (unless prefeeding serum levels are high): PO$_4$ 0.5–0.8 mmol/kg/day, K 1–2.2 mmol/kg/day, Mg 0.3–0.4 mmol/kg/day	Hypocaloric feeding, restricted fluid administration, electrolytes substitution according to the serum level	Yes
Eichelberger et al. 2014 [47]	Retrospective study	3b	37	Hypocaloric feeding, restricted fluid administration (0 fluid balance), thiamine 200–300 mg IV or PO for 3 days and multivitamin for 10 days, electrolyte supplementation (unless prefeeding serum levels are high): PO$_4$ 0.5–0.8 mmol/kg/day, K 1–2.2 mmol/kg/day, Mg 0.3–0.4 mmol/kg/day	Hypocaloric feeding, restricted fluid administration, electrolytes substitution according to the serum level	Yes
Terlevich et al. 2003 [31]	Prospective study	4	30	NR	50 mmol PO$_4$ over 24h	Yes
Gonzalez Aviva et al. 1996 [48]	Prospective study	3b	106	PO$_4$ supplementation	NR	Yes
Marvin et al. 2008 [49]	Case control study	3b	140	During the first 24 h slow PN regimen providing <70% of protein and calories but >12 mmol PO$_4$	NR	Yes
Garber et al. 2011 [50]	Retrospective study	4	40	No effective preventive measures found	NR	No
Coskun et al. 2014 [51]	Retrospective study	4	117	Lower energy intake	NR	No
Doig et al. 2015 [52]	RCT	1b	339	NR	Lower caloric intake	Yes
Whitelaw et al. 2010 [53]	Retrospective study	4	46	Prophylactic administration of PO$_4$, lower initial energy intake, monitoring of PO$_4$	Supplementation of PO4	Yes
Luque et al. 2007 [54]	Retrospective study	4	11	PO$_4$ supplementation, thiamine 3.51 mg/d	NR	Yes
Manning et al. 2014 [55]	Prospective study	2b	36	Repeated electrolyte testing	NR	No
Fan et al. 2004 [33]	Retrospective study	4	158	PO$_4$ supplementation	NR	Yes, if PO$_4$ <0.30
Gentile et al. 2010 [56]	Retrospective study	4	33	Prophylactic administration of PO$_4$ and K, cautious nutritional rehabilitation	NR	Yes
Vignaud et al. 2010 [38]	Retrospective study	4	68	For patients at risk for initial nutritional support 10 kcal/kg/day falling to as low as 5 kcal/kg/day	NR	Yes
Chen et al. 2014 [57]	Retrospective study	4	56	Thiamine and multivitamin supplementation, 15 kcal/kg/day	NR	Yes
Golden et al. 2013 [58]	Retrospective study	4	310	Lower caloric intake	NR	No
Leclerc et al. 2013 [59]	Retrospective study	4	29	Hypocaloric feeding	NR	No
Flesher et al. 2005 [60]	Retrospective study	4	51	Thiamine supplementation, cautious feeding	NR	No
Rio et al. 2013 [28]	Prospective	2b	243	Hypocaloric feeding	NR	No

IV: intravenous, NR: not reported, PO: per os, RCT: randomized controlled trial. Level of evidence after Level of evidence for clinical studies from the Oxford Centre for Evidence-based Medicine, http://www.cebm.net.

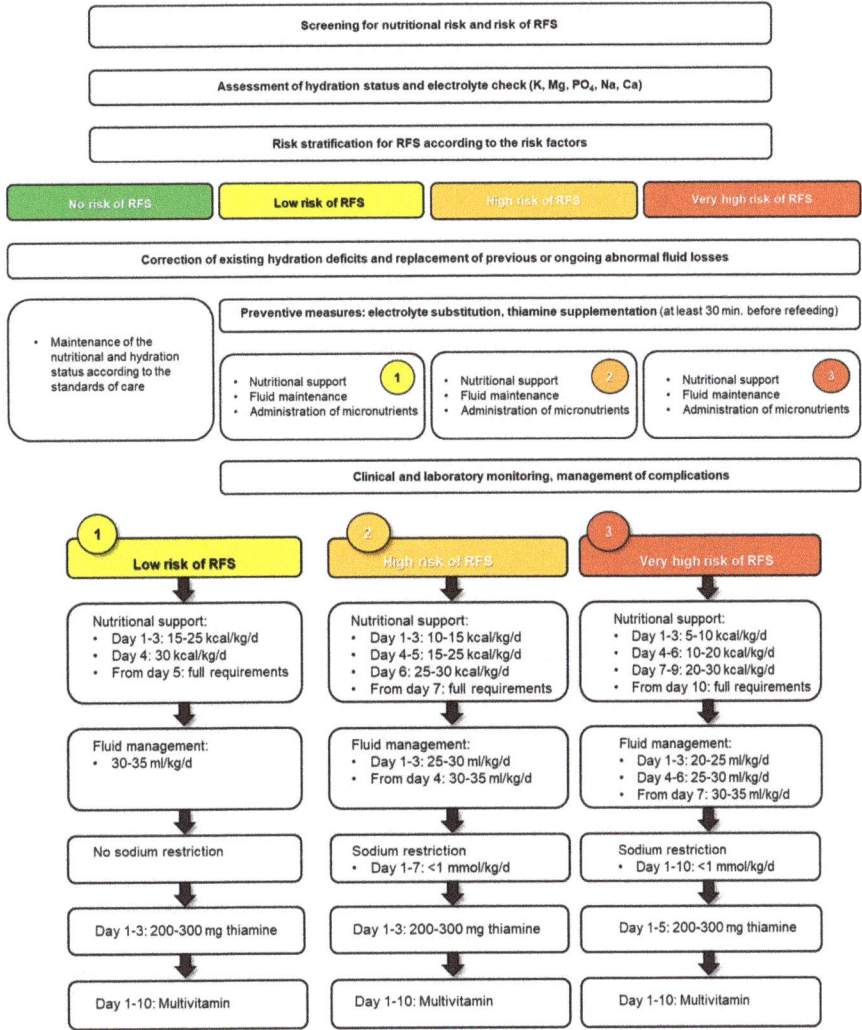

Figure 4. Management of nutritional therapy according to the risk for RFS, after [19]. Used by permission of the Division of Diabetes, Endocrinology, Nutritional Medicine and Metabolism, Prof. Dr. med. Zeno Stanga (2019) [22].

6.1. Macronutrients

Various studies and guidelines have shown a beneficial effect of starting energy intake at a lower rate than generally used, in order to prevent RFS in patients at high risk [12,16,23]. Based on a patient's individual risk for RFS, energy supply should be initiated at lower levels, starting with an initial amount of 5–15 kcal/kg/day, and increased stepwise depending on the laboratory parameters and clinical situation of the patient [8,19,20,23,52,61,62]. The full energy requirements should be met within 5 to 10 days, depending on the prior risk stratification, using a common nutritional macronutrients composition of 40–60% carbohydrates, 30–40% fats, and 15–20% proteins [12]. In clinically unstable critically ill patients with RFS, lowering the proportion of carbohydrates should be considered.

Nutritional rehabilitation of patients with risk to develop a RFS should be typically started with oral intake of regular food. If the patient cannot eat enough food to meet the energy targets, oral nutritional supplements may be prescribed. Enteral nutrition (tube feeding) is indicated for extremely malnourished patients (e.g., very low BMI) or patients who are unable to consume enough food to reach the energy targets. Parenteral nutrition is indicated when oral and/or enteral nutrition are insufficient or in the case of failure of the gut function. The risk of RFS may be greater with enteral or parenteral feeding compared to oral intake, thus artificial nutrition should be started cautiously at a reduced caloric rate [4,28,29,52,63–66].

Optimal nutritional support is still controversial and some experts and scientists recommend faster increase in nutritional support to counteract harm associated with malnutrition. Opinions on its management differ, because they are mostly based on personal experience in various populations. At this point, we would like to emphasize that the current review provides important insights into RFS based on a comprehensive literature research and critical appraisal of the evidence. In the light of the current scientific knowledge, it is very likely that there is a need for different intervention approaches adapted to the specific pathologies, e.g., anorexia nervosa.

6.2. Fluids

Disturbance of the acid-base balance may cause hypophosphatemia. Acute respiratory alkalosis is for example the most common clinical situation in which hypophosphatemia should be expected in hospitalized patients. The often uncritical use of diuretics (loop and thiazide diuretics) promotes the development of alkalosis through volume reduction and loss of electrolytes (chloride, potassium, magnesium). A decreased volume generates metabolic alkalosis in two ways. The reduction of phosphate is much more pronounced in respiratory alkalosis than in metabolic alkalosis of comparable severity [67,68].

RFS may occur regardless of energy restrictions if fluid balance is disregarded [39]. Hydration deficiencies and abnormal losses (e.g., fever, vomiting, diarrhea) should be addressed at the start of a replenishment phase. The choice of replacement fluid is thereby especially relevant. Balanced solutions should be the preferred option, except when replacing gastric and/or fistula losses over stoma. The fluid prescription should include the daily maintenance requirements plus the water and electrolytes replacement of any losses [69]. In general, fluid intake of 25–35 mL/kg/day is sufficient to maintain an adequate hydration state [69]. The fluid intake through artificial nutrition, infusions, and intravenously administered drugs (mainly antibiotics) should also be taken into account, as well as the salt content (up to 155.2 mmol of Na^+ in one liter of Ringer's lactate (Hartmann) solution and 154 mmol of Na^+ in one liter of isotonic 0.9% NaCl solution). Fluid balance should be corrected cautiously and checked daily. Diuretics, especially specific competitive aldosterone antagonists regulating sodium transport in the kidney, may be useful in case of fluid excess [69].

Particular attention should be paid to the sodium concentration of fluids/products given to patients at (very) high risk for RFS. Sodium restriction (<1 mmol/kg/day) should be considered in the first days after the start of the nutritional therapy in order to avoid fluid overload [12,19,25,47].

6.3. Micronutrients

Malnourished patients have depleted intracellular micronutrient stores. After the initiation of nutritional therapy, the intracellular flux of vitamins and electrolytes increases, causing serum levels to drop. It is therefore essential to correct electrolyte levels before initiation of the replenishment phase, with the supplementation of phosphate and thiamine being particularly important [15,19,20]. Prophylactic phosphate supplementation should be undertaken in patients at very high risk for RFS even in the case of normal serum levels to avoid or alleviate the occurrence of RFS, as hypophosphatemia plays a key role in RFS. During starvation, body stores of phosphate decrease, despite normal serum levels. As long as the energy metabolism depends on fat oxidation, phosphate is not required; as soon as the patient resumes carbohydrate intake, the metabolism of glucose uses large amounts of phosphate, thus leading to a drop in serum levels [12,15,64].

The prophylactic supplementation of high-dose thiamine (200–300 mg) at least 30 min before beginning refeeding is fundamental. Vitamins should be supplemented to 200% and the trace elements to 100% of the recommended daily intakes. Electrolytes, especially phosphate, potassium, and magnesium, must be closely monitored and supplemented throughout the refeeding period [12,19,25,47]. Hypokalemia is worsened by concomitant hypomagnesemia, since magnesium is necessary for the sodium-potassium-pump activity and therefore an important factor in the tubular resorption of potassium. Potassium supplementation alone is thus insufficient, and persistently low potassium values despite supplementation can subsequently be rectified only with simultaneous magnesium substitution [70]. Hypocalcemia may cause or further worsen hypophosphatemia [71].

Iron should not be supplemented in the first week after the start of the nutritional therapy, even in the case of manifest iron deficiency. As blood production requires high amounts of potassium, hypokalemia may worsen further. Moreover, parenteral iron supplementation must be considered with caution in malnourished catabolic patients, as it may induce and/or prolong hypophosphatemia [7].

7. Monitoring

RFS generally occurs within the first 72 h after initiation of nutritional therapy and may progress very rapidly. In the vulnerable phase (up to 10 days), intensive clinical monitoring of vital signs and hydration status, as well as analysis of laboratory parameters, is essential to detect early signs of RFS such as fluid overload and organ failure (mainly kidney) (Figure 5). Body weight and hydration status should be checked on a daily basis, as an increase of 0.3–0.5 kg/day may be an initial sign of pathological fluid retention [12,19,25,47].

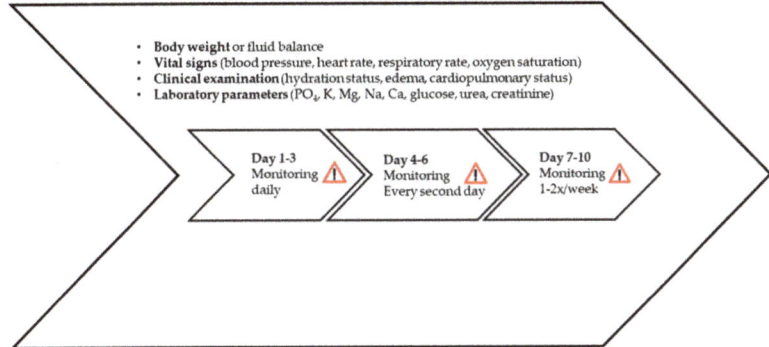

Figure 5. Monitoring of RFS, based on [19]. Used by permission of the Division of Diabetes, Endocrinology, Nutritional Medicine and Metabolism, Prof. Dr. med. Zeno Stanga (2019) [22].

Electrocardiogram monitoring is recommended only during the first three days in patients at very high risk of RFS or affected by severe electrolyte imbalances prior to refeeding (K < 2.5 mmol/L, PO_4 < 0.32 mmol/L, Mg < 0.5 mmol/L), as they may exhibit severe arrhythmia and QT-prolongation, up to Torsades de Pointes [8,12,19,20,23].

Electrolyte substitution respectively supplementation should be initiated or reinforced in case of extracellular electrolyte levels dropping (Table 4). In the case of edema, tachycardia, or tachypnea, symptoms should be treated individually and nutritional therapy should be continued according to the algorithm for the highest risk category [15,19,20].

Table 4. Suggested supplementation regimen [8,12,72–76].

	Potassium	Magnesium	Phosphate
Mild deficiency	3.1–3.5 mmol/L Oral replacement with 20 mmol (as KCl or other salts) OR i.v. replacement with 20 mmol KCl over 4 to 8 h. Check levels the next day.	0.5–0.7 mmol/L Oral replacement with 10–15 mmol $MgCl_2$ or Mg-citrate or Mg-L-aspartate Oral Mg should be given in divided doses to minimize diarrhea (absorption process is saturated at about 5–10 mmol Mg)	0.61–0.8 mmol/L Oral replacement with 0.3 mmol/kg/day PO_4 (divided doses to minimize diarrhea) OR i.v. replacement with 0.3 mmol/kg/day PO_4 (as K_3PO_4 or Na_3PO_4) over 8–12 h. Check levels the next day.
Moderate deficiency	2.5–3.0 mmol/L i.v. replacement with 20–40 mmol KCl over 4–8 h. Check levels after 8 h; if not normal, give an additional 20 mmol KCl.		0.32–0.6 mmol/L i.v. replacement with 0.6 mmol/kg/day PO_4 (as K_3PO_4 or Na_3PO_4) over 8–12 h. Check levels after 8–12 h and repeat infusion if necessary (max. of 50 mmol PO_4 in 24 h).
Severe deficiency	<2.5 mmol/L i.v. replacement with 40 mmol KCl over 4–8 h. Check levels after 8 h; if not normal, give an additional 40 mmol KCl.	<0.5 mmol/L i.v. replacement with 20–24 mmol $MgSO_4$ (4–6 g) over 4–8 h. Reassess every 8 to 12 h.	<0.32 mmol/L Same replacement therapy as for moderate deficiency.

8. Important Clinical Sequelae of Refeeding Syndrome and Management of Complications

RFS may increase rates of morbidity and mortality in severely catabolic patients (Table 5). Malnutrition may result from reduced food intake, reduced absorption of nutrients (e.g., coeliac disease, pancreatitis), or hypermetabolism (e.g., cancer, critical illness, surgery). Mild metabolic imbalances of electrolytes, fluid, and micronutrients are however often asymptomatic but may cause organ dysfunctions and become potentially lethal. Peripheral edema, tachypnea, and tachycardia are the most commonly observed clinical symptoms in patients suffering RFS. It is mandatory to treat these symptoms if they occur, ruling out an eventual lung embolism.

The first step in the management of RFS-related pathological conditions is to anticipate with preventive measures and closely monitor the at-risk patients. The overall objectives in the treatment of RFS complications are to stabilize the patient's general clinical state, to reverse the medical complications, as well as to restore nutritional needs and weight. The sooner the RFS complications are treated, the lower the risk of damage to patient's vital organs. The patients with RFS are often dehydrated and require correction of existing hydration deficits and replacement of abnormal fluid losses. Furthermore, electrolytes and vitamins have to be supplemented adequately, as well as any deficiency corrected. The nutritional rehabilitation should be started slowly and adapted to each individual patient. The introduction of carbohydrates in the replenishment phase leads to a quick decrease in renal excretion of sodium and water [21,77]. Patients require a close monitoring of the fluid balance to prevent fluid overload. Such uncontrolled clinical situations may lead quickly to congestive cardiac failure, pulmonary and brain edema, as well as cardiac arrhythmia [78,79]. Too much delivering of glucose in this vulnerable phase leads to hyperglycemia and consequently to osmotic diuresis, dehydration metabolic acidosis, hyperosmotic coma, and ketoacidosis, as well as increased carbon dioxide, hypercapnia, and respiratory failure [77,80–82]. Severely malnourished patients may suffer from hematological disorders and moderate to high increase of liver enzymes. The first pathophysiological changes are associated with bone marrow hypoplasia and with gelatinous marrow transformation [83,84]; the second seems to be multicausal and related to an ischemic hepatitis secondary to liver hypoperfusion, to oxidant stress from low glutathione levels, and to starvation-induced autophagy [83,85]. Both pathologies show a marked decrease after a few days during the replenishment phase (hydration and nutritional therapy) and possibly will normalize after the refeeding period [86]. In all these clinical situations, a complications-centric approach to RFS-related complications identifies patients who will benefit most from individual specific interventions and optimizes patient outcomes.

Table 5. Important symptoms and clinical sequelae of RFS (adapted from [15]).

System	Symptoms
Cardiovascular	Tachycardia Arrhythmias Hypotension Congestive heart failure Shock Edemas Sudden death
Gastrointestinal	Maldigestion and malabsorption Vomiting Constipation Abdominal pain
Musculoskeletal	Weakness Myalgia Rhabdomyolysis Osteomalacia
Respiratory	Tachypnea Dyspnea Respiratory failure Ventilator dependency Diaphragm muscle weakness
Neurologic	Anorexia Paresthesia Tremor Wernicke encephalopathy Korsakoff syndrome Ataxia Tetany Delirium Seizures Coma
Metabolic	Hyperglycemia Metabolic alkalosis Metabolic acidosis Respiratory alkalosis Insulin resistance
Hematologic	Thrombocytopenia Hemolysis Anemia Leukocyte dysfunction Decreased 2,3-DPG
Renal	Acute tubular necrosis
Hepatological	Acute liver failure

9. Outlook

Due to the lack of large randomized trials, the current literature confirms the clinical consequences but not the efficacy of measures used to prevent and treat RFS. A recent secondary analysis of the EFFORT trial showed that RFS has a significant impact on mortality and readmission rate [5,6]. Therefore, prevention, detection, and early treatment of malnourished catabolic medical patients at risk of RFS is essential [25,47,52]. As mentioned before, clinical manifestation can vary from mild to severe, and lethal complications are possible. Therefore, an implementation of the nutritional and fluid intake as proposed in Figure 4 seems opportune. Still, it remains unclear whether RFS is a physiological response or a problem of adaptation to nutritional therapy [19,20]. Thus, further research is needed to determine the optimal rate of energy and fluid increase during refeeding, as well as associated factors.

Many other unresolved issues have not yet been clarified. Does hypoglycemia or hyperglycemia play an important role in the clinical manifestation of RFS? Does insulin therapy influence the risk of RFS? Is RFS caused and/or influenced by the underlying disease [87]? Is there a difference between nutrition-induced hypophosphatemia and RFS? Are there reliable predictors of RFS [31]? For example, increased IGF-1 combined with increased leptin levels is associated with a 30% decrease in the phosphate level within the first 12–36 h after the start of parenteral nutrition [88]. Cytokines may also play an important role in the pathophysiology. Many studies have shown the importance of thiamine supplementation to avoid beriberi disease, whereas the potential action of other vitamins and trace elements in this context is much less investigated [78,89,90].

10. Conclusions

Nutritional therapies have shown to be efficacious and efficient, despite the overall low level of evidence. It however hides the risk of RFS in catabolic malnourished patients. RFS is a highly challenging metabolic situation, leading to potentially life-threatening complications with fluid and electrolyte disturbances. RFS should therefore be timely and adequately treated. As nutritional risk is associated with the risk of RFS, awareness of both conditions must be increased among the medical staff in daily clinical practice.

Author Contributions: Conceptualization, E.R. and Z.S.; writing—original draft preparation, E.R.; writing—review and editing, N.F., M.F.V., P.S., and Z.S.; supervision: Z.S.

Funding: The APC was funded by the Research Found of the Department of Diabetes, Endocrinology, Nutritional medicine and Metabolism and in part by Nestlé Health Science (grant to the institution).

Conflicts of Interest: The authors declare no conflicts of interest.

References

1. Keys, A.; Brožek, J.; Henschel, A.; Mickelsen, O.; Taylor, H.L. *The Biology of Human Starvation. (2 Vols)*; University of Minnesota Press: Minneapolis, MN, USA, 1950.
2. Schnitker, M.A.; Mattman, P.E.; Bliss, T.L. A clinical study of malnutrition in Japanese prisoners of war. *Ann. Intern. Med.* **1951**, *35*, 69–96. [PubMed]
3. Burger, G.; Drummond, J.; Sandstead, H. *Appendices to Malnutrition and Starvation in Western Netherlands, September 1944–July 1945 (Part II)*; The Hague General State Printing Office: The Hague, The Netherlands, 1948.
4. Hernandez-Aranda, J.C.; Gallo-Chico, B.; Luna-Cruz, M.L.; Rayon-Gonzalez, M.I.; Flores-Ramirez, L.A.; Ramos Munoz, R.; Ramirez-Barba, E.J. Malnutrition and total parenteral nutrition: A cohort study to determine the incidence of refeeding syndrome. *Rev. Gastroenterol. M.* **1997**, *62*, 260–265.
5. Schuetz, P.; Fehr, R.; Baechli, V.; Geiser, M.; Gomes, F.; Kutz, A.; Tribolet, P.; Bregenzer, T.; Hoess, C.; Pavlicek, V.; et al. Individualized nutritional support in medical inpatients at nutritional risk: A randomized clinical trial. *Lancet* **2019**, *393*, 2312–2321. [CrossRef]
6. Friedli, N.; Baumann, J.; Hummel, R.; Kloter, M.; Odermatt, J.; Fehr, R.; Felder, S.; Baechli, V.; Geiser, M.; Deiss, M.; et al. Refeeding Syndrome is associated with increased mortality in malnourished medical inpatients: Secondary Analysis of a Randomized Trial. *Medicine* **2019**, in press.
7. Fierz, Y.C.; Kenmeni, R.; Gonthier, A.; Lier, F.; Pralong, F.; Coti Bertrand, P. Severe and prolonged hypophosphatemia after intravenous iron administration in a malnourished patient. *Eur. J. Clin. Nutr.* **2014**, *68*, 531–533. [CrossRef]
8. Crook, M.; Hally, V.; Panteli, J. The Importance of the refeeding syndrome. *Nutrition* **2001**, *17*, 632–637. [CrossRef]
9. Felder, S.; Braun, N.; Stanga, Z.; Kulkarni, P.; Faessler, L.; Kutz, A.; Steiner, D.; Laukemann, S.; Haubitz, S.; Huber, A.; et al. Unraveling the Link between Malnutrition and Adverse Clinical Outcomes: Association of Acute and Chronic Malnutrition Measures with Blood Biomarkers from Different Pathophysiological States. *Ann. Nutr. Metab.* **2016**, *68*, 164–172. [CrossRef]

10. Preiser, J.C.; van Zanten, A.R.; Berger, M.M.; Biolo, G.; Casaer, M.P.; Doig, G.S.; Griffiths, R.D.; Heyland, D.K.; Hiesmayr, M.; Iapichino, G.; et al. Metabolic and nutritional support of critically ill patients: Consensus and controversies. *Crit. Care* **2015**, *19*, 35. [CrossRef]
11. Solomon, S.M.; Kirby, D.F. The refeeding syndrome: A review. *J. Parenter. Enter. Nutr.* **1990**, *14*, 90–97. [CrossRef]
12. Stanga, Z.; Brunner, A.; Leuenberger, M.; Grimble, R.F.; Shenkin, A.; Allison, S.P.; Lobo, D.N. Nutrition in clinical practice-the refeeding syndrome: Illustrative cases and guidelines for prevention and treatment. *Eur. J. Clin. Nutr.* **2008**, *62*, 687–694. [CrossRef]
13. Cahill, G.F., Jr. Fuel metabolism in starvation. *Annu. Rev. Nutr.* **2006**, *26*, 1–22. [CrossRef] [PubMed]
14. McCray, S.; Walker, S.; Parrish, C.R. Much ado about refeeding. *Pract. Gastroenterol.* **2005**, *29*, 26–44.
15. Boateng, A.A.; Sriram, K.; Meguid, M.M.; Crook, M. Refeeding syndrome: Treatment considerations based on collective analysis of literature case reports. *Nutrition* **2010**, *26*, 156–167. [CrossRef] [PubMed]
16. Mehanna, H.M.; Moledina, J.; Travis, J. Refeeding syndrome: What it is, and how to prevent and treat it. *BMJ* **2008**, *336*, 1495–1498. [CrossRef] [PubMed]
17. Brooks, M.J.; Melnik, G. The refeeding syndrome: An approach to understanding its complications and preventing its occurrence. *Pharmacotherapy* **1995**, *15*, 713–726.
18. Mehler, P.S.; Krantz, M. Anorexia nervosa medical issues. *J. Women's Health* **2003**, *12*, 331–340. [CrossRef]
19. Friedli, N.; Stanga, Z.; Culkin, A.; Crook, M.; Laviano, A.; Sobotka, L.; Kressig, R.W.; Kondrup, J.; Mueller, B.; Schuetz, P. Management and prevention of refeeding syndrome in medical inpatients: An evidence-based and consensus-supported algorithm. *Nutrition* **2018**, *47*, 13–20. [CrossRef]
20. Friedli, N.; Stanga, Z.; Sobotka, L.; Culkin, A.; Kondrup, J.; Laviano, A.; Mueller, B.; Schuetz, P. Revisiting the refeeding syndrome: Results of a systematic review. *Nutrition* **2017**, *35*, 151–160. [CrossRef]
21. DeFronzo, R.A. The effect of insulin on renal sodium metabolism. A review with clinical implications. *Diabetologia* **1981**, *21*, 165–171. [CrossRef]
22. Department of Diabetes, Endocrinology, Nutritional Medicine and Metabolism, Inselspital, Bern University Hospital, and University of Bern. Available online: http://www.udem.insel.ch/de/lehre-und-forschung/forschung/wichtige-abbildungen/ (accessed on 12 December 2019).
23. National Institute for Health and Clinical Excellence. Nutrition Support for Adults: Oral Nutrition Support, Enteral Tube Feeding and Parenteral Nutrition (Clinical Guidance 32). Available online: https://www.nice.org.uk/Guidance/CG32 (accessed on 12 December 2019).
24. Schuetz, P.; Zurfluh, S.; Stanga, Z. Mortality due to refeeding syndrome? You only find what you look for, and you only look for what you know. *Eur. J. Clin. Nutr.* **2018**, *72*, 307–308. [CrossRef]
25. Hofer, M.; Pozzi, A.; Joray, M.; Ott, R.; Hahni, F.; Leuenberger, M.; von Kanel, R.; Stanga, Z. Safe refeeding management of anorexia nervosa inpatients: An evidence-based protocol. *Nutrition* **2014**, *30*, 524–530. [CrossRef]
26. Nightingale, J. Nutrition support teams: How they work, are set up and maintained. *Frontline Gastroenterol.* **2010**, *1*, 171–177. [CrossRef]
27. Ten Dam, S.; Droop, A.; Arjaans, W.; de Groot, S.; van Bokhorst-de van der Schueren, M. Module 11.1 Organisation of a nutritional support team. In *Organisation of Nutritional Care. Ethical and Legal Aspects*; ESPEN: Luxembourg, 2012.
28. Rio, A.; Whelan, K.; Goff, L.; Reidlinger, D.P.; Smeeton, N. Occurrence of refeeding syndrome in adults started on artificial nutrition support: Prospective cohort study. *BMJ Open* **2013**, *3*, e002173. [CrossRef]
29. Zeki, S.; Culkin, A.; Gabe, S.M.; Nightingale, J.M. Refeeding hypophosphataemia is more common in enteral than parenteral feeding in adult in patients. *Clin. Nutr.* **2011**, *30*, 365–368. [CrossRef]
30. Goyale, A.; Ashley, S.L.; Taylor, D.R.; Elnenaei, M.O.; Alaghband-Zadeh, J.; Sherwood, R.A.; le Roux, C.W.; Vincent, R.P. Predicting refeeding hypophosphataemia: Insulin growth factor 1 (IGF-1) as a diagnostic biochemical marker for clinical practice. *Ann. Clin. Biochem.* **2015**, *52*, 82–87. [CrossRef]
31. Terlevich, A.; Hearing, S.D.; Woltersdorf, W.W.; Smyth, C.; Reid, D.; McCullagh, E.; Day, A.; Probert, C.S. Refeeding syndrome: Effective and safe treatment with Phosphates Polyfusor. *Aliment. Pharmacol. Ther.* **2003**, *17*, 1325–1329. [CrossRef]
32. Brown, C.A.; Sabel, A.L.; Gaudiani, J.L.; Mehler, P.S. Predictors of hypophosphatemia during refeeding of patients with severe anorexia nervosa. *Int. J. Eat. Disord.* **2015**, *48*, 898–904. [CrossRef]

33. Fan, C.G.; Ren, J.A.; Wang, X.B.; Li, J.S. Refeeding syndrome in patients with gastrointestinal fistula. *Nutrition* **2004**, *20*, 346–350. [CrossRef]
34. Gaudiani, J.L.; Sabel, A.L.; Mehler, P.S. Low prealbumin is a significant predictor of medical complications in severe anorexia nervosa. *Int. J. Eat. Disord.* **2014**, *47*, 148–156. [CrossRef]
35. Kagansky, N.; Levy, S.; Koren-Morag, N.; Berger, D.; Knobler, H. Hypophosphataemia in old patients is associated with the refeeding syndrome and reduced survival. *J. Intern. Med.* **2005**, *257*, 461–468. [CrossRef]
36. Kraaijenbrink, B.; Lambers, W.; Mathus-Vliegen, E.; Siegert, C. Incidence of RFS in internal medicine patients. *Ned. J. Med.* **2016**, *74*, 116–121.
37. Pourhassan, M.; Cuvelier, I.; Gehrke, I.; Marburger, C.; Modreker, M.K.; Volkert, D.; Willschrei, H.P.; Wirth, R. Risk factors of refeeding syndrome in malnourished older hospitalized patients. *Clin. Nutr.* **2018**, *37*, 1354–1359. [CrossRef]
38. Vignaud, M.; Constantin, J.M.; Ruivard, M.; Villemeyre-Plane, M.; Futier, E.; Bazin, J.E.; Annane, D.; AZUREA group (AnorexieRea Study Group). Refeeding syndrome influences outcome of anorexia nervosa patients in intensive care unit: An observational study. *Crit. Care* **2010**, *14*, R172. [CrossRef]
39. Tsiompanou, E.; Lucas, C.; Stroud, M. Overfeeding and overhydration in elderly medical patients: Lessons from the Liverpool Care Pathway. *Clin. Med.* **2013**, *13*, 248–251. [CrossRef]
40. Hearing, S.D. Refeeding syndrome. *BMJ* **2004**, *328*, 908–909. [CrossRef]
41. Marik, P.E.; Bedigian, M.K. Refeeding hypophosphatemia in critically ill patients in an intensive care unit. A prospective study. *Arch. Surg.* **1996**, *131*, 1043–1047. [CrossRef]
42. Dewar, H.; Horvath, R. *Refeeding Syndrome: Guidelines*; Oxford Radcliffe Hospital NHS Trust: Oxford, UK, 1996.
43. Stroud, M.; Duncan, H.; Nightingale, J. Guidelines for enteral feeding in adult hospital patients. *Gut* **2003**, *52* (Suppl. 7), vii1–vii12. [CrossRef]
44. Kraft, M.D.; Btaiche, I.F.; Sacks, G.S. Review of the refeeding syndrome. *Nutr. Clin. Pract.* **2005**, *20*, 625–633. [CrossRef]
45. Stanga, Z.; Sobotka, L.; Schuetz, P. Refeeding Syndrome. In *Basics in Clinical Nutrition*, 5th ed.; Sobotka, L., Ed.; Galen: Prag, Czech Republic, 2019; in press.
46. Crook, M.A. Refeeding syndrome: Problems with definition and management. *Nutrition* **2014**, *30*, 1448–1455. [CrossRef]
47. Eichelberger, M.; Joray, M.L.; Perrig, M.; Bodmer, M.; Stanga, Z. Management of patients during hunger strike and refeeding phase. *Nutrition* **2014**, *30*, 1372–1378. [CrossRef]
48. Gonzalez Avila, G.; Fajardo Rodriguez, A.; Gonzalez Figueroa, E. The incidence of the refeeding syndrome in cancer patients who receive artificial nutritional treatment. *Nutr. Hosp.* **1996**, *11*, 98–101. [PubMed]
49. Marvin, V.A.; Brown, D.; Portlock, J.; Livingstone, C. Factors contributing to the development of hypophosphataemia when refeeding using parenteral nutrition. *Pharm. World Sci.* **2008**, *30*, 329–335. [CrossRef] [PubMed]
50. Garber, A.K.; Michihata, N.; Hetnal, K.; Shafer, M.A.; Moscicki, A.B. A prospective examination of weight gain in hospitalized adolescents with anorexia nervosa on a recommended refeeding protocol. *J. Adolesc. Health* **2012**, *50*, 24–29. [CrossRef] [PubMed]
51. Coskun, R.; Gundogan, K.; Baldane, S.; Guven, M.; Sungur, M. Refeeding hypophosphatemia: A potentially fatal danger in the intensive care unit. *Turk. J. Med. Sci.* **2014**, *44*, 369–374. [CrossRef]
52. Doig, G.S.; Simpson, F.; Heighes, P.T.; Bellomo, R.; Chesher, D.; Caterson, I.D.; Reade, M.C.; Harrigan, P.W. Restricted versus continued standard caloric intake during the management of refeeding syndrome in critically ill adults: A randomised, parallel-group, multicentre, single-blind controlled trial. *Lancet Respir. Med.* **2015**, *3*, 943–952. [CrossRef]
53. Whitelaw, M.; Gilbertson, H.; Lam, P.Y.; Sawyer, S.M. Does aggressive refeeding in hospitalized adolescents with anorexia nervosa result in increased hypophosphatemia? *J. Adolesc. Health* **2010**, *46*, 577–582. [CrossRef]
54. Luque, S.; Berenguer, N.; Mateu de Antonio, J.; Grau, S.; Morales-Molina, J.A. Patients at risk of malnutrition: Assessment of 11 cases of severe malnutrition with individualised total parenteral nutrition. *Farm. Hosp.* **2007**, *31*, 238–242. [CrossRef]
55. Manning, S.; Gilmour, M.; Weatherall, M.; Robinson, G.M. Refeeding syndrome is uncommon in alcoholics admitted to a hospital detoxification unit. *Intern. Med. J.* **2014**, *44*, 512–514. [CrossRef]

56. Gentile, M.G.; Pastorelli, P.; Ciceri, R.; Manna, G.M.; Collimedaglia, S. Specialized refeeding treatment for anorexia nervosa patients suffering from extreme undernutrition. *Clin. Nutr.* **2010**, *29*, 627–632. [CrossRef]
57. Chen, L.J.; Chen, H.L.; Bair, M.J.; Wu, C.H.; Lin, I.T.; Lee, Y.K.; Chu, C.H. Refeeding syndrome in Southeastern Taiwan: Our experience with 11 cases. *World J. Gastroenterol.* **2014**, *20*, 10525–10530. [CrossRef]
58. Golden, N.H.; Keane-Miller, C.; Sainani, K.L.; Kapphahn, C.J. Higher caloric intake in hospitalized adolescents with anorexia nervosa is associated with reduced length of stay and no increased rate of refeeding syndrome. *J. Adolesc. Health* **2013**, *53*, 573–578. [CrossRef] [PubMed]
59. Leclerc, A.; Turrini, T.; Sherwood, K.; Katzman, D.K. Evaluation of a nutrition rehabilitation protocol in hospitalized adolescents with restrictive eating disorders. *J. Adolesc. Health* **2013**, *53*, 585–589. [CrossRef] [PubMed]
60. Flesher, M.E.; Archer, K.A.; Leslie, B.D.; McCollom, R.A.; Martinka, G.P. Assessing the metabolic and clinical consequences of early enteral feeding in the malnourished patient. *J. Parenter. Enter. Nutr.* **2005**, *29*, 108–117. [CrossRef] [PubMed]
61. Henderson, S.; Boyce, F.; Sumukadas, D.; Witham, M.D. Changes in serum magnesium and phosphate in older hospitalised patients—Correlation with muscle strength and risk factors for refeeding syndrome. *J. Nutr. Health Aging* **2010**, *14*, 872–876. [CrossRef]
62. Winter, T.A.; O'Keefe, S.J.; Callanan, M.; Marks, T. The effect of severe undernutrition and subsequent refeeding on whole-body metabolism and protein synthesis in human subjects. *J. Parenter. Enter. Nutr.* **2005**, *29*, 221–228. [CrossRef]
63. Olthof, L.E.; Koekkoek, W.; van Setten, C.; Kars, J.C.N.; van Blokland, D.; van Zanten, A.R.H. Impact of caloric intake in critically ill patients with, and without, refeeding syndrome: A retrospective study. *Clin. Nutr.* **2018**, *37*, 1609–1617. [CrossRef]
64. Knochel, J.P. Hypophosphatemia. *Clin. Nephrol.* **1977**, *7*, 131–137.
65. Pantoja, F.; Fragkos, K.C.; Patel, P.S.; Keane, N.; Samaan, M.A.; Barnova, I.; Di Caro, S.; Mehta, S.J.; Rahman, F. Refeeding syndrome in adults receiving total parenteral nutrition: An audit of practice at a tertiary UK centre. *Clin. Nutr.* **2019**, *38*, 1457–1463. [CrossRef]
66. Walmsley, R.S. Refeeding syndrome: Screening, incidence, and treatment during parenteral nutrition. *J. Gastroenterol. Hepatol.* **2013**, *28* (Suppl. 4), 113–117. [CrossRef]
67. Hoppe, A.; Metler, M.; Berndt, T.J.; Knox, F.G.; Angielski, S. Effect of respiratory alkalosis on renal phosphate excretion. *Am. J. Physiol.* **1982**, *243*, F471–F475. [CrossRef]
68. Mostellar, M.E.; Tuttle, E.P., Jr. Effects of alkalosis on plasma concentration and urinary excretion of inorganic phosphate in man. *J. Clin. Investig.* **1964**, *43*, 138–149. [CrossRef] [PubMed]
69. Lobo, D.; Lewington, A.; Allison, S. *Basic Concepts of Fluid and Electrolyte Therapy*; Bibliomed. Medizinische Verlagsgesellschaft mbH: Melsungen, Germany, 2013.
70. Huang, C.L.; Kuo, E. Mechanism of hypokalemia in magnesium deficiency. *J. Am. Soc. Nephrol.* **2007**, *18*, 2649–2652. [CrossRef] [PubMed]
71. Md Ralib, A.; Mat Nor, M.B. Refeeding hypophosphataemia after enteral nutrition in a Malaysian intensive care unit: Risk factors and outcome. *Asia Pac. J. Clin. Nutr.* **2018**, *27*, 329–335. [PubMed]
72. Brannan, P.G.; Vergne-Marini, P.; Pak, C.Y.; Hull, A.R.; Fordtran, J.S. Magnesium absorption in the human small intestine. Results in normal subjects, patients with chronic renal disease, and patients with absorptive hypercalciuria. *J. Clin. Investig.* **1976**, *57*, 1412–1418. [CrossRef] [PubMed]
73. Gennari, F.J. Hypokalemia. *N. Engl. J. Med.* **1998**, *339*, 451–458. [CrossRef]
74. Marinella, M.A. Refeeding syndrome in cancer patients. *Int. J. Clin. Pract.* **2008**, *62*, 460–465. [CrossRef]
75. Thatte, L.; Oster, J.R.; Singer, I.; Bourgoignie, J.J.; Fishman, L.M.; Roos, B.A. Review of the literature: Severe hyperphosphatemia. *Am. J. Med. Sc.* **1995**, *310*, 167–174. [CrossRef]
76. Weisinger, J.R.; Bellorin-Font, E. Magnesium and phosphorus. *Lancet* **1998**, *352*, 391–396. [CrossRef]
77. Btaiche, I.F.; Khalidi, N. Metabolic complications of parenteral nutrition in adults, part 1. *Am. J. Health Syst. Pharm.* **2004**, *61*, 1938–1949. [CrossRef]
78. Heymsfield, S.B.; Bethel, R.A.; Ansley, J.D.; Gibbs, D.M.; Felner, J.M.; Nutter, D.O. Cardiac abnormalities in cachectic patients before and during nutritional repletion. *Am. Heart J.* **1978**, *95*, 584–594. [CrossRef]
79. Kohn, M.R.; Golden, N.H.; Shenker, I.R. Cardiac arrest and delirium: Presentations of the refeeding syndrome in severely malnourished adolescents with anorexia nervosa. *J. Adolesc. Health* **1998**, *22*, 239–243. [CrossRef]

80. Havala, T.; Shronts, E. Managing the complications associated with refeeding. *Nutr. Clin. Pract.* **1990**, *5*, 23–29. [CrossRef] [PubMed]
81. Patel, U.; Sriram, K. Acute respiratory failure due to refeeding syndrome and hypophosphatemia induced by hypocaloric enteral nutrition. *Nutrition* **2009**, *25*, 364–367. [CrossRef] [PubMed]
82. Weinsier, R.L.; Krumdieck, C.L. Death resulting from overzealous total parenteral nutrition: The refeeding syndrome revisited. *Am. J. Clin. Nutr.* **1981**, *34*, 393–399. [CrossRef]
83. De Filippo, E.; Marra, M.; Alfinito, F.; Di Guglielmo, M.L.; Majorano, P.; Cerciello, G.; De Caprio, C.; Contaldo, F.; Pasanisi, F. Hematological complications in anorexia nervosa. *Eur. J. Clin. Nutr.* **2016**, *70*, 1305–1308. [CrossRef]
84. Yawata, Y.; Hebbel, R.P.; Silvis, S.; Howe, R.; Jacob, H. Blood cell abnormalities complicating the hypophosphatemia of hyperalimentation: Erythrocyte and platelet ATP deficiency associated with hemolytic anemia and bleeding in hyperalimented dogs. *J. Lab. Clin. Med.* **1974**, *84*, 643–653.
85. Kheloufi, M.; Boulanger, C.M.; Codogno, P.; Rautou, P.E. Autosis occurs in the liver of patients with severe anorexia nervosa. *Hepatology* **2015**, *62*, 657–658. [CrossRef]
86. Giordano, F.; Arnone, S.; Santeusanio, F.; Pampanelli, S. Brief elevation of hepatic enzymes due to liver ischemia in anorexia nervosa. *Eat. Weight Disord.* **2010**, *15*, e294–e297. [CrossRef]
87. Bally, M.R.; Blaser Yildirim, P.Z.; Bounoure, L.; Gloy, V.L.; Mueller, B.; Briel, M.; Schuetz, P. Nutritional Support and Outcomes in Malnourished Medical Inpatients: A Systematic Review and Meta-analysis. *JAMA Intern. Med.* **2016**, *176*, 43–53. [CrossRef]
88. Elnenaei, M.O.; Alaghband-Zadeh, J.; Sherwood, R.; Awara, M.A.; Moniz, C.; le Roux, C.W. Leptin and insulin growth factor 1: Diagnostic markers of the refeeding syndrome and mortality. *Br. J. Nutr.* **2011**, *106*, 906–912. [CrossRef]
89. Alaei Shahmiri, F.; Soares, M.J.; Zhao, Y.; Sherriff, J. High-dose thiamine supplementation improves glucose tolerance in hyperglycemic individuals: A randomized, double-blind cross-over trial. *Eur. J. Nutr.* **2013**, *52*, 1821–1824. [CrossRef] [PubMed]
90. Francini-Pesenti, F.; Brocadello, F.; Manara, R.; Santelli, L.; Laroni, A.; Caregaro, L. Wernicke's syndrome during parenteral feeding: Not an unusual complication. *Nutrition* **2009**, *25*, 142–146. [CrossRef] [PubMed]

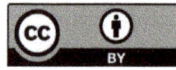

© 2019 by the authors. Licensee MDPI, Basel, Switzerland. This article is an open access article distributed under the terms and conditions of the Creative Commons Attribution (CC BY) license (http://creativecommons.org/licenses/by/4.0/).

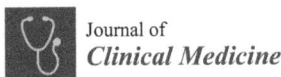

Review

Pharmaceutical Aspects of Artificial Nutrition

Emilie Reber [1,*], Markus Messerli [2], Zeno Stanga [1] and Stefan Mühlebach [3]

1. Department for Diabetes, Endocrinology, Nutritional Medicine and Metabolism, Bern University Hospital and University of Bern, 3010 Bern, Switzerland; zeno.stanga@insel.ch
2. Department of Pharmaceutical Sciences, Pharmaceutical Care Research Group, University of Basel, 4050 Basel, Switzerland; markus.messerli@unibas.ch
3. Department of Pharmaceutical Sciences, Division of Clinical Pharmacy & Epidemiology/Hospital Pharmacy, University of Basel, 4050 Basel, Switzerland; stefan.muehlebach@viforpharma.com
* Correspondence: emilie.reber@insel.ch

Received: 1 October 2019; Accepted: 15 November 2019; Published: 19 November 2019

Abstract: Artificial nutrition, including enteral (EN) and parenteral (PN) nutrition, is indicated whenever adequate oral nutrition fails to sufficiently supply the necessary nutrients to the body. It is a convenient, efficacious, safe, and well-tolerated form of clinical nutrition in the hospital and home setting. EN is administered via nasogastric tube or ostomies while PN usually requires a central venous access for administration, straight into the blood stream. The infused nutrients can then be taken up directly by the different organs. PN is targeted as a single daily portion formulated as an oil-in-water emulsion providing the necessary substrates for the catabolic and anabolic metabolism including macro- and micronutrients and fluids. PN has a complex pharmaceutical composition—all-in-one admixture—and its compounding or ready-to-use preparation. The use of PN is more challenging and more expensive compare to the use of EN, commercially available as ready-to-use formulations. EN and concomitant medication is highly challenging. Upon incorrect handling and administration, PN is associated with potentially severe or even fatal complications, mostly relating to the central venous access (e.g., catheter-related sepsis) or to a metabolic intolerance (e.g., hyperglycemia, refeeding syndrome) because of inappropriate administration. A correct order of admixing, correct dosing, and administration of the artificial is crucial for safety and efficacy; clinical and biochemical monitoring of the patient and treatment regimen adaption are necessary. The high number of reactive solutes allow only limited stability of a ready-to-use PN admixture. The potential for numerous incompatibilities and interactions renders PN admixtures generally unsuitable as drug vehicle. Laboratory compatibility and stability testing and pharmaceutical expertise are a prerequisite to define the PN composition including nutrients or even drugs admixed to define the appropriate and individualized nutrition and medication regimen. The aim of this narrative review is to present the actual state-of-the-art to deliver best quality artificial nutrition with special regard on pharmaceutical aspects such as instabilities, incompatibilities, and concomitant co-medication.

Keywords: parenteral nutrition; enteral nutrition; artificial nutrition; all-in-one parenteral admixture; compatibility; stability; pharmaceutical expertise; drug admixing; drug administration

1. Introduction

Enteral nutrition (EN) is used whenever the gastrointestinal tract is functioning and when oral access is impaired (e.g., chewing and/or swallowing issues). In patients with partial or total intestinal failure, nutrients may not or not be sufficiently absorbed from the intestine. Hence, parenteral nutrition (PN) has to be administered as a formulation, containing the necessary substrates, ready to be used in the intermediate metabolism. Intestinal failure may result from an extensive surgical bowel resection or a disease leading to reduced function of the intestine and/or impairment of motility, digestive or absorptive capacity (e.g., mesenteric infarction, laparoschisis, Morbus Hirschsprung). Table 1 shows recently published data from Pironi et al. regarding epidemiology of intestinal failure in 3239 patients across the world [1]. PN allows quantity- and quality-wise a full or partial nutritional support and can guarantee survival and good quality of life. EN and PN are the two forms of artificial nutrition, developed and introduced in the 1960s. EN and PN, or their combination, require an adapted and individualized nutrition regimen respecting the specific condition and requirements of the patient. Nowadays and in contrast to the early beginnings, EN and PN are mostly based on physico–chemically fully defined, balanced and stable products, manufactured in industry. While EN products can be delivered as stable ready-to-use formulations, total or partial PN has to be compounded or prepared ready-to-use for administration compliant with pharmaceutical good manufacturing practice (GMP) requirements. The available industrial PN premixes contain stable nutritional components mechanically separated from each other in chambers with breakable sealing. Upon ready-to-use preparation as all-in-one (AiO) admixture in a convenient, single container and for single line daily PN treatment, the sealing is mechanically broken and the content manually shaken. For safety and tolerance of administration of the usually hypertonic PN admixtures showing an osmolality exceeding 2000 mosm/kg, an inserted/implanted central intravenous access is required [2]. Consequently, PN and its prerequisites are more challenging, more expensive, and more prone for complications compared to EN. Nevertheless, a well-indicated PN according to existing guidelines shows good efficacy and safety in patients, also in long lasting home PN and if assisted by a nutrition support team (NST) [3–8].

Table 1. Epidemiologic data from 3239 patients with chronic intestinal failure in countries around the world, from Pironi et al. [1].

Type of Chronic Intestinal Failure	Underlying Disease
Benign chronic intestinal failure (n = 2919, 90.1%)	Crohn's disease (22.4%) Mesenteric ischemia (17.7%) Surgical complications (15.8%) Primary chronic intestinal pseudo-obstruction (9.7%) Post-radiation enteritis (7.3%) Others (21.3%, with <3% each-one) Not reported (5.9%)
Malignant chronic intestinal failure (n = 320, 9.9%)	Type of active cancer not specified (62%) Gastrointestinal cancer (28%) Extra-abdominal cancer (10%) Concurrent enteritis due to radio- or chemotherapy (5%) Peritoneal carcinomatosis (12%)

Databases such as PubMed and Cochrane were searched for guidelines, recommendations and registries, using filters for human studies in English only, and excluding children, as well as homepages from national and international nursing and nutritional societies. The aim of this narrative review is to present the actual state-of-the-art for artificial nutrition delivery with special regard on pharmaceutical aspects. This review aims to provide nutritionists dealing with artificial nutrition knowledge to deliver best quality PN, understanding of the concept and benefits of the AiO, and the pharmaceutical challenges of artificial nutrition (instabilities and incompatibilities, drug admixture).

2. Accesses for Artificial Nutrition

PN should be initiated at the latest after five to seven days of insufficient oral and/or enteral feeding. This may be initiated even earlier in case of severe malnutrition [5]. Preoperative PN and also EN have been for example been shown to improve surgical outcome in patients affected by Crohn's disease undergoing abdominal surgery [9,10]. The beneficial value of supplemental PN in critically ill patients has also been demonstrated in recent prospective studies [11]. EN may be administered via nasogastric tubes, nasojejunal tubes or percutaneous gastrostomy/jejunostomy (endoscopic or radiologic), Witzel fistulas or fine needle catheter jejunostomy, depending on the anticipated duration of the EN therapy and of the indication. The need for a central venous access for PN is obvious when for example calculating the individual daily requirements for electrolytes, which have to be contained in an AiO PN admixture. These alone increase the tonicity by more than 600–800 mosmol/kg, which is the maximal value for a peripherally administered intravenous infusion [5]. In long-term PN, tunneled subclavian or jugular catheters (e.g., Hickman catheters), implanted port systems or peripherally inserted central venous catheter (PICC) are used [6]. For short period of supplemental PN, the administration of peripheral PN admixtures through peripheral venous catheter is possible. Peripheral PN may be indicated for short-term use or as a supplement typically to maintain a previously well-nourished, patient or to serve as a bridge to centrally administered infusions or until adequate enteral feedings can be established [12,13]. The risk of microbial contamination and following growth is greater with peripheral PN than with PN, mainly due to the lower osmolarity in peripheral PN [14]. Moreover, the risk of phlebitis and extravasation is high and causes catheter removal [15].

3. Handling of Feeding Tubes and Catheters

The handling of feeding tubes is much less demanding than the catheter handling, as it does not require asepsis. It however largely depends on the type of tube. Regular dressing changes and slights moves of the tubes are however mandatory.

To minimize PN-associated complications, the appropriate central intravenous device has to be selected, placed, and inserted by a trained surgical team with experience. Together with good and regularly trained catheter handling, these are the two most important factors to keep the main intravenous access related complications in PN low. A rigorous aseptic technique is required for the manipulation and care of the catheters and the connections [2]. Blood drawing including aspiration through the central venous catheter has to be avoided. Suited trainings for patients and caregivers to learn the defined rules and best practices are essential and must be documented and evaluated [16]. Such education includes aseptic handling of the PN bag, of catheters, and its connections including also a rigorous handwashing procedure. Alcoholic chlorhexidine (0.5–2%) is recommended for skin disinfection; there are possible disinfectant alternatives in case of contraindications [2]. When a port system is used for PN, the giving set must be changed daily and in addition, the gripper needle has to be changed every three to seven days according to accepted standards. Evidence-based policies also apply for dressings of the exit sites [2]. The rinsing and plugging of the catheter with defined solutions are of critical importance and saline (0.9%) is the standard solution to be used. Heparin, initially recommended for port system rinsing, is still often used despite lacking appropriate compatibility documentation. Bozetti et al. showed a significant increase of catheter-related complication using heparin rinse compared to saline in HPN patients [17]. A recent Cochrane update analysis comparing saline against heparin for intermittent catheter locking in adults showed no evidence for a heparin benefit, as known from previous studies in children [18]. Heparin is prone to incompatibility reactions with many PN components, e.g., lipids, potentially leading to occlusion and/or infection of catheters. The use of heparin to rinse catheters lacks evidence regarding its effectiveness in reducing blood clotting. Moreover, it is prone to incompatibilities with lipids and emulsifiers from the PN admixtures. Even short and at low dose, heparin exposure in an intravenous line has shown emulsion cracking [19]. As a consequence of the cracking, lipid deposits form in catheters increasing risk for infectious complication and obstruction, possibly leading to catheter removal [6]. The potential risk to induce heparin hypersensitivity has also to be considered. In the actual PN guidelines, heparin is not more recommended for catheter rinsing and plugging [2,6,18]. A lock solution with taurolidine, a synthetic antimicrobial agent, might be considered in PN patients with repeated catheter-associated infections but should not be routinely used [20]. Other antibiotic lock solutions (vancomycin, gentamycin) are also used although the evidence for a preventing effect is low. Ethanol locks may be considered for secondary prevention in some cases. The use of in-line filters is not supported by the necessary evidence, similarly to heparin use or antibiotic prophylaxis [2]. Therefore, these methods are not considered as universal and compulsory preventive measures for all PN patients [5–7]. In-line filters may be used to (1) filter out precipitates or particles (reduce risk of embolism), (2) prevent pathogenic microorganisms to enter the bloodstream (reduce risk of infection), (3) hinder air to be infused into blood circulation (air embolization). In-line filters may however also create new problems [21]. They may themselves release particles or cause adsorption of nutrients or drugs reducing their systemic availability. In-line filters may thus also potentially be blocked and impair the PN administration. A fatality has even been associated with the use of in-line filters, as calcium phosphate precipitation occurred in the filtered admixture after warming up in the line [22]. There are no general recommendations for the use of in-line filters. German guidelines on PN settle beneficial effects of in-line filters in specific risk patient populations (e.g., children and immune-compromised patients) [23]. The ASPEN however recommends the use of 0.22 micron filter for lipid-free PN admixtures, and 1.2 micron filter for AiO admixtures [24]. The filter should be placed as close to the patient as possible and should be exchanged with each new PN container, as well as the administration set.

4. Complications of Enteral Nutrition

EN is generally efficient, safe and well tolerated. Small bore tubes made of more flexible materials, careful nursing and therapy monitoring contribute to decrease the complication rates. Risk factors for complications are among others neurological impairment, anatomical abnormalities, and advanced age [25]. Systematic antibiotic therapy before tube placement to prevent infectious complications (wounds and systemic infect) is controversially discussed. There is however good evidence for at-risk patients (e.g., immunocompromised patients) and placement of gastroscopic accesses [25]. Administration of a single dose of broad spectrum antibiotic half an hour before EN device placement has been shown to reduce peristomal infects by 22%. Complications rates vary according to the type of access, e.g., 0.3–15% for nasoenteric tubes, 1–4% for major and 13–40% for minor complications for endoscopic accesses. Complications rates are very low for surgical needle catheter jejeunostomies.

4.1. Gastrointestinal Complications

Gastrointestinal complications are frequent with enteral feeding [26]. Diarrhea may be the most common one, probably caused by adaption of the intestine after fasting period, by antibiotic therapy, or administration of too cold solutions. Delivery sites and rates influence may also influence the occurrence of diarrhea. Misplacement (too low) may be a further cause of diarrhea. Obstipation may also occur with enteral feeding solutions containing low or no dietary fibers, due to dehydration, immobility, or as a side effect of opiate therapy.

Nausea and vomiting may be due to tube dislocation, too fast administration or administration of too high volume. It may also be caused by the underlying disease or the related treatments, or due to medication containing sugar substitutes. Delayed gastric emptying and subsequent feeling of fullness are risk factor for aspiration and may also cause vomiting [25].

Reflux esophagitis and early dumping are further complications of EN.

4.2. Mechanical Complications

Feeding tubes may be misplaced, dislocate, or cause perforation (trachea or gastrointestinal tract), and nasal/gastrointestinal bleeding. Further, feeding tubes may be obstructed. Obstruction may be prevented by sufficient and consequent rinsing procedures, and by avoiding drug administration (as far as possible). There are various possibilities to re-open a tube, from warm water rinsing to rinsing with pancreatic enzymes and bicarbonate solutions. Feeding tubes may also cause irritation, and consecutive changes in the oral mucosa. Leaks or buried bumper syndrome may occur with PEG devices [25].

Aspiration is a rare complication (1–4%), causing fever and possibly pneumonia [25]. It may be silent or manifest with symptoms such as tachypnoea, tachycardia, and wheezing. Aspiration is however a great issue in critically ill patients [26]. It may be prevented elevating the head by 30–45° when lying [25].

4.3. Infectious Complications

Different infectious complications may occur during the EN therapy, such as pneumonia (arising from aspiration pneumonia), sinusitis, or bacterial contamination of the nutritional solution [26]. Some complications are related to the device, e.g., wound infection at the entry site with PEG devices and peritonitis with gastroenterostomies. Infections mostly require tube change/removal [25].

4.4. Metabolic Complication

The metabolic complications of the enteral nutrition are similar to the one of parenteral nutrition (e.g., the refeeding syndrome described in Section 5.3.1) but with much lower incidence and severity [25].

5. Complications of Parenteral Nutrition

5.1. Mechanical Complications

Catheters may sometimes dislocate or occlude, mainly due to incorrect manipulations. Reasons for catheter occlusions are manifold: PN admixture instabilities, incompatibilities with rinsing solutions and/or with other intravenous solutes administered through the catheter, etc. Taking blood samples through the central venous access must be prohibited since it is almost impossible to completely clear the line and the device afterwards. Moreover, blood samples from catheters often provide erroneous results because of residues of the PN in the catheters with high electrolyte or lipid concentrations. Blood clots may form and eventually mechanically occlude the catheter, being a possible origin of microbial colonization. Occluded catheters may be rinsed with saline solutions (10–20 mL) in a first step, applying slight pressure. If this is not successful, acidic or alkaline solutions may be applied according to defined procedures [2]. Reopening of occluded catheters is however discussed very controversially by the experts. It can be dangerous since clots may be microbially colonized. Blood stream infection may consecutively occur. Lipid deposits may be eliminated with ethanol or diluted sodium hydroxide. Thrombolytics are administered to eliminate an assumed blood clot [5,6]. Administration of PN with infusion pumps also helps to prevent catheter occlusions since the flow rate is kept constant [7].

5.2. Infectious Complications

In the beginning of PN history, infections and sepsis were frequent (affecting up to 40% of the patients) and thus a limitation to PN use [8]. By reducing the number of manipulations (e.g., AiO admixture administration), the incidence of catheter sepsis radically dropped (Table 1). Catheter-related sepsis occur at rates of 0.5–1 per catheter year in hospitals inpatients and 0.1–0.5 per catheter year in patients on home PN [5]. Gram-positive microbes (from the skin) are the mostly encountered microorganisms identified [2,27]. Catheter exit site-related or bloodstream infections are predominant complications and are associated with increased morbidity and mortality rates. Moreover, infectious complications contribute substantially to PN costs, causing additional hospitalizations and catheter removals.

5.3. Metabolic Complications

5.3.1. Refeeding Syndrome

The refeeding syndrome is a potentially life-threatening metabolic condition occurring in seriously malnourished patients or in patients recovering from severe catabolic diseases (e.g., sepsis, diabetic ketoacidosis) after start of a nutritional therapy. From a pathophysiological point of view, refeeding syndrome is an exaggerated response of the malnourished catabolic body to a nutritional therapy, indeed to anabolism [28,29]. Refeeding syndrome is characterized by severe electrolyte shifts (mainly hypophosphatemia, hypomagnesemia, and hypokalemia), vitamin deficiency (mainly thiamine), fluid overload and salt retention leading to organ dysfunction including cardiac arrhythmias up to death. Symptoms such as heart failure, peripheral edema and neurologic disorders can occur. The refeeding syndrome is most likely to appear within the first 72 h after initiation of the nutritional therapy. A risk stratification of patients before prior to start a nutritional intervention is recommended and can then by adapted according to the risk category [28,29]. Full energy requirements are targeted within five to ten days after initiation of the nutritional therapy depending on the risk category, starting at a low energy rate (5–15 kcal/kg/day) and increasing stepwise. Fluid management and sodium restriction may be necessary in patients belonging to higher risk categories. Thiamine (vitamin B1) has to be administrated as a 200–300 mg dose daily for three days, 30 min before the initiation of nutritional support. Finally, provision of trace elements and vitamins in the single and double recommended daily amounts of micronutrients, respectively, are recommended. Intensive clinical monitoring is mandatory to detect early signs of refeeding syndrome, such as organ failure and fluid overload. It should include vital signs, hydration status, and determinations of serum electrolyte levels.

5.3.2. Hyperglycemia

Hyperglycemia is another early and frequent complication affecting up to 50% of the patients upon PN initiation. Appropriate and initially frequent glycaemia testing is mandatory, since hyperglycemia has been linked with increased morbidity and mortality, especially in critically ill patients [30]. The targeted blood glucose level lies between 7.8 and 10.0 mM, (normoglycemia: 4.4–8.1 mM; 80–145 mg/100 mL) [31]. Insulin administration, optimally pump-assisted and in parallel to PN, may be necessary to control glycaemia (there is a dedicated specific article on this topic in this special issue [30]).

5.3.3. Liver-Associated Complications

Liver-associated PN complications are seen in up to 40% of the patients, especially in those with short bowel with less than 150 cm of remaining small intestine and in absence of colon (Table 2) [2]. In case of occurring liver-associated PN complications (e.g., hypertriglyceridemia, cholelithiasis, and cholestasis), it is recommended to administer PN formulations with reduced triglyceride (TG) content and a better fatty acids (FA) mix (e.g., by a higher monounsaturated FA (MUFA) content or an increased Ω-3 to Ω-6 ratio of the polyunsaturated FA (PUFA)) [2].

Table 2. Catheter- and parenteral nutrition (PN)-related complications [2].

Type	Rates Measures Per Catheter Year (95% Confidence Interval)
Catheter sepsis	0.34 (0.32–0.37)
Catheter occlusion	0.07 (0.06–0.08)
Central vein thrombosis	0.03 (0.02–0.03)
Liver/biliary issues	
Mild	0.42 (0.27–0.63)
Severe	0.02 (0.01–0.06)
Metabolic bone disease	0.05 (0.01–0.15)

5.3.4. Thrombosis

Central venous thrombosis is a common issue in PN patients with central venous access (up to 50% of PN patients) associated with high morbidity and mortality rates (Table 2). The localization is mostly proximal to the catheter. The frequency of thrombosis is linked to the experience and skills of the catheter insertion team as well as to the diameter of the catheter; small bore central venous catheters are therefore recommended. Low dose oral anticoagulants may be used in high-risk patients [6].

6. The Role of the Pharmacist and Specificities of Pharmaceutical Management

NSTs have multi-professional composition consisting of at least a physician, a specialized nurse, a dietician and a pharmacist, skilled to manage PN, and to deliver best nutritional support [16]. Pharmacists within the NST have an important role to play in selecting, preparing and instructing on the safe handling of nutritional products, especially PN. They have however also a clear role in optimizing medication for patients with EN (BN Group). Pharmacists provide medicinal products, care, and when necessary education and training related to artificial nutrition to the other NST members, to patients and their caregivers. Pharmacists are in charge for the logistic of the products and of their quality assurance. They check the drug and nutrients prescriptions from a pharmaceutical point of view, advising on the most effective and safe administration of drugs in order to prevent interactions and incompatibilities, in EN (administration via feeding tube) as well as in PN (admixture) [32]. Pharmacists are also in charge of the documentation and clarification of drug related adverse events, to increase treatment safety. Most patients on artificial nutrition also require drug treatment for their underlying diseases. This further complicates the overall treatment regimen aiming in given cases to combine the parenteral administration of nutrients and drugs, e.g., as the indication for (home) PN is extended to malignant chronic diseases or severe functional deficiency, often requiring additional complex medication in parallel to the artificial nutrition. This is a complicated endeavor, which needs a careful check of compatibility primarily respecting correct and suited dosing over time of both nutrition and medication to ensure safe and efficacious treatment requesting pharmaceutical skills [6,8,33]. Drug admixing issues are one of the main tasks of the pharmacist within the NST, who has to face and assess PN- and drug-related problems from the pharmaceutical perspective [32]. The pharmacist also contributes to define an appropriate nutritional and medical care plan, to avoid medication errors, and finally keeps responsibility that the right patient gets the right products administered in the right way [5,6,34].

7. Components of Artificial Nutrition

Standard commercial nutritional solutions for enteral use contain between 1 (isocaloric) and 2 kcal/mL (hypercaloric), with 15–20% proteins, 25–30% fats, and 50–60% carbohydrate, which represents a suitable macronutrients distribution for most patients. They may contain dietary fibers or not. Macromolecular and low-molecular weight solutions are available depending on the functionality of the gastrointestinal tract. Additionally, metabolically adapted solutions (e.g., high protein, low electrolyte content for kidney failure patients) or immunomodulating solutions (containing e.g., arginine or glutamine) are available. Organic amino acids (AA; protein), glucose (carbohydrate), different TG of FA (fat), and inorganic/organic electrolytes/nutrients together with water are the small molecular components of a PN [2]. Micronutrients, vitamins and trace elements have mostly to be added for a total PN as they are not necessarily included in industrial multi-chamber bags. Energy requirement in adults is 25–30 kcal/kg/day given as a mix of the most important universal fuel glucose and high caloric lipids. In contrast to EN, the AA content of PN is not calculated as energy as AA are primarily intended building components for protein synthesis which has to be considered when assessing the balance of EN and PN. The basic protein need in adults is 0.8–1 g/kg/day increasing to 1.2–1.5 g/kg/day in malnourished patients and even higher in special situations (e.g., 2.5 g/kg/day in burned patients or children). The energy need mainly depends the resting energy expenditure and on disease activity and severity (possibly increasing the requirements by 50%).

7.1. Amino Acids

In a severe catabolic state, glucose may be produced from AA over the formation of acetyl-CoA and through the Krebs cycle or over the pyruvate gluconeogenesis pathway (for glucose-dependent organs, e.g., brain), yielding in 1 g AA = 4 kcal. The protein (AA) breakdown may be estimated through the urine output, since nitrogen from the AA is eliminated as urea. One gram of urea contained in the urine matches 7.34 g of AA (0.47 g nitrogen). This calculation can be used for an intake-output estimate e.g., in well-monitored critically ill patients.

From the 21 AA, there are seven essential (isoleucine, leucine, lysine, methionine, phenylalanine, threonine, tryptophan, and valine) and four conditionally essential AA (histidine, tyrosine, cytosine, glutamine, and taurine). When AA show additional pharmacological effects, the term pharmaconutrition is used. This applies to glutamine, although the evidence for effectiveness is still debated. Commercial AA solutions for PN are traditionally crystalline solutions of L-AA (10%), despite differences between the manufacturers in the conditionally essential AA content (mainly glycine) [2]. AA in solutions are filled in airtight containers and protected by the antioxidant nitrogen gas, since oxygen oxidation (ambient air) is very likely to occur. AA and glucose put together in vitro can react and undergo Maillard reaction, which may influence their availability. Thus, a yellow to brownish colored product is then visible upon exposition to ambient conditions as e.g., beyond 24–48 h hanging time of ready-to-use AiO admixtures. The AA content in a daily dose of AiO PN admixture reaches 1.2–1.5 g/kg (100–150 g AA). In order to reverse catabolism (AA breakdown), AA should be administered together with fat/carbohydrates (mainly glucose). The suggested caloric intake is 20–27 kcal/g AA [5,7]. Optional admixtures of pharmaconutrients (e.g., 0.2 g glutamine/kg/day in trauma or burned patients) are dosed additionally to the necessary AA amount of the PN regimen and have to be taken into account in the nutrient balance.

7.2. Glucose

Around 66% of the body's energy fuel is normally provided by carbohydrates (1 g = 4 kcal), mainly by glucose, the primary and physiological energy substrate in the intermediate metabolism. It is prone to oxidative degradation when in solution. Some organs (e.g., blood and brain) fully depend on glucose for meet their energy requirements. Hence, mechanism such as gluconeogenesis ensures a minimal necessary glucose production (37 g/day) when external supply is insufficient or lacking and the restricted glycogen stores (150–300 g) empty [2]. Highly concentrated, hypertonic glucose solution is used to restrict the volume of an AiO PN admixtures and primarily contributing to their hyperosmolarity. Maximal infusion rate in adults is 3–6 g glucose/kg over 24 h. This rate is limiting the maximal infusion rate since the rate of glucose oxidation to pyruvate/acetyl-CoA/Krebs cycle in adults is limited to 5–7 mg/kg/min [2]. The level of blood glucose during PN has to be kept <10 mM and has to be regularly monitored, especially in the beginning of PN [31,35].

7.3. Lipids

Commercial intravenous lipid oil-in-water emulsions contain 100–200 g lipid/L [2]. The TG used are composed of different (PU)FA. The oil-in-water emulsion is stabilized with soya or egg yolk lecithin (12 g/L), a phosphatidylcholine with a negative surface charge resulting from the phosphate groups [36]. The surface charge is negative from the anionic phosphate moiety of the emulsifier at the surface of the oil droplets. This negative zeta potential keeps the emulsified oil droplets separated. The anionic charge of the phosphate lecithin moiety at the surface is critical for destabilizing incompatibilities, e.g., with (mainly polyvalent) cations. Intravenous lipid emulsions are nearly isotonic and contribute to decrease the osmolarity of an AiO PN admixture, e.g., in PN administered peripherally. Important to know, about 15 mmol phosphate are delivered from the emulsifier per liter of a commercial parenteral lipid emulsion [2]. TG are important energy fuels providing 9 kcal/g through the beta-oxidation of FA and the subsequent acetyl-CoA metabolism. Different FA types are contained in intravenous lipid emulsions, depending on the lipid sources. Nowadays, "structured lipids" are mostly being used, like SMOF lipids containing 30% soybean FA, 30% MCT, 25% olive oil FA, and 15% fish oil FA. Lipid emulsions dose in PN reaches 0.5–1.0 g/kg/day to cover about 33% of the patients' energy requirements. Lipids may be used to a higher extend in critically ill patients (up to 50%) to avoid insulin resistance issues [2]. Since they are partially essential FA, PUFAs must be included in AiO PN admixtures in the required doses. Ω-3 PUFAs like EPA (eicosatetraenoic acid) or DHA (docosahexaenoic acid) show anti-inflammatory effects through the synthesis of prostaglandins and leukotrienes and may be considered as pharmaconutrients. On the contrary, Ω-6 PUFAs shows pro-inflammatory effects forming arachidonic acid over the prostaglandins and leukotrienes pathways. Ω-9 MUFA have no action on these pathways and thus are neutral. Middle chain triglycerides (MCT) only contain non-essential saturated FA. They can be oxidized to produce energy directly in the mitochondria in absence of carnitine unlike long chain PUFAs. PUFAs are highly prone to peroxidation; resulting in toxic reaction products (e.g., radicals and aldehydes) contributing to the systemic inflammation and the oxidative stress of patients. Light and oxygen protection for storage and transport are therefore important to prevent peroxidation [37,38]. The oil droplet characteristics and distribution in the oil-in-water emulsion is a critical parameter. It should mimic the physiologic chylomicrons or lipoproteins with a critical upper diameter size of 5 μm correlating to a small blood vessel diameter. Larger droplets may eventually cause lipid embolism, while degradation products of lipid peroxidation may as radicals free cause DNA damages and contribute to inflammation [2,16].

7.4. Fluids and Electrolytes

Sufficient water and electrolytes doses have also to be provided by a nutrition regimen. Additional oral fluid or infusions to PN may be needed to reach the basic fluid requirements in adults of 30–40 mL/kg/day, but also to cover abnormal losses such as fever, vomiting, diarrhea, or stoma losses, burns and severe wounds [39]. The combination compatible amounts of (di- and trivalent) cations and anions in AiO admixture preventing instabilities e.g., by harmful precipitations of salts or deteriorated oil-in-water characteristics by interactions with the emulsifier is a pharmaceutical challenge.

7.5. Micronutrients

Daily administration of EN > 1500 mL covers the daily recommended micronutrients intake. Since most micronutrients are hydrophilic and body stores are limited, total PN must also cover vitamins and trace elements requirements from its initiation. Trace elements (polyvalent cations) show relevant and concentration-dependent physicochemical interactions e.g., with the oil-in-water emulsifier; they may also be catalyzers of chemical degradation processes (e.g., oxidation) [2]. This may become an issue since vitamins and trace elements are both infused into AiO PN bags. As an example, iron or copper catalyze the oxidation of the ascorbic acid (vitamin C), which then degrades within minutes. From an evidence-based standpoint, trace elements and vitamins should be administrated separately, e.g., trace elements admixed to the AA portion, and vitamins only given at the end of a PN administration limiting the exposure time of combined physical presence in the admixture [4–6].

7.6. The All-In-One Concept as the Pharmaceutical Formulation of Choice

PN is a complex, meta-stable, high quality pharmaceutical formulation defined by the pharmacopoeia. In presence of lipid, it represents an oil-in-water emulsion and contains various, partially ionized, reactive solutes, prone for physicochemical interactions. PN is highly concentrated (hypertonic) and its components are often close to their solubility limits as the volume is restricted [32]. A PN regimen has to be practicable and convenient, efficacious and safe, also upon long term use (home PN). Central venous access is needed for the administration and aseptic techniques are needed during ready-to-use preparation of industrial premixes or tailor-made compounding since PN has to be sterile and pyrogen-free [6]. Correct conditions for transport and storage and finally for the administration and hanging time are required to provide the right and ready to be metabolized amount of nutrients to fulfil the nutritional needs and to prevent and/or correct metabolic/physicochemical disturbances.

The PN composition and if needed its individualization has always been and is a challenge to ensure safety and optimal efficiency. The increased knowledge of disease and stress metabolism has contributed to diminish complications and to increase tolerance of PN [2]. Historically, PN started from the difficult to handle multi bottle to a convenient single container AiO system delivered as a ready-to-use complete daily portion enabling individualized, more physiologic and well-tolerated 24 h or cyclic co-administration of the nutrients (mostly overnight) [4,40].

Total PN admixtures and regimens contain over 50 individual solutes, mostly representing reactive species (Figure 1). This explains the stability issues and the important potential for physicochemical interactions such as degradation of components, generation of toxic products like reactive aldehydes from fatty acid degradation or harming precipitates formed from interacting electrolytes [2]. Additionally, a critically reduced homogeneity of the oil-in-water fat emulsion with eventual oiling out may cause serious adverse effects. The control and avoidance of microbial contamination are key issues to reduce infectious complications. Nowadays, pharmaceutical GMP rules are established and require for example to work in a laminar airflow bench for aseptic compounding/ready-to-use preparation. There are guidelines for correct labelling, storage, hanging time (24 h after ready to use preparation), transport and storage (2–8 °C) of AiO PN admixtures [4]. The combined admixing of potentially interacting or even incompatible microelements like trace elements with vitamins are still debated. Trace elements can catalyze oxidation and radical formation of e.g., vitamins [4,6] or of PUFA [37]. An acceptable, appropriately documented compromise has to be defined for the appropriate quality of the AiO admixture administered and the provision of the necessary amount of nutrients. Individualized compounding or ready-to-use preparation of a complete PN results in an AiO admixture, which cannot to be sterilized anymore by an established heating procedure [2]. Hence, in many countries, ready-to-use AiO PN has to be prepared according to the GMP rules and regulatory authorization is needed. There are however countries where extemporaneous parenteral nutrition preparations do not need any specific regulatory authorizations. The industrial approach with serial manufacturing targeted stable and storable PN products to overcome the stability issues of individually compounded AiO PN admixtures. This resulted in the development of different forms of special multi-chamber bags, separating the lipid emulsion, the AA and the glucose solutions from each other by mechanically separated chambers or compartments [2]. The bags materials are innovative multi-layered foils allowing vapor sterilization of the filled and sealed chambers representing AiO PN premixes which are with the additional air-tight wrapping including oxygen absorbing materials stable up to years as the main chemical destabilization by oxidative degradation of the nutrients is almost eliminated [40]. Ready-to-use preparation of these commercial AiO PN premixes includes mechanical breaking of the chamber sealing and manual shaking of the combined content still in a closed container envelop thus in aseptic conditions. Admixing of other needed components (electrolytes, micronutrients, or other intravenous supplements according to need and compatibility) into individual chambers require suited stability data, and defined and validated admixing procedures. The major part of PN adult patients can be treated with commercialized products. Therefore, PN treatment is sensibly facilitated. Nevertheless, individual PN compounding remains needed in selected patients, especially in children or neonates with their body growth requirements but also adults with home PN and/or after mesenteric infarction. However, such a service is available only in particular and experienced hospital pharmacies or compounding centers often also challenged for an appropriate logistic [2]. The evidence is still lacking whether an individualized tailor-made PN regime provides better outcome in neonates, acute critically ill patients or for patients in the home setting compared to a standardized commercial AiO PN. The debate concerning the individual energy, macro- and micronutrient requirements is still ongoing [41,42].

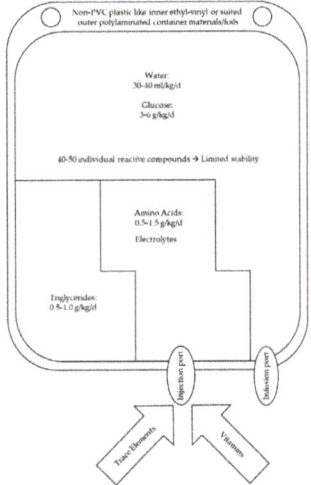

Figure 1. The all-in-one PN concept with adult nutrient requirement, adapted from [2].

8. Stability and Compatibility

Stability defines that the admixture components do not degrade in excess (e.g., <10%). Compatibility defines that these components do not physico–chemically interact with each other over a defined time. Stability and compatibility must last from compounding to delivery, up to the declared expiry date, and the administration under defined conditions. Both aspects are critical for the quality, efficacy and safety of the product [43] There are many physicochemical interactions occurring: instabilities (emulsion), solubility (precipitations), photo-induced (catalytic reactions), thermic reactions, material interactions (sorption, permeation), and chemical reactions (oxidation, reduction, hydrolysis, polymerization, decarboxylation, complexation, lipid peroxidation, Maillard reaction, etc.). A decrease in pH below 5.0 seriously compromises lipid emulsion stability. The first visible sign of decreased homogeneity of the oil-in-water emulsion is creaming (appearance of a white upper layer) [21]. Creaming is reversible by gentle mechanical shaking and occurs without a significant change in the mean particle size nor the particle size distribution. Such AiO PN admixture can be safely administered to the patient. The coalescence is the next deterioration step, which is not anymore reversible. Larger lipid droplets increasingly form over time and may be visible at the surface [21]. Coalescence may be measured by a light extinction method or validated microscopic analysis [44,45] Such emulsions should no more be administered to patients as they may induce adverse effects (e.g., inflammation from phagocytized fat globules, or embolism) [46]. The ultimate step of the on-going droplet enlargement is the emulsion breaking or cracking, where large fat globules separate from the dispersed oil-in-water phase [21]. Administration of such formulations is prohibited. These interactions occur between the components present in AiO PN admixture. They can become critical upon admixing and administration of higher amounts of electrolytes leading to precipitates when disrespecting the solubility product, which is influenced by specific conditions in the PN admixture (volume, pH, temperature, chelating components like AA for cations) [2]. Administration of parenterals containing precipitates may cause small vessels occlusion and consecutive organ damages, and may even become fatal when such precipitates are delivered e.g., into the lung [2]. Precipitates may as well occlude central venous catheter [2,16]. Critical concentrations of divalent cations (mainly Mg^{2+} and Ca^{2+}) in presence of inorganic phosphate lead to precipitation of insoluble phosphate salts. High requirements of such electrolytes exist in neonates but also in adults are incompatible in the amount needed since compatible concentrations for AiO PN admixture are overreached [2]. Such incompatibilities constitute medication errors and are preventable by careful expert proof and choice of appropriate formulations and dose of an individual AiO admixture by the pharmacist [34]. Replacing inorganic salts by organic ones may sometimes also prevent such insolubilities like organic (not hydrolyzed) glycerophosphates [6]. As a rule of thumb, monovalent (mainly Na^+ and K^+) and divalent (mainly Mg^{2+} and Ca^{2+}) cations concentrations in AiO admixtures should not exceed 130 mmol/L and 8 mmol/L, respectively (relative ratio of about 15 between mono- and divalent cations) [21,47].

Compatibility and stability of calcium and phosphate in PN admixtures depend on many factors, such as concentrations, pH, nature of the salts (inorganic or organic), presence/concentration of electrolytes, composition and concentration of the AA solution, lipid emulsion, mixing order, temperature, storage, and hanging time since admixing [21]. High concentrations of calcium and inorganic sodium or potassium phosphate (mono- or dibasic) salts show a greater risk of precipitation at room temperature due to the variation in solubility products at different pH (factor 60). The more acidic pH of peripheral PN admixtures (due to lower AA and/or glucose concentrations and increased lipid concentration) compared to central AiO PN admixtures (high osmolarity) also reduces calcium phosphate solubility [21]. Low infusion rates and room temperature, e.g., in PN admixtures for neonates, contribute to increase the risk of precipitation, eventually occurring during administration and consecutively causing severe organ damages, especially in the lungs. Calcium phosphate precipitation may also occur when iron dextran or bicarbonate are added to PN or infused through the same line without sufficient previous line rinsing [21]. Concentrations of organic calcium (e.g., gluconate) should not exceed 2.5 mmol/L in adult formulations with low osmolarity. Phosphate concentration (mono- and dibasic sodium phosphate salts) should not exceed 15 mmol/L [48]. Organic phosphate salts (e.g., glucoso-1-phosphate or glycerol phosphate) should be used in case of increased needs for calcium and phosphate (e.g., children or neonates). However, organic salts are prone to hydrolysis, possibly releasing highly incompatible inorganic phosphate [49].

Another critical reaction partner is the lipid emulsifier lecithin, a negatively charged natural, large molecular AiO PN component, important to control and stabilize the lipid droplet size, and their size distribution in intravenous formulations. Eventually, the stability of the emulsion is most decisive for the overall stability and safety of an individual AiO PN admixture. Polyvalent cations may react and neutralize the negatively charged phosphate moieties of lecithin at the lipid droplet surface (zeta potential) which is intended to hinder (reversible) aggregation of oil droplets (oil droplet agglomerates). Over time, agglomerates can further develop to irreversible oil droplet coalescence. The enlarged oil droplets (>5 µm diameter) are able to obstruct small blood vesicles (lipid embolism) [2]. Breaking apart of the emulsion and oiling out can occur, which has to be avoided strictly, whereas the initial oil droplet formation is potentially visible at the surface of an AiO PN admixture [2]. Their detection is challenging, and microscopic analysis might be a better approach [50]. Even though this microscopic technique is promising, it is not a recommended method to date. The United States pharmacopoeia recommends measuring the volume-weighted percent of fat droplets greater than 5 µm or PFAT5, must not exceed 0.05% of the total fat (PFAT5) [51] This measurement is usually performed by the manufacturer in an accredited laboratory and not in the daily analytical routine of hospital pharmacies [21]. Even small amounts of trace elements (µM concentration) or locally higher concentration upon admixing of components in a wrong order may influence the emulsion stability and safety. Solubilizers for lipophilic drugs used as vehicles in parenteral drug formulations when admixed or in contact with AiO PN may rise the emulsion stability. This negatively affects the lipid clearance in the body of administered TG from the AiO PN admixture since oil-in-water emulsion becomes meta-stable and thus resist to greater extent to enzymatic plasma lipid clearance [4].

8.1. Vitamin Stability

Some vitamins (e.g., vitamins A, B1, B2, B6, C and K) are chemically unstable and are easily oxidized with air and light. Vitamin A as a lipophilic compound may also interact with the PN container or the infusion set (absorption and/or adsorption). Vitamin B1 and B6 are unstable in presence of oxygen and in direct interaction with trace elements. Vitamin C is also easily degraded to oxalic acid reacting with calcium to form calcium oxalate precipitate [52]. Clinical deficiencies may occur due to such instabilities. Undesired degradation products (e.g., oxalate) may also be infused. Interactions between labile vitamins and PN components are manifold and therefore difficult to extrapolate in theory. Vitamins may only be added to PN AiO admixtures if specific and sufficient stability data are available. In best practice, vitamins should be added to AiO just before or at the very end of the PN administration [21]. This in order to reduce interaction time and eventual time-dependent degradation. Fat-soluble vitamins (A, D, E, K) can be added to lipid-containing AiO admixtures or into lipid infusions. They may be administered weekly or monthly (vitamin K) according to their storage in the body. Vitamins may be protected from light exposure and degradation by lipid emulsions, however, they are themselves prone to peroxidation. Light protection of AiO admixture containers containing vitamins is thus generally recommended during storage and administration [21]. Adding combined admixture of trace elements and vitamins hides high incompatibility potential (e.g., iron and vitamin C) and is therefore not recommended without specific stability data. Commercial multivitamin preparations can be safely administered as separate infusion or even as a slow bolus injection between daily administration of PN portions [53].

8.2. Trace Elements Compatibility

Copper cysteinate, iron phosphate, and formation of insoluble elemental selenium from selenite reduction with vitamin C are the best-known compatibility issues with trace elements [54]. Commercial trace elements solutions show very acidic pH (pH 2), which is critical for lipid stability. Emulsion stability and peroxidation are also negatively influenced by polyvalent cations (e.g., iron, copper, selenium, chrome and zinc) [38,49,55,56]. TG hydrolysis or admixing of trace elements may cause critical pH drop (below pH 5) hampering the emulsion stability. Trace elements should therefore never be added directly to lipid emulsion neither upon compounding nor in a multi-chamber bag. The pH of parenteral products may vary between manufacturers, making it difficult to extrapolate data from one brand to another. AA due to their pH buffering capacity may positively contribute to lipid emulsion stability. AA also have the ability to complex polyvalent cations like electrolytes or trace elements (chelation) avoiding bridging between negatively charged lipid droplets. During compounding or admixing, electrolytes and/or trace elements should therefore be added into the AA solution.

9. Artificial Nutrition and Drug Admixture

9.1. Drug Administration via Feeding Tube

Whenever drug administration occurs via a feeding tube, basic pharmaceutical questions arise to implement safe and efficient therapy: Can the tablet be crushed, or the capsule opened? How should a therapy plan ultimately be put into practice? Drug delivery via a feeding tube is an interprofessional challenge and requires special expertise from all involved stakeholders. Medical, nursing and pharmaceutical aspects have to be considered. The versatility of orally available drug formulations is large and includes specific forms with modified drug release or protective tablet coatings. Interactions between drugs, nutrients, and the human organism can lead to physicochemical reactions and pharmacological changes affecting treatment's efficacy and safety [57]. The prevention and handling of such interactions requires pharmaceutical advice and expertise. Incorrect administration of EN and/or medication due to improper handling must be considered as avoidable medication errors. While various international guidelines have been developed for the nutrition of patients, recommendations for the administration of drugs via feeding tubes are primarily based on empirical values [58]. Information on the accessibility of drugs to medications are not provided as standard information and therefore available only by means of extensive literature research. In 2012, Prohaska et al. found that information on the administration of antiretroviral drugs via feeding tube was only reported in 63% of the cases [59]. Significant problems may occur if drugs galenic is changed, e.g., when a tablet is crushed instead of swallowed. Fatalities have for example been reported after a retarded nifedipine preparation was repeatedly unduly crushed, and administered via feeding tube [60]. Enteral tubes are challenging for the caregivers, both during the hospital stay and after discharge. Resulting ambiguity in the care responsibility can endanger patient safety. Nowadays, tubes made of polyurethane or silicone should be used for EN. These materials guarantee a minimal foreign body sensation and good compatibility over a longer lying time. Polyvinyl chloride (PVC) should be used only for short periods because of the risk of pressure necrosis due to the washing out of the plasticizers [61,62]. Interactions between the tube material and the active ingredients of EN are common. PVC may for example retain relevant levels of carbamazepine, clonazepam, diazepam, phenytoin or tacrolimus, leading to treatment failure [63,64]. The position of the tube tip has a decisive influence on the release and absorption of active ingredients (pH stomach = 1–2, pH duodenum/jejunum = 7–8). Acid-sensitive drugs are destroyed in the acidic stomach environment. If a drug with an enteric coating is crushed and administered via a gastric tube, this leads to a loss of effect, since the drug is early degraded by the gastric acid. It is recommended to avoid administering medication through a jejunal or duodenal tube. In the case of jejunal feeding tube placement, the total amount of fluid used in drug administration should thus not exceed 50 mL. A time gap of 30 min should be kept between the individual bolus doses or the next application; otherwise, it can lead to diarrhea. It should further be taken into account that the tube tip does not have to be the site of the active ingredient intake, and that the passage time in the gastrointestinal tract differs significantly from the oral intake. Consequently, administration of drugs via feeding tube may result in a lower effectiveness or higher risk of side effects compared to the oral route. Blood/urine levels of drugs with narrow therapeutic range administered via a feeding tube should be regularly checked.

9.1.1. Administration of Drugs via Feeding Tube

From a methodical point of view, drug administration via feeding tube is challenging and offers the possibility of interprofessional medication review [65]. This is ideally be done before the final medication prescription, ensuring a safe and efficient administration. In the course of a visit on the ward or in the nursing home, the pharmacist clarify with the physician whether the patient really needs all prescribed drugs in his current situation. Any deprescribing relieves the patient and nursing staff, and reduces complications. Decision for the administration of drug via feeding tube is supported in a structured way as shown in Figure 2. The oral route should be preferred for the drug administration. The patient's ability to swallow has to be evaluated, and regularly promoted, as it may also depend on the form of the day. Depending on the patient's existing ability to swallow, solid dosage forms are replaced by sublingual, liquid, mouth-melting, or transdermal forms. If the patient can swallow liquids, medications should be offered in liquid form or as dispersible tablets (physiological route and less complication potential than via tube). Medicines in liquid dosage form are moreover uncomplicated to give over the tube than solid forms. Numerous interactions and reactions involving drug products, nutrients, and tube devices exist despite the use of solid drug formulation (lower reactivity compared to a dissolved drug delivery system).

Rectal, transdermal, nasal, sublingual or parenteral drug administration should be considered as alternatives to drug application via feeding tube [66]. If no alternative medication is available, an individualized formulation from the pharmacy may be considered. The tube system itself is equally crucial to further assessment. A PEG is more suitable for drug administration than a transnasal or a fine needle catheterized jejunostomy tube because of its brevity and width. The diameter and the location of the tip of the tube are just as important. The osmolality of enteral nutrition is on average 300 mosmol/kg and must not exceed 500–600 mosmol/kg. The stomach tolerates osmolality of up to 1000 mosmol/kg. Liquids with higher osmolality lead to diarrhea (due to a high volume of fluid and electrolyte that cannot be absorbed in the small intestine), nausea, flatulence (due to delayed gastric emptying), or vomiting. To prevent osmotic diarrhea or vomiting, drug formulations have to be diluted with water to isotonic or slightly hypertonic (<400–500 mosmol/kg) solutions to be given through the feeding tube. Even stricter isotonicity is required in case of small intestine tubes, due to the lack of dilution processes in the mouth, esophagus and stomach. Since the intestine, in contrast to the stomach has no storage function, no liquid amounts of more than 50 mL should be given as a bolus directly into the intestine. This significantly restricts the administration of several drugs with according tube position.

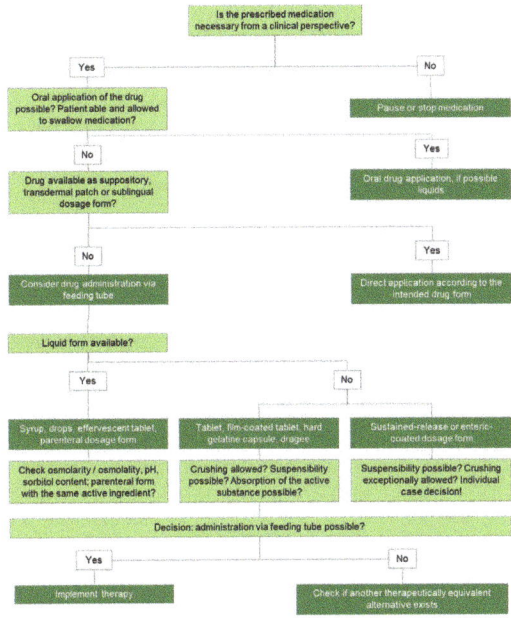

Figure 2. Algorithm for the evaluation of drug administration via feeding tube.

9.1.2. Safety Issues in the Administration of Drugs via Tube

The preparation and administration of carcinogenic, mutagenic drugs or drugs toxic to reproduction, so-called CMR drugs require special attention. Thus, the respective hazard risk handling with cytostatics, anti-infectives/virustatics, hormones, and immunosuppressants must be individually assessed. Work must then be carried out by trained staff, with the necessary protective measures (e.g., gloves, dust mask, protective googles). Patients' relatives and caregivers must be made aware of the relative risk potential. Pregnant or breastfeeding women have to be relieved of such activities. In addition, patients, relatives and caregivers must be informed about safer alternatives dosage forms as liquid dosage forms for example carry less risk than tablets that have to be divided or crushed. Open handling of CMR substances should always be avoided. Pharmacies having dedicated facilities may provide CMR drugs as capsules or pre-filled syringes to minimize drug exposure. The increasing number of oral cancer therapies on the drug market will lead to increased handling questions in the outpatient care.

9.2. Drug Admixture to PN

Extrapolation of AiO PN admixtures stability data from the literature is rarely possible because of the high number and concentration variabilities of components in an individual PN nutrition regimen (Table 3). This is even more complicated in case of drug admixing. The multitude and the concentration dependence of interactions create a multifactorial system not to be assessed by theoretical calculations only. Generation of pharmaceutical stability data may therefore be required for specific cases for documentation and reliability purposes. Sensitive and validated laboratory methods are available in tertiary care hospitals, which may be useful for components of an AiO PN admixtures and concomitant therapy but have to be adapted for the specific in vitro investigation. Such evaluation tools may help to assess the possibility to admix a specific item into a defined AiO PN composition or to check an individual nutrient and/or drug interaction upon request from the clinic in a reasonable and relative short time period [2]. Light microscopy may for example be applied to assess oil-in-water (oil droplet sizing) emulsions. Even though the admixing of drugs to AiO PN admixtures is not recommended, it may be needed in some cases. Compatibility and stability assessment of such combinations may be performed by means of defined drug analytic methods for quantification, adapted from blood plasma or serum to PN matrix [6,50]. Simple test methods have to be elaborated and validated to be used for stability and compatibility assessment of individual admixes to AiO PN regimens upon request [2,16,50].

Table 3. Advices to the possible drug admixture to AiO PN admixture.

Advice Not to Admix	<ul><li>lipophilic drugs with solubilizes such as cremophors, tweens, etc.</li><li>drugs with rapid chemical or physical instabilities</li><li>drugs with narrow therapeutic indices (cytotoxics, etc.)</li><li>macromolecular recombinant biotech drugs, (signaling proteins, monoclonal antibodies or fusion proteins)</li><li>synthetic non-biological complexes (nanomedicines)</li><li>drugs with short elimination half-lives and dosage intervals not adjusted to the PN administration period</li></ul>
Admixing May be Possible	<ul><li>stability documentation is sufficiently available</li><li>no ingredients with potential incompatibilities (CAVE polyvalent cations)</li><li>large therapeutic index drugs (analgesics, sedatives, H_2-antagonists, etc.)</li><li>simple stability testing is possible (pH, emulsion characterization and visual inspection)</li><li>well-established, often used, and physico–chemically fully characterized small-molecular drugs</li></ul>

The following points should be considered as good practice using concomitant parenteral drug therapy in PN patients [57,67]:

- Check if the medication is really needed.
- Ask for pharmaceutical advice, ideally from the nutrition support team when therapy regimen are complicated or when drug admixing to PN admixture is considered.
- Admix compatible drugs to PN only just before administration in order to minimize interactions.
- Document procedure, creating a database to control and reference drug-PN admixing interventions.
- If possible collect samples for later analysis and evaluation.
- Use alternative infusion lines (inclusive of other catheter lumen) for drug administration whenever possible. In absence of a separate line, intermittent intravenous drug administration in saline or glucose solutions may be considered. Sufficient catheter rinsing before and after drug administration is mandatory. Special attention is needed for metabolic adverse effects when stopping PN administration because of intermittent drug administration. Insulin stimulation induced by glucose infusion may for example be reduced by lowering the PN administration rates over the last half hour before stopping.

10. Monitoring of Artificial Nutrition

Regular, defined and appropriate assessment may help to avoid respectively decrease the metabolic complications of artificial nutrition. This should include the determination of (specific) individual nutrients, the monitoring and the course of the underlying disease and laboratory testing in addition to the routine clinical assessment. Specific laboratory tests of artificial nutrition-associated parameters include ([5–7]: Hematological testing, lipid status, liver and kidney function (especially in PN), glucose, sodium, potassium, calcium, magnesium, phosphate, CRP, and iron status. Monitoring of anthropometrics such as body weight, body mass index (BMI) and hydration status should as well be performed to ensure the metabolic tolerance of artificial nutrition. Extended and frequent monitoring is required at the initiation of PN for up to two months. Monitoring of long-term, clinically stable PN patients is recommended every 3 to 6 months [6].

11. Home Artificial Nutrition

Some patients require a long-term artificial nutrition, if possible performed in a home setting when no other hospital treatment is needed. The convenient and mostly nocturnal administration enables patients to have a nearly "normal" everyday life and in many cases to keep on working. Patients receiving home artificial nutrition show enhanced quality of life and better social integration [68]. Home artificial nutrition complications rates are lower than in hospital setting, possibly because of the highly trained aseptic handling skills and to the more stable health patients' situation [7]. Nevertheless, it should undergo regular supervision by NSTs and a reliable reporting on critical incidences or health problems has to be in place. European data show that home EN incidence is around 400 per million and home PN incidence around 5 per million people per year. These differences are most likely due to different healthcare systems and resources [3,5,68,69]. To draw conclusions how to better care these home artificial nutrition patients, national registries are necessary to improve and to benchmark the different national experiences [2].

12. Conclusions

The provision of artificial nutrition is a necessary when oral/enteral feeding is insufficient or impossible. With the development of artificial nutrition, administration of EN and mainly PN became convenient and safer, even possible in a home setting. Well-controlled procedures and steady monitoring of the patients by an experienced NST are key issues in the successful management of artificial nutrition, from the prescription (medical care) to through the validation (pharmaceutical care) to the implementation (nursing care) of the therapy. Proper handling, compounding and concomitant drug administration are of the highest relevance for therapeutic success and patient's safety, in EN as well as in PN therapy.

Author Contributions: Conceptualization, E.R. and S.M.; writing—Original draft preparation, E.R., M.M.; writing—Review and editing, Z.S. and S.M.

Funding: The APC was funded by the Research Found of the Department of Diabetes, Endocrinology, Nutritional medicine and Metabolism and in part by Nestlé Health Science (grant to the institution).

Conflicts of Interest: The authors declare no conflict of interest.

References

1. Pironi, L.; Steiger, E.; Brandt, C.; Joly, F.; Wanten, G.; Chambrier, C.; Aimasso, U.; Sasdelli, A.S.; Zeraschi, S.; Kelly, D.; et al. Home parenteral nutrition provision modalities for chronic intestinal failure in adult patients: An international survey. *Clin. Nutr.* **2019**. [CrossRef] [PubMed]
2. Mühlebach, S. Diets and Diet Therapy: Parenteral Nutrition. In *Encyclopedia of Food Security and Sustainablility (FOSS)*; Ferranti, P., Berry, E., Anderson, J., Eds.; Elsevier: Amsterdam, The Netherlands, 2019; pp. 131–142. [CrossRef]
3. National Collaborating Centre for Acute Care. *Nutrition Support in Adults Oral Nutrition Support, Enteral Tube Feeding and Parenteral Nutrition*; National Collaborating Centre for Acute Care: London, UK, 2006.
4. Mühlebach, S.; Driscoll, H.; Hardy, G. Pharmaceutical Aspects of Parenteral Nutrition Support. In *Basics in Clinical Nutrition*, 4th ed.; Sobotka, L., Ed.; Galen: Prague, Czech Republic, 2011; pp. 373–400.

5. Aeberhard, C.; Mühlebach, S. Parenteral Nutrition—Basics and Good Practice. *Aktuel Ernahr.* **2017**, *42*, 53–76. [CrossRef]
6. Bischoff, S.C.; Arends, J.; Dörje, F.; Engeser, P.; Hanke, G.; Köchling, K.; Leischkeret, A.H.; Mühlebach, S.; Schneider, A.; Seipt, A.; et al. S3-Leitlinie der Deutschen Gesellschaft für Ernährungsmedizin (DGEM) in Zusammenarbeit mit der GESKES und der AKE. *Aktuel Ernahrungsmed* **2013**, *38*, e101–e154. [CrossRef]
7. Wanten, G.; Calder, P.C.; Forbes, A. Managing adult patients who need home parenteral nutrition. *BMJ* **2011**, *342*, d1447. [CrossRef] [PubMed]
8. Dudrick, S.J. Early developments and clinical applications of total parenteral nutrition. *J. Parenter. Enter. Nutr.* **2003**, *27*, 291–299. [CrossRef]
9. Brennan, G.T.; Ha, I.; Hogan, C.; Nguyen, E.; Jamal, M.M.; Bechtold, M.L.; Nguyen, D.L. Does preoperative enteral or parenteral nutrition reduce postoperative complications in Crohn's disease patients: A meta-analysis. *Eur. J. Gastroenterol. Hepatol.* **2018**, *30*, 997–1002. [CrossRef]
10. Dreznik, Y.; Horesh, N.; Gutman, M.; Gravetz, A.; Amiel, I.; Jacobi, H.; Zmora, O.; Rosin, D. Preoperative Nutritional Optimization for Crohn's Disease Patients Can Improve Surgical Outcome. *Dig. Surg.* **2018**, *35*, 442–447. [CrossRef]
11. Heidegger, C.P.; Berger, M.M.; Graf, S.; Zingg, W.; Darmon, P.; Costanza, M.C.; Thibault, R.; Pichard, C. Optimisation of energy provision with supplemental parenteral nutrition in critically ill patients: A randomised controlled clinical trial. *Lancet* **2013**, *381*, 385–393. [CrossRef]
12. Anderson, A.D.; Palmer, D.; MacFie, J. Peripheral parenteral nutrition. *Br. J. Surg.* **2003**, *90*, 1048–1054. [CrossRef]
13. Gura, K.M. Is there still a role for peripheral parenteral nutrition? *Nutr. Clin. Pract.* **2009**, *24*, 709–717. [CrossRef]
14. Omotani, S.; Tani, K.; Nagai, K.; Hatsuda, Y.; Mukai, J.; Myotoku, M. Water Soluble Vitamins Enhance the Growth of Microorganisms in Peripheral Parenteral Nutrition Solutions. *Int. J. Med. Sci.* **2017**, *14*, 1213–1219. [CrossRef] [PubMed]
15. Sugrue, D.; Jarrell, A.S.; Kruer, R.; Davis, S.; Johnson, D.; Tsui, E.; Snyder, S.; Crow, J. Appropriateness of peripheral parenteral nutrition use in adult patients at an academic medical center. *Clin. Nutr. ESPEN* **2018**, *23*, 117–121. [CrossRef] [PubMed]
16. Hvas, C.L.; Farrer, K.; Donaldson, E.; Blackett, B.; Lloyd, H.; Forde, C.; Garside, G.; Paine, P.; Lal, S. Quality and safety impact on the provision of parenteral nutrition through introduction of a nutrition support team. *Eur. J. Clin. Nutr.* **2014**, *68*, 1294–1299. [CrossRef] [PubMed]
17. Bozzetti, F.; Mariani, L.; Bertinet, D.B.; Chiavenna, G.; Crose, N.; De Cicco, M.; Gigli, G.; Micklewright, A.; Moreno Villares, J.M.; Orban, A.; et al. Central venous catheter complications in 447 patients on home parenteral nutrition: An analysis of over 100.000 catheter days. *Clin. Nutr.* **2002**, *21*, 475–485. [CrossRef] [PubMed]
18. Lopez-Briz, E.; Ruiz Garcia, V.; Cabello, J.B.; Bort-Marti, S.; Carbonell Sanchis, R.; Burls, A. Heparin versus 0.9% sodium chloride locking for prevention of occlusion in central venous catheters in adults. *Cochrane Database Syst. Rev.* **2018**, *7*, Cd008462. [CrossRef] [PubMed]
19. Raupp, P.; von Kries, R.; Schmidt, E.; Pfahl, H.G.; Gunther, O. Incompatibility between fat emulsion and calcium plus heparin in parenteral nutrition of premature babies. *Lancet* **1988**, *1*, 700. [CrossRef]
20. Wouters, Y.; Theilla, M.; Singer, P.; Tribler, S.; Jeppesen, P.B.; Pironi, L.; Vinter-Jensen, L.; Rasmussen, H.H.; Rahman, F.; Wanten, G.J.A. Randomised clinical trial: 2% taurolidine versus 0.9% saline locking in patients on home parenteral nutrition. *Aliment. Pharmacol. Ther.* **2018**, *48*, 410–422. [CrossRef]
21. Muehlebach, S.; Driscoll, D.; Aeberhard, C.; Stanga, Z. Stability and compatibility of parenteral nutrition (PN) admixtures. In *Basics in Clinical Nutrition*, 5th ed.; Sobotka, L., Ed.; Galen: Prague, Czech Republic, 2019; pp. 354–361.
22. McKinnon, B.T. FDA safety alert: Hazards of precipitation associated with parenteral nutrition. *Nutr. Clin. Pract.* **1996**, *11*, 59–65. [CrossRef]
23. Jauch, K.W.; Schregel, W.; Stanga, Z.; Bischoff, S.C.; Brass, P.; Hartl, W.; Muehlebach, S.; Pscheidl, E.; Thul, P.; Volk, O. Access technique and its problems in parenteral nutrition—Guidelines on Parenteral Nutrition, Chapter 9. *GMS Ger. Med. Sci.* **2009**, *7*, Doc19. [CrossRef]

24. Ayers, P.; Adams, S.; Boullata, J.; Gervasio, J.; Holcombe, B.; Kraft, M.D.; Marshall, N.; Neal, A.; Sacks, G.; Seres, D.S. ASPEN parenteral nutrition safety consensus recommendations. *J. Parenter. Enter. Nutr.* **2014**, *38*, 296–333. [CrossRef]
25. Pirlich, M.; Bodoky, G.; Kent-Smith, L. Complications of enteral nutrition. In *Basics in Clinical Nutrition*, 5th ed.; Sobotka, L., Ed.; Galen: Prague, Czech Republic, 2019; pp. 319–323.
26. Montejo, J.C. Enteral nutrition-related gastrointestinal complications in critically ill patients: A multicenter study. The Nutritional and Metabolic Working Group of the Spanish Society of Intensive Care Medicine and Coronary Units. *Crit. Care Med.* **1999**, *27*, 1447–1453. [CrossRef] [PubMed]
27. Staun, M.; Pironi, L.; Bozzetti, F.; Baxter, J.; Forbes, A.; Joly, F.; Jeppesen, P.; Moreno, J.; Hebuterne, X.; Pertkiewicz, M.; et al. ESPEN Guidelines on Parenteral Nutrition: Home parenteral nutrition (HPN) in adult patients. *Clin. Nutr.* **2009**, *28*, 467–479. [CrossRef] [PubMed]
28. Aubry, E.; Friedli, N.; Schuetz, P.; Stanga, Z. Refeeding syndrome in the frail elderly population: Prevention, diagnosis and management. *Clin. Exp. Gastroenterol.* **2018**, *11*, 255–264. [CrossRef] [PubMed]
29. Friedli, N.; Stanga, Z.; Culkin, A.; Crook, M.; Laviano, A.; Sobotka, L.; Kressig, R.W.; Kondrup, J.; Mueller, B.; Schuetz, P. Management and prevention of refeeding syndrome in medical inpatients: An evidence-based and consensus-supported algorithm. *Nutrition* **2018**, *47*, 13–20. [CrossRef] [PubMed]
30. Laesser, C.; Cumming, P.; Reber, E.; Stanga, Z.; Muka, T.; Bally, L. Management of Glucose Control in Noncritically Ill, Hospitalized Patients Receiving Parenteral and/or Enteral Nutrition: A Systematic Review. *J. Clin. Med.* **2019**, *8*, 935. [CrossRef] [PubMed]
31. Umpierrez, G.E.; Hellman, R.; Korytkowski, M.T.; Kosiborod, M.; Maynard, G.A.; Montori, V.M.; Seley, J.J.; Van den Berghe, G. Management of hyperglycemia in hospitalized patients in non-critical care setting: An endocrine society clinical practice guideline. *J. Clin. Endocrinol. Metab.* **2012**, *97*, 16–38. [CrossRef] [PubMed]
32. Muehlebach, S.; Driscoll, D.F.; Hardy, G. How to prepare parenteral nutrition (PN) admixtures, and the role and function of the pharmacis. In *Basics in Clinical Nutrition*, 5th ed.; Sobotka, L., Ed.; Galen: Prague, Czech Republic, 2019; pp. 345–353.
33. Gales, B.J.; Riley, D.G. Improved total parenteral nutrition therapy management by a nutritional support team. *Hosp. Pharm.* **1994**, *29*, 469–470.
34. Taxis, K.; Barber, N. Ethnographic study of incidence and severity of intravenous drug errors. *BMJ* **2003**, *326*, 684. [CrossRef]
35. American Diabetes Association. 15. Diabetes Care in the Hospital: Standards of Medical Care in Diabetes-2019. *Diabetes Care* **2019**, *42*, S173–S181. [CrossRef]
36. Anez-Bustillos, L.; Dao, D.T.; Baker, M.A.; Fell, G.L.; Puder, M.; Gura, K.M. Intravenous Fat Emulsion Formulations for the Adult and Pediatric Patient: Understanding the Differences. *Nutr. Clin. Pract.* **2016**, *31*, 596–609. [CrossRef]
37. Steger, P.J.; Muhlebach, S.F. Lipid peroxidation of i.v. lipid emulsions in TPN bags: The influence of tocopherols. *Nutrition* **1998**, *14*, 179–185. [CrossRef]
38. Steger, P.J.; Muhlebach, S.F. Lipid peroxidation of intravenous lipid emulsions and all-in-one admixtures in total parenteral nutrition bags: The influence of trace elements. *J. Parenter. Enter. Nutr.* **2000**, *24*, 37–41. [CrossRef] [PubMed]
39. Lobo, D.; Lewington, A.; Allison, S. Basic Concepts of Fluid and Electrolyte Therapy. Available online: https://www.researchgate.net/publication/249625074_Basic_Concepts_of_Fluid_and_Electrolyte_Balance (accessed on 1 January 2013).
40. Muhlebach, S. Practical aspects of multichamber bags for total parenteral nutrition. *Curr. Opin. Clin. Nutr. Metab. Care* **2005**, *8*, 291–295. [CrossRef] [PubMed]
41. Evering, V.H.; Andriessen, P.; Duijsters, C.E.; Brogtrop, J.; Derijks, L.J. The Effect of Individualized Versus Standardized Parenteral Nutrition on Body Weight in Very Preterm Infants. *J. Clin. Med. Res.* **2017**, *9*, 339–344. [CrossRef]
42. Yailian, A.L.; Serre, C.; Fayard, J.; Faucon, M.; Thomare, P.; Filali, S.; Pivot, C.; Vetele, F.; Pirot, F.; Olivier, E. Production and stability study of a hospital parenteral nutrition solution for neonates. *J. Pharm. Anal.* **2019**, *9*, 83–90. [CrossRef]
43. Mühlebach, S. Incompatibility reactions in drug therapy–preventable medication errors. *Eur. Hosp. Pharm. J. Pract.* **2007**, *13*, 30–31.

44. Driscoll, D. Examination of selection of light-scattering and light-obscuration acceptance criteria for lipid injectable emulsions. *Pharm. Forum.* **2004**, *30*, 2244–2253.
45. Schmutz, C.W. Zubereitung Parenteraler Ernährungsmischungen in der Spitalapotheke: Untersuchungen zur Pharmazeutischen Qualität und Stabilität. Ph.D. Thesis, Universität Basel, Basel, Switzerland, 1993.
46. Washington, C. The stability of intravenous fat emulsions in total parenteral nutrition mixtures. *Int. J. Pharm.* **1990**, *66*, 1–21. [CrossRef]
47. Davis, S. The stability of fat emulsions for intravenous administration. In *Advances in Clinical Nutrition*; Springer: Berlin, Germany, 1983; pp. 213–239.
48. Newton, D.W.; Driscoll, D.F. Calcium and phosphate compatibility: Revisited again. *Am. J. Health Syst. Pharm.* **2008**, *65*, 73–80. [CrossRef]
49. Gräflein, C. Parenterale Ernährung mit Stabilitätsgeprüften, Modularen Standardlösungen in der Neonatologie. Ph.D. Thesis, Philosophisch-Naturwissenschaftliche Fakultät der Universität Basel, Basel, Switzerland, 2004.
50. Aeberhard, C.; Steuer, C.; Saxer, C.; Huber, A.; Stanga, Z.; Muhlebach, S. Physicochemical stability and compatibility testing of levetiracetam in all-in-one parenteral nutrition admixtures in daily practice. *Eur. J. Pharm. Sci.* **2017**, *96*, 449–455. [CrossRef]
51. Pharmacopea, U. Globule size distribution in lipid injectable emulsions. *U. S. Pharm. Rockv. MD US Pharm.* **2011**, *1*, 297–299.
52. Ribeiro, D.O.; Pinto, D.C.; Lima, L.M.; Volpato, N.M.; Cabral, L.M.; de Sousa, V.P. Chemical stability study of vitamins thiamine, riboflavin, pyridoxine and ascorbic acid in parenteral nutrition for neonatal use. *Nutr. J.* **2011**, *10*, 47. [CrossRef] [PubMed]
53. Muhlebach, S.; Franken, C.; Stanga, Z. Practical handling of AIO admixtures—Guidelines on Parenteral Nutrition, Chapter 10. *GMS Ger. Med. Sci.* **2009**, *7*, Doc18. [CrossRef] [PubMed]
54. Allwood, M.C.; Martin, H.; Greenwood, M.; Maunder, M. Precipitation of trace elements in parenteral nutrition mixtures. *Clin. Nutr.* **1998**, *17*, 223–226. [CrossRef]
55. Laborie, S.; Lavoie, J.C.; Pineault, M.; Chessex, P. Contribution of multivitamins, air, and light in the generation of peroxides in adult and neonatal parenteral nutrition solutions. *Ann. Pharmacother.* **2000**, *34*, 440–445. [CrossRef]
56. Allwood, M.C.; Kearney, C. Compatibility and stability of additives in parenteral nutrition admixtures. *Nutrition* **1998**, *14*, 697–706. [CrossRef]
57. Muehlebach, S.; Aeberhard, C.; Stanga, Z. Drugs and Nutritional Admixtures. In *Basics in Clinical Nutrition*; Sobotka, L., Ed.; Galen: Prague, Czech Republic, 2019; p. 362.
58. Volkert, D.; Beck, A.M.; Cederholm, T.; Cruz-Jentoft, A.; Goisser, S.; Hooper, L.; Kiesswetter, E.; Maggio, M.; Raynaud-Simon, A.; Sieber, C.C.; et al. ESPEN guideline on clinical nutrition and hydration in geriatrics. *Clin. Nutr.* **2019**, *38*, 10–47. [CrossRef]
59. Prohaska, E.S.; King, A.R. Administration of antiretroviral medication via enteral tubes. *Am. J. Health Syst. Pharm.* **2012**, *69*, 2140–2146. [CrossRef]
60. Schier, J.G.; Howland, M.A.; Hoffman, R.S.; Nelson, L.S. Fatality from administration of labetalol and crushed extended-release nifedipine. *Ann. Pharmacother.* **2003**, *37*, 1420–1423. [CrossRef]
61. Subotic, U.; Hannmann, T.; Kiss, M.; Brade, J.; Breitkopf, K.; Loff, S. Extraction of the plasticizers diethylhexylphthalate and polyadipate from polyvinylchloride nasogastric tubes through gastric juice and feeding solution. *J. Pediatr. Gastroenterol. Nutr.* **2007**, *44*, 71–76. [CrossRef]
62. Stein, J.; Dormann, A. Sonden-und Applikationstechniken. In *Praxishandbuch Klinische Ernährung und Infusionstherapie*; Springer: Berlin, Germany, 2003; pp. 291–310.
63. Treleano, A.; Wolz, G.; Brandsch, R.; Welle, F. Investigation into the sorption of nitroglycerin and diazepam into PVC tubes and alternative tube materials during application. *Int. J. Pharm.* **2009**, *369*, 30–37. [CrossRef] [PubMed]
64. Shibata, N.; Ikuno, Y.; Tsubakimoto, Y.; Hoshino, N.; Minouchi, T.; Yoshio, K.; Inoue, T.; Taga, T.; Ando, A.; Hodohara, K.; et al. Adsorption and pharmacokinetics of cyclosporin A in relation to mode of infusion in bone marrow transplant patients. *Bone Marrow Transplant.* **2000**, *25*, 633–638. [CrossRef] [PubMed]
65. Griese-Mammen, N.; Hersberger, K.E.; Messerli, M.; Leikola, S.; Horvat, N.; van Mil, J.W.F.; Kos, M. PCNE definition of medication review: Reaching agreement. *Int. J. Clin. Pharm.* **2018**, *40*, 1199–1208. [CrossRef] [PubMed]

66. Muehlebach, S.; Aeberhard, C.; Stanga, Z. Pharmaceutical aspects in enteral feeding and drugs. In *Basics in Clinical Nutrition*; Sobotka, L., Ed.; Galen: Prague, Czech Republic, 2019; p. 314.
67. Mühlebach, S. Basics in clinical nutrition: Drugs and nutritional admixtures. *E-SPEN Eur. E-J. Clin. Nutr. Metab.* **2009**, *3*, e134–e136. [CrossRef]
68. Bischoff, S.C.; Austin, P.; Boeykens, K.; Chourdakis, M.; Cuerda, C.; Jonkers-Schuitema, C.; Lichota, M.; Nyulasi, I.; Schneider, S.M.; Stanga, Z.; et al. ESPEN guideline on home enteral nutrition. *Clin. Nutr.* **2019**. [CrossRef] [PubMed]
69. Van Gossum, A.; Bakker, H.; De Francesco, A.; Ladefoged, K.; Leon-Sanz, M.; Messing, B.; Pironi, L.; Pertkiewicz, M.; Shaffer, J.; Thul, P.; et al. Home parenteral nutrition in adults: A multicentre survey in Europe in 1993. *Clin. Nutr.* **1996**, *15*, 53–59. [CrossRef]

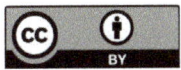

© 2019 by the authors. Licensee MDPI, Basel, Switzerland. This article is an open access article distributed under the terms and conditions of the Creative Commons Attribution (CC BY) license (http://creativecommons.org/licenses/by/4.0/).

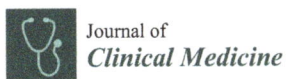

Review

Nutritional Challenges in Patients with Advanced Liver Cirrhosis

Jessica Stirnimann [1] and Guido Stirnimann [2,*]

[1] Division of Diabetology, Endocrinology, Nutritional Medicine and Metabolism, University Hospital Inselspital and University of Bern, 3010 Bern, Switzerland; jessica.stirnimann@insel.ch
[2] University Clinic for Visceral Surgery and Medicine, University Hospital Inselspital and University of Bern, 3010 Bern, Switzerland
* Correspondence: guido.stirnimann@dbmr.unibe.ch or guido.stirnimann@insel.ch; Tel.: +41-31-632-2111

Received: 24 September 2019; Accepted: 5 November 2019; Published: 9 November 2019

Abstract: Patients with advanced liver cirrhosis are at risk of malnutrition and nutrition-associated complications. Significant ascites, a frequent finding in these patients, has an especially negative impact on oral nutrition. A negative caloric and protein balance can further deteriorate the already impaired synthetic function of the cirrhotic liver. An important factor in this situation is the diminished capacity of glycogen production and storage in the cirrhotic liver and, consequently, a reduced tolerability for fasting episodes. These episodes are frequently observed in hospitalized patients, e.g., while waiting for investigations, interventions or surgery. A comprehensive work-up of patients with advanced liver cirrhosis should include not only a thorough assessment regarding nutritional deficits, but also a muscularity analysis to identify patients with sarcopenia. The overall nutritional treatment goal is to cover caloric deficits and assure a sufficiently high protein intake. Furthermore, vitamin and micronutrient deficiencies should be identified and corrective measures implemented where required. Ideally, optimal nutrition management can not only prevent the progression of malnutrition and sarcopenia in patients with advanced liver cirrhosis, but positively influence the evolution of the liver disease.

Keywords: cirrhosis; ascites; sarcopenia; sarcopenic obesity; nutrition; vitamins; micronutrients

1. Introduction

Liver cirrhosis is a common end stage of several liver diseases. The most prevalent aetiologies are chronic hepatitis B virus (HBV) and hepatitis C virus (HCV) infection, alcoholism, and nonalcoholic steatohepatitis [1]. As, with the introduction of direct acting antiviral therapy, HCV and HCV-related complications are rapidly declining, nonalcoholic steatohepatitis is now a growing burden of cirrhosis.

In patients with advanced liver cirrhosis, malnutrition and sarcopenia are not only related to alterations in the nutritional behavior, but also to changes in the GI-tract, the liver and the muscle. An increased protein loss, via the GI-tract, the kidneys or frequent paracenteses, can further aggravate the situation.

Patients with chronic advanced liver disease suffer from increased fatigue, nausea, bloating, and anorexia, which can result in a reduced food intake. In the presence of clinically relevant ascites, mechanical effects may further compromise nutrition by compression of the stomach, resulting in early satiety [2]. Inadequate appetite regulation and energy expenditure may be related to an elevation in bound leptin in patients with cirrhosis. Whereas free leptin correlates with fat mass in cirrhotic patients as well as in healthy controls, bound leptin was positively correlated with energy expenditure in patients with cirrhosis [3]. Increased serum concentrations of bound leptin could be associated with wasting in patients with liver cirrhosis, as has been shown in patients with symptomatic human immunodeficiency virus [4]. Furthermore, leptin is also a known contributor to fibrinogenesis in chronic liver disease [5]. Small bowel transit time is correlated with the severity of liver disease, and patients with decompensated cirrhosis or spontaneous bacterial peritonitis in the context of ascites have a slower transit time [6].

In patients with alcoholic cirrhosis, anorexia and irregular unbalanced nutrition uptake are common, and energy supply may be achieved through the consumption of alcohol rather than by a balanced food intake [7]. A low socioeconomic status is an additional risk factor for poor nutrition [2].

Dietary restrictions, e.g., an untasty, sodium-reduced diet, inadequate protein supply, or taste alterations, may further compromise the nutrition of patients with cirrhosis [2].

For the assessment of malnutrition and sarcopenia different tools, comprising clinical and laboratory parameters, physical assessments, image analysis and anthropometric measurements, are available. Clinical bedside assessments are easy to perform and inexpensive, but may lack precision in patients with advanced cirrhosis, especially if significant ascites is present. In contrast, muscularity analysis on cross-sectional images is precise but technically demanding and may require special software tools and trained personnel.

2. Comprehensive Assessment of Patients with Advanced Liver Cirrhosis

2.1. Malnutrition

To assess the nutritional status of patients, the subjective global assessment (SGA) is a well-established and widely used bedside tool. Patients are assigned to one of the three different risk categories: A (well nourished), B (mildly/moderately malnourished), and C (severely malnourished), based on five items that can be derived from the patient's history and three items that are based on clinical examinations. SGA is an independent predictor of outcome in liver transplant recipients [8,9]. However, especially in decompensated patients with ascites or peripheral fluid accumulation, the performance of SGA is limited [10].

2.2. Liver Function

Unfortunately, a simple test to assess the main dimensions of liver function (synthetic function, metabolic capacity and excretion function) does not exist. In the context of malnutrition, the synthetic function of the liver is of special interest. Albumin levels are frequently tested in patients with liver disease, and albumin is part of the widely used Child–Pugh–Turcotte (CPT) score to determine the stage of liver disease [11]. However, albumin levels do not solely reflect endogenous albumin production, but may also be low due to infection/inflammation, or an increased albumin loss or high in the case of albumin substitution, for instance, in patients that frequently require large volume paracenteses. In recent years, functional aspects, like the binding of lipopolisaccharides or other bacterial products and qualitative alterations (oxidation and glycation) of albumin, have been investigated in more detail. However, to date, it is not clear what the impact of these findings is [12].

Prealbumin (transthyretin) is an alternative parameter to assess the synthetic function in patients with liver cirrhosis. Prealbumin plasma levels decrease progressively from CPT stage A to C and correlate with galactose elimination capacity, a test to assess functional liver capacity [13]. A major advantage of this parameter compared to albumin is the fact that it is not influenced by exogenous albumin administration, a frequent treatment in patients with decompensated liver cirrhosis. The addition of prealbumin to the Model for End-stage Liver Disease (MELD) score improved outcome prediction in patients with decompensated liver cirrhosis [14], and prealbumin was a predictive factor regarding postoperative liver insufficiency and survival in CPT A patients with hepatocellular carcinoma-related surgery [15–17]. In clinical practice, prealbumin is an inexpensive and easy to determine functional liver parameter that helps to assess the synthetic liver function in cirrhotic patients. However, compared to albumin, the available evidence is limited in patients with liver cirrhosis.

Prothrombin time (PT) is the second parameter reflecting synthetic liver function that is an integral part of the CPT score (all coagulation factors, with the exception of factor VIII, are produced in the liver). However, production of coagulation factors may be preserved even in advanced cirrhosis and patients may still present with a normal or only slightly decreased PT in this situation. In contrast, patients with acute liver failure frequently have markedly decreased PT values.

2.3. Sarcopenia

Although sarcopenia is usually a visual diagnosis in malnourished patients with cirrhosis, diagnosis may be more challenging in obese patients, e.g., in patients with non-alcoholic fatty liver disease (NAFLD). To obtain an objective measure of sarcopenia, a quantitative analysis of the patient's muscularity should be performed.

The most-validated method to date is the muscle assessment on cross-sectional CT or MR images. Several methods have been proposed, e.g., area of the psoas muscle at the level of the 4th lumbar vertebra without and with normalization by height [18,19], the skeletal muscles index at the level of the 3rd lumbar vertebra (SMI) [19,20], or transversal psoas thickness at the level of the umbilicus [21]. Importantly, by using the SMI with the gender specific cut-offs (42 cm^2/m^2 for women and 50 cm^2/m^2 for men), muscle wasting was not limited to underweight patients, but could be detected in cirrhotic patients with a normal or even elevated BMI [20]. Regarding mortality risk in patients with cirrhosis, the skeletal muscle index (SMI) seems to be superior to the psoas index, especially in men with cirrhosis [22].

Special attention is required for patients with advanced liver cirrhosis who have a BMI >25 kg/m^2. Sarcopenia in obese patients is frequently overlooked, since it is less expected than in underweight or normal-weight patients with malnutrition. It is important to note that sarcopenic obesity, as well as myosteatosis, characterized by an increased proportion of muscular fat, are independent risk factors regarding long-term mortality [23].

Apart from simple measurements, like psoas muscle diameter, the assessment of cross-sectional image analysis is technically demanding and may require special image analysis software and trained personnel. Therefore, image analysis is mainly used in the context of clinical research projects.

In clinical practice, bio impedance analysis (BIA), dual-energy X-ray absorptiometry (DEXA) and anthropometric measurements are easier to perform. However, DEXA and BIA results may be altered in patients with significant ascites and general fluid overload, limiting their use in decompensated patients [24]. Restricting DEXA to the upper limb lean mass, and therefore excluding the body parts that are most prone to fluid overload, resulted in a good sarcopenia-related prediction of mortality in men with advanced cirrhosis [25]. Mid-arm muscle circumference (MAMC) measurement is easy to perform, but its relevance in clinical practice is limited [26].

Unfortunately, the most frequently used scores in patients with cirrhosis, CPT and MELD score [27], do not contain specific information about the nutritional status of a given patient. Therefore, new scores have been developed and evaluated, with a focus on outcome, in patients awaiting liver transplantation. The MELD-psoas score includes transversal psoas muscle thickness normalized by height at the level of the umbilicus. This score was significantly associated with mortality, especially in patients with refractory ascites [21].

The addition of the skeletal muscle index (SMI), as a measure of sarcopenia, to the MELD score resulted in an improved prediction of mortality in patients with cirrhosis [20,28]. Especially in low MELD patients on a liver transplant list, the inclusion of sarcopenia resulted in a better association with mortality [21].

2.4. Deficiencies of Vitamins and Micronutrients

2.4.1. Vitamin D

Vitamin D is synthesized in the skin from 7-dehydrocholesterol. An alternative source is food-derived vitamin D that is absorbed in the gastrointestinal tract with the help of bile acids. Vitamin D subsequently undergoes two hydroxylation steps, 25-hydroxylation in the liver and 1α-hydroxylation in the kidney. Whereas vitamin D is considered biologically inactive, 25-hydroxy(OH)-vitamin D is the main circulating metabolite. Conversion to 1,25-dihydroxy-vitamin D in the kidney increases the affinity for the vitamin D receptor (VDR).

The main purpose of vitamin D is the regulation of mineral and bone homeostasis. However, several other functions in different tissues (kidney, intestine, skin, immune cells and non-parenchymal hepatic cells) are known, too [29].

Vitamin D deficiency is common in liver cirrhosis. Whereas liver function correlates with vitamin D deficiency, aetiology of the liver disease seems to be of minor importance [30,31]. Decreased vitamin D levels are associated with an unfavorable outcome in patients with chronic advanced liver disease. The relative risk for hepatic decompensation and for mortality was 6.37 (95% confidence interval (CI) 1.75–23.2) and 4.31 (95% CI 1.38–13.5), respectively, for patients in the lowest OH-vitamin D level group, compared to patients in the highest OH-vitamin D level group [31].

2.4.2. Vitamin A

The liver is the organ where most (>90%) of the body vitamin A is stored. Plasma contains only a fraction (1%) of the total amount of vitamin A. While normal and high vitamin A concentrations do not show a linear correlation with liver vitamin A reserves, low retinol plasma levels do correlate [32]. In patients with chronic liver disease, vitamin A levels are frequently reduced, and the concentration progressively decreases with the progression of liver disease. Importantly, patients with hepatocellular carcinoma have the lowest levels, independent of the stage of liver disease [33]. While, in patients with CPT A cirrhosis, severe deficiency was absent, 52.8% of Child–Pugh C patients presented with a severe vitamin A deficiency (<0.35 µmol/L) [34]. It is important to note that chronic high dose supplementation over a period of several years has been associated with relevant liver damage [35].

2.4.3. Zinc

Zinc deficiency is a common finding in patients with advanced chronic liver disease. Reasons for low zinc levels are inadequate dietary intake and an increased zinc loss in the urine that is related to severe muscle catabolism, diuretic therapy in patients with cirrhosis and ascites [36], alcohol-induced impaired absorption, and changes in the protein and amino acid metabolism. Furthermore, endotoxins and cytokines (IL6) may play a role [37].

Since the liver is the key organ in the metabolism of zinc, liver disease can affect zinc levels and, vice versa, zinc deficiency can affect the liver. Reduced zinc levels can have a negative impact on several liver functions and impair the regeneration capacity of the liver. However, independent of the stage of cirrhosis, zinc stores in in liver, bone and muscle can be replenished over the course of six or more months [37]. In patients with cirrhosis, supplementation of zinc in combination with branched-chain amino acids (BCAA) for six months with [38] and without [39] hepatic encephalopathy has demonstrated a positive effect on blood ammonia levels. However, an increase in albumin could be demonstrated only in one of the two studies [38].

2.4.4. Selenium

The essential micronutrient selenium is incorporated in at least 25 selenoproteins. Deficiency of selenium can be found in some patients with advanced chronic liver disease. In addition to a nutritional deficit, reduced selenium levels may reflect an impaired metabolism of selenomethionine to selenide in the liver. In a study by Burk et al., selenoprotein P, a protein that is mainly formed in the liver and that transports selenium to extrahepatic tissues, was reduced in parallel with the severity of the liver disease [40].

2.5. Bone Disease

Osteopenia and osteoporosis are common findings in patients with cirrhosis, with a prevalence of up to 68% for osteopenia and a range from 11% to 55% for osteoporosis [41]. Consequently, fractures are common in patients with chronic liver disease, and occur in up to 40% of patients with cirrhosis [42].

The pathophysiology is complex and, in addition to an altered vitamin D and calcium metabolism, other factors may be important. Hypogonadism is associated with an increased osteoclast activity, leading to accelerated bone loss. An excess of unconjugated bilirubin negatively affects the differentiation of primary osteoblasts into their primary function. Chronic glucocorticoid therapy in patients with autoimmune hepatitis is associated with osteoporosis, and environmental factors, such as chronic alcohol consumption, smoking, low BMI, sedentary lifestyle and poor nutrition have an additional negative effect on bone turnover [43].

Screening for osteopenia and osteoporosis should be considered in all patients suffering from liver cirrhosis, and be part of the standard procedure in patients that are evaluated for liver transplantation. A timely diagnosis is important to prevent fractures as typical osteoporosis-related complications. Bone mineral density screening should be repeated on a yearly basis in patients with cholestatic liver disease and/or multiple risk factors and every two to three years in other patients with liver cirrhosis [41].

3. Therapeutic Approach to Treat Nutritional Deficits

3.1. Caloric, Protein and Lipid Supplementation

In patients with advanced cirrhosis, nutrition is of paramount importance. A nutritional assessment should be performed on a regular basis and corrective measures implemented as soon as a deficit is observed. If available, a clinical nutrition specialist should perform the nutritional assessment. The aim is to identify daily deficits and to define daily nutritional requirements. This assessment should include caloric and protein intake as well as vitamins and micronutrients.

In patients with cirrhosis, a daily intake of 30–35 kcal and of 1.2 to 1.5 g protein per kg body weight (BW) is recommended [44,45]. In obese patients with liver cirrhosis, a moderately hypocaloric diet (−500–800 kcal/d), respectively a reduced daily caloric intake of 20–25 kcal/kg BW, should be combined with an increase in protein intake (>1.5 g, up to 2.5 g/kg BW) [44–46], Table 1.

Regarding lipids, no specific recommendations are provided in the guidelines for patients with liver cirrhosis [44,45]. Compared to the glucose and protein metabolism, alterations in the lipid metabolism seem to be of minor importance in patients with liver cirrhosis. This is illustrated by the finding that the elimination of lipid emulsions containing long-chain or long-chain and medium-chain triglycerides, and the release of free fatty acids thereof were not altered in patients with chronic hepatic failure compared to healthy controls [47,48].

Table 1. Nutrition management in patients with advanced liver cirrhosis.

	Cirrhosis with Malnutrition	Cirrhosis with Sarcopenic Obesity
Caloric intake	30–35 kcal/kg BW	20–25 kcal/kg BW
Protein intake	1.2 to 1.5 g/kg BW	>1.5 g, up to 2.5 g/kg BW
Lipid intake	No specific recommendation	No specific recommendation
Vitamins		
Vitamin A *	Supplement if decreased	Supplement if decreased
Vitamin D	Supplement if decreased	Supplement if decreased
Micronutrients		
Zinc	Supplement if decreased	Supplement if decreased
Selenium	Supplement if decreased	Supplement if decreased

BW: body weight. * avoid oversubstitution.

Ideally, the nutritional goals can be achieved by regular meals, if required, by reducing the size and increasing the frequency of meals. A late evening snack is recommended to compensate for the reduced glycogen production and storage, and to prevent muscle proteolysis in patients with advanced cirrhosis [49]. The snack should comprise at least 50 g of complex carbohydrates [46]. If required, protein-enriched oral drinks can be added.

In patients that cannot achieve the nutritional goals with oral substitution, placement of an enteral tube should be considered. The presence of non-bleeding esophageal varices is not a contraindication for enteral tube feeding [44,45]. In contrast, a percutaneous enteral gastrostomy (PEG) is associated with an elevated risk of complications, especially bleeding, and is therefore not recommended in patients with chronic advanced liver disease [44,45].

Periods of prolonged fasting should be avoided whenever possible. Risk situations are prolonged waiting time for interventions or surgery, and situations in which a patient is temporarily not able to maintain oral nutrition, e.g., during a stay in the intensive care unit. If oral or enteral feeding is not possible, parenteral nutrition should be considered early [44,45], Figure 1.

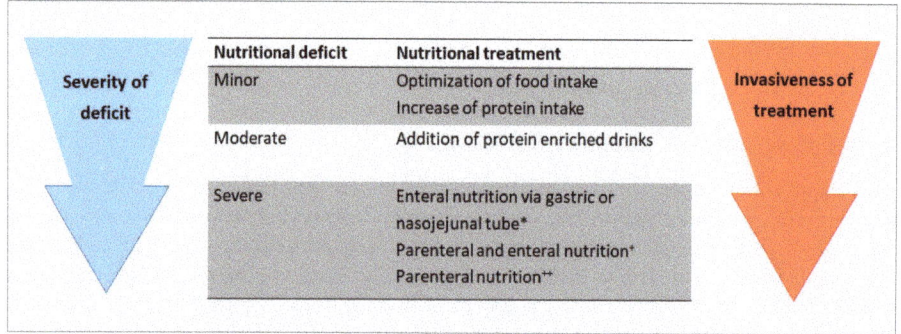

Figure 1. Nutrition management in malnourished patients with liver cirrhosis. * Non-bleeding esophageal varices are not a contraindication for enteral tube feeding, + if enteral nutrition is insufficient, ++ if enteral nutrition is not possible.

In patients with liver cirrhosis, restriction of protein intake is not indicated [44,45], since this promotes muscle proteolysis [50] and increased the risk of mortality on the waiting list for liver transplants [51]. Intolerance of mixed proteins with consecutive development of hepatic encephalopathy is very rare. In this specific situation, a diet with vegetable proteins may be beneficial [44], since vegetable proteins are rich in BCAA compared to animal proteins, and BCAA remove one mole of ammonia per mole of BCAA [52]. Alternatively, BCAA or leucine-enriched BCAA supplementation can be considered, the latter showing a stimulatory, and therefore beneficial, effect on mTORC1 in the skeletal muscle of patients with alcoholic liver cirrhosis [53]. After an episode of overt hepatic encephalopathy, BCAA supplementation improved muscle mass and minimal HE, but did not decrease recurrence of overt hepatic encephalopathy [45,54].

3.2. Albumin

From a nutritionist point of view, there is no indication for the substitution of albumin in patients with liver cirrhosis. However, albumin is used in patients with refractory ascites to prevent the circulatory dysfunction syndrome following paracentesis, in the setting of hepatorenal syndrome and in case of infection, especially spontaneous bacterial peritonitis (SBP) [55]. Whether long-term albumin infusions have a significant effect on morbidity and mortality in patients with advanced liver cirrhosis is currently being debated. In the ANSWER study, patients receiving albumin on a weekly basis had a lower mortality and complication rate than patients in the placebo group [56]. However, there were some concerns regarding the methodology of this trial (open label study, different management of the two treatment arms). No effect on the complication rate in patients with cirrhosis awaiting liver transplantation was found in the MACHT trial, that investigated the addition of midodrine and albumin to the standard of care treatment [57].

3.3. Vitamins and Micronutrients

Vitamin D has a broad impact not only on bone metabolism, but also on several hepatic cells and functions. Therefore, supplementation in case of reduced levels (<20 ng/mL) is indicated to prevent the risk of fractures that is increased in patients with cirrhosis [42], and to maintain Vitamin D related liver functions. A level of >30 ng/mL should be the therapeutic target [58,59].

For vitamin A, there is no generally accepted opinion regarding supplementation. Due to the negative effect on the liver in case of long-term high-dose substitution (>40,000 IU per day), some authors recommend against supplementation of vitamin A [34]. Taking into account the linear relationship between low serum retinol and vitamin A storage, and the association of HCC with very low vitamin A levels [33], low level substitution for a limited period of time in case of reduced vitamin A levels can be considered.

Zinc deficiency is frequent in patients with chronic liver disease and has been associated with insulin resistance, hepatic steatosis, iron overload and hepatic encephalopathy. Consequently, zinc levels should be measured in patients with cirrhosis and zinc supplemented in case of reduced levels [37,60].

Since cirrhosis causes functional selenium deficit in some patients, and, taking into account that the prevalence of selenium deficit rises with the severity of cirrhosis, supplementation in case of a confirmed deficit can be considered. However, to date, data regarding positive or negative effects of selenium substitution in patients with advanced liver cirrhosis are missing and, consequently, no general recommendation is possible. If selenium is supplemented, selenite and not selenomethionine should be prescribed, due to the altered metabolism in patients with cirrhosis [61].

3.4. General Management

Patients with malnutrition and sarcopenia should be followed on a regular basis by a clinical nutrition specialist, and nutritional status as well as measures to correct malnutrition and sarcopenia should be periodically reassessed. Furthermore, nutritional aspects should be integrated in the assessment and the clinical decision-making process by the multidisciplinary medical team treating patients with advanced chronic liver disease.

4. Conclusions

Patients with advanced liver cirrhosis are prone to malnutrition. Reasons for malnutrition are a reduced intake of food and especially proteins, a decreased synthetic function of the liver, impaired glycogen production and storage, proteolysis in the muscle, and loss of proteins via paracenteses, the kidneys or the GI tract.

A comprehensive management of patients with advanced chronic liver disease should aim at the identification of malnutrition in general and selective nutritional deficits in particular. Due to ascites and general fluid overload, body weight and body mass index may be misleading in cirrhotic patients, and a more in-depth analysis of body composition and function is indicated. SGA is an easy to perform nutritional assessment in patients with liver cirrhosis. However, in overweight and obese patients, its performance is limited, due to a weak concordance with sarcopenia [10].

Sarcopenia, a common complication in patients with advanced liver cirrhosis, is at least partially the consequence of malnutrition. Ideally, it can be diagnosed from cross-sectional abdominal images. Sarcopenic obese patients need special attention, since nutritional and muscularity deficits may be overlooked.

Treatment of patients with advanced liver cirrhosis should be comprehensive and address the individual patients' caloric and protein requirements, as well as the correction of vitamin and micronutrient deficits. Whether continuous administration of albumin is helpful in malnourished cirrhotic patients is currently not clear, since study results are discordant.

There is certainly a need for more randomized studies, to better assess the effect of a comprehensive nutritional management on mortality and morbidity, and, in particular, on the evolution of sarcopenia and other cirrhosis-associated complications.

Author Contributions: Conceptualization, J.S. and G.S.; methodology, J.S and G.S.; writing—original draft preparation, J.S. and G.S.; writing—review and editing, J.S. and G.S.

Conflicts of Interest: The authors declare no conflict of interest.

References

1. Ge, P.S.; Runyon, B.A. Treatment of Patients with Cirrhosis. *N. Engl. J. Med.* **2016**, *375*, 767–777. [CrossRef] [PubMed]
2. Cheung, K.; Lee, S.S.; Raman, M. Prevalence and mechanisms of malnutrition in patients with advanced liver disease, and nutrition management strategies. *Clin. Gastroenterol. Hepatol.* **2012**, *10*, 117–125. [CrossRef] [PubMed]
3. Ockenga, J.; Bischoff, S.C.; Tillmann, H.L.; Rifai, K.; Widjaja, A.; Boker, K.H.; Manns, M.P.; Brabant, G. Elevated bound leptin correlates with energy expenditure in cirrhotics. *Gastroenterology* **2000**, *119*, 1656–1662. [CrossRef] [PubMed]
4. Ockenga, J.; Widjaja, A.; Holtmannspotter, M.; Schmidt, R.E.; Brabant, G. Bound leptin is regulated by tumour necrosis factor-alpha in HIV-infected patients: A potential mediator of wasting? *AIDS* **1998**, *12*, 2233–2235.
5. Buechler, C.; Haberl, E.M.; Rein-Fischboeck, L.; Aslanidis, C. Adipokines in Liver Cirrhosis. *Int. J. Mol. Sci.* **2017**, *18*, 1392. [CrossRef]
6. Chander Roland, B.; Garcia-Tsao, G.; Ciarleglio, M.M.; Deng, Y.; Sheth, A. Decompensated cirrhotics have slower intestinal transit times as compared with compensated cirrhotics and healthy controls. *J. Clin. Gastroenterol.* **2013**, *47*, 888–893. [CrossRef]
7. Bergheim, I.; Parlesak, A.; Dierks, C.; Bode, J.C.; Bode, C. Nutritional deficiencies in German middle-class male alcohol consumers: Relation to dietary intake and severity of liver disease. *Eur. J. Clin. Nutr.* **2003**, *57*, 431–438. [CrossRef]
8. Merli, M.; Giusto, M.; Gentili, F.; Novelli, G.; Ferretti, G.; Riggio, O.; Corradini, S.G.; Siciliano, M.; Farcomeni, A.; Attili, A.F.; et al. Nutritional status: Its influence on the outcome of patients undergoing liver transplantation. *Liver Int.* **2010**, *30*, 208–214. [CrossRef]
9. Stephenson, G.R.; Moretti, E.W.; El-Moalem, H.; Clavien, P.A.; Tuttle-Newhall, J.E. Malnutrition in liver transplant patients: Preoperative subjective global assessment is predictive of outcome after liver transplantation. *Transplantation* **2001**, *72*, 666–670. [CrossRef]
10. Moctezuma-Velazquez, C.; Ebadi, M.; Bhanji, R.A.; Stirnimann, G.; Tandon, P.; Montano-Loza, A.J. Limited performance of subjective global assessment compared to computed tomography-determined sarcopenia in predicting adverse clinical outcomes in patients with cirrhosis. *Clin. Nutr.* **2018**. [CrossRef]
11. Child, C.G.; Turcotte, J.G. Surgery and portal hypertension. *Major Prob. Clin. Surg.* **1964**, *1*, 1–85.
12. Arroyo, V.; Garcia-Martinez, R.; Salvatella, X. Human serum albumin, systemic inflammation, and cirrhosis. *J. Hepatol.* **2014**, *61*, 396–407. [CrossRef]
13. Rondana, M.; Milani, L.; Merkel, C.; Caregaro, L.; Gatta, A. Value of prealbumin plasma levels as liver test. *Digestion* **1987**, *37*, 72–78. [CrossRef] [PubMed]
14. Liu, F.; Cai, L.Y.; Zhong, L.; Chen, C.; Xu, F.; Zhao, Z.X.; Chen, X.M. Model for end-stage liver disease combined with serum prealbumin to predict the prognosis of patients with decompensated liver cirrhosis. *J. Dig. Dis.* **2010**, *11*, 352–357. [CrossRef] [PubMed]
15. Huang, L.; Li, J.; Yan, J.J.; Liu, C.F.; Wu, M.C.; Yan, Y.Q. Prealbumin is predictive for postoperative liver insufficiency in patients undergoing liver resection. *World J. Gastroenterol.* **2012**, *18*, 7021–7025. [CrossRef]
16. Wen, X.; Yao, M.; Lu, Y.; Chen, J.; Zhou, J.; Chen, X.; Zhang, Y.; Lu, W.; Qian, X.; Zhao, J.; et al. Integration of Prealbumin into Child-Pugh Classification Improves Prognosis Predicting Accuracy in HCC Patients Considering Curative Surgery. *J. Clin. Trans. Hepatol.* **2018**, *6*, 377–384. [CrossRef] [PubMed]
17. Alberino, F.; Gatta, A.; Amodio, P.; Merkel, C.; Di Pascoli, L.; Boffo, G.; Caregaro, L. Nutrition and survival in patients with liver cirrhosis. *Nutrition* **2001**, *17*, 445–450. [CrossRef]

18. Englesbe, M.J.; Patel, S.P.; He, K.; Lynch, R.J.; Schaubel, D.E.; Harbaugh, C.; Holcombe, S.A.; Wang, S.C.; Segev, D.L.; Sonnenday, C.J. Sarcopenia and mortality after liver transplantation. *J. Am. Coll. Surg.* **2010**, *211*, 271–278. [CrossRef]
19. Golse, N.; Bucur, P.O.; Ciacio, O.; Pittau, G.; Sa Cunha, A.; Adam, R.; Castaing, D.; Antonini, T.; Coilly, A.; Samuel, D.; et al. A new definition of sarcopenia in patients with cirrhosis undergoing liver transplantation. *Liver Transpl.* **2017**, *23*, 143–154. [CrossRef]
20. Montano-Loza, A.J. Muscle wasting: A nutritional criterion to prioritize patients for liver transplantation. *Curr. Opin. Clin. Nutr. Metab. Care* **2014**, *17*, 219–225. [CrossRef]
21. Durand, F.; Buyse, S.; Francoz, C.; Laouenan, C.; Bruno, O.; Belghiti, J.; Moreau, R.; Vilgrain, V.; Valla, D. Prognostic value of muscle atrophy in cirrhosis using psoas muscle thickness on computed tomography. *J. Hepatol.* **2014**, *60*, 1151–1157. [CrossRef] [PubMed]
22. Ebadi, M.; Wang, C.W.; Lai, J.C.; Dasarathy, S.; Kappus, M.R.; Dunn, M.A.; Carey, E.J.; Montano-Loza, A.J.; From the Fitness, Life Enhancement, and Exercise in Liver Transplantation (FLEXIT) Consortium. Poor performance of psoas muscle index for identification of patients with higher waitlist mortality risk in cirrhosis. *J. Cachexia Sarcopenia Muscle* **2018**, *9*, 1053–1062. [CrossRef] [PubMed]
23. Montano-Loza, A.J.; Angulo, P.; Meza-Junco, J.; Prado, C.M.M.; Sawyer, M.B.; Beaumont, C.; Esfandiari, N.; Ma, M.; Baracos, V.E. Sarcopenic obesity and myosteatosis are associated with higher mortality in patients with cirrhosis. *J. Cachexia Sarcopenia Muscle* **2016**, *7*, 126–135. [CrossRef] [PubMed]
24. Romeiro, F.G.; Augusti, L. Nutritional assessment in cirrhotic patients with hepatic encephalopathy. *World J. Hepatol.* **2015**, *7*, 2940–2954. [CrossRef]
25. Sinclair, M.; Hoermann, R.; Peterson, A.; Testro, A.; Angus, P.W.; Hey, P.; Chapman, B.; Gow, P.J. Use of Dual X-ray Absorptiometry in men with advanced cirrhosis to predict sarcopenia-associated mortality risk. *Liver Int.* **2019**, *39*, 1089–1097. [CrossRef]
26. Giusto, M.; Lattanzi, B.; Albanese, C.; Galtieri, A.; Farcomeni, A.; Giannelli, V.; Lucidi, C.; Di Martino, M.; Catalano, C.; Merli, M. Sarcopenia in liver cirrhosis: The role of computed tomography scan for the assessment of muscle mass compared with dual-energy X-ray absorptiometry and anthropometry. *Eur. J. Gastroenterol. Hepatol.* **2015**, *27*, 328–334. [CrossRef]
27. Kamath, P.S.; Wiesner, R.H.; Malinchoc, M.; Kremers, W.; Therneau, T.M.; Kosberg, C.L.; D'Amico, G.; Dickson, E.R.; Kim, W.R. A model to predict survival in patients with end-stage liver disease. *Hepatology* **2001**, *33*, 464–470. [CrossRef]
28. Montano-Loza, A.J.; Duarte-Rojo, A.; Meza-Junco, J.; Baracos, V.E.; Sawyer, M.B.; Pang, J.X.Q.; Beaumont, C.; Esfandiari, N.; Myers, R.P. Inclusion of Sarcopenia Within MELD (MELD-Sarcopenia) and the Prediction of Mortality in Patients with Cirrhosis. *Clin. Trans. Gastroenterol.* **2015**, *6*, e102. [CrossRef]
29. Zuniga, S.; Firrincieli, D.; Housset, C.; Chignard, N. Vitamin D and the vitamin D receptor in liver pathophysiology. *Clin. Res. Hepatol. Gastroenterol.* **2011**, *35*, 295–302. [CrossRef]
30. Konstantakis, C.; Tselekouni, P.; Kalafateli, M.; Triantos, C. Vitamin D deficiency in patients with liver cirrhosis. *Ann. Gastroenterol.* **2016**, *29*, 297–306. [CrossRef]
31. Putz-Bankuti, C.; Pilz, S.; Stojakovic, T.; Scharnagl, H.; Pieber, T.R.; Trauner, M.; Obermayer-Pietsch, B.; Stauber, R.E. Association of 25-hydroxyvitamin D levels with liver dysfunction and mortality in chronic liver disease. *Liver Int.* **2012**, *32*, 845–851. [CrossRef] [PubMed]
32. Olson, J.A. Serum levels of vitamin A and carotenoids as reflectors of nutritional status. *J. Natl. Cancer Inst.* **1984**, *73*, 1439–1444. [PubMed]
33. Newsome, P.N.; Beldon, I.; Moussa, Y.; Delahooke, T.E.; Poulopoulos, G.; Hayes, P.C.; Plevris, J.N. Low serum retinol levels are associated with hepatocellular carcinoma in patients with chronic liver disease. *Aliment. Pharmacol. Ther.* **2000**, *14*, 1295–1301. [CrossRef] [PubMed]
34. Chaves, G.V.; Peres, W.A.; Goncalves, J.C.; Ramalho, A. Vitamin A and retinol-binding protein deficiency among chronic liver disease patients. *Nutrition* **2015**, *31*, 664–668. [CrossRef]
35. Geubel, A.P.; De Galocsy, C.; Alves, N.; Rahier, J.; Dive, C. Liver damage caused by therapeutic vitamin A administration: Estimate of dose-related toxicity in 41 cases. *Gastroenterology* **1991**, *100*, 1701–1709. [CrossRef]
36. Barry, M.; Keeling, P.W.; Feely, J. Tissue zinc status and drug elimination in patients with chronic liver disease. *Clin. Sci.* **1990**, *78*, 547–549. [CrossRef]
37. Grungreiff, K.; Reinhold, D.; Wedemeyer, H. The role of zinc in liver cirrhosis. *Ann. Hepatol.* **2016**, *15*, 7–16. [CrossRef]

38. Takuma, Y.; Nouso, K.; Makino, Y.; Hayashi, M.; Takahashi, H. Clinical trial: Oral zinc in hepatic encephalopathy. *Aliment. Pharmacol. Ther.* **2010**, *32*, 1080–1090. [CrossRef]
39. Hayashi, M.; Ikezawa, K.; Ono, A.; Okabayashi, S.; Hayashi, Y.; Shimizu, S.; Mizuno, T.; Maeda, K.; Akasaka, T.; Naito, M.; et al. Evaluation of the effects of combination therapy with branched-chain amino acid and zinc supplements on nitrogen metabolism in liver cirrhosis. *Hepatol. Res.* **2007**, *37*, 615–619. [CrossRef]
40. Burk, R.F.; Early, D.S.; Hill, K.E.; Palmer, I.S.; Boeglin, M.E. Plasma selenium in patients with cirrhosis. *Hepatology* **1998**, *27*, 794–798. [CrossRef]
41. Patel, N.; Munoz, S.J. Bone disease in cirrhosis. *Clin. Liver Dis.* **2015**, *6*, 96–99. [CrossRef] [PubMed]
42. Nakchbandi, I.A. Osteoporosis and fractures in liver disease: Relevance, pathogenesis and therapeutic implications. *World J. Gastroenterol.* **2014**, *20*, 9427–9438. [PubMed]
43. Handzlik-Orlik, G.; Holecki, M.; Wilczynski, K.; Dulawa, J. Osteoporosis in liver disease: Pathogenesis and management. *Ther. Adv. Endocrinol. Metab.* **2016**, *7*, 128–135. [CrossRef] [PubMed]
44. Plauth, M.; Bernal, W.; Dasarathy, S.; Merli, M.; Plank, L.D.; Schutz, T.; Bischoff, S.C. ESPEN guideline on clinical nutrition in liver disease. *Clin. Nutr.* **2019**, *38*, 485–521. [CrossRef]
45. EASL. Clinical Practice Guidelines on nutrition in chronic liver disease. *J. Hepatol.* **2019**, *70*, 172–193. [CrossRef]
46. Amodio, P.; Bemeur, C.; Butterworth, R.; Cordoba, J.; Kato, A.; Montagnese, S.; Uribe, M.; Vilstrup, H.; Morgan, M.Y. The nutritional management of hepatic encephalopathy in patients with cirrhosis: International Society for Hepatic Encephalopathy and Nitrogen Metabolism Consensus. *Hepatology* **2013**, *58*, 325–336. [CrossRef]
47. Druml, W.; Fischer, M.; Pidlich, J.; Lenz, K. Fat elimination in chronic hepatic failure: Long-chain vs medium-chain triglycerides. *Am J Clin Nutr.* **1995**, *61*, 812–817. [CrossRef] [PubMed]
48. Xu, Z.; Li, Y.; Wang, J.; Wu, B.; Li, J. Effect of omega-3 polyunsaturated fatty acids to reverse biopsy-proven parenteral nutrition-associated liver disease in adults. *Clin. Nutr.* **2012**, *31*, 217–223. [CrossRef] [PubMed]
49. Tsien, C.D.; McCullough, A.J.; Dasarathy, S. Late evening snack: Exploiting a period of anabolic opportunity in cirrhosis. *J. Gastroenterol. Hepatol.* **2012**, *27*, 430–441. [CrossRef]
50. Cordoba, J.; Lopez-Hellin, J.; Planas, M.; Sabin, P.; Sanpedro, F.; Castro, F.; Esteban, R.; Guardia, J. Normal protein diet for episodic hepatic encephalopathy: Results of a randomized study. *J. Hepatol.* **2004**, *41*, 38–43. [CrossRef]
51. Ney, M.; Abraldes, J.G.; Ma, M.; Belland, D.; Harvey, A.; Robbins, S.; Den Heyer, V.; Tandon, P. Insufficient Protein Intake Is Associated with Increased Mortality in 630 Patients with Cirrhosis Awaiting Liver Transplantation. *Nutr. Clin. Pract.* **2015**, *30*, 530–536. [CrossRef] [PubMed]
52. Dasarathy, S.; Merli, M. Sarcopenia from mechanism to diagnosis and treatment in liver disease. *J. Hepatol.* **2016**, *65*, 1232–1244. [CrossRef]
53. Tsien, C.; Davuluri, G.; Singh, D.; Allawy, A.; Ten Have, G.A.; Thapaliya, S.; Schulze, J.M.; Barnes, D.; McCullough, A.J.; Engelen, M.P.; et al. Metabolic and molecular responses to leucine-enriched branched chain amino acid supplementation in the skeletal muscle of alcoholic cirrhosis. *Hepatology* **2015**, *61*, 2018–2029. [CrossRef] [PubMed]
54. Les, I.; Doval, E.; Garcia-Martinez, R.; Planas, M.; Cardenas, G.; Gomez, P.; Flavià, M.; Jacas, C.; Mínguez, B.; Vergara, M.; et al. Effects of branched-chain amino acids supplementation in patients with cirrhosis and a previous episode of hepatic encephalopathy: A randomized study. *Am. J. Gastroenterol.* **2011**, *106*, 1081–1088. [CrossRef] [PubMed]
55. EASL. Clinical Practice Guidelines for the management of patients with decompensated cirrhosis. *J. Hepatol.* **2018**, *69*, 406–460. [CrossRef]
56. Caraceni, P.; Riggio, O.; Angeli, P.; Alessandria, C.; Neri, S.; Foschi, F.G.; Levantesi, F.; Airoldi, A.; Boccia, S.; Svegliati-Baroni, G.; et al. Long-term albumin administration in decompensated cirrhosis (ANSWER): An open-label randomised trial. *Lancet* **2018**, *391*, 2417–2429. [CrossRef]
57. Sola, E.; Sole, C.; Simon-Talero, M.; Martin-Llahi, M.; Castellote, J.; Garcia-Martinez, R.; Moreira, R.; Torrens, M.; Márquez, F.; Fabrellas, N.; et al. Midodrine and albumin for prevention of complications in patients with cirrhosis awaiting liver transplantation. A randomized placebo-controlled trial. *J. Hepatol.* **2018**, *69*, 1250–1259. [CrossRef]

58. Holick, M.F.; Binkley, N.C.; Bischoff-Ferrari, H.A.; Gordon, C.M.; Hanley, D.A.; Heaney, R.P.; Murad, M.H.; Weaver, C.M.; Endocrine Society. Evaluation, treatment, and prevention of vitamin D deficiency: An Endocrine Society clinical practice guideline. *J. Clin. Endocrinol. Metab.* **2011**, *96*, 1911–1930. [CrossRef]
59. Elangovan, H.; Chahal, S.; Gunton, J.E. Vitamin D in liver disease: Current evidence and potential directions. *Biochim. Biophys. Acta* **2017**, *1863*, 907–916. [CrossRef]
60. Grungreiff, K. Branched Amino Acids and Zinc in the Nutrition of Liver Cirrhosis. *J. Clin. Exp. Hepatol.* **2018**, *8*, 480–483. [CrossRef]
61. Burk, R.F.; Hill, K.E.; Motley, A.K.; Byrne, D.W.; Norsworthy, B.K. Selenium deficiency occurs in some patients with moderate-to-severe cirrhosis and can be corrected by administration of selenate but not selenomethionine: A randomized controlled trial. *Am. J. Clin. Nutr.* **2015**, *102*, 1126–1133. [CrossRef] [PubMed]

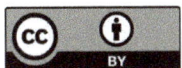

© 2019 by the authors. Licensee MDPI, Basel, Switzerland. This article is an open access article distributed under the terms and conditions of the Creative Commons Attribution (CC BY) license (http://creativecommons.org/licenses/by/4.0/).

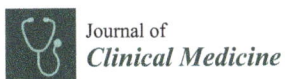

Review

Management of Dehydration in Patients Suffering Swallowing Difficulties

Emilie Reber [1,*], Filomena Gomes [2], Ilka A. Dähn [3], Maria F. Vasiloglou [4] and Zeno Stanga [1]

1. Department for Diabetes, Endocrinology, Nutritional Medicine and Metabolism, Bern University Hospital, and University of Bern, Freiburgstrasse 15, 3010 Bern, Switzerland; zeno.stanga@insel.ch
2. The New York Academy of Sciences, 250 Greenwich Sweet, 40th floor, New York, NY 10007, USA; filomenisabel@hotmail.com
3. Cereneo Schweiz AG, Center for Neurology and Rehabilitation, Seestrasse 18, 6354 Vitznau, Switzerland; ilka.daehn@cereneo.ch
4. AI in Health and Nutrition Laboratory, ARTORG Center for Biomedical Engineering Research, University of Bern, Murtenstrasse 50, 3008 Bern, Switzerland; maria.vasiloglou@artorg.unibe.ch
* Correspondence: emilie.reber@insel.ch

Received: 24 September 2019; Accepted: 5 November 2019; Published: 8 November 2019

Abstract: Swallowing difficulties, also called dysphagia, can have various causes and may occur at many points in the swallowing process. The treatment and rehabilitation of dysphagia represent a major interdisciplinary and multiprofessional challenge. In dysphagic patients, dehydration is frequent and often accelerated as a result of limited fluid intake. This condition results from loss of water from the intracellular space, disturbing the normal levels of electrolytes and fluid interfering with metabolic processes and body functions. Dehydration is associated with increased morbidity and mortality rates. Dysphagic patients at risk of dehydration thus require close monitoring of their hydration state, and existing imbalances should be addressed quickly. This review gives an overview on dehydration, as well as its pathophysiology, risk factors, and clinical signs/symptoms in general. Available management strategies of dehydration are presented for oral, enteral, and parenteral fluid replacement.

Keywords: dehydration; dysphagia; fluid intake; water

1. Introduction

Dysphagia is a dysfunction of the digestive system, consisting of a difficulty in swallowing. It affects the proper transit of the bolus in the upper digestive tract, preventing a safe oral feeding process. The main complications of dysphagia are aspiration (i.e., the passage of solid and liquid food into the respiratory tract, which can be "silent" in the absence of the protective cough reflex), aspiration pneumonia (pneumonia caused by food in the lungs), malnutrition, and dehydration. Because symptoms are very unspecific, dysphagia is frequently undetected, and either untreated or undertreated. Nevertheless, prevalence of dysphagia is high, especially among older patients with neurological disorders due to multifactorial changes of swallowing physiology, affecting at least 50% of the acute stroke population and 60% of those who suffer a severe traumatic brain injury [1,2]. In a recent systematic review with six high quality studies, the average prevalence of dysphagia in the community dwelling elderly population was 15% [3]. The same authors defined the risk factors for dysphagia as a history of clinical disease, physical frailty, and reduced ability to accomplish activities of daily living [3]. Dysphagia and the subsequent reduction of the coordination of pharyngeal muscles increase the risk of dehydration, malnutrition, pneumonia, and mortality [2]. Consequently, dysphagia may lead to dehydration—a shortage of body water due to either insufficient drinking or excess losses, or a combination of both [4]. Water and electrolyte balance is crucial for body homeostasis and is one of the most protected mechanisms in the body. Organisms can survive months without eating, but not many days without drinking, as fluid and electrolytes play major regulatory roles in many mechanisms, for example, transport systems, signal transduction, and body temperature [5].

This review highlights and discusses dehydration, as well as its pathophysiology, risk factors, and clinical signs/symptoms, focusing on dysphagic patients in particular. Possible management strategies of dehydration are presented for oral, enteral and parenteral fluid replacement.

2. Dysphagia

Swallowing is an essential and highly complex process of movements. This physiological process requires an exact coordination of nerval and muscular structures as well as an intact sensitivity of the mouth and throat area. The deglutition can be divided into five phases (preoral, two oral phases, pharyngeal, and oesophageal), whereby the phases run smoothly into each other and work together as muscle chains. Normally, the act of swallowing proceeds unnoticed and highly automated [6,7]. The muscle strength and the temporal orientation of the movement sequence are regulated in relation to the food/drink in the mouth (consistency and quantity). The system can be severely disturbed by diseases such as strokes, degenerative diseases, traumas, or tumours. A swallowing disorder (dysphagia) can occur in different forms. A healthy person swallows about 1,000 to 2,000 times a day [8]. The adaptation of food/drink, for example, balanced soft food or thickened liquids, may be needed to enable the patient to eat orally without an additional risk of aspiration.

Motor and cognitive performance decreases with increasing age [9,10]. Changes in the age-related swallowing disorder (presbyphagia) are the reduction of the sense of taste and smell, a reduced chewing function due to lack of oral hygiene/prosthesis, and the loss of strength to swallow food and liquids effectively and safely [10]. More than 40% of muscle mass is lost in old age [11]. Cancer patients are also severely impaired in their food intake owing to severe surgery, subsequent chemotherapy, and/or radiation. All these factors make the patients highly dependent [9,12], which leads to further health problems such as dehydration, malnutrition, anorexia, sarcopenia, and pneumonia. Older people and patients with dementia are more susceptible to stroke, pneumonia, and dehydration, which are among the most common causes of death in this population [9].

Dysphagia is associated with malnutrition, dehydration, pneumonia, reduced functional outcome, and mortality [13]. Therefore, similarly to nutritional management, populations at risk should regularly be screened for dysphagia and, when needed, further assessed by a clinical specialist (e.g., a speech-language pathologist). Patients suspected to have dysphagia after a screening test undergo assessment to determine the degree of severity of dysphagia and further treatment. Individual screening tests are performed by speech-language pathologists or trained nursing staff. They serve to identify symptoms and differentiate dysphagic patients from non-dysphagic patients. This procedure is non-invasive and can be performed quickly (in 10–15 min) while the patient is sitting in an upright position. There are several criteria that indicate that the screening test should be ceased in order to minimize the risk of aspiration (i.e., the involuntary passage of food or liquid through the vocal folds, to the lungs). Nonetheless, this test shows a sensitivity and specificity between 50% and 80% and fails to detect a significant number of aspirations [14,15].

The clinical swallowing examination is performed by speech-language pathologists. The patient sits upright at 90°. The inspection of the facial-oral structures, the oral skills, and sensitivity, as well as the oral motor arbitrary movements; the oral reflexes in the pharynx area (gag reflex, palata reflex, and so on); and the existing protective mechanisms, such as coughing and deliberate coughing, are included [16]. According to Daniels et al., liquid is gradually swallowed, thus single sips ≤20 mL of water up to 100 ml are examined (timed test) [17]. Soft and solid consistencies are also examined. Pathomechanisms like leaking anterior, nasal penetration, signs of aspiration, and residuals in the oral cavity are observed and described. Finally, an inspection of the oral cavity and a longer phonation sample are performed to clarify a sizzling voice and possibly the suspicion of penetration with aspiration [16]. In addition, instrumental examinations such as, for example, fiber optic endoscopic evaluation of swallowing (FEES; a transnasal procedure) and the video fluoroscopic swallowing study (a radiographic procedure), can be carried out.

FEES is a reportable procedure that may be completed in an outpatient clinic setting or at the bedside by passing an endoscope transnasally. It requires minimal positioning of the patient, and is thus commonly used [18]. In contrast, the video-fluoroscopy swallowing study, the gold standard for diagnosis of dysphagia, is a radiographic procedure that provides a direct, dynamic view of oral, pharyngeal, and upper oesophageal function. It, however, requires the use of a radiology suite (which can be very costly) and includes radiation exposure of the patient, who must be able to follow verbal commands (i.e., requires adequate cognitive functioning) [18]. All results will be brought together and the individual therapy plan will be defined. Regular repetitive examinations are needed to adapt swallowing treatment and the nutrition and hydration care plan.

Dysphagia therapy may be split into two categories: compensatory and rehabilitative therapies. Compensative strategies aim to maintain patient's safety when eating, while rehabilitative strategies aim to speed up the recovery process (e.g., swallowing training). Patients may be treated first with compensatory therapy and later with rehabilitation treatments. Functional oriented swallowing therapy, defined and applied by a trained speech-language pathologist, aims to create muscular conditions for largely normal swallowing and, therefore, to recover the physiological swallowing function, maintaining or improving quality of life by reducing morbidity and mortality associated with chest infections (pneumonia) and reduced nutritional status. There are also several supportive technical stimulation treatment methods available such as thermal tactile stimulation, transcranial magnetic stimulation, or transcranial direct current stimulation [19].

On the basis of the severity of dysphagia complaints and the level of alertness, the adequate food support with modified texture diets and thickened fluids will be proposed. The change of food consistency is mandatory in dysphagia, in order to reduce the need of oral manipulation, to make the swallowing process slower and safer, and to increase food and fluid intake [20]. Nevertheless, such diets lean towards less acceptance by patients, less nutritionally dense meals, less food choices, and less appealing meals than normal, leading to insufficient nutritional and fluid intake [21,22]. That is why it makes sense to make use of food fortification as well as supplemental enteral feed and fluids in these patients. Thickening agents, which are used to thicken a variety of fluids (e.g., water, tea, coffee, fruit juice), are supposed to induce a "coating feeling" in the mouth, suppressing flavour without reducing the sensation of thirst [23]. Hence, swallowing safety may be improved, but fluid intake does not substantially improve [1]. Liquid thickening is recommended in patients with dysphagia aspirating on liquids, as a way to slow the flow of the swallowed liquids, which should allow more time for airway closure and eventually reduce the risk of aspiration [24,25]. However, thickening fluids significantly decreases of the acceptance of the beverages, and thus is a practice that needs to be closely monitored. Whelan et al. showed in their study of 24 acute stroke patients with dysphagia that the intake of thickened fluids per day amounted to only 30% of the recommended 1500 mL/day [22]. The other 70% of the hydration needs had to be met through supplementary (parenteral and enteral) fluids. The group of patients who received pre-thickened fluids consumed almost double the amount of fluids than the group of patients receiving powder-thickened fluids, suggesting that the commercially available pre-thickened ready-to-drink beverages have better acceptability and can be used as a strategy to increase fluid intake among dysphagic patients (although the costs may he higher) [22].

Different food consistencies have been defined and numerous guidelines exist in many countries describing the various types of texture-modified diets and thickened fluids. These recommendations, aiming to improve patient's safety and nutritional status while avoiding aspiration pneumonia, are, however, based on best practice and are not evidence-based [26,27]. Modification of food texture and liquid thickness is a mainstay of dysphagia management. As there are only a few high-quality studies, the evidence is weak [28]. A couple of years ago, the "International Dysphagia Diet Standardisation Initiative" (IDDSI) published new global standardized definitions describing texture-modified foods and thickened liquids [29]. This terminology allows the use of a common language on multiprofessional teams (therapists, nurses, chiefs, patients, and relatives), which will support scientists working in this field, thus generating comparable research data worldwide. When applying the IDDSI definitions in each clinical setting, the food and drinks should always be tested under serving conditions. Drinks and liquidized foods are evaluated by a gravity flow test with a 10 ml syringe. This classifies beverages based on their flow rate, representing the process of drinking through a straw [29].

It is important to note that thickened liquids and adapted food consistencies are only a start to increase the quality of life of the dysphagic patients, as they work as a motivation tool and prepare them to eventually swallow food and fluid with normal consistency. Given the disadvantages of the use of thickened fluids and adapted food consistencies (which may lead to insufficient nutritional and fluid intake), it is important to control the progression of the dysphagia in order to adapt the food/drink consistency and protect the patient from being restricted to a certain consistency for too long [30].

3. Dehydration

Adequate water supply is indispensable to maintain cellular homeostasis and several physiological functions. Historically, total body water loss is differentiated into two types: dehydration and volume depletion [31]. Dehydration occurs when the body water losses, mostly from the intracellular volume (ICV), are higher than the intake. Low-intake dehydration is a shortage of pure water, leading to loss of both intracellular and extracellular fluid, and to raised osmolality in both compartments. Volume depletion is the result of excess losses of fluid and salts (especially sodium and sometimes other components), primarily related to a loss of extracellular volume (ECV), and clinically affecting the interstitial compartment; the fluid is lost primarily, not intracellular fluid, and serum osmolality will be normal or low. From the physiological view point, it makes sense that many physicians tend to use the term of dehydration for any loss of total body water in daily clinical practice [32].

There are numerous definitions for dehydration hampering the diagnosis. The best diagnostic approach for this complex condition thus includes history, clinical observations, laboratory tests, and physical assessment [33]. From a clinical point of view, dehydration may be defined as the rapid decrease of >3% of body weight [34]. Pathophysiologically, however, dehydration is a loss of water, resulting in a relative deficit of body water referring to sodium [35]. Consequently, increased sodium values cause the plasma osmolality to rise, reducing the ICV. This is often referred to as hypovolemic hypernatremia or hypertonic dehydration. Even if commonly used, "isotonic dehydration" and "hypotonic dehydration" differ from a pathophysiologic point of view, rather characterizing a volume depletion (loss of sodium from the ECV) than dehydration [35]. This distinction is especially relevant for the therapeutic approach [33].

If the fluid intake is too low, fluid in and around body cells concentrates, raising plasma and serum osmolality [36]. This consecutively triggers protection mechanisms (e.g., thirst and increased urine concentration by the kidney). In the elderly, with kidney function being mostly low, renal parameters do not truthfully indicate dehydration [36]. The U.S. Panel on Dietary Reference Intakes for Electrolytes and Water hence considers the plasma or serum osmolality as the main factor of hydration status, thus setting the reference standard for dehydration in older adults [37]. This is based on physiological and biochemical considerations and is accepted by experts [36]. Extracellular water loss due to diarrhoea, vomiting, or renal sodium loss (volume depletion) is, however, linked to normal or decreased plasma osmolality. While severe dehydration is not exactly defined, there are indicators of a distinctive lack of water: serum osmolality ≥ 300 mOsm/kg, serum sodium concentration ≥ 150 mmol/L, or blood urea nitrogen (BUN) to creatinine ratio ≥ 20. In the case of hypernatremia, free water shortage may be estimated with the following formula [35]:

$$\text{free water shortage (L)} = 0.6 \times \text{body weight (kg)} \times ((\text{plasma sodium (mmol/L)}/140) - 1)$$

3.1. Adequate Intake

The recommendations for adequate fluid intake show great variation (from 1.0 L/day in the Nordic countries to 2.2 L/day in the USA in women, 1.0–3.0 L/day in men) [36]. The European Food Safety Authority recommends an adequate intake of 2.0 L/day for women and 2.5 L/day for men of all ages [38]. Because 80% of the fluids come from beverages, adequate intake is 1.6 L/day in women and 2.0 L/day in men. Fluid requirements need to be adapted individually, for example, increased with higher activity level, fever, diarrhoea, and vomiting, or decreased in the case of heart and renal failure.

3.2. Prevalence

As dehydration is not properly defined, it is problematic to accurately assess its prevalence. Dehydration is, however, especially common in the elderly (up to 60%), depending on the definition used [39]. Bennett et al. showed that laboratory parameters indicated dehydration in 48% of elderly people admitted to an emergency department, while proper assessment of dehydration was documented only in 26% [40]. Dehydration is one of the ten most frequent diagnoses for hospital admission in older adults [41], and has been reported to be the most common fluid and electrolyte imbalance in older adults [42]. A study showed that 6.7% of inpatients aged ≥65 years were diagnosed with dehydration, with it being the principal diagnosis in 1.4% [43]. Among those suffering from swallowing difficulties, the prevalence of dehydration ranges from 44% [44] to 75% depending on the patient population, setting, and criteria used to define dehydration [45]. Nevertheless, Thomas et al. revealed that physicians misdiagnose dehydration in at least 30% of older adult inpatients [46].

3.3. Impact and Risk Factors

Elderly people tend to have diminished feeling of thirst owing to the decrease of sensitivity to the antidiuretic hormone (ADH) [47]. Numerous studies showed that adequate hydration status is normally maintained in healthy older people. Nevertheless, mental and/or physical illnesses, trauma, or operation, among others, may increase the risk of dehydration [48]. A six-month study among nursing home residents found 31% to be dehydrated during that period, and thereof, two-thirds had prior episodes of dehydration [49]. Risk factors for dehydration in dysphagic nursing home residents were, among others, severe impairment of the functional and/or cognitive function, speech disorders [45], and insufficient support at mealtime [50]. Inadequate nursing staff training, multiple medication, and being of female gender have also further been shown to increase the risk of dehydration [51]. Elderly people affected by acute infections and or chronic diseases (cardiovascular disease, diabetes, cancers), especially polymorbid patients, are at high risk of dehydration [40,41,43,51]. Dysphagia was shown to be directly linked with dehydration [4]. Evidence has shown that the clinical outcome of elderly people is worse in the presence of dysphagia [36]. High serum osmolality (>300 mOsm/kg) has been linked to an increased disability and mortality risk [36].

There are many physiological age-related alterations increasing the risk of dehydration (Figure 1) [36]. Growing age seems to dampen the two main physiological answers to reduced fluid intake: thirst and primary urine concentration (through the kidney) [36]. Moreover, fluid reserves are decreased, as body water decreases with age. In addition, common drug therapies in older people may further aggravate fluid loss, such as diuretics and laxatives therapies [36]. However, the severity of cognitive and functional impairment appears to be more relevant than only older age [36]. A study with patients suffering from dysphagia and receiving thickened fluids assessed water supply, including that from food and drinks (thickened beverages), as well as from artificial nutrition (enteral and parenteral nutrition). This study showed that estimated fluid requirements were not met for any of the patients without the use of enteral or parenteral fluids [4]. Another surprising finding of this study is that food, not thickened beverages, provided the greatest contribution to oral fluid intake, which probably reflects the general low level of acceptance of and compliance with thickened fluids. It is very important for the medical and nursing staff to be aware not only of the risk of dehydration in patients with dysphagia, but also of its clinical signs and symptoms. In collaboration with speech-language pathologists and dietitians, an individual nutrition and hydration care plan must be placed in a timely manner, as dehydration may cause severe complications and increase medical costs, morbidity, and the mortality rate [43].

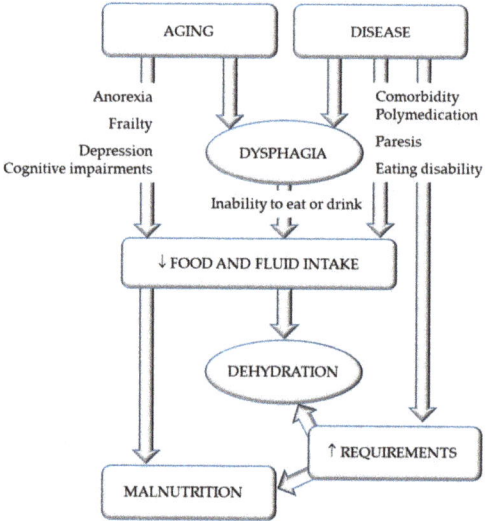

Figure 1. Risk factors for dehydration in dysphagia, modified after the work of [8].

4. Pathophysiological Considerations

4.1. Body Compartments

Water distribution into the different body compartments in healthy individuals is shown in Figure 2. Body water fulfils many physiological functions: it regulates body temperature and absorbs shocks, it is a solvent for chemical reactions, it serves as transport medium, and it contributes to the removal of waste products. Water accounts for about 60% of body weight. This proportion may vary according to gender and age. Body water is generally somewhat less in women than in men owing to differences in body composition. The body water is divided intracellular (two-thirds of body water) and extracellular (one-third of body water) space. The water within the extracellular space is further divided into intravascular (1/12 of body water) and extravascular (3/4 of body water) fluid by the capillary wall. The extravascular compartment may be further divided into interstitial/transcellular fluids.

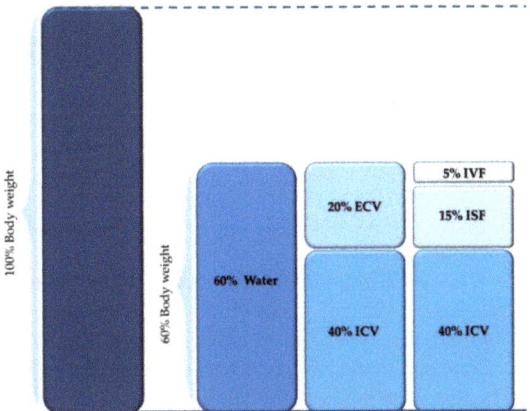

Figure 2. The repartition of body water within the different compartments as percentage of body weight [35]. ICV: Intracellular volume; ECV: Extracellular volume; ISF: Interstitial fluid; IVF: Intravascular fluids.

4.2. External Fluid Balance

Fluid balance is a complex interplay of numerous organs (e.g., skin, respiratory tract, kidneys, and gastrointestinal tract). The typical daily fluid turnover amounts to approximately 2600 mL (30–40 mL/kg body weight). Liquids represent about 1500 mL of daily input; 800 mL comes from liquids within solid food and a further 300 mL comes from oxidation water (Figure 3). The main water output (1500 mL) passes through the kidneys. The insensible perspiration composed of water losses from respiration and transpiration accounts for a substantial loss (Figure 3), while faeces alone represent a loss of 100–150 mL per day. The regulation of the sodium balance is essential for the maintenance of normal blood volume. The regulation of the water balance, however, relies on the maintenance of osmolarity. Volume maintenance has priority at any time on osmolality. The regulation of water balance also strongly relies on the capability of the kidney to excrete urine with an osmolality different from plasma, as kidneys are very efficacious in retaining sodium, but only hardly evacuate its surplus.

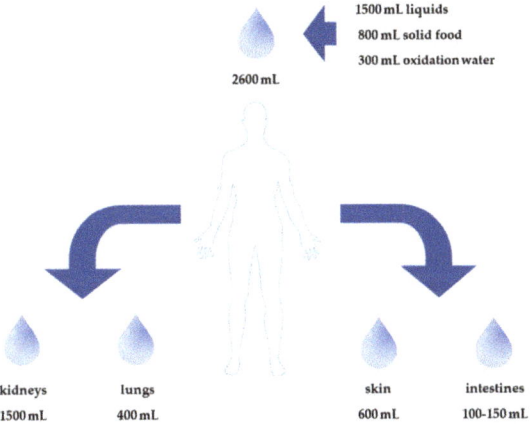

Figure 3. Fluid balance [35]. This figure shows the sites involved in fluid loss.

4.3. Internal Fluid Balance

The distribution of water within the body compartments undergoes strict control. Semipermeable cell membranes separating the intracellular and extracellular space enable the passage of water and selected molecules. The quantity of solutes per kilogram of solution is referred to as osmolality and usually fluctuates around 275 to 290 mOsm/kg. It may be directly measured or calculated with the following equation:

$$2 \times (\text{serum sodium (mmol/L)}) + \text{BUN (mg/dL)}/2.8 + \text{plasma glucose (mg/dL)}/18.$$

Tonicity is defined by the solutes determining the transcellular distribution of water, referred to as effective osmoles. Inactive osmole (e.g., urea) can freely pass the membrane and their rise in serum does not trigger water movement toward extracellular space. Nevertheless, inactive osmoles contribute to osmolality. Plasma osmolality is mostly determined by sodium (extracellular) and potassium (intracellular). Potassium in the extracellular fluid reaches 2% of the total body potassium. Anions such as chloride and bicarbonate and proteins grant the electroneutrality (Table 1). The first determining factor for the distribution of body water is the osmotic forces. Osmotic changes will immediately trigger the movement of water from lower to higher osmolarity, which has to be similar on both sides of the cell membrane.

Table 1. Electrolyte concentrations in the human body [5,52].

Electrolyte	Plasma (mmol/L)	Extracellular Volume (mmol/L)	Intracellular Volume (mmol/L)
Sodium	135–145	142–155	10–18
Potassium	3.5–5.3	4.0–5.5	120–145
Calcium	2.2–2.6	2.2–2.5	1.5
Chloride	95–105	98–108	2–6
Magnesium	0.8–1.2	0.7–1.2	15–25
Phosphate	0.81–1.45	0.7–1.3	8–20
Bicarbonate	22–30	22–30	10

5. Disorders of Fluid Balance

5.1. Isotonic and Hypotonic Dehydration

The term "isotonic dehydration" may be confusing to a certain degree as it in fact more refers to volume depletion than to dehydration. Isotonic dehydration occurs when the loss of water and solutes is balanced, reducing the volume of extracellular fluid, leading to reduced perfusion of the tissues, while osmolality and thus the intracellular fluid volume are kept normal (Figure 4). The reasons for this are manifold: fasting, haemorrhage, burns, gastrointestinal symptoms (vomiting, diarrhoea), drugs (sedative, diuretics), and so on. Renal perfusion is decrease owing to volume depletion and the renin–angiotensin–aldosterone system is thus activated, resulting in greater reabsorption of sodium and water. Secretion of ADH moreover causes water retention, aiming to correct volume depletion.

When sodium losses are greater than water losses, causing serum osmolality >270 mOsm/kg and sodium concentration >135 mmol/L in serum, "hypotonic dehydration" occurs. When fluids and sodium losses are partly replaced using hypotonic fluids, the extracellular space is reduced, owing to the low serum osmolality (Figure 4).

Both forms must be treated by means of isotonic fluids.

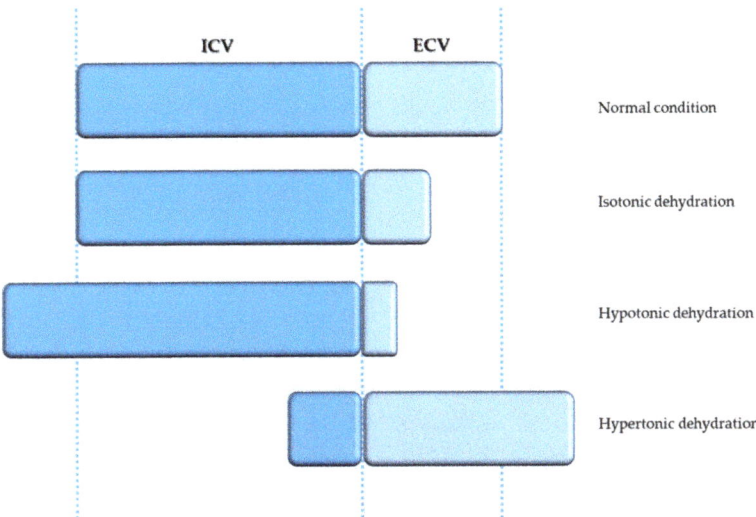

Figure 4. Water balance disturbances.

5.2. Hypertonic Dehydration

"Hypertonic dehydration" represents the pathophysiologic type of dehydration, where BUN to creatinine ratio is ≥20 and serum sodium concentrations exceed ≥150 mmol/L. Loss of water is higher than loss of sodium. The succeeding rise of sodium concentration in serum induces a rise in osmolality, which consecutively causes water to move towards the extracellular compartment, causing acute hypernatremia (Figure 4). Theses water movements also affect the brain, possibly causing a diminution in brain volume, and eventually causing rupture of veins and subsequent intracerebral or subarachnoid haemorrhage. Brain cells initially accumulate sodium and potassium, and later osmolytes (mainly myoinositol, glutamine, and glutamate), to compensate for water loss and restore volume [53,54]. As in dysphagia, hypertonic dehydration happens because of decreased water intake or as a result of either excessive (extra) renal water losses. Many factors may cause renal water losses such as renal or central diabetes insipidus, polyuric phase of acute renal failure, loop or osmotic diuretics, post obstructive disease, and so on. Extra renal water losses are the result of transcutaneous losses (e.g., sweat, fever, burns) or losses over the respiratory tract (e.g., hyperventilation). The consecutive rise in osmolality activates ADH release, and thus thirst (Figure 5). ADH secretion may be triggered by non osmolar volume-depending receptors or by supraoptic and paraventricular nuclei of the thalamus. The latest causes a reduced free water excretion. Above the threshold for ADH secretion in humans, which is 280–285 mOsm/kg, ADH secretion rises in a linear manner with rising osmolality (Figure 6). The threshold value for thirst, the major protective physiological mechanism of the body to compensate for hypernatremia, is higher than the ADH threshold [55].

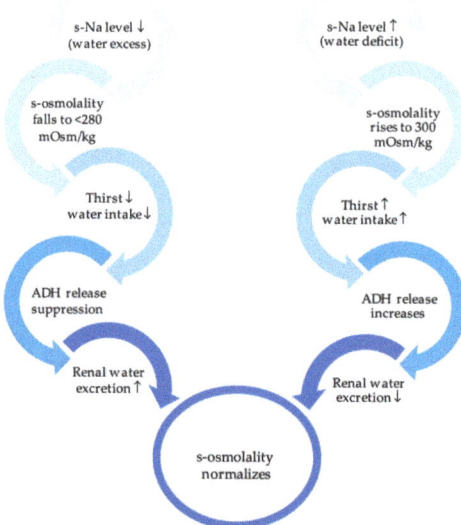

Figure 5. Regulation mechanisms of sodium and water. s-Na: Serum sodium; s-osmolarity: Serum osmolarity; ADH: Antidiuretic hormone.

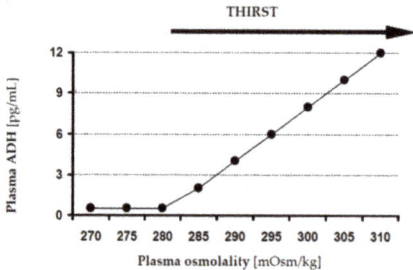

Figure 6. ADH release and thirst [56]. ADH: Antidiuretic hormone.

Hypotonic fluids represent the best treatment option for hypertonic dehydration.

6. Clinical and Biochemical Diagnostic Features

The sensitivity and specificity of dehydration signs largely depend on the volume of blood loss, where the clearest signs are heart rates changes (30 beats per minute) or severe postural dizziness leading to a lack of ability to stand [57]. Medication (e.g., beta-blockers) and older age may further influence sensitivity and specificity of these signs. Signs consecutive to fluid and electrolyte losses (e.g., due to vomiting or diarrhoea) are less clear.

Clinical signs taken alone are not very useful. A combination of at least four signs described hereafter indicates moderate to severe volume depletion. Typical clinical signs of dehydration with high scientific value are listed in Table 2. Absence of tears, transpiration, and/or thirst are among others symptoms of dehydration [33,58,59]. Clinical features with poor sensitivity and specificity are as follows: dry mucous membrane, low skin turgor, long nail bed refill time, altered respiratory pattern, changes in heart rate, dry or furrowed tongue, dry axilla, absence of tears, sunken eyes, high palpated ocular pressure, and weight loss [33,57]. The highest diagnostic utility was given by systolic blood pressure <100 mmHg in a clinical trial [58]. Owing to the loss of subcutaneous tissue with aging skin, turgor is not reliable in the elderly population. If present, dry axilla is fairly used with an appositive likelihood ratio of 2.8 (sensitivity 50%, specificity 82%) [60]. Symptoms that have a sensitivity over 80% are furrows on the tongue, dry mucous membranes, speech incoherence, extremity weakness, and orthostasis. Sunken eyes show a specificity greater than 80% and a sensitivity of 62% [32]. Central nervous system symptoms like confusion, speech difficulty, or weakness in the extremities are manifest when dehydration results in a 1% loss of body weight and are more notable at a 5% loss [32,58,61]. The development of neurologic effects is more likely to occur in acute hypernatremia developing within 48 hours than in chronic cases. Severe dehydration may cause hypotension, including the related risk of falls, reduced cardiac output, as well as consecutive reduced blood flow through organs and tissues. It may also escalate to hypovolemic shock. The risk for chronic renal disease, morbidity, and mortality are increased in the case of chronic dehydration (mild to severe) if not treated [62–64].

Table 2. Single signs, symptoms, and laboratory tests to identify dehydration [33,58,59].

Assessment of Hydration Status	Feasibility of Test	Scientific Value
Signs and symptoms		
Seated systolic blood pressure ≤100 mmHg	H	H
Blood pressure change supine/standing ≥20 mmHg	H	H
Thirst sensation	H	M
Dark urine colour	H	M
Laboratory tests		
Urine specific gravity ≥1.025	H	H
Blood urea nitrogen/creatinine ratio ≥20	M	H
Blood osmolality calculated ≥300 mmol/kg	M	H
Haematocrit/haemoglobin ratio	M	M
Mean corpuscular volume	M	M
Serum sodium concentration >150 mmol/L	M	M
Additional measurements (mainly for scientific purposes)		
Total body water (isotope dilution)	L	M
Total body water (bioelectrical impedance analysis)	H	M
Fluid volumes and ionic content (neutron activation analysis)	L	M
Blood osmolality (measured)	M	H
Urine osmolality	H	H
Salivary osmolality	H	H
Tear osmolality	M	M
Intraocular pressure (measured)	M	L

H = high; M = medium; L = low.

Although the patient's history and physical examination may indicate the appearance of dehydration (symptoms and signs), it is obvious that medical staff should not only rely on these clinical data, but also have to integrate biochemical parameters to enable the diagnosis (Table 2) [33,58,59]. Plasma osmolarity ≥300 mOsm/kg, plasma sodium, urine specific gravity, tear, and saliva osmolality have all been shown to be suitable to diagnose dehydration [58,65,66]. For an optimal diagnostic strategy, you need at least calculate or measure BUN, glucose, creatinine, sodium, bicarbonate, and osmolality [32].

7. Management of Dehydration

7.1. General Recommendations

The identification of acute situations potentially leading to dehydration, as well as the monitoring of vital parameters, clinical signs and symptoms, and laboratory parameters (Table 2), are of utmost importance. Fluid balance (including intake and output) should additionally be monitored. Skin integrity (including mucous membranes) and drug treatments (mainly diuretics) may impact the water and electrolyte balance, as well as diseases or conditions affecting renal perfusion (e.g., heart failure, chronic kidney disease) [33,67,68]. The evidence suggests that multicomponent interventions (including increased staff awareness, assistance with drinking, support using the toilet, and a greater variety of drinks on offer) may be effective [69]. Fluid therapy may be used for resuscitation, replacement, or maintenance of the fluid balance depending on the stage of illness. The National Institute for Health and Care Excellence (NICE) provides a set of interrelated algorithms for assessment, fluid resuscitation, routine intravenous maintenance, and replacement and redistribution of fluid and electrolytes [70]. Resuscitation may be needed in the case of considerable blood loss (e.g., surgery, injury) or plasma loss (e.g., burns, acute pancreatitis). Fluids are then immediately needed to maintain circulation and organ vital function [70]. Fluid maintenance may be initiated once the vital signs and urine output are normalized.

The maintenance of fluid and electrolyte balance is the key to prevent and treat dehydration. Maintenance aims to restore insensible losses and provide sufficient water and electrolytes to maintain the normal status of body fluid compartments and sufficient water to enable the kidneys to excrete waste products. Maintenance fluid prescriptions should target the daily requirements and replace ongoing abnormal losses. Requirements of patients receiving artificial nutrition are mostly covered though the artificial nutrition itself. Special attention is needed regarding overhydration, particularly in patients suffering congestive heart failure. The best route/method/fluid for administration depends on the severity/nature/acuteness of dehydration. Oral administration should be the preferred option, although parenteral administration of fluids may be mandatory in some cases. Such prescriptions must be changed to oral administration as soon as possible, as fluids prescriptions are often maintained too long, causing infects and oedema, especially in the postoperative phase. Subcutaneous infusions should be considered to manage chronic problems, particularly in the elderly [5]. A calculation of fluids requirements has been proposed by Chidester et al. [71], suggesting the prescription of 100 mL per kilogram body weight for first 10 kg, 50 mL per kilogram for next 10 kg, and 15 mL for the remaining kilograms of body weight. When body temperature is higher than 37 °C, 100–150 mL should additionally be given.

7.2. Oral/Enteral Replacement

Fluid and electrolyte requirements should be met via oral or enteral routes as far as possible when fluid resuscitation is not needed [70]. The first measure to replace fluid loss should be offering thickened liquids or food with high fluids content, whereas sodium-containing food and liquids must be avoided. As previously mentioned, the evidence level for such interventions is, however, weak [72]. Enteral liquid administration (via feeding tube) may be appropriate in the case of severe dysphagia or if maintaining fluid balance is not possible. Moderate dehydration (loss of 1.5–2% body weight) may easily be corrected with the administration of oral or enteral fluids, but already alters moods and causes decreased physical and cognitive performance [62,63,73,74]. Treatment for low-intake dehydration involves administration of hypotonic fluids [36], which will help correct the fluid deficit while diluting the raised osmolality. Oral rehydration therapy (aiming the replacement of electrolytes lost in volume depletion by diarrhoea or vomiting) and sports drinks are not indicated. Hydration status should be reassessed regularly until corrected, and then regularly monitored.

7.3. Parenteral Replacement

The parenteral administration of (low sodium-containing) fluids is the method of choice in the case of severe dehydration (high amounts of fluid needed) or when intravenous access is anyway given for administration of medication or nutrition [36,70]. Intravenous hydration must, however, always be regarded to as a medical treatment and not as basic care. The risk and benefit balance must be cautiously considered. Figure 7 illustrates the distribution of different fluids within body compartments after infusion. Deficits in free water must be substituted quickly if hypernatremia lasts for shorter than 48 hours. To avoid oedemas, caused by fluids shifts, high-rate administration of intravenous hypotonic solutions must be prevented. As its cells accumulate osmolytes to maintain normal cell volume, the brain is especially endangered. Brain oedema may develop as a result of hasty administration of hypotonic solutions. Fluids must hence be administered progressively, over 12 to 48 h. Hyponatraemia lasting for more than 48 h have to be corrected slowly. Not more than half of the replacement should occur in the first 24 hours of treatment, during which one should look out extremely cautiously for brain oedema, the symptoms of which may be headache or seizures. The residual replacement may occur within the next 48 to 72 h. In the case of hypernatremia, fluid replacement is considered adequate when the urine sodium concentration is over 25 mmol/L.

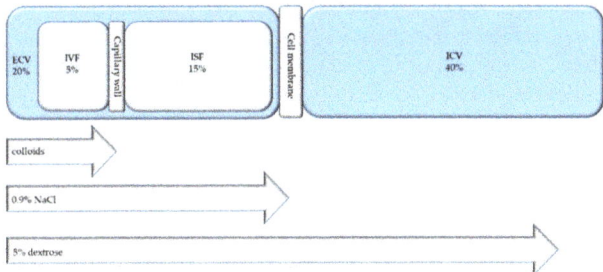

Figure 7. Infused fluids across the body compartments. ECV: Extracellular volume, ICV: Intracellular volume, IVF: Intravascular fluids, ISF: Interstitial fluids, NaCl: Sodium chloride.

8. Hypodermoclysis

Evidence has shown that adequate volumes of subcutaneous infusions are an effective treatment for dehydration, showing comparable rates of adverse effects to parenteral administration [36,75]. Many clinical trials have shown the safety and effectiveness of fluid infusion into the subcutaneous space using a fine cannula, called hypodermoclysis (HDC), making it a possible alternative to parenteral administration. HDC is particularly useful for the rehydration of patients with mild to moderate dehydration, who are cannot keep their fluid balance via the oral route [76–78]. Preferred sites for HDC are, for example, the anterior chest wall, lateral abdominal wall, inner tight, and back above or below shoulder blade. Recommendations for fluid infusion rates differ; that is, using gravity, up to 1,500 mL may be infused over 24 h at one site (rate of 20–80 mL/h), while rates of 82–148 mL/h have been recommended as well [32,79–81]. The authors' clinical experience indicates the safety of infusion of 500 mL per hour. A study using radioactive labelled injection showed that absorption into the blood occurs within one hour [82]. Infusion solutions are chosen regarding the clinical condition of the patient (balanced solutions, saline solutions, dextrose solutions, or their combination). A study among dement nursing home residents suffering dehydration showed more agitation (80%) in subjects receiving parenteral fluids compared with those receiving subcutaneous fluids (37%), regardless of the volume of administered fluid or the improvement of dehydration [83].

Subcutaneous infusions with hyaluronidase (useful enzyme to break down hyaluronic acid, thus opening the interstitial space) usually permit a more rapid infusion rate, lower rate of moderate oedema, and more comfort for the patient. Even though there are no systematic studies available, administering up to 20 mmol/L potassium chloride appears unproblematic. Local adverse effects (e.g., oedema, erythema, and cellulitis) and systemic adverse effects (e.g., heart failure or hyponatremia) occur rarely and at similar rates compared with parenteral administration [78]. The effectiveness of both methods appears to be the same. The expense for HDC is about four times less than intravenous administration and demands reduced nursing care [83,84]. HDC use may be easily used in a community setting (nursing home or home), by patients and/or their caregivers [77]. HDC is suitable to prevent dehydration or to treat mild to moderate dehydration. Intravenous fluid replacement remains mandatory, however, to treat hypovolemic shock or severe dehydration.

Colloids and (Balanced) Crystalloids

The volume of distribution and the metabolization of the solute are the two main factors to determine the plasma expansion capacity of a solution. Colloids are principally distributed within the intravascular space, while dextrose solutions are first metabolized and then distributed within the whole body water. Their volume expansion ability is hence limited and temporary. Resuscitation should thus be undertaken using colloids. Intravascular volume expansion is mostly done using crystalloids. If appropriated, dextrose solutions (5% or combined with saline) are used to provide free water. The expansion capacity of isotonic crystalloids, distributed within the extracellular fluids, is 20% to 25%. The remaining crystalloid volume is kept within the interstitial space. This overload of interstitial fluid has to be eliminated after the acute phase of the disease is over. Even if the use of crystalloid solutions is effective, the price to pay remains quite high. Additionally, the excessive use of sodium-containing crystalloids may cause oedema and further impair the clinical outcome. Dextrose solutions may cause potential harmful effects as well (e.g., hyponatraemia <130 mM). Hypochloraemic acidosis may occur as a result of the administration of saline, as they contain much higher concentrations of chloride compared with plasma. This may seriously impair the kidney function (reduced perfusion and glomerular filtration rates), the gastrointestinal function (mucosal acidosis, ileus), or other cellular dysfunction including impairment of mitochondrial function. Recent studies have shown the superiority of balanced electrolyte solutions (Hartmann's or Ringer's) on saline solutions replacing water and salt deficits, except for cases of gastric juice losses, where chloride losses are high [5]. Isotonic dextrose solutions should be used to replace deficits in free water. Colloid solutions such as albumin or hydroxyethyl starch should be used to expand volume, as they induce less salt/water overloads and oedemas than crystalloid solutions (e.g., dextrose 5%, 0.9% NaCl, and balanced crystalloids). The combination of both in varying proportions may be used in the clinical practice, depending on the patient's condition. Newly published trials show balanced crystalloids to be superior on saline solutions in critical and non-critical care [85,86]. These trials showed a lower rate of the composite outcome of death from any cause, new renal-replacement therapy, or persistent renal dysfunction with balanced crystalloids than with saline (number needed to treat 1/94).

9. Conclusions

Dehydration is a relevant clinical problem with severe consequences, particularly in patients suffering from dysphagia, whose fluids' intake is very restricted by the use of thickeners. At least in one-third of inpatients, dehydration is misdiagnosed and thus underestimated as well as undertreated. It is very important for the medical and nursing staff dealing with patients suffering dysphagia to be aware of dehydration, and work closely with speech-language pathologists and dietitians to place a nutrition and hydration care plan tailored to the needs and condition of each patient. Volume depletion, treated with isotonic fluids, and dehydration treated with hypotonic fluids, must be clearly taken apart. Rehydration should be treated by the oral (or enteral) route whenever possible. Parenteral rehydration must be used in severe cases. The use of HDC may be considered in the case of mild dehydration when there are contraindications for oral/enteral treatment. It represents an effective and safe treatment option, especially in patients with dysphagia.

Author Contributions: Conceptualization, E.R. and Z.S.; writing—original draft preparation, E.R.; writing—review and editing, F.G., I.A.D., M.F.V. and Z.S.; supervision, Z.S.

Funding: The APC was funded by the Research Found of the Department of Diabetes, Endocrinology, Nutritional Medicine, and Metabolism and in part by Nestlé Health Science.

Conflicts of Interest: The authors declare no conflict of interest.

References

1. Burgos, R.; Breton, I.; Cereda, E.; Desport, J.C.; Dziewas, R.; Genton, L.; Gomes, F.; Jesus, P.; Leischker, A.; Muscaritoli, M.; et al. ESPEN guideline clinical nutrition in neurology. *Clin. Nutr.* **2018**, *37*, 354–396. [CrossRef] [PubMed]
2. Geeganage, C.; Beavan, J.; Ellender, S.; Bath, P.M. Interventions for dysphagia and nutritional support in acute and subacute stroke. *Cochrane. Database Syst. Rev.* **2012**. [CrossRef] [PubMed]
3. Madhavan, A.; LaGorio, L.A.; Crary, M.A.; Dahl, W.J.; Carnaby, G.D. Prevalence of and Risk Factors for Dysphagia in the Community Dwelling Elderly: A Systematic Review. *J. Nutr. Health Aging* **2016**, *20*, 806–815. [CrossRef] [PubMed]
4. Vivanti, A.P.; Campbell, K.L.; Suter, M.S.; Hannan-Jones, M.T.; Hulcombe, J.A. Contribution of thickened drinks, food and enteral and parenteral fluids to fluid intake in hospitalised patients with dysphagia. *J. Hum. Nutr. Diet* **2009**, *22*, 148–155. [CrossRef] [PubMed]
5. Lobo, D.; Lewington, A.; Allison, S. Basic concepts of fluid and electrolyte therapy. *Clin. Med.* **2013**. [CrossRef]
6. Bartolome, G.; Schröter-Morasch, H. *Schluckstörungen: Diagnostik und Rehabilitation*; Elsevier, Urban & Fischer: Munich, Germany, 2013.
7. Prosiegel, M.; Weber, S. *Dysphagie: Diagnostik und Therapie: Ein Wegweiser für Kompetentes Handeln*; Springer: Berlin, Germany, 2018.
8. Wirth, R.; Dziewas, R.; Beck, A.M.; Clave, P.; Hamdy, S.; Heppner, H.J.; Langmore, S.; Leischker, A.H.; Martino, R.; Pluschinski, P.; et al. Oropharyngeal dysphagia in older persons—From pathophysiology to adequate intervention: A review and summary of an international expert meeting. *Clin. Interv. Aging* **2016**, *11*, 189–208. [CrossRef]
9. Amella, E.J. Feeding and hydration issues for older adults with dementia. *Nurs. Clin. North Am.* **2004**, *39*, 607–623. [CrossRef]
10. Kolb, C. *Nahrungsverweigerung bei Demenzkranken: PEG-Sonde-Ja oder Nein?* Mabuse-Verlag: Frankfurt am Main, Germany, 2004.
11. Schreier, M.M.; Bartholomeyczik, S. *Mangelernährung bei Alten und Pflegebedürftigen Menschen: Ursachen und Prävention aus Pflegerischer Perspektive-Review/Literaturanalyse*; Schlütersche: Hannover, Germany, 2004.
12. Baijens, L.W.; Clave, P.; Cras, P.; Ekberg, O.; Forster, A.; Kolb, G.F.; Leners, J.C.; Masiero, S.; Mateos-Nozal, J.; Ortega, O.; et al. European society for swallowing disorders—European union geriatric medicine society white paper: Oropharyngeal dysphagia as a geriatric syndrome. *Clin. Interv. Aging* **2016**, *11*, 1403–1428. [CrossRef]
13. Tagliaferri, S.; Lauretani, F.; Pela, G.; Meschi, T.; Maggio, M. The risk of dysphagia is associated with malnutrition and poor functional outcomes in a large population of outpatient older individuals. *Clin. Nutr.* **2018**. [CrossRef]
14. Logemann, J.A.; Veis, S.; Colangelo, L. A screening procedure for oropharyngeal dysphagia. *Dysphagia* **1999**, *14*, 44–51. [CrossRef]
15. Sonies, B.C. Swallowing disorders and rehabilitation techniques. *J. Pediatr. Gastroenterol. Nutr.* **1997**, *25*, S32–S33. [CrossRef] [PubMed]
16. Ickenstein, G.; Hofmayer, A.; Lindner-Pfleghar, B.; Pluschinski, P.; Riecker, A.; Schelling, A.; Prosiegel, M. Standardisierung des Untersuchungsablaufs bei neurogener oropharyngealer Dysphagie (NOD). *Neurol. Rehabil.* **2009**, *15*, 290–300.
17. Wu, M.-C.; Chang, Y.-C.; Wang, T.-G.; Lin, L.-C. Evaluating swallowing dysfunction using a 100-mL water swallowing test. *Dysphagia* **2004**, *19*, 43–47. [CrossRef] [PubMed]
18. Marcotte, P. Critical Review: Effectiveness of FEES in Comparison to VFSS at Identifying Aspiration. Available online: https://www.uwo.ca/fhs/lwm/teaching/EBP/2006_07/Marcotte.pdf (accessed on 7 November 2007).

19. Yamamura, K.; Kurose, M.; Okamoto, K. Guide to Enhancing Swallowing Initiation: Insights from Findings in Healthy Subjects and Dysphagic Patients. *Curr. Phys. Med. Rehabil. Rep.* **2018**, *6*, 178–185. [CrossRef] [PubMed]
20. Dennis, M.; Lewis, S.; Cranswick, G.; Forbes, J. FOOD: A multicentre randomised trial evaluating feeding policies in patients admitted to hospital with a recent stroke. *Health Technol. Assess.* **2006**, *10*, 1–120. [CrossRef]
21. Foley, N.; Finestone, H.; Woodbury, M.G.; Teasell, R.; Greene Finestone, L. Energy and protein intakes of acute stroke patients. *J. Nutr. Health Aging* **2006**, *10*, 171–175.
22. Whelan, K. Inadequate fluid intakes in dysphagic acute stroke. *Clin. Nutr.* **2001**, *20*, 423–428. [CrossRef]
23. Cichero, J.A. Thickening agents used for dysphagia management: Effect on bioavailability of water, medication and feelings of satiety. *Nutr. J.* **2013**. [CrossRef]
24. Clave, P.; de Kraa, M.; Arreola, V.; Girvent, M.; Farre, R.; Palomera, E.; Serra-Prat, M. The effect of bolus viscosity on swallowing function in neurogenic dysphagia. *Aliment. Pharmacol. Ther.* **2006**, *24*, 1385–1394. [CrossRef]
25. Steele, C.M.; Alsanei, W.A.; Ayanikalath, S.; Barbon, C.E.; Chen, J.; Cichero, J.A.; Coutts, K.; Dantas, R.O.; Duivestein, J.; Giosa, L.; et al. The influence of food texture and liquid consistency modification on swallowing physiology and function: A systematic review. *Dysphagia* **2015**, *30*, 2–26. [CrossRef]
26. Cichero, J.A.; Lam, P.; Steele, C.M.; Hanson, B.; Chen, J.; Dantas, R.O.; Duivestein, J.; Kayashita, J.; Lecko, C.; Murray, J.; et al. Development of international terminology and definitions for texture-modified foods and thickened fluids used in dysphagia management: The IDDSI framework. *Dysphagia* **2017**, *32*, 293–314. [CrossRef] [PubMed]
27. Marcason, W. What is the international dysphagia diet standardisation initiative? *J. Acad. Nutr. Diet* **2017**. [CrossRef] [PubMed]
28. Cichero, J.A.; Steele, C.; Duivestein, J.; Clave, P.; Chen, J.; Kayashita, J.; Dantas, R.; Lecko, C.; Speyer, R.; Lam, P.; et al. The need for international terminology and definitions for texture-modified foods and thickened liquids used in dysphagia management: Foundations of a global initiative. *Curr. Phys. Med. Rehabil. Rep.* **2013**, *1*, 280–291. [CrossRef] [PubMed]
29. International Dysphagia Diet Standardisation Committee. Complete International Dysphagia Diet Standardisation Initiative (IDDSI) Framework: Detailed Definitions. Available online: https://iddsi.org/Documents/IDDSIFramework-CompleteFramework.pdf (accessed on 29 July 2019).
30. Lippert, W.C.; Chadha, R.; Sweigart, J.R. Things We Do for No Reason: The Use of Thickened Liquids in Treating Hospitalized Adult Patients with Dysphagia. *J. Hosp. Med.* **2019**, *14*, 315–317. [CrossRef] [PubMed]
31. Mange, K.; Matsuura, D.; Cizman, B.; Soto, H.; Ziyadeh, F.N.; Goldfarb, S.; Neilson, E.G. Language guiding therapy: The case of dehydration versus volume depletion. *Ann. Intern. Med.* **1997**, *127*, 848–853. [CrossRef]
32. Thomas, D.R.; Cote, T.R.; Lawhorne, L.; Levenson, S.A.; Rubenstein, L.Z.; Smith, D.A.; Stefanacci, R.G.; Tangalos, E.G.; Morley, J.E. Understanding clinical dehydration and its treatment. *J. Am. Med. Dir. Assoc.* **2008**, *9*, 292–301. [CrossRef]
33. Armstrong, L.E.; Kavouras, S.A.; Walsh, N.P.; Roberts, W.O. Diagnosing dehydration? Blend evidence with clinical observations. *Curr. Opin. Clin. Nutr. Metab. Care* **2016**, *19*, 434–438. [CrossRef]
34. Weinberg, A.D.; Minaker, K.L. Dehydration. Evaluation and management in older adults. Council on Scientific Affairs, American Medical Association. *JAMA* **1995**, *274*, 1552–1556. [CrossRef]
35. Stanga, Z.; Aubry, E. Dehydration in Dysphagia. In *Dysphagia: Diagnosis and Treatment*; Ekberg, O., Ed.; Springer International Publishing: Cham, Switzerland, 2019; pp. 859–871.
36. Volkert, D.; Beck, A.M.; Cederholm, T.; Cruz-Jentoft, A.; Goisser, S.; Hooper, L.; Kiesswetter, E.; Maggio, M.; Raynaud-Simon, A.; Sieber, C.C.; et al. ESPEN guideline on clinical nutrition and hydration in geriatrics. *Clin. Nutr.* **2019**, *38*, 10–47. [CrossRef]
37. Institute of Medicine; Food and Nutrition Board; Panel on Dietary Reference Intakes for Electrolytes and Water; Standing Committee on the Scientific Evaluation of Dietary Reference Intakes. *DRI, Dietary Reference Intakes for Water, Potassium, Sodium, Chloride, and Sulfate*; The National Academy Press: Washington, DC, USA, 2005.
38. EFSA Panel on Dietetic Products; Nutrition; Allergies (NDA). Scientific opinion on dietary reference values for water. *EFSA J.* **2010**. [CrossRef]

39. Stookey, J.D.; Pieper, C.F.; Cohen, H.J. Is the prevalence of dehydration among community-dwelling older adults really low? Informing current debate over the fluid recommendation for adults aged 70+years. *Public Health Nutr.* **2005**, *8*, 1275–1285. [CrossRef] [PubMed]
40. Bennett, J.A.; Thomas, V.; Riegel, B. Unrecognized chronic dehydration in older adults: Examining prevalence rate and risk factors. *J. Gerontol. Nurs.* **2004**, *30*, 22–28. [CrossRef] [PubMed]
41. Xiao, H.; Barber, J.; Campbell, E.S. Economic burden of dehydration among hospitalized elderly patients. *Am. J. Health Syst. Pharm.* **2004**, *61*, 2534–2540. [CrossRef] [PubMed]
42. Martin, J.H.; Larsen, P.D. Dehydration in the elderly surgical patient. *AORN J.* **1994**, *60*, 666–671. [CrossRef]
43. Warren, J.L.; Bacon, W.E.; Harris, T.; McBean, A.M.; Foley, D.J.; Phillips, C. The burden and outcomes associated with dehydration among US elderly, 1991. *Am. J. Public Health* **1994**, *84*, 1265–1269. [CrossRef]
44. Murray, J.; Doeltgen, S.; Miller, M.; Scholten, I. A Descriptive Study of the Fluid Intake, Hydration, and Health Status of Rehabilitation Inpatients without Dysphagia Following Stroke. *J. Nutr. Gerontol. Geriatr.* **2015**, *34*, 292–304. [CrossRef]
45. Leibovitz, A.; Baumoehl, Y.; Lubart, E.; Yaina, A.; Platinovitz, N.; Segal, R. Dehydration among long-term care elderly patients with oropharyngeal dysphagia. *Gerontology* **2007**, *53*, 179–183. [CrossRef]
46. Thomas, D.R.; Tariq, S.H.; Makhdomm, S.; Haddad, R.; Moinuddin, A. Physician misdiagnosis of dehydration in older adults. *J. Am. Med. Dir. Assoc.* **2003**, *4*, 251–254. [CrossRef]
47. Phillips, P.A.; Johnston, C.I.; Gray, L. Disturbed fluid and electrolyte homoeostasis following dehydration in elderly people. *Age Ageing* **1993**, *22*, S26–S33. [CrossRef]
48. Luckey, A.E.; Parsa, C.J. Fluid and electrolytes in the aged. *Arch. Surg.* **2003**, *138*, 1055–1060. [CrossRef]
49. Mentes, J. Oral hydration in older adults: Greater awareness is needed in preventing, recognizing, and treating dehydration. *Am. J. Nurs.* **2006**, *106*, 40–49. [CrossRef] [PubMed]
50. Kayser-Jones, J.; Schell, E.S.; Porter, C.; Barbaccia, J.C.; Shaw, H. Factors contributing to dehydration in nursing homes: Inadequate staffing and lack of professional supervision. *J. Am. Geriatr. Soc.* **1999**, *47*, 1187–1194. [CrossRef] [PubMed]
51. Lavizzo-Mourey, R.; Johnson, J.; Stolley, P. Risk factors for dehydration among elderly nursing home residents. *J. Am. Geriatr. Soc.* **1988**, *36*, 213–218. [CrossRef] [PubMed]
52. Lubos, S.; Simon, A.; Zeno, S. Water and electrolytes in health and disease. In *Basics in Clinical Nutrition*, 5th ed.; Luboš, S., Ed.; Galen: Belfast, Ireland, 2019.
53. Heilig, C.W.; Stromski, M.E.; Blumenfeld, J.D.; Lee, J.P.; Gullans, S.R. Characterization of the major brain osmolytes that accumulate in salt-loaded rats. *Am. J. Physiol.* **1989**, *257*, F1108–F1116. [CrossRef]
54. Lien, Y.H.; Shapiro, J.I.; Chan, L. Effects of hypernatremia on organic brain osmoles. *J. Clin. Invest.* **1990**, *85*, 1427–1435. [CrossRef]
55. Robertson, G.L. Physiology of ADH secretion. *Kidney Int. Suppl.* **1987**, *21*, S20–S26.
56. Robertson, G.L.; Aycinena, P.; Zerbe, R.L. Neurogenic disorders of osmoregulation. *Am. J. Med.* **1982**, *72*, 339–353. [CrossRef]
57. McGee, S.; Abernethy, W.B., 3rd; Simel, D.L. The rational clinical examination. Is this patient hypovolemic? *JAMA* **1999**, *281*, 1022–1029. [CrossRef]
58. Fortes, M.B.; Owen, J.A.; Raymond-Barker, P.; Bishop, C.; Elghenzai, S.; Oliver, S.J.; Walsh, N.P. Is this elderly patient dehydrated? Diagnostic accuracy of hydration assessment using physical signs, urine, and saliva markers. *J. Am. Med. Dir. Assoc.* **2015**, *16*, 221–228. [CrossRef]
59. Hooper, L.; Abdelhamid, A.; Attreed, N.J.; Campbell, W.W.; Channell, A.M.; Chassagne, P.; Culp, K.R.; Fletcher, S.J.; Fortes, M.B.; Fuller, N.; et al. Clinical symptoms, signs and tests for identification of impending and current water-loss dehydration in older people. *Cochrane. Database Syst. Rev.* **2015**. [CrossRef]
60. Eaton, D.; Bannister, P.; Mulley, G.P.; Connolly, M.J. Axillary sweating in clinical assessment of dehydration in ill elderly patients. *BMJ* **1994**. [CrossRef] [PubMed]
61. Lieberman, H.R. Hydration and cognition: A critical review and recommendations for future research. *J. Am. Coll. Nutr.* **2007**, *26*, 555–561. [CrossRef] [PubMed]
62. Armstrong, L.E. Challenges of linking chronic dehydration and fluid consumption to health outcomes. *Nutr. Rev.* **2012**, *70*, S121–S127. [CrossRef] [PubMed]

63. Armstrong, L.E.; Ganio, M.S.; Casa, D.J.; Lee, E.C.; McDermott, B.P.; Klau, J.F.; Jimenez, L.; Le Bellego, L.; Chevillotte, E.; Lieberman, H.R. Mild dehydration affects mood in healthy young women. *J. Nutr.* **2012**, *142*, 382–388. [CrossRef]
64. Cowen, L.E.; Hodak, S.P.; Verbalis, J.G. Age-associated abnormalities of water homeostasis. *Endocrinol. Metab. Clin. North Am.* **2013**, *42*, 349–370. [CrossRef] [PubMed]
65. Cheuvront, S.N.; Kenefick, R.W.; Charkoudian, N.; Sawka, M.N. Physiologic basis for understanding quantitative dehydration assessment. *Am. J. Clin. Nutr.* **2013**, *97*, 455–462. [CrossRef] [PubMed]
66. Sollanek, K.J.; Kenefick, R.W.; Walsh, N.P.; Fortes, M.B.; Esmaeelpour, M.; Cheuvront, S.N. Assessment of thermal dehydration using the human eye: What is the potential? *J. Therm. Biol.* **2012**, *37*, 111–117. [CrossRef]
67. Clark, W.F.; Sontrop, J.M.; Huang, S.H.; Moist, L.; Bouby, N.; Bankir, L. Hydration and Chronic Kidney Disease Progression: A Critical Review of the Evidence. *Am. J. Nephrol.* **2016**, *43*, 281–292. [CrossRef]
68. Sontrop, J.M.; Dixon, S.N.; Garg, A.X.; Buendia-Jimenez, I.; Dohein, O.; Huang, S.H.; Clark, W.F. Association between water intake, chronic kidney disease, and cardiovascular disease: A cross-sectional analysis of NHANES data. *Am. J. Nephrol.* **2013**, *37*, 434–442. [CrossRef]
69. Bunn, D.; Jimoh, F.; Wilsher, S.H.; Hooper, L. Increasing fluid intake and reducing dehydration risk in older people living in long-term care: A systematic review. *J. Am. Med. Dir. Assoc.* **2015**, *16*, 101–113. [CrossRef]
70. National Clinical Guideline Centre (UK). Intravenous Fluid Therapy: Intravenous Fluid Therapy in Adults in Hospital. Available online: https://www.nice.org.uk/guidance/cg174 (accessed on 10 December 2013).
71. Chidester, J.C.; Spangler, A.A. Fluid intake in the institutionalized elderly. *J. Am. Diet Assoc.* **1997**, *97*, 23–28. [CrossRef]
72. Beck, A.M.; Kjaersgaard, A.; Hansen, T.; Poulsen, I. Systematic review and evidence based recommendations on texture modified foods and thickened liquids for adults (above 17 years) with oropharyngeal dysphagia—An updated clinical guideline. *Clin. Nutr.* **2018**, *37*, 1980–1991. [CrossRef] [PubMed]
73. Bardis, C.N.; Kavouras, S.A.; Kosti, L.; Markousi, M.; Sidossis, L.S. Mild hypohydration decreases cycling performance in the heat. *Med. Sci. Sports Exerc.* **2013**, *45*, 1782–1789. [CrossRef] [PubMed]
74. Watson, P.; Whale, A.; Mears, S.A.; Reyner, L.A.; Maughan, R.J. Mild hypohydration increases the frequency of driver errors during a prolonged, monotonous driving task. *Physiol. Behav.* **2015**, *147*, 313–318. [CrossRef] [PubMed]
75. Turner, T.; Cassano, A.M. Subcutaneous dextrose for rehydration of elderly patients–An evidence-based review. *BMC Geriatr.* **2004**. [CrossRef] [PubMed]
76. Dasgupta, M.; Binns, M.A.; Rochon, P.A. Subcutaneous fluid infusion in a long-term care setting. *J. Am. Geriatr. Soc.* **2000**, *48*, 795–799. [CrossRef]
77. Remington, R.; Hultman, T. Hypodermoclysis to treat dehydration: A review of the evidence. *J. Am. Geriatr. Soc.* **2007**, *55*, 2051–2055. [CrossRef]
78. Slesak, G.; Schnurle, J.W.; Kinzel, E.; Jakob, J.; Dietz, P.K. Comparison of subcutaneous and intravenous rehydration in geriatric patients: A randomized trial. *J. Am. Geriatr. Soc.* **2003**, *51*, 155–160. [CrossRef]
79. Jain, S.; Mansfield, B.; Wilcox, M.H. Subcutaneous fluid administration–Better than the intravenous approach? *J. Hosp. Infect.* **1999**, *41*, 269–272. [CrossRef]
80. Sasson, M.; Shvartzman, P. Hypodermoclysis: An alternative infusion technique. *Am. Fam. Physician.* **2001**, *64*, 1575–1578.
81. Walsh, G. Hypodermoclysis: An alternate method for rehydration in long-term care. *J. Infus. Nurs.* **2005**, *28*, 123–129. [CrossRef] [PubMed]
82. Lipschitz, S.; Campbell, A.J.; Roberts, M.S.; Wanwimolruk, S.; McQueen, E.G.; McQueen, M.; Firth, L.A. Subcutaneous fluid administration in elderly subjects: Validation of an under-used technique. *J. Am. Geriatr. Soc.* **1991**, *39*, 6–9. [CrossRef] [PubMed]
83. O'Keeffe, S.T.; Lavan, J.N. Subcutaneous fluids in elderly hospital patients with cognitive impairment. *Gerontology* **1996**, *42*, 36–39. [CrossRef] [PubMed]
84. Pershad, J. A systematic data review of the cost of rehydration therapy. *Appl. Health Econ. Health Policy* **2010**, *8*, 203–214. [CrossRef]

85. Self, W.H.; Semler, M.W.; Wanderer, J.P.; Wang, L.; Byrne, D.W.; Collins, S.P.; Slovis, C.M.; Lindsell, C.J.; Ehrenfeld, J.M.; Siew, E.D.; et al. Balanced Crystalloids versus Saline in Noncritically Ill Adults. *N. Engl. J. Med.* **2018**, *378*, 819–828. [CrossRef]
86. Semler, M.W.; Self, W.H.; Wanderer, J.P.; Ehrenfeld, J.M.; Wang, L.; Byrne, D.W.; Stollings, J.L.; Kumar, A.B.; Hughes, C.G.; Hernandez, A.; et al. Balanced Crystalloids versus Saline in Critically Ill Adults. *N. Engl. J. Med.* **2018**, *378*, 829–839. [CrossRef]

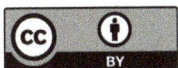

© 2019 by the authors. Licensee MDPI, Basel, Switzerland. This article is an open access article distributed under the terms and conditions of the Creative Commons Attribution (CC BY) license (http://creativecommons.org/licenses/by/4.0/).

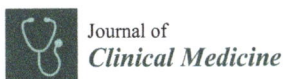 Journal of *Clinical Medicine*

Review

Challenges and Perspectives in Nutritional Counselling and Nursing: A Narrative Review

Maria F. Vasiloglou [1], Jane Fletcher [2] and Kalliopi-Anna Poulia [3],*

1. Diabetes Technology Research Group, ARTORG Center for Biomedical Engineering Research, University of Bern, Murtenstrasse 50, 3008 Bern, Switzerland; maria.vasiloglou@artorg.unibe.ch
2. Nutrition Nurses, Queen Elizabeth Hospital Birmingham, University Hospitals Birmingham NHS Foundation Trust, Mindelsohn Way, Edgbaston, Birmingham B15 2WG, UK; jane.fletcher@uhb.nhs.uk
3. Department of Nutrition and Dietetics, Laiko General Hospital of Athens, 11527 Athens, Greece
* Correspondence: lpoulia@gmail.com; Tel.: +30-213-206-1666

Received: 15 July 2019; Accepted: 12 September 2019; Published: 18 September 2019

Abstract: Nutritional counselling has been recognised as the first line approach in the management of numerous chronic diseases. Though usually carried out by dietitians, nutritional counselling may be used by nurses, or other healthcare professionals to improve nutritional status and meet healthcare goals. Healthcare professionals require training and education to facilitate a patient centred approach to effective counselling. Advances in digital technology have the potential to improve access to nutritional counselling for some patients such as those in primary care. However, caution is required to ensure that valuable interpersonal relationships are not lost, as these form the cornerstone of effective nutritional counselling. The aim of this narrative review is to explore aspects of effective nutritional counselling, including advances in e-counselling and areas where nursing input in nutritional counselling might enhance overall nutritional care.

Keywords: nutritional counselling; nursing; interventions; e-counselling

1. Introduction

Nutrition related chronic diseases—i.e., cancer, diabetes mellitus, chronic kidney disease, inflammatory bowel disease and so forth—and health problems that have significant implications on nutritional status, mainly by affecting digestion and absorption of food, place a significant burden on the overall health of a population and health care systems. As dietary modification can have a significant impact on biomarkers of non-communicable diseases and on symptoms of different clinical conditions, nutritional counselling has been recognised as the first line approach for their management [1]. Furthermore nutrition counselling is recommended as a key intervention in the management of malnutrition in older adults [2,3], and has been proven to be effective in chronic kidney disease, cancer and other clinical conditions [4–6].

Nutrition counselling is a two-way interaction through which a patient and the member of the medical team interpret the results of a nutritional assessment, identify patient's nutritional problems, needs and goals, discuss ways to meet these goals, and agree on future steps and the frequency of monitoring. It aims to help patients understand important information about the impact of nutrition on their health status and focuses on practical measures to cover nutritional needs. Moreover, it strengthens the importance of behavioural change [7–10]. However, nutrition counselling may present a time burden to patients, with high drop-out rates being a key challenge likely to affect outcomes [1], and face to face counselling having a significant impact on the use of resources in terms of clinic space and facilities. The development of new technology in e-counselling seeks to address these issues and expand access for patients.

Most of the time, nutrition counsellors are nutritionists or dietitians. However, other healthcare professionals such as nurses, community health workers or volunteers [3,7,11] play an essential role in nutritional counselling. The role of the nurse is recognised in nutrition screening but there is little evidence regarding the impact or effectiveness of the nurses' role in nutrition counselling. However, nurses form a core part of the team providing direct care to patients and as such are in a position to make positive behaviour changes [12], improving the effectiveness of nutritional interventions.

To meet the needs of an ever-changing healthcare environment, there is a need to explore the benefits of new technology in providing nutritional counselling to a wider audience. Although dietitians are key professionals in the nutritional counselling of patients, expanding the roles of other healthcare professionals may improve the impact and effectiveness of both counselling and interventions.

Aims

In this narrative review we aim to explore aspects of effective nutritional counselling including advances in technology and the role of the nurse in enhancing nutritional care.

2. Methodology

An electronic search was implemented in PubMed, Google Scholar Medline and Cinahl databases. Search terms included: 'Nutritional counselling', 'nurs* AND nutrition counselling' 'dietary counselling', 'patient education', 'nutrition education', 'nutrition AND nurse AND specialist' 'nursing', 'e-counselling', 'mHealth', 'eHealth', 'nutrition nurse specialist', 'patient-centred approach', 'nutritional care', 'remote nutrition counselling'. Publications were only included in the analysis if they were written in English and were related to humans. Articles were searched from January 2000 till May 2019. Non-peer reviewed literature, letters to the editor and studies performed on animals were excluded. From the articles retrieved in the first search round, additional references were identified by a manual search among the cited references. Moreover, additional references including characteristic and cornerstone references on nutrition counselling were added in introductory parts. As the review is narrative and not systematic, the references were selected according to the relevance to the subject of the manuscript.

3. Basic Characteristics of Effective Nutritional Counselling

As nutrition counselling can enhance health and nutrition outcomes, ideally it should be performed in a way that ensures patients' privacy and that the counsellor and the patient are feeling comfortable. This may be challenging in the hospital setting and measures should be taken towards this direction. Moreover, counsellors should be trained and use appropriate materials to enhance understanding and documentation, such as illustrations, food models, take-home brochures, data collection forms and referral forms.

Moreover, respecting the ethical aspects of nutritional counselling improves its outcomes. The main ethical values that should be followed are described in Table 1:

Table 1. Ethical values that underpin effective counselling [4].

Ethical Values	Rationale
The provision of accurate information	Patients should develop a relation of trust with the counsellor, based on the fact that the words and actions are true and reliable.
Confidentiality	All information shared should be kept confidentially, except as needed for the nutritional treatment and recovery.
Respect of patients' autonomy	Patients, as long as they are mentally stable, keep the right to decide for themselves, without coercion.
Do no harm	Nutritional interventions in the hospital setting should always be based on evidence-based medicine. Any intervention that could harm or exploit patients emotionally, financially or medically should always be avoided.
Be fair	All patients should receive the same level of attention, according to their needs, without discrimination. Patient's rights dignity and differences should be respected.

Patient-Centered Approach in Nutrition Counselling

The implementation of changes on nutrition behaviour is a complex procedure, as it combines elements of psychology, physiological needs, socioeconomic status and the level of the counsellor's ability to firstly identify the needs of the patients, and then to work co-operatively with them [3]. The patient-centred approach is generally accepted as efficient in managing nutritional counselling. It has been developed based on theoretical models developed in the late 40's by Rogers [13]. According to this theoretical model the patient has to identify the diet related problems and the nutritional counsellor will guide him towards the possible solutions.

The nutritionist/dietitian is the expert in the medical nutrition team, able to translate and combine the most current scientific information on food and health, food composition, psychological and physiological factors that could have an impact on dietary choices, and the relationship of those with health and diseases. He/she is the nutrition communicator, a skilled listener and a translator of emotions and abstract ideas on specific actions and steps towards dietary modification needed to enhance nutritional status, based on the individuals' life and biomedical requirements [14–16]. Gaining a better understanding of patients' preferences, attitudes and beliefs regarding their state of health and nutrition would allow interventions to be more focused, appropriate, sustainable and therefore, more effective [17]. The clinician–patient relationship has been associated with better patient attendance and adherence and greater patient satisfaction with care and treatment [18]. Moreover, patients' recall understanding, treatment adherence, and psychological wellbeing have been associated with effective doctor–patient communication. Therefore, an effective counselor refers not only to the expert nutrition knowledge but also to the privilege of having good communication skills. In this way, the development of a therapeutic relationship, characterized by mutual respect with the clients, will be easier to manage. However, this mode of practice requires organizational support and time, which are not always available to the dietitian in clinical practice. These dimensions may also be important in nutrition interventions, and future research should focus on the efficacy of nutritional counselling with these limitations in mind [19].

Under this spectrum, the main aim, and yet a great challenge, is to ensure that the patient has a full understanding of the relevant information of the nutritional problem and can work towards the development of specific skills to deal with the health challenges and their personal goals [20]. In order to have a successful outcome in patients receiving nutritional counselling, it is important to assess not only the patients' food choices and behavior, but also their access to health, environmental and social support systems. Therefore, the challenge is to be able to achieve essential and meaningful clinical outcomes, enhance the quality of life of the patient and, at the same time, encourage positive attitudes towards behavioral changes [21].

4. Challenges in Nutritional Counselling

Health professionals should always have in mind that patients are members of the community at large. At the community level, they receive multiple messages from different sources regarding nutritional behaviors that could enhance their wellbeing, their quality of life and improve health outcomes. Although health outcomes can be estimated by objective measurements, in terms of biochemical and physiological responses to interventions, the main issue is to identify what patients consider important as endpoints of quality of life and wellbeing [21]. Under the spectrum of the patient-centered approach, the bridging of biomedical imperatives and individual perspectives on health, quality of life and wellbeing is of paramount importance.

According to a recent systematic review by Mitchell et al. [1] of 26 randomized controlled studies (RCTs), representing 5500 adults, dietetic consultation in primary care appeared to be effective for the improvement of diet quality, the glycaemic control, and body weight control. One major limitation in analyzing RCTs that deals with nutrition consultations and dietary interventions though, is the fact that dietary assessment is subjected to errors and the available dietary assessment tools may not be too specific to identify qualitative improvements to the diet. Moreover, as nutrition is a factor influencing patients' life to a great extent, and at the same time is being influenced by personal, economic, psychological and emotional reasons, dietary interventions are usually characterized by high dropout rates and limited compliance. Therefore, measures to enhance adherence to dietetic interventions should always be considered [1].

Moving to more clinical settings, dietary interventions have been studied in environments that compromised health has a negative impact on nutritional status and raised the risk of malnutrition. In clinical cases health professionals providing nutrition consultations should always follow evidence-based medicine and established guidelines. As nutrition can be used as a complementary treatment that could be even harmful in some cases, i.e., in cancer patients, nutrition counselling should always be provided by specialized and qualified nutrition and dietetics professionals, to ensure the validity of the provided information. Lack of knowledge and misconceptions should be pointed out and scientific evidence should be provided. All non-justified and not scientific-based dietary theories should be addressed, under the spectrum of the individual perception of wellbeing [22,23].

In order to enhance compliance and adherence to nutritional interventions, other factors that could have an impact on the effectiveness of the intervention must be considered. The duration and the frequency of the consultations, the aims set on each consultation, the feedback that was given to the patients about their improvement or the achievement of the set goals can have an impact on the adherence to the nutritional intervention. More focused, clearly defined and measurable objectives increase effectiveness, whereas the use of vague objectives may limit the effectiveness of nutrition education due to the fact that it creates confusion and does not provide answers to the questions of the patients. Therefore, the design of the interventions should be clear and continued training for the trainers, with an emphasis on targeted interventions, should be available [24,25].

5. Nursing and Nutritional Care

Where studies have shown that patients benefit from receiving counselling and an individualised nutrition plan from a registered dietitian [26,27], the nurses' role is essential in reinforcing and facilitating nutritional plans and interventions in hospitalised patients. Observations suggest that nutritional outcomes may be enhanced with collaborative input from both dietitians and nurses [28]. As the daily providers of care, ward-based nurses are responsible for the direct delivery of nutritional interventions [29]. Additionally, nurses have a responsibility to pay special attention to promoting wellbeing, with nutrition being one of the fundamentals of care [30].

5.1. Ward-Based Nurses

Perry et al. [31] report a systematic review identifying the range of nursing interventions implemented to improve nutritional outcomes in patients who have suffered a stroke. The review included 27 papers from 26 studies with five RCT's and five clinical trials. Due to the heterogeneity and poor quality of reported data, few interventions showed statistical significance. However, this review is important in highlighting the diversity of nursing activities in nutritional care. The Alliance to Advance Patient Nutrition [32] stresses the importance of multidisciplinary involvement in nutrition, with a focus on all stakeholders valuing nutritional care interventions. Important points for nursing intervention include nutrition screening, implementing early nutritional measures in those at risk and developing strategies to ensure patient compliance. Where dietitians carry out comprehensive assessment and patient education, the nurse's role is to reinforce this information and answer patient questions [32]. In this way, collaborative working between disciplines is essential.

Nevertheless, one of the key challenges in practice is the level of importance that nurses place on nutritional care. A study of the attitudes of 106 nurses found respondents felt strongly that it was the role of the nurse to carry out nutrition counselling [33]. Key nursing nutritional interventions were significantly positively associated with the overall nutrition knowledge score: Patient counselling ($r = 0.23$, $p = 0.02$) and nutrition screening/assessment ($r = 0.23$, $p = 0.02$). This finding indicated that the higher the overall nutrition knowledge score among nurses, the higher these tasks were ranked [4].

However, the same study found that nurses ranked tasks associated with nutrition lower than other nursing tasks, such as giving medication and carrying out wound dressings. A small ($n = 22$) focus group study of staff working in an acute medical ward found that nurses struggled to put nutritional priorities in to practice, with competing activities being a particular issue at mealtimes [34]. A nursing survey carried out in Canadian hospitals ($n = 346$) reported nurses' perceptions as one of the reasons for insufficient nutrition [35]. The study found that 17% of the respondents thought that a lack of assistance at mealtimes was a major contributor, and 14% thought that assisting with nutrition was time consuming [35].

Though nursing interventions such as screening and assistance with eating and drinking are crucial, there appears to be little recorded evidence of nurses carrying out nutritional counselling at the ward level in internal medicine. Studies suggest successful nurse involvement in nutritional counselling in other settings including cancer care [36,37], primary care [38] and community care [39,40]. This then suggests that nurses working in internal medicine may be missing a valuable opportunity to improve patient care and compliance with nutritional interventions.

5.2. Nutrition Nurse Specialist

Specialist nurses have an important part to play in empowering ward-based nurses to deliver evidence-based care within their speciality, bridging the gap between research and bedside practice [41]. The nutrition nurse specialist (NNS) role may be known by numerous titles including 'nutrition support nurse', 'nutrition nurse practitioner/advanced practitioner' and 'nutrition support consultant nurse' [42]. Regardless of title, NNSs generally form a core part of hospital nutrition support teams, caring for patients with complex nutritional requirements. Though it is difficult to ascertain the exact value that individual members of the multidisciplinary teams bring to nutritional support, input from NNSs have been shown to reduce catheter related sepsis and other complications of parenteral nutrition [43].

However, the NNS role reaches far beyond this. The NNS may coordinate patient education on self-management of enteral or parenteral nutrition and provide training and educational programmes for other healthcare professionals [42]. Yordy et al. [44] report outcomes of a NNS-led quality improvement project. The project included a program of nutritional education for ward nurses with an audit of practice before and after education. In observations of mealtime interactions ($n = 100$), patient interruptions at mealtimes were shown to have reduced by 59% following the education program. Nursing documentation of nutritional risk factors and screening showed some improvement after education, although no statistical significance was described. The authors suggest that following targeted education, the nursing culture had changed to recognize nutrition as an essential part of the patients' treatment [35].

Some NNSs may be involved at a strategic and organisational level with the provision of nutritional services within their institution. Depending on the nature and requirements of the healthcare setting, NNSs may expand their skills to include technical procedures such as central venous catheter insertion [45] or gastrostomy insertion. Their scope is expanding further to include independent non-medical prescribing [46]. However, there is a lack of evidence regarding the function of NNSs in nutritional counselling. Given the nature of the role, it is reasonable to expect that NNSs play an important part in counselling patients with complex nutritional needs and particularly those that require artificial nutrition support. For these reasons NNSs must develop effective counselling skills. Fundamentally, the overall purpose of the NNS should be an improvement in quality of nutritional care, and nutritional counselling must be a core activity in this.

Further research is required to measure the improvements that the enhanced skills of the NNS brings to nutritional care. Nevertheless, NNSs are key participants in the wider nutrition support team and have an important function in supporting and educating ward-based nurses to deliver excellent care and reinforcing multidisciplinary nutritional treatment goals.

6. Nutritional Counselling with the Use of Modern Technology

Nutritional counselling is usually a time- and resource-demanding procedure that requires commitment by the patient [47]. The dropout rate of up to 35% of patients enrolled in dietetic consultation interventions shows the challenge of adhering to numerous counselling sessions [1]. Modern technology, including electronic health (eHealth) and mobile health (mHealth) may help keep patients engaged in their goals [48]. According to the European Commission's definition, eHealth is the "digital health and care which refers to tools and services that use information and communication technologies (ICTs) to improve prevention, diagnosis, treatment, monitoring and management of health and lifestyle". mHealth is a subcategory of eHealth, used mainly for describing healthcare management conducted by smartphones [49].

Electronic or e-counselling, i.e., remote counselling, can reduce barriers related to patient disengagement, geographical distance, time constraints [48], socioeconomic status [50], and also low need or desire for in-person contact [47]. In addition, the integration of eHealth and mHealth technologies could render the flexibility of dietetic services administered to patients [51,52]. Smartphone applications (apps) have been used of late to improve nutrition knowledge and contribute to behavioural change (beyond weight loss) [53], while presenting positive effects on measured nutritional outcomes in chronic diseases [47]. Artificial Intelligence (AI)-based smartphone apps can provide accurate and almost real-time dietary assessments [54–59]. However, even though there is an abundance of nutrition and diet apps, the majority of them focus on diet monitoring and nutrient content estimation. There is only a limited number of studies investigating the long-term impacts of apps focusing on nutritional e-counselling [52].

E-counselling through web-based apps has also already produced some positive effects, in comparison to in-person treatment for both delivery and dissemination [60]. Weight loss of approximately 4–6 kg can be reliably achieved with web programs that involve some form of weekly human e-counselling or constant feedback from behavioural lifestyle counsellors via email, group chat, etc. [61]. The results of this study also suggest that using a hybrid approach (in-person and online) may be an effective way to reach larger and more diverse populations [61]. Weight loss targeted web applications, where participants also received e-counselling via weekly e-mails, resulted in weight loss of 4.4 kg after one year of intervention in people at risk of type 2 diabetes [62]. Providing automated, computer-tailored feedback by a weight loss targeted web application for three months was as effective as human counselling via e-mail [63]. Clinically significant weight loss could be achieved through a combination of tailored goals and the use of a mobile app, whereas people interested in lower-intensity weight loss approaches could consider stand-alone digital health treatments [64]. Furthermore, Haas et al. [50] concluded that an app which complemented the dietitians' professional skills, can provide effective support towards behavioural change and sustainable weight reduction in overweight and obese individuals. Moreover, traditional consultations delivered by dietitians were compared against remote ones delivered by eHealth technologies, using theoretical cost in weight management as the outcome measure [52]. The eHealth approach needed an initial higher investment but was less costly in the long-term than in-person counselling [52].

In a qualitative study, healthcare professionals stated that it was challenging to establish and maintain an empathetic relationship with their clients (which is one of the most crucial factors for coaching) when conducting eHealth counselling [65]. Hence, e-counselling should include specific attributes that ensure it simulates—as closely as possible—a face-to face consultation [50], tailored to the individual patient [65].

Finally, including innovative technologies into dietetic practice could assist nutritional counselling by not only enhancing the efficiency and quality of nutrition care but also increasing adherence to self-monitoring of patient-centred goals [66]. Currently there is no evidence on the most effective use of apps in a clinical setting. Thus, it is suggested that the apps are used alongside individualized dietetic support, while performance for long-term weight management is being assessed [67]. End-users (patients) should be involved in the design process concerning health advice since it increases app efficacy and usability [68]. Future research, preferably in the form of randomized controlled trials, should investigate the clinical efficacy, feasibility and cost-effectiveness of e-counselling and eHealth technologies on dietetic practice.

7. Conclusions

Nutritional counselling has been recognised as the first line approach in the management of numerous chronic diseases. A patient-centred approach has been identified as the best way of providing nutritional counselling. Ideally, it is carried out by dietitians and nutritionists, but other members of the medical nutrition team such as nurses and other healthcare professionals can also play an important role. Nutrition nurse specialists have a particularly key part to play in both the carrying out of nutritional counselling as well as encouraging other nurses to participate in nutritional counselling. However, research is required to fully understand the benefits that the NNS brings to nutritional counselling and care.

It is important to stress that effective counselling needs training and education, and at the same time the use of eHealth technology has the potential to improve access for some patients. However, caution is required to ensure that valuable interpersonal relationships are not lost, as these form the cornerstone of effective nutritional counselling.

Author Contributions: Conceptualization, M.F.V., J.F. and K.-A.P.; writing—original draft preparation, M.F.V., J.F. and K.-A.P.; writing—review and editing, M.F.V., J.F. and K.-A.P.

Funding: The APC was funded by the Research Foundation of the Department of Diabetes, Endocrinology, Nutritional medicine and Metabolism, Bern University Hospital, Switzerland, and in parts by Nestlé Health Science (grant to the institution).

Conflicts of Interest: The authors declare no conflict of interest.

Abbreviations

The following abbreviations are used in this manuscript:

NNS	Nutrition nurse specialist
eHealth	Electronic health
mHealth	Mobile health
e-counselling	Electronic counselling
ICTs	Information and communication technologies

References

1. Mitchell, L.; Ball, L.; Ross, L.; Barnes, K.; Williams, L. Effectiveness of Dietetic Consultations in Primary Health Care: A Systematic Review of Randomized Controlled Trials. *J. Acad. Nutr. Diet.* **2017**, *117*, 1941–1962. [CrossRef] [PubMed]
2. Volkert, D.; Beck, A.M.; Cederholm, T.; Cruz-Jentoft, A.; Goisser, S.; Hooper, L.; Kiesswetter, E.; Maggio, M.; Raynaud-Simon, A.; Sieber, C.C.; et al. ESPEN guideline on clinical nutrition and hydration in geriatrics. *Clin. Nutr.* **2019**, *38*, 10–47. [CrossRef]
3. Rosal, M.; Ebbeling, C.; Lofgren, I.; Ockene, J.; Ockene, L.; Herbert, J. Facilitating dietary change: The patient centered counseling model. *J. Am. Diet. Assoc.* **2001**, *101*, 332–341. [CrossRef]
4. Ravasco, P.; Monteiro-Grillo, I.; Vidal, P.M.; Camilo, M.E. Dietary counseling improves patient outcomes: A prospective, randomized, controlled trial in colorectal cancer patients undergoing radiotherapy. *J. Clin. Oncol.* **2005**, *23*, 1431–1438. [CrossRef] [PubMed]
5. Ravasco, P.; Monteiro-Grillo, I.; Camilo, M. Individualized nutrition intervention is of major benefit to colorectal cancer patients. *Am. J. Clin. Nutr.* **2012**, *96*, 1346–1353. [CrossRef] [PubMed]
6. Orell, H.; Schwab, U.; Saarilahti, K.; Österlund, P.; Ravasco, P.; Mäkitie, A. Nutritional Counseling for Head and Neck Cancer Patients Undergoing (Chemo) Radiotherapy—A Prospective Randomized Trial. *Front. Nutr.* **2019**, *6*, 1–12. [CrossRef] [PubMed]

7. Scarlet, S. Dietary Counseling. In *Essentials of Human Nutrition*; Mann, J., Truswell, A.S., Eds.; Oxford University Press: New York, NY, USA, 1998.
8. MacLellan, D.; Berenbaum, S. Client-centred nutrition counseling: Do we know what it means? *Can. J. Diet. Pract. Res.* **2003**, *64*, 12–15. [CrossRef] [PubMed]
9. MacLellan, D.; Berenbaum, S. Dietitians' opinions and experiences of client-centred nutrition counseling. *Can. J. Diet. Pract. Res.* **2006**, *67*, 119–124. [CrossRef]
10. Lee, R.; Garvin, T. Moving from information transfer to information exchange in health and health care. *Soc. Sci. Med.* **2003**, *56*, 449–464. [CrossRef]
11. Mahan, K.; Raymond, J. *Krause's Food and Nutrition Care Process*, 14th ed.; Elsevier: St. Louis, MO, USA, 2017.
12. National Institute for Health and Care Excellence: Making Every Contact Count. Available online: https://stpsupport.nice.org.uk/mecc/index.html (accessed on 5 September 2019).
13. Rogers, C. *Client-Centered Therapy: Its Current Practice, Implications and Theory*; Houghton Mifflin: Boston, MA, USA, 1951.
14. Lu, A.; Dollahite, J. Assessment of dietitians' nutrition counselling self-efficacy and its positive relationship with reported skill usage. *J. Hum. Nutr. Diet.* **2010**, *23*, 144–153. [CrossRef]
15. Academy of Nutrition and Dietetics. Nutrition Intervention. Prescription. Nutrition Care Process Model 2015. Available online: https://bit.ly/2lTiFCo (accessed on 15 May 2019).
16. Holli, B.B.; Calabrese, R.J.; Maillet, J.O.S. *Communication and Education Skills for Dietetic Professionals*; Lippincott Williams and Wilkins: Philadelphia, PA, USA, 2009.
17. Sladdin, I.; Ball, L.; Bull, C.; Chaboyer, W. Patient-centred care to improve dietetic practice: An integrative review. *J. Hum. Nutr. Diet.* **2017**, *30*, 453–470. [CrossRef] [PubMed]
18. Hall, A.M.; Ferreira, P.H.; Maher, C.G.; Latimer, J.; Ferreira, M.L. The influence of the therapist-patient relationship on treatment outcome in physical rehabilitation: A systematic review. *Phys. Ther.* **2010**, *90*, 1099–1110. [CrossRef] [PubMed]
19. Street, R.L., Jr.; Makoul, G.; Arora, N.K.; Epstein, R.M. How does communication heal? Pathways linking clinician-patient communication to health outcomes. *Patient Educ. Couns.* **2009**, *74*, 295–301. [CrossRef]
20. MacLellan, D.; Berenbaum, S. Canadian Dietitians' Understanding of the Client-Centered Approach to Nutrition Counseling. *J. Am. Diet. Assoc.* **2007**, *107*, 1414–1417. [CrossRef] [PubMed]
21. McMahon, A.-T.; Tay, P.C.; Tapsell, L.; Williams, P. Building bridges in dietary counselling: An exploratory study examining the usefulness of wellness and wellbeing concepts. *J. Hum. Nutr. Diet.* **2016**, *29*, 75–85. [CrossRef]
22. Huebner, J.; Marienfeld, S.; Abbenhardt, C.; Ulrich, C.; Muenstedt, K.; Micke, O.; Muecke, R.; Loeser, C. Counseling patients on cancer diets: A review of the literature and recommendations for clinical practice. *Anticancer. Res.* **2014**, *34*, 39–48.
23. Shofield, P.; Diggens, J.; Charleson, C.; Mariglanie, R.; Jefford, M. Effectively discussing complementary and alternative medicine in a conventional oncology setting: Communication recommendations for clinicians. *Patient Educ. Couns.* **2010**, *79*, 143–151. [CrossRef]
24. Hand, R.; Abram, J.; Brown, K.; Ziegler, P.; Scott Parrott, J.; Steiber, A. Development and Validation of the Guide for Effective Nutrition Interventions and Education (GENIE): A tool for assessing the quality of proposed nutrition education programs. *J. Nutr. Educ. Behav.* **2015**, *47*, 308–316. [CrossRef]
25. Murimi, M.; Kanyi, M.; Mupfudze, T.; Amin, M.; Mbogori, T.; Aldubayan, K. Factors Influencing Efficacy of Nutrition Education Interventions: A Systematic Review. *J. Nutr. Educ. Behav.* **2017**, *49*, 142–165. [CrossRef]
26. Rüfenacht, U.; Rühlin, M.; Wegmann, M.; Imoberdorf, R.; Ballmer, P.E. Nutritional counseling improves quality of life and nutrient intake in hospitalized undernourished patients. *Nutrition* **2010**, *26*, 53–60. [CrossRef]
27. Singh, S.; Midha, S.; Singh, N.; Joshi, Y.K.; Garg, P.K. Dietary Counseling Versus Dietary Supplements for Malnutrition in Chronic Pancreatitis: A Randomized Controlled Trial. *Clin. Gastroenterol. Hepatol.* **2008**, *6*, 353–359. [CrossRef] [PubMed]
28. Johansen, N.; Kondrup, J.; Plum, L.M.; Bak, L.; Nørregaard, P.; Bunch, E.; Bærnthsen, H.; Andersen, J.R.; Larsen, I.H.; Martinsen, A. Effect of nutritional support on clinical outcome in patients at nutritional risk. *Clin. Nutr.* **2004**, *23*, 539–550. [CrossRef]
29. Xu, X.; Parker, D.; Ferguson, C.; Hickman, L. Where is the nurse in nutritional care? *Contemp. Nurse* **2017**, *53*, 267–270. [CrossRef] [PubMed]

30. Patience, S. Advising patients on nutrition and healthy eating. *Br. J. Nurs.* **2016**, *25*, 1182–1186. [CrossRef] [PubMed]
31. Perry, L.; Hamilton, S.; Williams, J.; Jones, S. Nursing Interventions for Improving Nutritional Status and Outcomes of Stroke Patients: Descriptive Reviews of Processes and Outcomes. *Worldviews Evid. Based Nurs.* **2013**, *10*, 17–40. [CrossRef] [PubMed]
32. Tappenden, K.A.; Quatrara, B.; Parkhurst, M.L.; Malone, A.M.; Fanjiang, G.; Ziegler, T.R. Critical Role of Nutrition in Improving Quality of Care. *J. Parenter. Enter. Nutr.* **2013**, *37*, 482–497. [CrossRef] [PubMed]
33. Boaz, M.; Rychani, L.; Barami, K.; Houri, Z.; Yosef, R.; Siag, A.; Berlovitz, Y.; Leibovitz, E. Nurses and nutrition: A survey of knowledge and attitudes regarding nutrition assessment and care of hospitalized elderly patients. *J. Contin. Educ. Nurs.* **2013**, *44*, 357–364. [CrossRef]
34. Ross, L.J.; Mudge, A.M.; Young, A.M.; Banks, M. Everyone's problem but nobody's job: Staff perceptions and explanations for poor nutritional intake in older medical patients. *Nutr. Diet.* **2011**, *68*, 41–46. [CrossRef]
35. Duerksen, D.R.; Keller, H.H.; Vesnaver, E.; Laporte, M.; Jeejeebhoy, K.; Payette, H.; Gramlich, L.; Bernier, P.; Allard, J.P. Nurses' Perceptions Regarding the Prevalence, Detection, and Causes of Malnutrition in Canadian Hospitals: Results of a Canadian Malnutrition Task Force Survey. *JPEN J. Parenter. Enter. Nutr.* **2016**, *40*, 100–106. [CrossRef] [PubMed]
36. Hopkinson, J.B. Nutritional support of the elderly cancer patient: The role of the nurse. *Nutrition* **2015**, *31*, 598–602. [CrossRef] [PubMed]
37. Hopkinson, J.B.; Fenlon, D.R.; Okamoto, I.; Wright, D.N.M.; Scott, I.; Addington-Hall, J.M.; Foster, C. The Deliverability, Acceptability, and Perceived Effect of the Macmillan Approach to Weight Loss and Eating Difficulties: A Phase II, Cluster-Randomized, Exploratory Trial of a Psychosocial Intervention for Weight- and Eating-Related Distress in People with Advanced Cancer. *J. Pain Symptom Manag.* **2010**, *40*, 684–695.
38. Van Dillen, S.M.E.; Noordman, J.; van Dulmen, S.; Hiddink, G.J. Quality of weight-loss counseling by Dutch practice nurses in primary care: An observational study. *Eur. J. Clin. Nutr.* **2014**, *69*, 73. [CrossRef] [PubMed]
39. Ahn, J.-A.; Park, J.; Kim, C.-J. Effects of an individualised nutritional education and support programme on dietary habits, nutritional knowledge and nutritional status of older adults living alone. *J. Clin. Nurs.* **2018**, *27*, 2142–2151. [CrossRef] [PubMed]
40. Young, K.; Bunn, F.; Trivedi, D.; Dickinson, A. Nutritional education for community dwelling older people: A systematic review of randomised controlled trials. *Int. J. Nurs. Stud.* **2011**, *48*, 751–780. [CrossRef] [PubMed]
41. Gurzick, M.; Kesten, K.S. The impact of clinical nurse specialists on clinical pathways in the application of evidence-based practice. *J. Prof. Nurs. Off. J. Am. Assoc. Coll. Nurs.* **2010**, *26*, 42–48. [CrossRef] [PubMed]
42. Boeykens, K.; Van Hecke, A. Advanced practice nursing: Nutrition Nurse Specialist role and function. *Clin. Nutr. ESPEN* **2018**, *26*, 72–76. [CrossRef]
43. Sutton, C.D.; Garcea, G.; Pollard, C.; Berry, D.P.; Dennison, A.R. The introduction of a nutrition clinical nurse specialist results in a reduction in the rate of catheter sepsis. *Clin. Nutr.* **2005**, *24*, 220–223. [CrossRef]
44. Yordy, B.M.; Roberts, S.; Taggart, H.M. Quality Improvement in Clinical Nutrition: Screening and Mealtime Protection for the Hospitalized Patient. *Clin. Nurse Spec. CNS* **2017**, *31*, 149–156. [CrossRef]
45. Hamilton, H.C. Advantages of a nurse-led central venous vascular access service. *J. Vasc. Access.* **2004**, *5*, 109–112. [CrossRef]
46. Guenter, P.; Boullata, J.I.; Ayers, P.; Gervasio, J.; Malone, A.; Raymond, E.; Holcombe, B.; Kraft, M.; Sacks, G.; Seres, D. Standardized Competencies for Parenteral Nutrition Prescribing. *Nutr. Clin. Pract.* **2015**, *30*, 570–576. [CrossRef]
47. Fakih El Khoury, C.; Karavetian, M.; Halfens, R.; Crutzen, R.; Khoja, L.S. A systematic review of the effect of dietary mobile apps on nutritional indicators in adults with a chronic illness. *J. Acad. Nutr. Diet.* **2019**, *119*, 626–651. [CrossRef] [PubMed]
48. Stein, K. Remote Nutrition Counseling: Considerations in a New Channel for Client Communication. *J. Acad. Nutr. Diet.* **2015**, *115*, 1561–1576. [CrossRef] [PubMed]
49. European Commission. mHealth. Available online: https://ec.europa.eu/digital-single-market/en/mhealth (accessed on 24 May 2019).
50. Haas, K.; Hayoz, S.; Maurer-Wiesner, S. Effectiveness and Feasibility of a Remote Lifestyle Intervention by Dietitians for Overweight and Obese Adults: Pilot Study. *JMIR MHealth UHealth* **2019**, *7*, e12289. [CrossRef] [PubMed]

51. Rollo, M.E.; Hutchesson, M.J.; Burrows, T.L.; Krukowski, R.A.; Harvey, J.R.; Hoggle, L.B.; Collins, C.E. Video Consultations and Virtual Nutrition Care for Weight Management. *J. Acad. Nutr. Diet.* **2015**, *115*, 1213–1225. [CrossRef] [PubMed]
52. Rollo, M.E.; Burrows, T.; Vincze, L.J.; Harvey, J.; Collins, C.E.; Hutchesson, M.J. Cost evaluation of providing evidence-based dietetic services for weight management in adults: In-person versus eHealth delivery. *Nutr. Diet.* **2018**, *75*, 35–43. [CrossRef] [PubMed]
53. DiFilippo, K.N.; Huang, W.H.; Andrade, J.E.; Chapman-Novakofski, K.M. The use of mobile apps to improve nutrition outcomes: A systematic literature review. *J. Telemed. Telecare* **2015**, *21*, 243–253. [CrossRef] [PubMed]
54. Vasiloglou, M.F.; Mougiakakou, S.; Aubry, E.; Bokelmann, A.; Fricker, R.; Gomes, F.; Guntermann, C.; Meyer, A.; Studerus, D.; Stanga, Z. A Comparative Study on Carbohydrate Estimation: GoCARB vs. Dietitians. *Nutrients* **2018**, *10*, 741. [CrossRef]
55. Bally, L.; Dehais, J.; Nakas, C.T.; Anthimopoulos, M.; Laimer, M.; Rhyner, D.; Rosenberg, G.; Zueger, T.; Diem, P.; Mougiakakou, S.; et al. Carbohydrate Estimation Supported by the GoCARB System in Individuals with Type 1 Diabetes: A Randomized Prospective Pilot Study. *Diabetes Care* **2017**, *40*, e6–e7. [CrossRef]
56. Rhyner, D.; Loher, H.; Dehais, J.; Anthimopoulos, M.; Shevchik, S.; Botwey, R.H.; Duke, D.; Stettler, C.; Diem, P.; Mougiakakou, S. Carbohydrate Estimation by a Mobile Phone-Based System Versus Self-Estimations of Individuals with Type 1 Diabetes Mellitus: A Comparative Study. *J. Med. Internet Res.* **2016**, *18*, e101. [CrossRef]
57. Dehais, J.; Anthimopoulos, M.; Shevchik, S.; Mougiakakou, S. Two-view 3D reconstruction for food volume estimation. *IEEE Trans. Multimed.* **2017**, *19*, 1090–1099. [CrossRef]
58. Anthimopoulos, M.; Dehais, J.; Shevchik, S.; Ransford, B.H.; Duke, D.; Diem, P.; Mougiakakou, S. Computer vision-based carbohydrate estimation for type 1 patients with diabetes using smartphones. *J. Diabetes Sci. Technol.* **2015**, *9*, 507–515. [CrossRef] [PubMed]
59. Reber, E.; Gomes, F.; Vasiloglou, M.F.; Schuetz, P.; Stanga, Z. Nutritional Risk Screening and Assessment. *J. Clin. Med.* **2019**, *8*, 1065. [CrossRef] [PubMed]
60. Harvey-Berino, J.; West, D.; Krukowski, R.; Prewitt, E.; VanBiervliet, A.; Ashikaga, T.; Skelly, J. Internet delivered behavioral obesity treatment. *Prev. Med.* **2010**, *51*, 123–128. [CrossRef] [PubMed]
61. Tate, D.F.; Valle, C.G.; Crane, M.M.; Nezami, B.T.; Samuel-Hodge, C.D.; Hatley, K.E.; Diamond, M.; Polzien, K. Randomized trial comparing group size of periodic in-person sessions in a remotely delivered weight loss intervention. *Int. J. Behav. Nutr. Phys. Act.* **2017**, *14*, 144. [CrossRef] [PubMed]
62. Tate, D.F.; Jackvony, E.H.; Wing, R.R. Effects of Internet behavioral counseling on weight loss in adults at risk for type 2 diabetes: A randomized trial. *JAMA* **2003**, *289*, 1833–1836. [CrossRef] [PubMed]
63. Tate, D.F.; Jackvony, E.H.; Wing, R.R. A randomized trial comparing human e-mail counseling, computer-automated tailored counseling, and no counseling in an Internet weight loss program. *Arch. Intern. Med.* **2006**, *166*, 1620–1625. [CrossRef] [PubMed]
64. Patel, M.L.; Hopkins, C.M.; Brooks, T.L.; Bennett, G.G. Comparing Self-Monitoring Strategies for Weight Loss in a Smartphone App: Randomized Controlled Trial. *JMIR Mhealth Uhealth* **2019**, *7*, e12209. [CrossRef] [PubMed]
65. Brandt, C.J.; Sogaard, G.I.; Clemensen, J.; Sondergaard, J.; Nielsen, J.B. Determinants of Successful eHealth Coaching for Consumer Lifestyle Changes: Qualitative Interview Study Among Health Care Professionals. *J. Med. Internet Res.* **2018**, *20*, e237. [CrossRef]
66. Chen, J.; Gemming, L.; Hanning, R.; Allman-Farinelli, M. Smartphone apps and the nutrition care process: Current perspectives and future considerations. *Patient Educ. Couns.* **2018**, *101*, 750–757. [CrossRef]
67. Rollo, M.E.; Collins, C.E.; MacDonald-Wicks, L. Evaluation of the Introduction of an e-Health Skills Component for Dietetics Students. *Telemed. J. e-Health* **2017**, *23*, 930–933. [CrossRef]
68. Apinaniz, A.; Cobos-Campos, R.; Saez de Lafuente-Moringo, A.; Parraza, N.; Aizpuru, F.; Pérez, I.; Goicoechea, E.; Trápaga, N.; García, L. Effectiveness of randomized controlled trial of a mobile app to promote healthy lifestyle in obese and overweight patients. *Fam. Pract.* **2019**. [CrossRef] [PubMed]

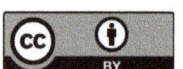

© 2019 by the authors. Licensee MDPI, Basel, Switzerland. This article is an open access article distributed under the terms and conditions of the Creative Commons Attribution (CC BY) license (http://creativecommons.org/licenses/by/4.0/).

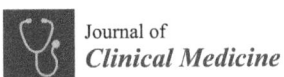

Review

Medical Nutrition Therapy in Critically Ill Patients Treated on Intensive and Intermediate Care Units: A Literature Review

Andrea Kopp Lugli [1],*, Aude de Watteville [2],†, Alexa Hollinger [3],†, Nicole Goetz [4] and Claudia Heidegger [2],*

1. Intensive Care Unit and Intermediate Care Unit, Intensive Care Medicine and Department of Anesthesiology, University Hospital Basel, 4031 Basel, Switzerland
2. Division of Intensive Care, Department of Acute Medicine, Geneva University Hospitals, 1205 Geneva, Switzerland
3. Intensive Care Unit and Intermediate Care Unit, Intensive Care Medicine and Department of Anesthesiology, University Hospital Basel, 4031 Basel, Switzerland
4. Endocrinology, Diabetes and Metabolism, University Hospital Basel, 4031 Basel & Department of Anesthesiology, University Hospital Basel, 4031 Basel, Switzerland
* Correspondence: andrea.kopplugli@usb.ch (A.K.L.); claudia.heidegger@hcuge.ch (C.H.)
† Equally contributed.

Received: 4 August 2019; Accepted: 3 September 2019; Published: 6 September 2019

Abstract: Medical nutrition therapy in critically ill patients remains challenging, not only because of the pronounced stress response with a higher risk for complications, but also due to their heterogeneity evolving from different phases of illness. The present review aims to address current knowledge and guidelines in order to summarize how they can be best implemented into daily clinical practice. Further studies are urgently needed to answer such important questions as best timing, route, dose, and composition of medical nutrition therapy for critically ill patients and to determine how to assess and to adapt to patients' individual needs.

Keywords: nutritional support; medical nutrition therapy; intensive care unit; intermediate care unit; critically ill patients

---

1. Introduction

The critical importance, complexity, and challenge of clinical nutrition for critically ill patients is best understood when recapitulating the evolution of this complex patient group and, consequently, the proposed guidelines and clinical practice strategies during the last decades, as follows: (1) Adult critically ill patients present as a heterogeneous group with regard to diagnosis, severity of illness, and the number of (pre-)existing comorbidities. (2) Critically ill patients are treated not only on intensive care units (ICU), but increasingly in smooth transition on so-called step-down or intermediate care units (IMC-U) depending on the severity of illness, the available facilities, and hospital internal regulations. Still, these patients should not be systematically divided into separate categories. From a metabolic point of view, all patients requiring intensive or intermediate care suffer from a relevant catabolic stress response, which parallels the severity of injury or illness. From an institutional point of view, IMC-Us are relatively new facilities treating patients who require less care than standard intensive care, but more than that which is available from ward care [1]. Taking these two points into account, an overlap of IMC-U and ICU treatment is owed to the organization and available facilities of each individual hospital, as follows: Patients with the same severity of illness may be treated in one hospital on the ICU and in another hospital on the IMC-U. Since IMC-Us are an emerging type of treatment facility, IMC-U specific randomized clinical trials (RCTs) and guidelines are still missing and should be a field of future research. Therefore, patients in both of these groups are considered to be critically ill patients throughout this review article as their nutritional needs, first and foremost, parallel the course of illness and are not defined by the treating facility per se. (3) The ICU population suffers from a high prevalence of malnutrition when admitted to hospital (up to 60%) and during the intensive care treatment phase [2–5]. (4) The diagnosis of malnutrition and the assessment of nutritional needs are complex and ask for systematic re-evaluation and adaptation. (5) Some study data from recent years have highlighted the association between protein and caloric deficiency and higher morbidity and mortality rates [2,6–9]. These findings have introduced the conversion from "nutritional support" as an adjunctive care to "nutrition therapy", which not only covers micro- and macronutrient needs, but also intends to blunt the metabolic response, cellular injury, and immunological alteration. However, several further studies showed no clinical benefit [10–13] for higher protein and calorie administration in the ICU or reported harmful results, such as increased adjusted mortality at 6 months for mechanically ventilated patients [10] and less gastrointestinal tolerance in patients with acute lung injury [13]. Additionally, the idea of pharmaco-nutrition was abandoned after several neutral and one lethal trial [14–16]. On these grounds, the current European Society for Clinical Nutrition and Metabolism (ESPEN) guideline defines the term "medical nutrition therapy" (MNT), which encompasses oral nutritional supplements, enteral, and parenteral nutrition. Furthermore, ESPEN underlines the need for well conducted trials on optimal protein intake since currently available studies are not comparable in terms of patient selection and calorie and protein intake, as well as timing and route of administration. Yet, ESPEN evokes the possibility that it is possible that, similar to caloric targets, optimal protein targets change over time in the ICU and that a high protein intake is only beneficial if not associated with overfeeding [17]. However, so far this hypothesis is not yet confirmed by RCTs.

To date, nutritional practices are widely diverse [18] and many studies, reviews, and guidelines address only one or some of the relevant aspects of MNT [7,17,19–47]. The ESPEN guidelines [17] and those of the American Society on Parenteral and Enteral Nutrition (ASPEN) [27], as well as the Canadian Critical Care Practice Guidelines (CCPG) [48], are among the most regularly updated evidence-based guidelines. All three underline the relevance of the points stated above and the need for further carefully planned randomized trials. The present review aims to address current knowledge and guidelines in order to summarize how they can best be implemented into daily clinical practice. We specified the different guidelines' recommendation grades. The ESPEN guidelines use standard operation procedure (grade A, B, 0, or good practice point (GPP)) [49] and the ASPEN guidelines grade the study evidence level, from high to very low for RCTs and low to very low for observational studies; the good practice statement is ungraded [50].

2. Screening

A high prevalence of malnutrition is observed at ICU admission [5], with a further energy and protein deficit (50% and 60%, respectively) occurring during ICU stay [51,52]. Indeed, an international multicenter observational study revealed an association between the increase of energy and protein intake and the decrease of mortality in patients with a body mass index (BMI) <25 or >35 kg/m^2 [6]. The same research group failed to validate this concept in the TOP-UP trial [53]. More generally, no nutritional intervention reduced mortality in critically ill patients, except withholding early glutamine in patients with multiorgan failure [14].

On the other hand, some recent RCTs investigating the timing of initiation as well as the quantity and the route of MNT showed contradictory results [7,54–57]. Waiting for more conclusive studies, actual guidelines suggest that all critically ill patients should be routinely screened with the aim of preventing malnutrition [17,27].

Many different screening tools to identify the malnutrition risk are available. Some scores are widely used, such as (1) the Nutrition Risk Screening (NRS) 2002 [58], focusing on nutritional state, illness severity, and age; (2) the Nutrition Risk in the Critically Ill (NUTRIC) score [59], including a severity score, comorbidities, and the number of hospital days; (3) the Subjective Global Assessment (SGA), combining historical data and a clinical examination [60]; and (4) the Mini-Nutrition Assessment (MNA) [61], which is specific for the elderly population. Despite the large number of existing scores, none has been validated for the critically ill thus far [62] and none have been able to identify patients who improve with enhanced feeding.

Laboratory data, such as albumin and pre-albumin, are frequently used as markers of nutritional status, but cannot be clearly interpreted during critical illness, as low albumin and prealbumin levels occur as a response to increased inflammation [63].

Weight changes are also difficult to interpret considering the relevant amounts of fluid administration and depletion during the ICU and IMC-U stay. Thus, weight loss does not reflect loss of lean body mass. Nevertheless, this aspect is an important issue for the detection of malnutrition, as the loss of lean body mass has been associated with longer hospitalization and reduced quality of life and functional abilities [60]. Some methods, such as ultrasound [64] or computerized tomography (CT) scan [65], are promising tools that can help to determine the extent of lean body mass loss. However, these methods still need to be validated in clinical practice. Moreover, the way in which they influence therapy is not yet clear. Bioelectrical impedance to assess body composition and lean body mass may be useful, but its interpretation is complicated by important fluid changes that occur in the critically ill [66].

Concerning these screening tools, ASPEN [27] and ESPEN [17] have taken different positions. While the current ASPEN guidelines recommend using either the NRS 2002 or the NUTRIC-Score for nutritional risk determination [27], the new ESPEN guidelines propose a more general clinical assessment including anamnesis, evaluation of muscle mass and strength, unintentional weight loss, and body composition (GPP). Furthermore, all critically ill patients with a length of stay of more than 48 h should be considered at risk for malnutrition (GPP) [17].

3. Assessment of Medical Nutrition Therapy

3.1. Energy Needs

It is extremely challenging to assess energy requirements of the critically ill, as the requirements depend on many factors and may be dynamic over time [67].

Initially, critical illness provokes an acute early phase [17] characterized by a major metabolic instability with hypermetabolism, insulin resistance, glycemia perturbation, and increased catabolism with the production of endogenous substrates [68]. This is followed by an acute late period with a certain degree of stabilization but persistent catabolism. Finally, when the inflammatory state and critical conditions decrease, the late phase or chronic phase sets in, with the beginning of anabolism and rehabilitation [43]. Moreover, energy expenditure (EE) is also modulated by many other conditions such as underlying illness, inflammatory state, medications, body composition, and nutritional status prior to admission [67].

While predictive formulas to estimate EE are widely used for MNT, many studies have shown them to be inaccurate and imprecise [69–72]. Up to now, no predictive equation has been validated for the critically ill [17,27]. If predictive formulas are used, hypocaloric MNT (<70% of the estimated EE) should be preferred over isocaloric nutrition during the first week of the ICU and IMC-U stay in order to avoid overnutrition [17].

For some time, the ESPEN guidelines have recommended the use of indirect calorimetry (IC) to determine EE as the best standard practice [73,74]. This attitude is reiterated in the current ASPEN (grade very low) and ESPEN guidelines (grade B) [17,27]. Furthermore, the ESPEN guidelines suggest that if IC is used, an isocaloric nutrition can be progressively implemented after the early phase of acute illness (grade 0). However, during the early phase of acute illness, hypocaloric nutrition (not exceeding 70% of EE) should be administered (grade B). Still, the exact way to use IC measurements to guide MNT needs to be validated by further studies.

The IC measurement is based on O_2 and CO_2 concentrations as well as the volume of expired gas/minute [67]. The EE is then calculated directly by the calorimeter according to the Weir's equation [75]. This measurement can be performed either in mechanically ventilated or spontaneously breathing patients. Measurements are influenced by several factors such as medications, stress, body temperature, mechanical ventilation, agitation, etc. [76,77]. The currently available IC devices are expensive, time consuming, and not always accurate; thus, IC measurements cannot be performed regularly. The International Multicentric Study Group for Indirect Calorimetry (ICALIC) recently developed a new IC aimed at meeting clinical needs [67].

The ICALIC study group suggests IC measurements on day 3 to 4 after admission [67], which should be repeated as soon as clinical conditions change. They suggest adapting energy targets to the result of the last IC measurement with the aim of optimizing nutritional management [67].

If IC is not available, energy expenditure calculated from the carbon dioxide production (VCO2) extracted from the ventilator or oxygen consumption (VO2) from pulmonary arterial catheter are recommended by the new ESPEN guidelines [17]. However, these methods were not shown to be accurate compared to IC measurements [78–80] and can only be obtained with invasive monitoring.

3.2. Protein Needs

Although the coverage of energy needs is an area that has been studied for several years, the importance of the protein needs has only recently become a subject of focus. Indeed, critical illness causes protein catabolism resulting in important muscle loss, which influences a patient's survival and clinical outcome [81]. Current recommendations on protein intake for critically ill patients are based mainly on observational data and only a few RCTs having different designs. Thus, it is difficult to draw definitive conclusions.

Various recent observational studies have focused on the association between protein intake and patients' clinical outcomes, suggesting an association between mortality reduction and protein intake [82–84]. For instance, decreased mortality has been related to protein intake ≥1.2 g/kg/day in non-septic and non-overfeed critically ill patients [84] by achieving ≥80% of the prescribed protein intake [82] and to a protein intake of >1 g/kg/day [83].

Conversely, recent RCTs on protein needs have shown contradictory results and up-to-date no mortality benefit with higher amino acid intake could be shown by RCTs. In the Ferrie study ($n = 120$), the administration of 1.2 g/kg parenteral amino acids (AA) compared to 0.8 g/kg was associated with attenuated muscle wasting, less fatigue, and better nitrogen balance, but no difference in mortality or length of stay was observed [85].

The Nephro-Protective trial ($n = 474$), with higher AA administration in the intervention group, did not affect the duration of renal dysfunction but only showed an improved estimated glomerular filtration rate (eGFR) and daily urinary output. Furthermore, serum urea was significantly higher, with a trend toward increased renal replacement therapy (RTT) in patients receiving AA therapy, which was not present after controlling for baseline imbalance in terms of renal failure at the time of study enrollment [86].

Other recent RCTs, such as the EAT-ICU ($n = 203$) and the TOP-UP trial ($n = 125$) on protein needs, have confirmed no differences on clinical outcomes including mortality, hospital stay, days of ventilation, nosocomial infections, or organ failure rates [53,56]. However, the EAT-ICU trial also showed a prolonged ICU length of stay (post-hoc analysis) as well as a trend to increased plasma urea levels in the Early Goal-directed Nutrition group [56].

The EPaNIC trial ($n = 4640$) showed that early initiation of parenteral nutrition (PN) was associated with a longer course of RTT and a longer ICU stay. Similar functional status was observed in the early and late PN group [54]. A prospectively planned subanalysis of the EPaNIC trial found an increased incidence of ICU-acquired muscle weakness with slower recovery in the early-PN group [87]. Apart from this, in another post hoc analysis of the EPaNIC trial, delayed recovery was also attributed to the early administration of amino acids by PN [88].

The results of the recent RCTs underline the urgent need for further studies to provide answers to questions still outstanding, such as the right amount of protein to administer and the best timing.

Based on the available results and without the possibility to assess individual protein needs during a protein-loss phase, ESPEN guidelines [17] suggest a progressive provision of 1.3 g/kg/day of protein equivalent during critical illness (grade 0). In contrast, the ASPEN guidelines [27] propose a protein intake of 1.2–2.0 g/kg/day (grade very low).

Exercise in combination with achieving protein targets has also been suggested to maximally maintain muscle mass [17,89,90].

4. Practical Implementation

4.1. Special Risk Groups

A few distinct patient subgroups, consisting of critically ill surgical and medical patients at particular risk for malnutrition, are defined and discussed below.

4.1.1. Obese and Bariatric Patients

One steadily growing sub-population consists of patients who are already metabolically challenged (i.e., diabetic, severely obese, and post-bariatric/obese surgery patients) [91].

As the number of bariatric operations increases, one must keep in mind that approximately 30% of bariatric patients develop nutritional complications [91]. Furthermore, the proportion of obese critically ill patients is growing parallel to the increasing prevalence in the general population [92]. The ASPEN guidelines suggest to additionally focus the nutritional assessment of these patients on biomarkers of metabolic syndrome, evaluation of comorbidities, and the level of inflammation [27].

In order to estimate patient nutritional needs, resting EE is best assessed by IC [20]. If not available, energy intake can be guided by adjusted body weight (BW) and protein delivery by urinary nitrogen losses or lean body mass determination (using CT or other tools), according to the ESPEN guidelines [17].

Several existing predictive scores, such as the Mifflin-St Jeor (MSJ) and the Harris–Benedict equations [93,94], can be applied if IC is not available in the case of complicated bariatric patients [20,94]. However, it is important to consider that these scores are not specifically validated for post-bariatric patients and IC is recommended in the first place [17].

The ESPEN guidelines recommend an isocaloric high protein diet including a protein intake of 1.3 g/kg adjusted BW/day (GPP) [17]. On the other hand, the ASPEN guidelines [27] suggest a hypocaloric high-protein feeding protocol, with 65%–70% of measured energy requirements using IC or weight-based equations (calories: BMI 30–50 kg/m^2 = 11–14 kcal/kg actual BW/day, BMI > 50 kg/m^2 = 22–25 kcal/kg ideal BW/day; protein: BMI 30–40 kg/m^2 = 2 g/kg ideal BW/day, BMI ≥ 40 kg/m^2 = 2.5/kg ideal BW/day), for all classes of obesity.

In order to avoid micronutrient (iron, calcium, vitamin D, vitamin B$_{12}$, folate) deficiency after bariatric surgery, life-long multivitamin supplementation is necessary for post-bariatric patients. Since many patients show malabsorption for iron, a documented deficiency is best supplemented intravenously [91].

4.1.2. Geriatric Patients

Patients aged ≥65 years comprise a large portion of the critically ill population and often struggle with nutritional intake and risk of malnutrition. In the ICU and IMC-U setting, additional acute illness on top of an already frail state often leads to poor outcomes [95]. The assessment of the frailty score in this subgroup might be a valuable addition to malnutrition screening [21].

A state of sarcopenia in acutely ill elderly patients is associated with increased short-term mortality [22]. The course of elderly patients according to their nutritional status (BMI and albumin levels) was evaluated and resulted in a higher prognostic value than their absolute age [23].

However, a recent review emphasized the importance of additional parameters such as energy intake, weight loss, and grip strength, whereas biochemical markers were susceptible to the underlying disease process and were not always reliable [96].

Swallowing and chewing problems may be an important issue affecting oral intake in geriatric patients. Therefore, smaller and more frequent meals completed by oral nutritional supplements (ONS) are suggested [96]. Evaluation of swallowing, dental status, oral health, and potential drug side effects that might impair oral feeding should be conducted systematically [95].

About 20% of older critically ill patients have sarcopenia before hospitalization [22,97] and are subjected to various antianabolic and procatabolic factors during critical illness. An ESPEN expert working group recommends 1.2–1.5 g protein/kg/day in elderly patients suffering or at risk for malnutrition, since they have acute or chronic illness. Even higher protein intakes are recommended for this patient population in case of severe illness or injury [98]. In a recent review of older ICU patients, besides the provision of at least 1.2–1.5 g protein/kg usual BW/day, a combination including regular and early ambulation (if possible) and/or physical therapy and follow-up rehabilitation are prudently recommended to counteract muscle loss [97]. These recommendations are based on observational data or studies in non-critically ill patients [99,100]. Therefore, this review acknowledges the need of further research to consolidate the most efficacious in-unit and post-discharge nutrition and physical activity strategies with well conducted clinical trials [97].

Vitamin D deficiency is common in the elderly and the critically ill and is associated with increased mortality. According to the 2019 ESPEN guidelines, vitamin D can be supplemented (GPP) with a single dose of 500,000 IU vitamin D3 within one week after admission (grade 0) in case of measured low plasma levels (25-hydroxy vitamin D <12.5 ng/mL, or <50 nmol/L) [17].

4.1.3. Other Risk Groups

With the development of advanced medicine, the new patient group of so-called chronic critically ill patients has emerged and is often treated in the step-down unit. A recent review provides a thorough discussion of the nutritional approach for these patients [101]. The ASPEN guidelines, based on expert consensus, define chronic critically ill patients as having persistent organ dysfunction requiring ICU treatment >21 days and suggest management with aggressive high-protein EN therapy and, when feasible, use of a resistance exercise program [27].

Patients with renal failure can be placed on a standard enteral formula following the recent ICU recommendations for protein administration [17,27]. According to the ASPEN guidelines, a special formula might be indicated in case of significant electrolyte or volume abnormalities. Renal replacement therapy may require increased protein support (≤2.5 g/kg/day) (grade very low) and adapted micronutrient support [17,27]. Importantly, protein support should not be restricted in order to avoid or delay initiation of dialysis therapy [27].

The ESPEN Society provides separate nutritional management recommendations for severe burn patients [102] and for patients with acute or chronic liver failure [103].

Patients with alcohol abuse are particularly at risk for thiamine deficiency, as are patients with severe sepsis, congestive heart failure, or burn injuries [104]. Recommended daily doses for alcoholic patients are substantially higher than for non-alcoholic patients, reaching up to 500 mg thiamine three times daily [105]. Another review underlines the importance of additive therapies such as correction of electrolyte disturbances and malnourishment [106].

4.2. International Guidelines on Nutrition in Critically Ill Patients

In this review on most recent practices to provide adequate nutrition in the critically ill, we concentrated on three widely used and regularly updated international guidelines issued by the Canadian Critical Care Society/Canadian Critical Care Trials Group (CCCS/CCCTG) [48] in 2015, by ASPEN [27] in 2016, and, most recently, by ESPEN [17]. These three guidelines discuss main and subtopics of critical care nutrition in which most recommendations are based on expert consensus

(Table S1). As such, ESPEN guidelines include the most recent studies and meta-analyses from robust RCTs. Moreover, recommendations have been well separated into grade A, B, level 0, or GPP, according to the strength of the evidence [107]. The ASPEN guidelines include the largest number of recommendations, whereas certain aspects of the guidelines are not exclusively covered by the European and Canadian societies (ESPEN; CCCS/CCTG) (e.g., non-intubated patients (ESPEN), ornithine ketoglutarate in burn patients or specific mentioning of vitamin C supplementation (CCCS/CCTG), or recommendation on insulin administration (ESPEN; CCCS/CCTG). Many recommendations in the ASPEN guidelines target a certain group of critically ill, whereas the ESPEN and CCCS/CCCTG guidelines address the critically ill in general (e.g., vitamin D supplementation). Notably, ASPEN proposes a higher number of recommendations for subgroups of critically ill patients by labelling with a grade of expert consensus due to the lack of solid evidence. Moreover, the concept of ALI (acute lung injury), not part of the 2013 Berlin definition of acute respiratory distress syndrome (ARDS), is not mentioned in the ESPEN guidelines [28]. ASPEN and ESPEN offer recommendations for frequent diseases seen in critical care, such as sepsis and acute pancreatitis and statements for trauma and burn patients. In addition, the American society includes a chapter on end-of-life care.

4.3. Medical Nutrition Therapy: EN, PN, ONS, and Combinations

Routes, quantity, and timing of nutritional delivery have been widely discussed over recent decades. With the increasing administration of parenteral nutrition (PN) to the critically ill, some studies have shown more infectious complications in comparison to enteral nutrition (EN) [29,30]. Enteral feeding was subsequently used in first line with an important reduction in the use of PN [108]. However, achieving energy and protein targets with EN alone is difficult during the ICU and IMC-U stay and may result in undernutrition in most patients [31,32]. Recent RCTs have shown no increase in the rate of complications independent of the chosen route of nutrition [57,109]. Avoiding under- or overnutrition is more important than the feeding route [108].

The SPN study (n = 305) showed that the use of supplemental parenteral nutrition (SPN) (when EN was insufficient to match the energy targets at day 4 after ICU admission) could reduce nosocomial infections after the end of the intervention and until the end of the observation period (days 9 to 28), as well as antibiotic use during the ICU stay [7]. However, no impact on infections was shown when counting the infection rate from the randomization day onward. The TICACOS pilot study (n = 130) [55] showed, based on prospective intention to treat analysis of the data, that IC-guided nutrition therapy provoked an increase in complications with more infections, longer duration of ventilation, and prolonged ICU stays. A per protocol analysis, on the contrary, suggested a short-lived survival benefit [55].

Some other studies (e.g., EAT-ICU (n = 203) [56], TARGET (n = 3957) [11], EDEN (n = 1000) [13]) showed no difference between the early versus standard initiation groups in primary clinical outcomes, but secondary outcomes revealed hyperglycemia [13,56] and decreased gastric tolerance [11,13] in the early nutrition intervention group. The PermiT trial (n = 894) group studied permissive underfeeding (40–60% of calculated caloric requirements) compared to standard enteral feeding (70–100%) with similar protein intake. The results showed no difference in 90-day mortality and no differences in other significant outcomes between the groups [12]. The results of the EPaNIC trial (n = 4640) revealed no difference in 90-day mortality but an increased complication rate with early initiation of parenteral support (i.e., infections, longer mechanical ventilation, and length of stay) [54].

The divergence of results may be related to the heterogeneous patient population and highly variable study designs with differences such as the amount of calories administered, the timing of EN or PN initiation, and the use of IC or predictive formulas.

Considering these contradictory findings, expert guidelines agree on the following indications for MNT [17,27]: (1) Oral nutrition should be preferred over EN or PN in patients able to eat voluntarily (GPP). (2) If needed, oral nutritional supplements (ONS) can be given with the aim to achieve energy and protein needs [34]. (3) Early EN (within 48 h) is suggested for all patients with a functional digestive tract who cannot eat voluntarily (grade B). Enteral feeding can be performed progressively after the early phase of the critical illness and, after 3 days, caloric delivery can be increased up to 80–100% of the measured EE (grade 0). (4) In patients who do not tolerate full EN during the first week, initiation of SPN should be considered on a case-by-case basis and should only be started after all strategies to maximize EN tolerance have been attempted (GPP). (5) In case of impossible oral feeding and EN contraindications, PN must also be started progressively during the first week of the ICU stay.

The timing of PN initiation is a highly debated topic. ESPEN experts propose an early implementation of PN within 3–7 days in case of contraindications to oral feeding or EN (grade B). SPN should be considered for patients who do not tolerate full-dose EN during the first week of ICU or IMC-U stay (GPP). In contrast, the ASPEN guidelines recommend SPN in case of insufficient early EN (<60% of energy and protein requirements) only after 7–10 days. Further, the ESICM guidelines extensively discuss clinical states and medications that warrant delayed EN initiation [17,27,110].

4.4. Adaptation/Reassessment and Monitoring

Monitoring is an essential part of nutritional management and is central to achieving high-quality nutritional care. The quantity of prescribed and received nutrition in terms of volume, energy, and protein must be assessed including non-nutritional calories (e.g., Propofol®, citrate) [35] in order to avoid under- or overfeeding. Gastric tolerance must be monitored, including clinical abdominal examination and evaluation of stools, gastric residual volume, or vomit [111]. Laboratory monitoring of glycemia, electrolytes, liver parameters, and triglycerides is necessary to assess MNT tolerance [35]; prealbumin can be helpful to assess the efficacy of the MNT [36].

4.5. Role of the Intensive Care Unit Dietician

Even if nutritional guidelines and local protocols have been shown to be helpful in standardizing and improving the quality of MNT in ICUs [37,38], physicians and nurses have reported a lack of knowledge, training, and time in nutrition management [39,40]. Dieticians, specialized in ICU nutrition, can provide valuable help concerning nutrition management for the ICU teams. It was suggested that the presence of dieticians in the ICU team was helpful to achieve the desired daily energy and protein targets during the ICU stay [39]. Their role should also include detection of too early aggressive nutrition support with the aim to prevent refeeding and overfeeding. To increase the quality of the care, we recommend working in a multidisciplinary team including intensivists, ICU nutritional specialists, dieticians, nurses, physiotherapists, and others if necessary. In addition, regular adaptation of local protocols to the current guidelines and facilitating protocol adherence is necessary [41]. These efforts should be extended to patients on the IMC-U.

4.6. Continuation of Medical Nutrition Therapy After Transfer or Discharge to Home

MNT is not only important during ICU/IMC-U stay, it is an essential part of both the post-ICU/IMC-U recovery phase and after hospital discharge [43]. While advances in medicine and improvements in the quality of care have reduced ICU mortality in recent years, the number of post-critically ill patients in rehabilitation has consequently increased [112]. Low oral intake (e.g., only 700 kcal/day for one week after extubation) has been reported to be an amount insufficient to cover the energy needs of 97% of patients [42,76]. In this context, most critically ill patients would need continuous medium-length or long-term MNT (ONS, EN, PN, and SPN) coupled with exercise for rehabilitation. MNT can also be continued at home after hospital discharge. However, it is also important to consider the physical and mental abilities of patients and their relatives, in addition to the patient's living conditions, with the aim of achieving a supportive environment [44]. Educating the patient and his/her close relatives should be proposed to achieve the highest level of independence possible [44]. Follow up involving a multidisciplinary nutrition team helps to increase the quality of care, facilitating the adaptation of the therapy and the support in case of possible complications [44].

5. Complications

5.1. Over- and Underfeeding

Over- and underfeeding frequently occur in critical care patients as nutritional substrates, whether given parenterally or enterally, do not have the same metabolic consequences in the critically ill. While overfeeding occurs more often with PN, underfeeding is more common in enterally fed patients. Patients most at risk for energy excess or nutritional deficits are those with low caloric targets (e.g., due to small body size, non-nutritional energy (e.g., Propofol® for sedation) or geriatric patients) [113].

Overfeeding is defined as the administration of excess energy in relation to the body's need to maintain metabolic homeostasis when exceeding >110% of the EE [17] and can lead to a multitude of complications and increased mortality. Depending on the macro-nutrients delivered in excess, these complications include hypercapnia, refeeding syndrome (RFS) and liver disturbances, hyperglycemia and hypertriglyceridemia, as well as azotemia, hypertonic dehydration, and metabolic acidosis [114]. Therefore, higher protein amounts (1.3 g/kg/day) can be delivered progressively as long as these amounts are not associated with overfeeding (grade 0) [17].

The lower limit of optimal energy supplementation to the critically ill is not yet clearly defined and may vary depending on the underlying disease and nutritional status of the patient. Underfeeding (<70% of the defined target) [17] often occurs during EN due to feeding intolerance, airway management, or disruption of feeding due to elective procedures [115].

5.2. Refeeding Syndrome

RFS is recognized as a life-threatening cause-independent complication in severely malnourished patients. These patients may show severe adverse reactions involving the cardiac, respiratory, hematological, hepatic, and neuromuscular systems when refed too rapidly, especially with carbohydrates [46]. The difficulty to precisely define RFS limits screening and estimated numbers of unreported cases are presumably high. Therefore, assessing the risk of RFS before starting MNT in high-risk patients [46,47], including those with anorexia nervosa, chronic alcoholics, elderly patients with multiple comorbidities, patients with signs of chronic malnutrition (e.g., marasmus, severe inflammatory bowel disease, short bowel syndrome), the morbidly obese, and patients receiving PN, has been suggested [47]. Furthermore, an algorithm for RFS management has been proposed, including an initial risk assessment and recommendations for electrolyte and fluid repletion [116,117]. However, a more recent retrospective study [118] in critically ill patients with prolonged ventilation found no baseline characteristics predicting RFS. Patients developing RFS had a reduced 6-month mortality risk when receiving low caloric intake. These results confirm those of a previous trial proposing a caloric restriction in the context of RFS [119] as follows: (1) Reduced energy intake of 20 kcal/h for at least 2 days, (2) if serum phosphate concentrations did not need to be supplemented, as determined per protocol (as described in the Appendix S3 of [119]), energy intake should be returned to normal during 2–3 days, (3) a gradual return to 40 kcal/h for 24 h, then increased goals to 60 kcal/h for 24 h, followed by 80% of calculated energy goals for another 24 h, with 100% of goals achieved by day 4 [119].

According to the National Institute for Health and Care Excellence (NICE) guidelines, patients at risk should be nourished with regular control of electrolytes as follows: (1) Feeding starting at 10 kcal/kg/day, (2) increasing to full need over ≥4 days, and (3) supplementation of thiamine (vitamin B1, 200–300 mg/day) for the first 10 days [47,120].

5.3. Parenteral Nutrition

Complications attributed to the use of PN include mechanical complications with catheter obstruction, catheter infections, venous thrombosis, or pneumothorax [121]. Short-term metabolic complications can occur as well as fluid imbalance (overload or dehydration), electrolyte disturbances, glycemic abnormalities, and dyslipidemia [122]. These complications can be avoided by systematic and precise monitoring [122]. Major long-term metabolic complications include metabolic bone diseases and hepatobiliary disorders. It was shown that the frequency of osteoporosis and osteomalacia increases in patients with long-term PN [123]. In addition, intestinal failure-associated liver disease can occur during parenteral feeding, and cholestasis and hepatic steatosis in those with long-term PN. Hepatobiliary disorders have been attributed to overfeeding during PN [121,124].

Some recent studies suggest that, if provided in isocaloric doses, PN and EN result in similar clinical outcomes [7,57,109]. Therefore, PN is not in opposition to EN but can be used as an additional therapy as soon as a close monitoring of the MNT is assured [39,108]. However, PN should not be started before all strategies to maximize EN tolerance have been attempted (GPP) [17].

5.4. Enteral Nutrition

Two large randomized trials specifically designed to investigate the feeding route in critically ill patients [57,109] found more episodes of both hypoglycemia and vomiting with EN compared to PN. Furthermore, the NUTRIREA-2 trial assessing severely ill ICU patients under mechanical ventilation and on vasopressors detected a pronounced difficulty to reach protein and calorie targets and an increased risk for gastrointestinal complications (e.g., diarrhea, bowel ischemia, acute colonic pseudo-obstruction) with early EN [57].

Enteral Nutrition and Dysphagia: Risk of Aspiration, Swallowing Screening

Dysphagia occurs in 50–70% of the critically ill [125]. Risk factors include older age, congestive heart failure, sepsis, perioperative stroke, non-coronary bypass surgical procedures, transesophageal echocardiography, and previous stroke [125]. Patients suffering from dysphagia are at major risk for aspiration. Several high-quality swallowing tests (e.g., DePippo, Horner, Kidd) developed to thoroughly assess aspiration risk have been summarized in a recent review [126] in which the authors report the swallowing screening published by Daniels et al. in 1998 to be the most convenient. This assessment is also applicable for intubated patients for a certain period of time. Moreover, it is considered by non-speech therapists (i.e., nurses specialized in intensive care) to be the most suitable assessment.

In case of aspiration risk, feeding tubes are used to nourish the patient. Tube selection depends on the expected duration of feeding. Furthermore, the selection of a large bore tube (≥14 French) ensures gastric suctioning and decompression in case of gastroparesis and paralytic ileus, which are usually present during the early postoperative period.

The measurement of gastric residual volume (GRV) for the assessment of gastrointestinal function is commonly used and may help to detect intolerance to EN during initiation and progression of EN, especially in patients who underwent abdominal procedures or major surgery. However, monitoring of GRV in case of established EN may not be necessary. The ESPEN guidelines suggest that EN should be delayed when GRV is >500 mL/6 h, and prokinetic treatment should be considered if acute abdominal complications are excluded [17]. ASPEN and the Surviving Sepsis Initiative support the use of prokinetics (e.g., metoclopramide (three times 10 mg/day) and erythromycin (3–7 mg/kg/day)) in the case of feeding intolerance [27,127].

6. Financial Aspects

Disease-related malnutrition has relevant consequences on patient outcome, especially in the most severely ill patients treated on ICUs and IMC-Us. However, for several reasons it remains difficult to demonstrate the economic benefit related to improved outcome rooted in MNT. The comparison of different clinical practices in hospitals and countries, variable costs for hospital staff and MNT products, and heterogeneous accounting systems complicate any reliable comparison of cost and benefit. Furthermore, the acquisition of nationwide and international data is limited and explains why study data are scarce [128] and why cost-economic analyses show discrepancies in this important field of interest.

Relevant data for the critically ill exist concerning the potentially cost-saving introduction of the pre-mixed multi-chamber bag compared to compound PN. In a real-world analysis of PN use, potential savings of up to $1545 USD per patient using a multi-chamber bag could be achieved according to US data from the Premier Perspective™ database [129]. Patients on PN also benefit from a nutritional care team in order to assure adequate indication, application, and adaptation of PN, resulting in savings of 245,000 € EUR in one year per 100 treated patients in a Swiss university hospital [130]. A meta-analysis involving six clinical trials evaluating early EN in the ICU setting found a statistically significant reduction in mortality compared to standard timing of EN [131]. A cost-effectiveness analysis of these data showed a $14,462 USD reduction in total costs per patient for acute hospital care of patients receiving EN within 24 h after admission. These results were robust also when including sensitivity analysis with European cost data [132].

The Swiss SPN study added PN on days 4–8, whenever >60% of the caloric needs where not covered by EN on day 3. Based on the Swiss accounting system (Swiss DRG), a simulated calculation revealed a risk reduction for infection of 10%, resulting in savings of 63,048 CHF per infection [7,133]. The cost-analysis of the EPaNIC trial showed increased expenses with early-PN, mainly due to pharmacy-related costs and higher expenditures for PN and anti-infectious agents when compared to late PN patients who only received PN when EN remained insufficient after the first week of ICU treatment. Withholding early PN resulted in a net cost saving of 1210 Euro per patient [134].

The pronounced loss of lean body tissue, lack of mobilization, and increased protein energy needs all lead to higher complication rates with increased morbidity and mortality in this most fragile group of critically ill patients. Further studies, such as the recently published EFFORT study [135], should describe the effect of MNT not only in terms of clinical benefit but also with regard to monetary equivalent. Such data are of utmost interest to support and spread the relevance of MNT and linked-care teams.

7. Conclusions

MNT in all categories of critically ill patients remains a challenge, not only because these patients suffer from a pronounced stress response and are at higher risk for complications, but also due to their heterogeneity and their different illness phases (acute, subacute, chronic critically ill; pre- or post-resuscitation). Further studies are urgently needed to answer important questions such as the best timing, route, dose, and composition of MNT for the critically ill and to determine how to assess and to adapt to each patient's individual needs.

Current guidelines, as presented and discussed in this review, integrate actual knowledge and best clinical practice. Further steps would be to introduce them into (pre-existing) local feeding protocols. A MNT team offers an important additional value to optimize both patient care and education of hospital staff.

Supplementary Materials: The following are available online at http://www.mdpi.com/2077-0383/8/9/1395/s1, Table S1: Overview of current guidelines issued by ESPEN, ASPEN and CCCS/CCCTG.

Author Contributions: Conceptualization: A.K.L. and C.H. Writing, original draft preparation, review, and editing: A.K.L., A.d.W., A.H., N.G. and C.H.

Funding: This review received no external funding.

Acknowledgments: The authors would like to thank Allison Dwileski, BSc (Department of Anesthesiology, University Hospital Basel, Switzerland) for her editorial support.

Conflicts of Interest: The authors declare no conflict of interest.

References

1. Nasraway, S.A.; Cohen, I.L.; Dennis, R.C.; Howenstein, M.A.; Nikas, D.K.; Warren, J.; Wedel, S.K. Guidelines on admission and discharge for adult intermediate care units. American College of Critical Care Medicine of the Society of Critical Care Medicine. *Crit. Care Med.* **1998**, *26*, 607–610. [CrossRef]

2. Havens, J.M.; Columbus, A.B.; Seshadri, A.J.; Olufajo, O.A.; Mogensen, K.M.; Rawn, J.D.; Salim, A.; Christopher, K.B. Malnutrition at Intensive Care Unit Admission Predicts Mortality in Emergency General Surgery Patients. *JPEN J. Parenter. Enter. Nutr.* **2018**, *42*, 156–163. [CrossRef]
3. Imoberdorf, R.; Meier, R.; Krebs, P.; Hangartner, P.J.; Hess, B.; Stäubli, M.; Wegmann, D.; Rühlin, M.; Ballmer, P.E. Prevalence of undernutrition on admission to Swiss hospitals. *Clin. Nutr.* **2010**, *29*, 38–41. [CrossRef]
4. Kyle, U.G.; Genton, L.; Pichard, C. Hospital length of stay and nutritional status. *Curr. Opin. Clin. Nutr. Metab. Care* **2005**, *8*, 397–402. [CrossRef]
5. Mogensen, K.M.; Robinson, M.K.; Casey, J.D.; Gunasekera, N.S.; Moromizato, T.; Rawn, J.D.; Christopher, K.B. Nutritional Status and Mortality in the Critically Ill. *Crit. Care Med.* **2015**, *43*, 2605–2615. [CrossRef]
6. Alberda, C.; Gramlich, L.; Jones, N.; Jeejeebhoy, K.; Day, A.G.; Dhaliwal, R.; Heyland, D.K. The relationship between nutritional intake and clinical outcomes in critically ill patients: Results of an international multicenter observational study. *Intensiv. Care Med.* **2009**, *35*, 1728–1737. [CrossRef]
7. Heidegger, C.P.; Berger, M.M.; Graf, S.; Zingg, W.; Darmon, P.; Costanza, M.C.; Thibault, R.; Pichard, C. Optimisation of energy provision with supplemental parenteral nutrition in critically ill patients: A randomised controlled clinical trial. *Lancet* **2013**, *381*, 385–393. [CrossRef]
8. Rubinson, L.; Diette, G.B.; Song, X.; Brower, R.G.; Krishnan, J.A. Low caloric intake is associated with nosocomial bloodstream infections in patients in the medical intensive care unit. *Crit. Care Med.* **2004**, *32*, 350–357. [CrossRef]
9. Villet, S.; Chiolero, R.L.; Bollmann, M.D.; Revelly, J.-P.; Rn, M.-C.C.; Delarue, J.; Berger, M.M. Negative impact of hypocaloric feeding and energy balance on clinical outcome in ICU patients. *Clin. Nutr.* **2005**, *24*, 502–509. [CrossRef]
10. Van Zanten, A.R.; Sztark, F.; Kaisers, U.X.; Zielmann, S.; Felbinger, T.W.; Sablotzki, A.R.; De Waele, J.J.; Timsit, J.F.; Honing, M.L.; Keh, D.; et al. High-protein enteral nutrition enriched with immune-modulating nutrients vs. standard high-protein enteral nutrition and nosocomial infections in the ICU: A randomized clinical trial. *JAMA* **2014**, *312*, 514–524. [CrossRef]
11. Chapman, M.; Peake, S.L.; Bellomo, R.; Davies, A.; Deane, A.; Horowitz, M.; Hurford, S.; Lange, K.; Little, L.; Mackle, D.; et al. Energy-Dense versus Routine Enteral Nutrition in the Critically Ill. *N. Engl. J. Med.* **2018**, *379*, 1823–1834.
12. Arabi, Y.M.; Aldawood, A.S.; Haddad, S.H.; Al-Dorzi, H.M.; Tamim, H.M.; Jones, G.; Mehta, S.; McIntyre, L.; Solaiman, O.; Sakkijha, M.H.; et al. Permissive Underfeeding or Standard Enteral Feeding in Critically Ill Adults. *N. Engl. J. Med.* **2015**, *372*, 2398–2408. [CrossRef]
13. National Heart, Lung, and Blood Institute Acute Respiratory Distress Syndrome (ARDS) Clinical Trials Network; Rice, T.W.; Wheeler, A.P.; Thompson, B.T.; Steingrub, J.; Hite, R.D.; Moss, M.; Morris, A.; Dong, N.; Rock, P. Initial trophic vs. full enteral feeding in patients with acute lung injury: The EDEN randomized trial. *JAMA* **2012**, *307*, 795–803.
14. Heyland, D.; Muscedere, J.; Wischmeyer, P.E.; Cook, D.; Jones, G.; Albert, M.; Elke, G.; Berger, M.M.; Day, A.G.; Canadian Critical Care Trials Group. A randomized trial of glutamine and antioxidants in critically ill patients. *N. Engl. J. Med.* **2013**, *368*, 1489–1497. [CrossRef]
15. Andrews, P.J.; Avenell, A.; Noble, D.W.; Campbell, M.K.; Croal, B.L.; Simpson, W.G.; Vale, L.D.; Battison, C.G.; Jenkinson, D.J.; Cook, J.A.; et al. Randomised trial of glutamine, selenium, or both, to supplement parenteral nutrition for critically ill patients. *BMJ* **2011**, *342*, 1542. [CrossRef]
16. Wernerman, J.; Kirketeig, T.; Andersson, B.; Berthelson, H.; Ersson, A.; Friberg, H.; Guttormsen, A.B.; Hendrikx, S.; Pettilä, V.; Rossi, P.; et al. Scandinavian glutamine trial: A pragmatic multi-centre randomised clinical trial of intensive care unit patients. *Acta Anaesthesiol. Scand.* **2011**, *55*, 812–818. [CrossRef]
17. Singer, P.; Blaser, A.R.; Berger, M.M.; Alhazzani, W.; Calder, P.C.; Casaer, M.P.; Hiesmayr, M.; Mayer, K.; Montejo, J.C.; Pichard, C.; et al. ESPEN guideline on clinical nutrition in the intensive care unit. *Clin. Nutr.* **2019**, *38*, 48–79. [CrossRef]
18. Bendavid, I.; Singer, P.; Theilla, M.; Themessl-Huber, M.; Sulz, I.; Mouhieddine, M.; Schuh, C.; Mora, B.; Hiesmayr, M. NutritionDay ICU: A 7 year worldwide prevalence study of nutrition practice in intensive care. *Clin. Nutr.* **2017**, *36*, 1122–1129. [CrossRef]

19. Looijaard, W.; Denneman, N.; Broens, B.; Girbes, A.R.J.; Weijs, P.J.M.; Oudemans-van Straaten, H.M. Achieving protein targets without energy overfeeding in critically ill patients: A prospective feasibility study. *Clin. Nutr.* **2018**. [CrossRef]
20. Pompilio, C.E.; Pelosi, P.; Castro, M.G. The Bariatric Patient in the Intensive Care Unit: Pitfalls and Management. *Curr. Atheroscler. Rep.* **2016**, *18*, 55. [CrossRef]
21. Lorenzo-López, L.; Maseda, A.; De Labra, C.; Regueiro-Folgueira, L.; Rodríguez-Villamil, J.L.; Millán-Calenti, J.C. Nutritional determinants of frailty in older adults: A systematic review. *BMC Geriatr.* **2017**, *17*, 108. [CrossRef]
22. Cerri, A.P.; Bellelli, G.; Mazzone, A.; Pittella, F.; Landi, F.; Zambon, A.; Annoni, G. Sarcopenia and malnutrition in acutely ill hospitalized elderly: Prevalence and outcomes. *Clin. Nutr.* **2015**, *34*, 745–751. [CrossRef]
23. Onal, O.; Ozgun, G. Comparison of the Course and Prognosis of Geriatric Patients Admitted to the Intensive Care Unit According to BMI and Albumin Values. *Anesth. Pain Med.* **2016**, *6*, e32509. [CrossRef]
24. Grigoryan, K.V.; Javedan, H.; Rudolph, J.L. Ortho-Geriatric Care Models and Outcomes in Hip Fracture Patients: A Systematic Review and Meta-Analysis. *J. Orthop. Trauma* **2014**, *28*, e49–e55. [CrossRef]
25. Manzanares, W.; Hardy, G. Thiamine supplementation in the critically ill. *Curr. Opin. Clin. Nutr. Metab. Care* **2011**, *14*, 610–617. [CrossRef]
26. Nishimoto, A.; Usery, J.; Winton, J.C.; Twilla, J. High-dose Parenteral Thiamine in Treatment of Wernicke's Encephalopathy: Case Series and Review of the Literature. *In Vivo* **2017**, *31*, 121–124. [CrossRef]
27. McClave, S.A.; Taylor, B.E.; Martindale, R.G.; Warren, M.M.; Johnson, D.R.; Braunschweig, C.; McCarthy, M.S.; Davanos, E.; Rice, T.W.; Cresci, G.A.; et al. Guidelines for the Provision and Assessment of Nutrition Support Therapy in the Adult Critically Ill Patient: Society of Critical Care Medicine (SCCM) and American Society for Parenteral and Enteral Nutrition (A.S.P.E.N.). *JPEN J. Parenter. Enter. Nutr.* **2016**, *40*, 159–211. [CrossRef]
28. Fanelli, V.; Vlachou, A.; Ghannadian, S.; Simonetti, U.; Slutsky, A.S.; Zhang, H. Acute respiratory distress syndrome: New definition, current and future therapeutic options. *J. Thorac. Dis.* **2013**, *5*, 326–334.
29. Fong, Y.; Marano, M.A.; Barber, A.; He, W.; Moldawer, L.L.; Bushman, E.D.; Coyle, S.M.; Shires, G.T.; Lowry, S.F. Total Parenteral Nutrition and Bowel Rest Modify the Metabolic Response to Endotoxin in Humans. *Ann. Surg.* **1989**, *210*, 449–457. [CrossRef]
30. The Veterans Affairs Total Parenteral Nutrition Cooperative Study Group. Perioperative total parenteral nutrition in surgical patients. *N. Engl. J. Med.* **1991**, *325*, 525–532. [CrossRef]
31. Genton, L.; Dupertuis, Y.M.; Romand, J.-A.; Simonet, M.L.; Jolliet, P.; Huber, O.; Kudsk, K.A.; Pichard, C. Higher calorie prescription improves nutrient delivery during the first 5 days of enteral nutrition. *Clin. Nutr.* **2004**, *23*, 307–315. [CrossRef]
32. Spain, D.A.; McClave, S.A.; Sexton, L.K.; Adams, J.L.; Blanford, B.S.; Sullins, M.E.; Owens, N.A.; Snider, H.L. Infusion Protocol Improves Delivery of Enteral Tube Feeding in the Critical Care Unit. *J. Parenter. Enter. Nutr.* **1999**, *23*, 288–292. [CrossRef]
33. Simpson, F.; Doig, G.S. Parenteral vs. enteral nutrition in the critically ill patient: A meta-analysis of trials using the intention to treat principle. *Intensive Care Med.* **2005**, *31*, 12–23. [CrossRef]
34. Cawood, A.L.; Elia, M.; Stratton, R.J. Systematic review and meta-analysis of the effects of high protein oral nutritional supplements. *Ageing Res. Rev.* **2012**, *11*, 278–296. [CrossRef]
35. Berger, M.M.; Reintam-Blaser, A.; Calder, P.C.; Casaer, M.; Hiesmayr, M.J.; Mayer, K.; Montejo, J.C.; Pichard, C.; Preiser, J.C.; van Zanten, A.R.H.; et al. Monitoring nutrition in the ICU. *Clin. Nutr.* **2019**, *38*, 584–593. [CrossRef]
36. Delliere, S.; Cynober, L. Is transthyretin a good marker of nutritional status? *Clin. Nutr.* **2017**, *36*, 364–370. [CrossRef]
37. Barr, J.; Hecht, M.; Flavin, K.E.; Khorana, A.; Gould, M.K. Outcomes in critically ill patients before and after the implementation of an evidence-based nutritional management protocol. *Chest* **2004**, *125*, 1446–1457. [CrossRef]
38. Wøien, H.; Bjørk, I.T. Nutrition of the critically ill patient and effects of implementing a nutritional support algorithm in ICU. *J. Clin. Nurs.* **2006**, *15*, 168–177. [CrossRef]
39. Soguel, L.; Revelly, J.P.; Schaller, M.D.; Longchamp, C.; Berger, M.M. Energy deficit and length of hospital stay can be reduced by a two-step quality improvement of nutrition therapy: The intensive care unit dietitian can make the difference. *Crit. Care Med.* **2012**, *40*, 412–419. [CrossRef]

40. Mowe, M.; Bosaeus, I.; Rasmussen, H.H.; Kondrup, J.; Unosson, M.; Rothenberg, E.; Irtun, O.; Scandinavian Nutrition Group. Insufficient nutritional knowledge among health care workers? *Clin. Nutr.* **2008**, *27*, 196–202. [CrossRef]
41. Jones, N.E.; Suurdt, J.; Ouelette-Kuntz, H.; Heyland, D.K. Implementation of the Canadian Clinical Practice Guidelines for Nutrition Support: a multiple case study of barriers and enablers. *Nutr. Clin. Pract.* **2007**, *22*, 449–457. [CrossRef]
42. Wischmeyer, P.E. Are we creating survivors ... or victims in critical care? Delivering targeted nutrition to improve outcomes. *Curr. Opin. Crit. Care* **2016**, *22*, 279–284. [CrossRef]
43. Wischmeyer, P.E. Tailoring nutrition therapy to illness and recovery. *Crit. Care* **2017**, *21* (Suppl. 3), 316. [CrossRef]
44. Staun, M.; Pironi, L.; Bozzetti, F.; Baxter, J.; Forbes, A.; Joly, F.; Jeppesen, P.; Moreno, J.; Hebuterne, X.; Pertkiewicz, M.; et al. ESPEN Guidelines on Parenteral Nutrition: Home parenteral nutrition (HPN) in adult patients. *Clin. Nutr.* **2009**, *28*, 467–479. [CrossRef]
45. Reintam Blaser, A.; Berger, M.M. Early or Late Feeding after ICU Admission? *Nutrients* **2017**, *9*, 1278. [CrossRef]
46. Stanga, Z.; Brunner, A.; Leuenberger, M.; Grimble, R.F.; Shenkin, A.; Allison, S.P.; Lobo, D.N. Nutrition in clinical practice-the refeeding syndrome: Illustrative cases and guidelines for prevention and treatment. *Eur. J. Clin. Nutr.* **2008**, *62*, 687–694. [CrossRef]
47. Walmsley, R.S. Refeeding syndrome: Screening, incidence, and treatment during parenteral nutrition. *J. Gastroenterol. Hepatol.* **2013**, *28*, 113–117. [CrossRef]
48. The Canadian Critical Care Society (CCCS) and the Canadian Critical Care Trials Group (CCCTG). The 2015 Clinical Practice Guidelines on Critical Care Nutrition. Available online: https://www.criticalcarenutrition.com/resources/cpgs/past-guidelines/2015 (accessed on 31 May 2019).
49. Bischoff, S.C.; Singer, P.; Koller, M.; Barazzoni, R.; Cederholm, T.; Van Gossum, A. Standard operating procedures for ESPEN guidelines and consensus papers. *Clin. Nutr.* **2015**, *34*, 1043–1051. [CrossRef]
50. Atkins, D.; Best, D.; Briss, P.A.; Eccles, M.; Falck-Ytter, Y.; Flottorp, S.; Guyatt, G.H.; Harbour, R.T.; Haugh, M.C.; Henry, D.; et al. Grading quality of evidence and strength of recommendations. *BMJ* **2004**, *328*, 1490.
51. Cahill, N.E.; Dhaliwal, R.; Day, A.G.; Jiang, X.; Heyland, D.K. Nutrition therapy in the critical care setting: What is "best achievable" practice? An international multicenter observational study. *Crit. Care Med.* **2010**, *38*, 395–401. [CrossRef]
52. Kyle, U.G.; Genton, L.; Heidegger, C.P.; Maisonneuve, N.; Karsegard, V.L.; Huber, O.; Mensi, N.; Romand, J.A.; Jolliet, P.; Pichard, C. Hospitalized mechanically ventilated patients are at higher risk of enteral underfeeding than non-ventilated patients. *Clin. Nutr.* **2006**, *25*, 727–735. [CrossRef]
53. Wischmeyer, P.E.; Hasselmann, M.; Kummerlen, C.; Kozar, R.; Kutsogiannis, D.J.; Karvellas, C.J.; Besecker, B.; Evans, D.K.; Preiser, J.-C.; Gramlich, L.; et al. A randomized trial of supplemental parenteral nutrition in underweight and overweight critically ill patients: The TOP-UP pilot trial. *Crit. Care* **2017**, *21*, 142. [CrossRef]
54. Casaer, M.P.; Mesotten, D.; Hermans, G.; Wouters, P.J.; Schetz, M.; Meyfroidt, G.; Van Cromphaut, S.; Ingels, C.; Meersseman, P.; Müller, J.; et al. Early versus Late Parenteral Nutrition in Critically Ill Adults. *N. Engl. J. Med.* **2011**, *365*, 506–517. [CrossRef]
55. Singer, P.; Anbar, R.; Cohen, J.; Shapiro, H.; Shalita-Chesner, M.; Lev, S.; Grozovski, E.; Theilla, M.; Frishman, S.; Madar, Z. The tight calorie control study (TICACOS): A prospective, randomized, controlled pilot study of nutritional support in critically ill patients. *Intensiv. Care Med.* **2011**, *37*, 601–609. [CrossRef]
56. Allingstrup, M.J.; Kondrup, J.; Wiis, J.; Claudius, C.; Pedersen, U.G.; Hein-Rasmussen, R.; Bjerregaard, M.R.; Steensen, M.; Jensen, T.H.; Lange, T.; et al. Early goal-directed nutrition versus standard of care in adult intensive care patients: The single-centre, randomised, outcome assessor-blinded EAT-ICU trial. *Intensiv. Care Med.* **2017**, *43*, 1637–1647. [CrossRef]
57. Reignier, J.; Boisrame-Helms, J.; Brisard, L.; Lascarrou, J.B.; Ait Hssain, A.; Anguel, N.; Argaud, L.; Asehnoune, K.; Asfar, P.; Bellec, F.; et al. Enteral versus parenteral early nutrition in ventilated adults with shock: A randomised, controlled, multicentre, open-label, parallel-group study (NUTRIREA-2). *Lancet* **2018**, *391*, 133–143. [CrossRef]
58. Kondrup, J.; Rasmussen, H.H.; Hamberg, O.; Stanga, Z.; Ad Hoc, E.W.G. Nutritional risk screening (NRS 2002): A new method based on an analysis of controlled clinical trials. *Clin. Nutr.* **2003**, *22*, 321–336. [CrossRef]

59. De Vries, M.C.; Koekkoek, W.K.; Opdam, M.H.; van Blokland, D.; van Zanten, A.R. Nutritional assessment of critically ill patients: Validation of the modified NUTRIC score. *Eur. J. Clin. Nutr.* **2018**, *72*, 428–435. [CrossRef]
60. Detsky, A.S.; Baker, J.P.; Mendelson, R.A.; Wolman, S.L.; Wesson, D.E.; Jeejeebhoy, K.N. Evaluating the Accuracy of Nutritional Assessment Techniques Applied To Hospitalized Patients: Methodology and Comparisons. *J. Parenter. Enter. Nutr.* **1984**, *8*, 153–159. [CrossRef]
61. Vellas, B.; Guigoz, Y.; Garry, P.J.; Nourhashemi, F.; Bennahum, D.; Lauque, S.; Albarède, J.-L. The mini nutritional assessment (MNA) and its use in grading the nutritional state of elderly patients. *Nutrition* **1999**, *15*, 116–122. [CrossRef]
62. Kondrup, J. Nutrition risk screening in the ICU. *Curr. Opin. Clin. Nutr. Metab. Care* **2019**, *22*, 159–161. [CrossRef]
63. Shenkin, A. Serum prealbumin: Is it a marker of nutritional status or of risk of malnutrition? *Clin. Chem.* **2006**, *52*, 2177–2179. [CrossRef]
64. Wischmeyer, P.E.; San-Millan, I. Winning the war against ICU-acquired weakness: New innovations in nutrition and exercise physiology. *Crit. Care* **2015**, *19* (Suppl. 3), S6.
65. Looijaard, W.G.; Dekker, I.M.; Stapel, S.N.; Girbes, A.R.; Twisk, J.W.; Oudemans-van Straaten, H.M.; Weijs, P.J. Skeletal muscle quality as assessed by CT-derived skeletal muscle density is associated with 6-month mortality in mechanically ventilated critically ill patients. *Crit. Care* **2016**, *20*, 386. [CrossRef]
66. Lee, J.E. Increased intra-abdominal pressure in acute kidney injury: A cause or an effect? *Kidney Res. Clin. Pract.* **2015**, *34*, 67–68. [CrossRef]
67. Oshima, T.; Berger, M.M.; De Waele, E.; Guttormsen, A.B.; Heidegger, C.-P.; Hiesmayr, M.; Singer, P.; Wernerman, J.; Pichard, C. Indirect calorimetry in nutritional therapy. A position paper by the ICALIC study group. *Clin. Nutr.* **2017**, *36*, 651–662. [CrossRef]
68. Singh, R.; Cuervo, A.M. Autophagy in the Cellular Energetic Balance. *Cell Metab.* **2011**, *13*, 495–504. [CrossRef]
69. Anderegg, B.A.; Worrall, C.; Barbour, E.; Simpson, K.N.; DeLegge, M. Comparison of Resting Energy Expenditure Prediction Methods with Measured Resting Energy Expenditure in Obese, Hospitalized Adults. *J. Parenter. Enter. Nutr.* **2009**, *33*, 168–175. [CrossRef]
70. Boullata, J.; Williams, J.; Cottrell, F.; Hudson, L.; Compher, C. Accurate Determination of Energy Needs in Hospitalized Patients. *J. Am. Diet. Assoc.* **2007**, *107*, 393–401. [CrossRef]
71. Graf, S.; Pichard, C.; Genton, L.; Oshima, T.; Heidegger, C.P. Energy expenditure in mechanically ventilated patients: The weight of body weight! *Clin. Nutr.* **2017**, *36*, 224–228. [CrossRef]
72. Kross, E.K.; Sena, M.; Schmidt, K.; Stapleton, R.D. A Comparison of Predictive Equations of Energy Expenditure and Measured Energy Expenditure in Critically Ill Patients. *J. Crit. Care* **2012**, *27*, 321.e5–321.e12. [CrossRef]
73. Kreymann, K.G.; Berger, M.M.; Deutz, N.E.; Hiesmayr, M.; Jolliet, P.; Kazandjiev, G.; Nitenberg, G.; van den Berghe, G.; Wernerman, J.; Ebner, C.; et al. ESPEN Guidelines on Enteral Nutrition: Intensive care. *Clin. Nutr.* **2006**, *25*, 210–223. [CrossRef]
74. Singer, P.; Berger, M.M.; Berghe, G.V.D.; Biolo, G.; Calder, P.; Forbes, A.; Griffiths, R.; Kreyman, G.; Leverve, X.; Pichard, C. ESPEN Guidelines on Parenteral Nutrition: Intensive care. *Clin. Nutr.* **2009**, *28*, 387–400. [CrossRef]
75. Weir, J.B.D.V. New methods for calculating metabolic rate with special reference to protein metabolism. *J. Physiol.* **1949**, *109*, 1–9. [CrossRef]
76. Frankenfield, D.C.; Ashcraft, C.M. Estimating Energy Needs in Nutrition Support Patients. *J. Parenter. Enter. Nutr.* **2011**, *35*, 563–570. [CrossRef]
77. Psota, T.; Chen, K.Y. Measuring energy expenditure in clinical populations: Rewards and challenges. *Eur. J. Clin. Nutr.* **2013**, *67*, 436–442. [CrossRef]
78. Kagan, I.; Zusman, O.; Bendavid, I.; Theilla, M.; Cohen, J.; Singer, P. Validation of carbon dioxide production (VCO2) as a tool to calculate resting energy expenditure (REE) in mechanically ventilated critically ill patients: A retrospective observational study. *Crit. Care* **2018**, *22*, 186. [CrossRef]
79. Soussi, S.; Vallee, F.; Roquet, F.; Bevilacqua, V.; Benyamina, M.; Ferry, A.; Cupaciu, A.; Chaussard, M.; De Tymowski, C.; Boccara, D.; et al. Measurement of Oxygen Consumption Variations in Critically Ill Burns Patients: Are the Fick Method and Indirect Calorimetry Interchangeable? *Shock* **2017**, *48*, 532–538. [CrossRef]

80. Oshima, T.; Graf, S.; Heidegger, C.-P.; Genton, L.; Pugin, J.; Pichard, C. Can calculation of energy expenditure based on CO_2 measurements replace indirect calorimetry? *Crit. Care* **2017**, *21*, 13. [CrossRef]
81. Weijs, P.J.M. Route, early or energy? Protein improves protein balance in critically ill patients. *Crit. Care* **2018**, *22*, 91. [CrossRef]
82. Nicolo, M.; Heyland, D.K.; Chittams, J.; Sammarco, T.; Compher, C. Clinical Outcomes Related to Protein Delivery in a Critically Ill Population: A Multicenter, Multinational Observation Study. *JPEN J. Parenter. Enter. Nutr.* **2016**, *40*, 45–51. [CrossRef]
83. Weijs, P.J.; Mogensen, K.M.; Rawn, J.D.; Christopher, K.B. Protein Intake, Nutritional Status and Outcomes in ICU Survivors: A Single Center Cohort Study. *J. Clin. Med.* **2019**, *8*, 43. [CrossRef]
84. Weijs, P.J.; Looijaard, W.G.; Beishuizen, A.; Girbes, A.R.; Oudemans-van Straaten, H.M. Early high protein intake is associated with low mortality and energy overfeeding with high mortality in non-septic mechanically ventilated critically ill patients. *Crit. Care* **2014**, *18*, 701. [CrossRef]
85. Ferrie, S.; Allman-Farinelli, M.; Daley, M.; Smith, K. Protein Requirements in the Critically Ill: A Randomized Controlled Trial Using Parenteral Nutrition. *JPEN J. Parenter. Enter. Nutr.* **2016**, *40*, 795–805. [CrossRef]
86. Doig, G.S.; Simpson, F.; Bellomo, R.; Heighes, P.T.; Sweetman, E.A.; Chesher, D.; Pollock, C.; Davies, A.; Botha, J.; Harrigan, P.; et al. Intravenous amino acid therapy for kidney function in critically ill patients: A randomized controlled trial. *Intensiv. Care Med.* **2015**, *41*, 1197–1208. [CrossRef]
87. Hermans, G.; Casaer, M.P.; Clerckx, B.; Guiza, F.; Vanhullebusch, T.; Derde, S.; Meersseman, P.; Derese, I.; Mesotten, D.; Wouters, P.J.; et al. Effect of tolerating macronutrient deficit on the development of intensive-care unit acquired weakness: A subanalysis of the EPaNIC trial. *Lancet Respir. Med.* **2013**, *1*, 621–629. [CrossRef]
88. Casaer, M.P.; Wilmer, A.; Hermans, G.; Wouters, P.J.; Mesotten, D.; Van den Berghe, G. Role of disease and macronutrient dose in the randomized controlled EPaNIC trial: A post hoc analysis. *Am. J. Respir. Crit. Care Med.* **2013**, *187*, 247–255. [CrossRef]
89. Burtin, C.; Clerckx, B.; Robbeets, C.; Ferdinande, P.; Langer, D.; Troosters, T.; Hermans, G.; Decramer, M.; Gosselink, R. Early exercise in critically ill patients enhances short-term functional recovery. *Crit. Care Med.* **2009**, *37*, 2499–2505. [CrossRef]
90. Schaller, S.J.; Anstey, M.; Blobner, M.; Edrich, T.; Grabitz, S.D.; Gradwohl-Matis, I.; Heim, M.; Houle, T.; Kurth, T.; Latronico, N.; et al. Early, goal-directed mobilisation in the surgical intensive care unit: A randomised controlled trial. *Lancet* **2016**, *388*, 1377–1388. [CrossRef]
91. Fujioka, K.; DiBaise, J.K.; Martindale, R.G. Nutrition and metabolic complications after bariatric surgery and their treatment. *JPEN J. Parenter. Enter. Nutr.* **2011**, *35* (Suppl. 5), 52S–59S. [CrossRef]
92. Schindler, K.; Themessl-Huber, M.; Hiesmayr, M.; Kosak, S.; Lainscak, M.; Laviano, A.; Ljungqvist, O.; Mouhieddine, M.; Schneider, S.; De Van Der Schueren, M.; et al. To eat or not to eat? Indicators for reduced food intake in 91,245 patients hospitalized on nutritionDays 2006–2014 in 56 countries worldwide: A descriptive analysis. *Am. J. Clin. Nutr.* **2016**, *104*, 1393–1402. [CrossRef]
93. Amirkalali, B.; Hosseini, S.; Heshmat, R.; Larijani, B. Comparison of Harris Benedict and Mifflin-ST Jeor equations with indirect calorimetry in evaluating resting energy expenditure. *Indian J. Med. Sci.* **2008**, *62*, 283–290.
94. Beebe, M.L.; Crowley, N. Can Hypocaloric, High-Protein Nutrition Support Be Used in Complicated Bariatric Patients to Promote Weight Loss? *Nutr. Clin. Pract.* **2015**, *30*, 522–529. [CrossRef]
95. Volkert, D.; Beck, A.M.; Cederholm, T.; Cruz-Jentoft, A.; Goisser, S.; Hooper, L.; Kiesswetter, E.; Maggio, M.; Raynaud-Simon, A.; Sieber, C.C.; et al. ESPEN guideline on clinical nutrition and hydration in geriatrics. *Clin. Nutr.* **2019**, *38*, 10–47. [CrossRef]
96. Wade, C.E.; Kozar, R.A.; Dyer, C.B.; Bulger, E.M.; Mourtzakis, M.; Heyland, D.K. Evaluation of nutrition deficits in adult and elderly trauma patients. *JPEN J. Parenter. Enter. Nutr.* **2015**, *39*, 449–455. [CrossRef]
97. Phillips, S.M.; Dickerson, R.N.; Moore, F.A.; Paddon-Jones, D.; Weijs, P.J.M. Protein Turnover and Metabolism in the Elderly Intensive Care Unit Patient. *Nutr. Clin. Pract.* **2017**, *32*, 112S–120S. [CrossRef]
98. Deutz, N.E.P.; Bauer, J.M.; Barazzoni, R.; Biolo, G.; Boirie, Y.; Bosy-Westphal, A.; Cederholm, T.; Cruz-Jentoft, A.J.; Krznaric, Z.; Nair, K.S.; et al. Protein intake and exercise for optimal muscle function with aging: Recommendations from the ESPEN Expert Group. *Clin. Nutr.* **2014**, *33*, 929–936. [CrossRef]
99. Dickerson, R.N.; Maish, G.O., 3rd; Croce, M.A.; Minard, G.; Brown, R.O. Influence of aging on nitrogen accretion during critical illness. *JPEN J. Parenter. Enter. Nutr.* **2015**, *39*, 282–290. [CrossRef]

100. Loenneke, J.P.; Loprinzi, P.D.; Murphy, C.H.; Phillips, S.M. Per meal dose and frequency of protein consumption is associated with lean mass and muscle performance. *Clin. Nutr.* **2016**, *35*, 1506–1511. [CrossRef]
101. Schulman, R.C.; Mechanick, J.I. Metabolic and nutrition support in the chronic critical illness syndrome. *Respir. Care* **2012**, *57*, 958–977. [CrossRef]
102. Rousseau, A.-F.; Losser, M.-R.; Ichai, C.; Berger, M.M. ESPEN endorsed recommendations: Nutritional therapy in major burns. *Clin. Nutr.* **2013**, *32*, 497–502. [CrossRef]
103. Plauth, M.; Bernal, W.; Dasarathy, S.; Merli, M.; Plank, L.D.; Schütz, T.; Bischoff, S.C. ESPEN guideline on clinical nutrition in liver disease. *Clin. Nutr.* **2019**, *38*, 485–521. [CrossRef]
104. Dixit, D.; Endicott, J.; Burry, L.; Ramos, L.; Yeung, S.Y.A.; Devabhakthuni, S.; Chan, C.; Tobia, A.; Bulloch, M.N. Management of Acute Alcohol Withdrawal Syndrome in Critically Ill Patients. *Pharmacother. J. Hum. Pharmacol. Drug Ther.* **2016**, *36*, 797–822. [CrossRef]
105. Finoccchiaro, D.; Hook, J. Enteral Nutritional Support of the Critically Ill Older Adult. *Crit. Care Nurs. Q.* **2015**, *38*, 253–258. [CrossRef]
106. Vargas, N.; Tibullo, L.; Landi, E.; Carifi, G.; Pirone, A.; Pippo, A.; Alviggi, I.; Tizzano, R.; Salsano, E.; Di Grezia, F.; et al. Caring for critically ill oldest old patients: a clinical review. *Aging Clin. Exp. Res.* **2017**, *29*, 833–845. [CrossRef]
107. McClave, S.A.; Patel, J.J.; Weijs, P.J.M. Editorial: Introduction to the 2018 ESPEN guidelines on clinical nutrition in the intensive care unit: Food for thought and valuable directives for clinicians! *Curr. Opin. Clin. Nutr. Metab. Care* **2019**, *22*, 141–145. [CrossRef]
108. Berger, M.M.; Pichard, C. Parenteral nutrition in the ICU: Lessons learned over the past few years. *Nutrition* **2019**, *59*, 188–194. [CrossRef]
109. Harvey, S.E.; Parrott, F.; Harrison, D.A.; Bear, D.E.; Segaran, E.; Beale, R.; Bellingan, G.; Leonard, R.; Mythen, M.G.; Rowan, K.M.; et al. Trial of the route of early nutritional support in critically ill adults. *N. Engl. J. Med.* **2014**, *371*, 1673–1684. [CrossRef]
110. Reintam Blaser, A.; Starkopf, J.; Alhazzani, W.; Berger, M.M.; Casaer, M.P.; Deane, A.M.; Fruhwald, S.; Hiesmayr, M.; Ichai, C.; Jakob, S.M.; et al. Early enteral nutrition in critically ill patients: ESICM clinical practice guidelines. *Intensive Care Med.* **2017**, *43*, 380–398. [CrossRef]
111. Reintam Blaser, A.; Malbrain, M.L.; Starkopf, J.; Fruhwald, S.; Jakob, S.M.; De Waele, J.; Braun, J.P.; Poeze, M.; Spies, C. Gastrointestinal function in intensive care patients: Terminology, definitions and management. Recommendations of the ESICM Working Group on Abdominal Problems. *Intensive Care Med.* **2012**, *38*, 384–394. [CrossRef]
112. Wischmeyer, P.E.; Puthucheary, Z.; Millán, I.S.; Butz, D.; Grocott, M. Muscle Mass and Physical Recovery in ICU: Innovations for Targeting of Nutrition and Exercise. *Curr. Opin. Crit. Care* **2017**, *23*, 269–278. [CrossRef]
113. Taylor, S.; Dumont, N.; Clemente, R.; Allan, K.; Downer, C.; Mitchell, A. Critical care: Meeting protein requirements without overfeeding energy. *Clin. Nutr. ESPEN* **2016**, *11*, e55–e62. [CrossRef]
114. Klein, C.J.; Stanek, G.S.; Wiles, C.E., 3rd. Overfeeding macronutrients to critically ill adults: Metabolic complications. *J. Am. Diet. Assoc.* **1998**, *98*, 795–806. [CrossRef]
115. McClave, S.A.; Snider, H.L. Clinical Use of Gastric Residual Volumes as a Monitor for Patients on Enteral Tube Feeding. *J. Parenter. Enter. Nutr.* **2002**, *26*, S43–S50. [CrossRef]
116. Friedli, N.; Stanga, Z.; Culkin, A.; Crook, M.; Laviano, A.; Sobotka, L.; Kressig, R.W.; Kondrup, J.; Mueller, B.; Schuetz, P. Management and prevention of refeeding syndrome in medical inpatients: An evidence-based and consensus-supported algorithm. *Nutrition* **2018**, *47*, 13–20. [CrossRef]
117. Friedli, N.; Stanga, Z.; Sobotka, L.; Culkin, A.; Kondrup, J.; Laviano, A.; Mueller, B.; Schuetz, P. Revisiting the refeeding syndrome: Results of a systematic review. *Nutrition* **2017**, *35*, 151–160. [CrossRef]
118. Olthof, L.E.; Koekkoek, W.; van Setten, C.; Kars, J.C.N.; van Blokland, D.; van Zanten, A.R.H. Impact of caloric intake in critically ill patients with, and without, refeeding syndrome: A retrospective study. *Clin. Nutr.* **2018**, *37*, 1609–1617. [CrossRef]

119. Doig, G.S.; Simpson, F.; Heighes, P.T.; Bellomo, R.; Chesher, D.; Caterson, I.D.; Reade, M.C.; Harrigan, P.W.; Refeeding Syndrome Trial Investigators Group. Restricted versus continued standard caloric intake during the management of refeeding syndrome in critically ill adults: A randomised, parallel-group, multicentre, single-blind controlled trial. *Lancet Respir. Med.* **2015**, *3*, 943–952. [CrossRef]
120. Mehanna, H.M.; Moledina, J.; Travis, J. Refeeding syndrome: What it is, and how to prevent and treat it. *BMJ* **2008**, *336*, 1495–1498. [CrossRef]
121. Lappas, B.M.; Patel, D.; Kumpf, V.; Adams, D.W.; Seidner, D.L. Parenteral Nutrition: Indications, Access, and Complications. *Gastroenterol. Clin. N. Am.* **2018**, *47*, 39–59. [CrossRef]
122. Davila, J.; Konrad, D. Metabolic Complications of Home Parenteral Nutrition. *Nutr. Clin. Pract.* **2017**, *32*, 753–768. [CrossRef]
123. Pironi, L.; Labate, A.M.; Pertkiewicz, M.; Przedlacki, J.; Tjellesen, L.; Staun, M.; De Francesco, A.; Gallenca, P.; Guglielmi, F.W.; Van Gossum, A.; et al. Prevalence of bone disease in patients on home parenteral nutrition. *Clin. Nutr.* **2002**, *21*, 289–296. [CrossRef]
124. Grau, T.; Bonet, A.; Rubio, M.; Mateo, D.; Farre, M.; Acosta, J.A.; Blesa, A.; Montejo, J.C.; de Lorenzo, A.G.; Mesejo, A.; et al. Liver dysfunction associated with artificial nutrition in critically ill patients. *Crit. Care* **2007**, *11*, R10. [CrossRef]
125. Zhou, X.-D.; Dong, W.-H.; Zhao, C.-H.; Feng, X.-F.; Wen, W.-W.; Tu, W.-Y.; Cai, M.-X.; Xu, T.-C.; Xie, Q.-L. Risk scores for predicting dysphagia in critically ill patients after cardiac surgery. *BMC Anesthesiol.* **2019**, *19*, 7. [CrossRef]
126. Poorjavad, M.; Jalaie, S. Systemic review on highly qualified screening tests for swallowing disorders following stroke: Validity and reliability issues. *J. Res. Med. Sci.* **2014**, *19*, 776–785.
127. Dellinger, R.P.; Levy, M.M.; Rhodes, A.; Annane, D.; Gerlach, H.; Opal, S.M.; Sevransky, J.E.; Sprung, C.L.; Douglas, I.S.; Jaeschke, R.; et al. Surviving Sepsis Campaign: international guidelines for management of severe sepsis and septic shock, 2012. *Intensive Care Med.* **2013**, *39*, 165–228. [CrossRef]
128. Rice, N.; Normand, C. The cost associated with disease-related malnutrition in Ireland. *Public Health Nutr.* **2012**, *15*, 1966–1972. [CrossRef]
129. Turpin, R.S.; Canada, T.; Liu, F.X.; Mercaldi, C.J.; Pontes-Arruda, A.; Wischmeyer, P. Nutrition therapy cost analysis in the US: Pre-mixed multi-chamber bag vs. compounded parenteral nutrition. *Appl. Health Econ. Health Policy* **2011**, *9*, 281–292. [CrossRef]
130. Piquet, M.-A.; Bertrand, P.C.; Roulet, M. Role of a nutrition support team in reducing the inappropriate use of parenteral nutrition. *Clin. Nutr.* **2004**, *23*, 437. [CrossRef]
131. Doig, G.S.; Heighes, P.T.; Simpson, F.; Sweetman, E.A.; Davies, A.R. Early enteral nutrition, provided within 24 h of injury or intensive care unit admission, significantly reduces mortality in critically ill patients: A meta-analysis of randomised controlled trials. *Intensive Care Med.* **2009**, *35*, 2018–2027. [CrossRef]
132. Doig, G.S.; Chevrou-Séverac, H.; Simpson, F. Early enteral nutrition in critical illness: A full economic analysis using US costs. *Clin. Outcomes Res.* **2013**, *5*, 429–436. [CrossRef]
133. Pradelli, L.; Graf, S.; Pichard, C.; Berger, M.M.; Information, P.E.K.F.C. Supplemental parenteral nutrition in intensive care patients: A cost saving strategy. *Clin. Nutr.* **2018**, *37*, 573–579. [CrossRef]
134. Vanderheyden, S.; Casaer, M.P.; Kesteloot, K.; Simoens, S.; De Rijdt, T.; Peers, G.; Wouters, P.J.; Coenegrachts, J.; Grieten, T.; Polders, K.; et al. Early versus late parenteral nutrition in ICU patients: Cost analysis of the EPaNIC trial. *Crit. Care* **2012**, *16*, R96. [CrossRef]
135. Schuetz, P.; Fehr, R.; Baechli, V.; Geiser, M.; Deiss, M.; Gomes, F.; Kutz, A.; Tribolet, P.; Bregenzer, T.; Braun, N.; et al. Individualised nutritional support in medical inpatients at nutritional risk: A randomised clinical trial. *Lancet* **2019**, *393*, 2312–2321. [CrossRef]

© 2019 by the authors. Licensee MDPI, Basel, Switzerland. This article is an open access article distributed under the terms and conditions of the Creative Commons Attribution (CC BY) license (http://creativecommons.org/licenses/by/4.0/).

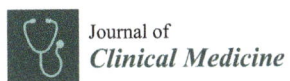

Review

Indirect Calorimetry in Clinical Practice

Marta Delsoglio [1], Najate Achamrah [2], Mette M. Berger [3] and Claude Pichard [1,*]

1. Clinical Nutrition, Geneva University Hospital (HUG), 1205 Geneva, Switzerland
2. Nutrition Department, Rouen University Hospital Center, 76000 Rouen, France
3. Service of Intensive Care Medicine & Burns, University of Lausanne Hospitals (CHUV), 1005 Lausanne, Switzerland
* Correspondence: Claude.Pichard@unige.ch; Tel.: +41-(0)22-372-9345; Fax: +41-(0)22-372-9363

Received: 9 August 2019; Accepted: 30 August 2019; Published: 5 September 2019

Abstract: Indirect calorimetry (IC) is considered as the gold standard to determine energy expenditure, by measuring pulmonary gas exchanges. It is a non-invasive technique that allows clinicians to personalize the prescription of nutrition support to the metabolic needs and promote a better clinical outcome. Recent technical developments allow accurate and easy IC measurements in spontaneously breathing patients as well as in those on mechanical ventilation. The implementation of IC in clinical routine should be promoted in order to optimize the cost–benefit balance of nutrition therapy. This review aims at summarizing the latest innovations of IC as well as the clinical indications, benefits, and limitations.

Keywords: indirect calorimetry; indirect calorimeter; resting energy expenditure; nutrition therapy

1. Introduction

The accurate determination of patients' energy needs is required to optimize nutritional support and to reduce the deleterious effects of under- and over-feeding [1]. However nutritional requirements may be difficult to predict, especially in patients with acute or chronic conditions where many factors (e.g., stress, brain activity, endocrine profile, inflammation status, feeding state, drugs, etc.) affect their resting energy expenditure (REE). REE represents the energy expended by the body during a 24 h non-active period to maintain involuntary functions such as substrate turnover, respiration, cardiac output, and body temperature regulation [2]. In healthy sedentary adult subjects REE constitutes two-thirds of the total energy expenditure (TEE) which includes energy needed for nonobligatory expenses such as physical activity and diet-induced thermogenesis. This assumption is probably not entirely correct in sick patients where continuous nutrition, treatments and diseased-related stress increase, or decrease REE: extreme variations among individuals can be observed within the same day [3].

Indirect calorimetry (IC) is considered as the gold standard to measure REE, by measuring oxygen consumption (VO_2) and carbon dioxide production (VCO_2). Apart from REE, other parameters can be derived from IC, such as substrate (carbohydrates, fat, and protein) utilization. Indeed, the ratio between VCO_2 and VO_2 ($\frac{VCO_2}{VO_2}$) defines the respiratory quotient (RQ) that corresponds to the substrate use. The complete oxidation of glucose generates a RQ value of 1.0, while a RQ of 0.7 is indicative of a mixed substrate oxidation [2].

Recent technical developments of indirect calorimeters allow accurate, non-invasive, and easy IC measurements in spontaneously breathing patients as well as in those on mechanical ventilation. Recent trials have shown IC allows clinicians to personalize the prescription of nutrition support to the metabolic needs and to monitor the metabolic response to nutrition therapy promoting a better clinical outcome in acutely ill patients [4–8]. These results have increased the interest for IC as a tool for improving the routine nutritional evaluation and prescription.

This review aims to summarize the latest innovations of IC as well as the clinical indications, benefits, and limitations of the technique.

2. Indications

Equations predicting REE are relatively reliable in healthy subjects. Contrariwise, in case of disease or trauma, REE is influenced by many factors with synergic or antagonist impact (Table 1) [1,2,9]. In these conditions, predictive equations are largely inaccurate [10]. As a consequence, IC is mainly indicated in three different scenarios: (a) clinical conditions significantly modifying REE; (b) failure of a nutrition support based on predicted energy needs to maintain or restore body weight; (c) acute critical illness associated with large and dynamic changes of metabolic stress level [11]. The latter indication requires special caution, as the IC results will reflect the patient's instability: repeated IC studies are required to observe the evolution of the metabolic response to hemodynamic instability, fever, surgery, weaning from mechanical ventilation, etc. A single IC is rarely sufficient, thereby repeated measurements every second or third day are needed in patients with rapid changes of their clinical status [12–14].

Table 1. Factors influencing resting energy expenditure. Adapted from [1,2,9].

Effects on REE	Factors	
↑	<ul><li>Burns</li><li>Hyperventilation</li><li>Hyperthermia</li><li>Hyperthyroidism, pheochromocytoma</li><li>Inflammation (interleukins, interferons, tumor necrosis factors etc.)</li><li>Metabolic acidosis</li></ul>	<ul><li>Morbid obesity</li><li>Overfeeding</li><li>Physical agitation</li><li>Sepsis</li><li>Stress (epinephrine, cortisol, glucagon etc.)</li></ul>
↓	<ul><li>Coma/deep sleep</li><li>General anesthesia</li><li>Heavy sedation</li><li>Hypothermia</li><li>Hypothyroidism</li><li>Hypoventilation</li></ul>	<ul><li>Gluconeogenesis</li><li>Metabolic alkalosis</li><li>Paralysis</li><li>Sarcopenia, cachexia</li><li>Starvation/underfeeding/ketosis</li></ul>

Performing IC in clinical routine is recommended not only to set an optimal nutrition therapy, but also to monitor the results of the nutritional interventions, in order to avoid complications of inappropriate nutrition, i.e., of under- or over-feeding.

3. Practicalities

IC allows measuring REE in both mechanically ventilated and spontaneously breathing patients (Figure 1). In mechanically ventilated patients, the respiratory gas sampling is acquired by the circuit connecting the endotracheal tube to the ventilator and measured by 'breath-by-breath' or mixing chamber analyses. In spontaneously breathing subjects, a ventilated canopy hood or a fitted face-mask is used to collect inspired and expired gas. In canopy system the patient's head is surrounded by a clear rigid hood and a pump pulls air through the canopy at a constant rate. In both ventilator and canopy mode, respiratory gases are analyzed by the indirect calorimeter and used to calculate REE through Weir's equation [1]. As will be detailed below, acutely and chronically ill patients at high risk of malnutrition are the ones who benefit most from IC.

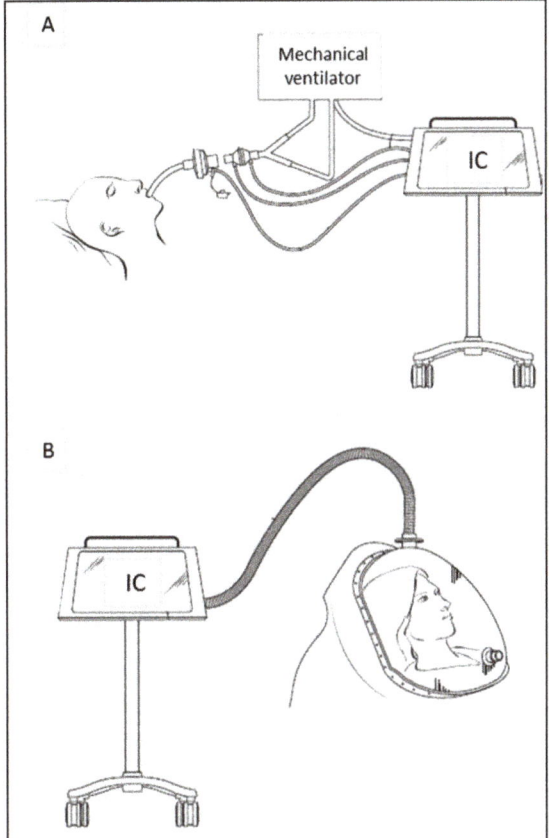

Figure 1. Indirect calorimetry on mechanically ventilated patient (**A**) and on spontaneous breathing patient in canopy mode (**B**). In mechanical ventilation the gas sampling is acquired by the circuit connecting the endotracheal tube to the ventilator and measured by 'breath-by-breath' or mixing chamber analyses. In spontaneous breathing mode, the subject is placed under a clear canopy with a plastic drape to avoid air leakage. Breath exchanges are collected by the calorimeter for gas analysis and enable calculation of REE using Weir's equation (REE (kcal/day) = [(VO$_2$ × 3.941) + (VCO$_2$ × 1.11)] × 1440).

3.1. Acute Diseases

Metabolic responses to shock and injury were first described by Sir Cuthbertson [15]. According to his investigations, there is a short ebb phase starting immediately after a traumatic shock and followed by a flow phase of longer duration after 3 to 10 days (Figure 2) [16]. The ebb phase is characterized by a decrease in metabolic rate, oxygen consumption, body temperature, and enzymatic activity. The flow phase, on the contrary, is marked by an increased catabolism, with a high oxygen consumption and an elevated REE rate.

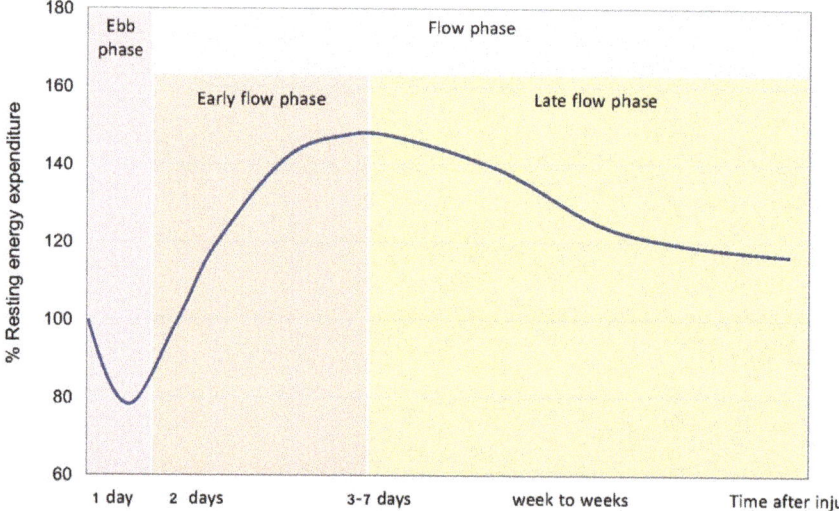

Figure 2. Metabolic response to injury proposed by Cuthbertson et al. A short ebb phase characterized by hypometabolism occurs immediately after the injury and is characterized by a decrease in metabolic rate, oxygen consumption, body temperature, and enzymatic activity. The ebb phase is followed by a longer hypermetabolic flow phase marked by an increased catabolism, with a high oxygen consumption and an elevated REE rate. Reused with permission from [16].

Recent studies have supported this pattern of longitudinal changes in REE in acutely ill patients [17–19]. The degree of increase from normal REE may reflect the severity of the metabolic response to the injury. However, the interaction between natural course of disease, individual inflammatory and immune system response, and medical treatments make it difficult for the clinician to evaluate caloric needs. For these reasons, IC is the only available tool enabling the individual assessment of the patients' energy needs, and to ensure precise nutritional interventions in acute conditions such as post-surgery period, pancreatitis, kidney injury, and sepsis.

The post-operative period of uncomplicated surgery has been associated with a modest 7% increase in energy metabolism as the effect of the surgical operation itself, that cannot be predicted by static equations [20]. Non-septic patients with acute pancreatitis presented a hypermetabolic state with a REE increase of 120 ± 11% compared to predicted [21]. Energy metabolism in patients with renal failure has been studied as well. Acute kidney injury (AKI) has not been shown to affect REE, but concomitant conditions, such as sepsis, mostly play role in the hypermetabolism found in these patients [22,23]. The presence of hypermetabolism has also been associated with lower age and higher vasoactive drug dose [24] and no predictive formula was able to correctly calculate energy needs in AKI patients compared to IC [25]. Sepsis is characterized by a hyperdynamic cardiovascular response against infection and has been reported to increase REE differently among patients with uncomplicated sepsis, sepsis syndrome, and septic shock (mean REE +55 ± 14%, +24 ± 12%, and +2 ± 24%) [26]. A higher REE in severe sepsis adult patients has also been associated with higher mortality [27], however further studies should investigate the effect of specific individual factors on metabolic evolution during sepsis and patient outcome.

Critical Illness

Critical illness is frequently associated with a hypermetabolic state related to the activation of catabolic hormones and resulting in elevated REE compared to healthy subjects. However, iatrogenic factors such as beta-blockers, analgesics, and sedatives may attenuate the response and even induce a hypometabolic state. Prolonged bed rest, atrophy of the metabolically active lean body mass, and mechanical ventilation have also been reported to decrease REE [1]. In patients with multiple organ failure, the loss of lean body mass is very rapid and resulted in 22% loss in 10 days [28] and no predictive equation showed good agreement compared to REE measured by IC [29].

Trauma patients showed hypermetabolism even when heavily sedated or medically paralyzed, however those with head injury on neuromuscular blockade or in a barbiturate coma showed reduced REE compared to similar patients without these agents [30]. Brain trauma was found to increase REE with high variability among different studies, ranging from 87% to 200% compared to predicted during the first 30 days post-injury; surprisingly, in patients admitted with a brain death diagnosis, the value ranged from 75% to 200% compared to predicted during the first 7 days [31].

Similarly, post-burn hypermetabolism was shown to increase REE as high as 100% above normal as consequence of a strong catabolic response mediated by endogenous catecholamines and inflammatory cytokines. Nevertheless, this hypermetabolic state is a direct effect of burn trauma, its persistence leads to severe septic complications, multiple organ failure, and higher mortality [16]. Nutritional follow up in burn patients shows a highly dynamic and variable REE up to 160 days after injury (Figure 3) [32].

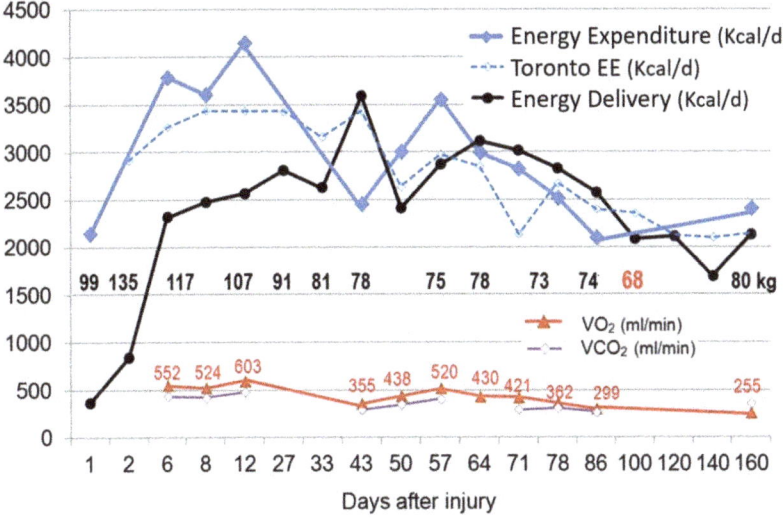

Figure 3. Evolution of measured REE by IC (blue), Toronto predictive equation (dashed blue), delivered energy (black), VO_2 (red △), and VCO_2 (purple ◆) in a young man weighing 99 kg upon admission with major burns covering 85% body surface over 160 days. The REE variations were important over time particularly during the early phase (weight gain due to fluid resuscitation was 36 kg by day 3), and paralleled the loss of body weight, i.e., of lean body mass (−31 kg after 3 months, with slow recovery). The REE value on day 1 corresponds to the Harris & Benedict prediction of basal EE. The figure also shows the reasonable precision of the Toronto equation, and how difficult it is to feed to measured IC value during the first 14 days. Adapted from [32].

The accurate determination of energy needs and the prevention of energy imbalance are essential in critically ill patients to avoid the harmful consequences of inadequate feeding. Underfeeding has been shown to increase hospital length of stay, infections, organ failure, to prolong mechanical ventilation, and to increase mortality, while overfeeding has been associated with hyperglycemia, hypertriglyceridemia, hepatic steatosis, azotemia, hypercapnia, and increased mortality [33]. In long staying patients with dynamic clinical conditions, IC should be repeated to monitor their nutritional requirements and avoid energy imbalance [34,35]. Optimal energy delivery targeting REE measured by IC seems to be significantly associated with reduced mortality, stressing the importance of this technique to assess caloric needs in ICU patients (Figure 4) [17].

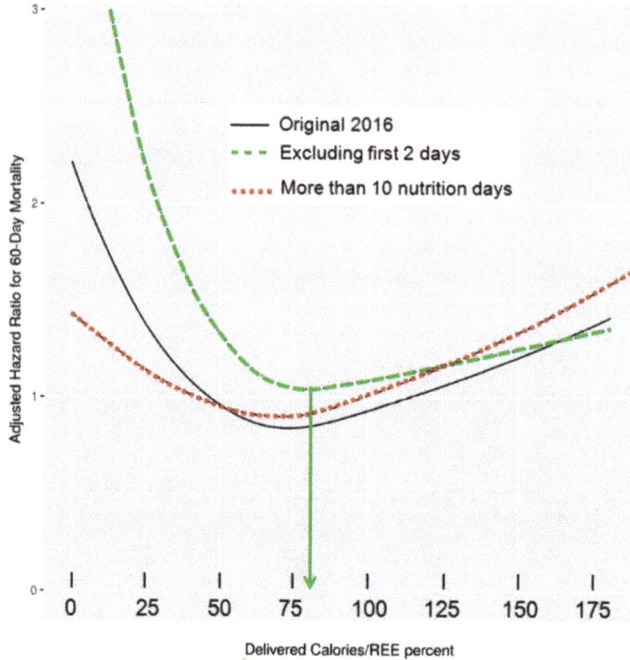

Figure 4. Association of delivered calories/resting energy expenditure (REE) percent by indirect calorimetry (IC) with 60-day mortality in different models: the authors recalculated their original 2016 data to integrate the fact that energy delivery increased progressively during the initial 2–3 days, reducing the mean value in stays <5 days. The lowest ICU mortality was observed when percent of delivered calories by REE obtained by IC was 80% (excluding first two feeding days) and 75% (with >10 evaluable nutrition days) ($p < 0.05$). On the contrary, increments of the ratio above that point—specifically >110%—were associated with increasing mortality ($p < 0.05$). Reproduced with permission (http://creativecommons.org/licenses/by/4.0/) [17].

The question which remains debated is the timing from which the measured REE should be prescribed as energy goal. Considering the importance of the early endogenous energy production, which is not suppressed by nutrition in the critically ill [36], feeding to measured value may result in overfeeding (Figure 5) [1]. Moreover, during the early phase of disease, catecholamines and the multiple treatments needed in these patients generate high instability and directly impact on measured REE. Tappy et al. showed that, in young starved trauma patients, the endogenous glucose production (EGP) was about 310 g/day (Figure 6), while the measured REE in these patients was 1830 kcal: feeding to the mean measured REE would clearly result in early overfeeding [37]. The figure also shows that endogenous glucose production continues in the sickest patients for many days even during feeding [8] (Figure 6). Therefore, the crude REE value provided by IC requires a careful interpretation to adequately prescribe exogenous energy supply.

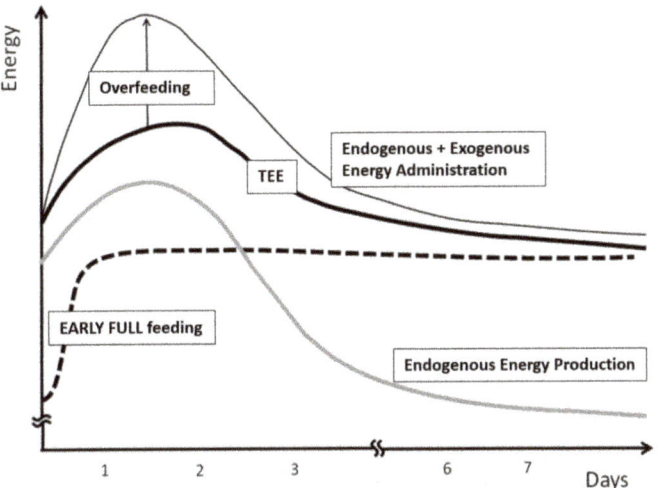

Figure 5. Conceptual representation of the relative overfeeding commonly resulting from early full feeding during the first days of critical illness. During this phase, the endogenous glucose production (EGP) is increased, covering up to two-thirds of total energy expenditure (TEE—solid black bold line). Full feeding in this phase will results in overfeeding, as the EGP is not attenuated by energy administration (different form healthy): exogenous feeding adds to the EGP resulting in an excessive energy availability, superior to TEE. (Solid black bold line: TEE; grey bold line: adapted endogenous energy production; dotted bold line: early energy administration; thin line: combined endogenous and exogenous energy administration). Reproduced with permission from [1].

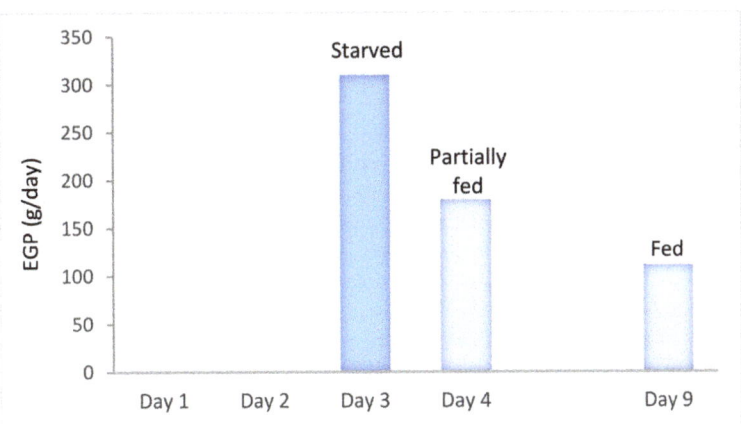

Figure 6. Evolution of the endogenous glucose production (EGP) over time in critically ill patients. EGP was shown to be 310 g/day in 40 years old starved trauma patients at day 3 of ICU admission (blue) [37] and then decreased to 180 and 111 g/day in older fed patients at day 4 and 9 respectively (light blue) [8]. EGP has to be considered as source of energy in order to avoid overfeeding by extrinsic energy during the first days of ICU stay. Data combined from [8,37].

There is also a debate regarding the optimal timing to cover the energy value determined by IC and the capacity of the critically ill intestine to accommodate and absorb the delivered feeding. Gastrointestinal intolerance is frequent in ICU patients and may preclude the achievement of the predefined calorie target due to the incapability of absorbing supplied nutrition [38]. The best feeding route for each patient has to be assessed in order to limit the risk of stressing the intestine and cumulative caloric deficit [39].

3.2. Chronic Diseases

Energy requirements may be even more difficult to predict in patients with chronic conditions due to the large individual variations in REE. Both hyper- and hypo-metabolism have been shown in chronic pathologies due to alterations in metabolism, lean body mass, organ function, and presence of inflammation. The most common pathologies with important REE alterations are described below and summarized in Table 2.

Table 2. Common chronic pathologies with effects on resting energy expenditure

Condition		Effect on REE
Anorexia nervosa	↓	Low energy intake and reduced lean body mass
Cancer	↑ ↓	Cancer growth and inflammation Progressive reduction of lean body mass
Chronic kidney diseases	↑ ↓	Metabolic acidosis and inflammation Acute and chronic renal failure
Chronic obstructive pulmonary disease	↑	Increased respiratory efforts
Diabetes	↑	Increased metabolism
Obesity	↑ ↓	Increased lean body mass Sarcopenia
Neuromuscular degenerative diseases	↑ ↓	Inflammation and endocrine disorders Dysfunction of muscle tissue

Both hyper- and hypo-metabolism, with respectively increased or decreased REE, have been observed in cancer patients. Several factors such as type, location, and size of tumor and presence of liver metastasis may contribute to this variability [16]. Similarly some studies showed increased REE in patients with chronic kidney disease, while others reported equal or even lower REE than those of matched healthy controls [40,41]. Renal replacement therapy such as hemodialysis or peritoneal dialysis also seem to affect REE, but results are contrasted [42,43]. Neurological diseases, such as Alzheimer's, Parkinson's, Huntington's, and amyotrophic lateral sclerosis significantly affect patients' REE as consequence of motor, endocrine, and metabolic abnormalities [44]. Diabetes is known to alter macronutrient metabolism, and increase the sympathetic activity leading to 5–10% augmentation of REE. On the contrary, the administration of anti-diabetic treatments is associated with a REE decrease [45]. Patients with chronic obstructive pulmonary disease feature an increased REE associated together with the progression of the disease severity, but a decreased TEE mainly due to a reduction of physical activity [46]. Both obesity and anorexia nervosa have been associated with altered REE mainly due to the different pattern of body composition compared to normal weight subjects. Obese patients showed significantly higher REE compared to non-obese patients; however, in most cases this difference disappeared after adjusting for fat-free mass [47]. Underweight and anorectic patients showed hypometabolic status with lower REE compared to predicted as a consequence of adaptation to starvation, loss of fat, and fat-free mass [48]. Conducting IC together with body composition measurement is useful to further optimize the nutrition prescription in these patients.

4. Benefits

The major benefit of performing IC in clinical practice is the prevention of both under- and over-feeding among patients with different conditions, thanks to the precise assessment and control of their energy needs. Inappropriate feeding has been associated with increased risk of infectious and non-infectious complications, length of hospitalization, more frequent readmission, and mortality, especially in ICU patients. Patients at risk of malnutrition were also found to be more likely to go to rehabilitation or nursing facilities rather than home after discharge [49]. In addition to negative outcomes in hospitalized patients, malnutrition also represents an economic burden for hospitals and the society [50]. In the ICU setting, supplemental parenteral nutrition (SPN) guided by IC has been shown to allow personalized and optimal nutrition in patients intolerant to full enteral nutrition. A reduction of nosocomial infections in the patients on SPN versus those on exclusive and insufficient enteral nutrition has been reported [5]. In depth analysis has further shown that the provision of SPN compared to exclusive enteral nutrition turned out to be a cost saving strategy [51,52]. Up to now, only four studies based their nutritional intervention on measured REE by IC [53]. A meta-analysis of available studies nevertheless shows that interventions guided by IC versus equations have significantly better clinical outcomes [34]. Promoting a systematic use of IC to individually optimize nutrition support among in- and out-patients, should result in meaningful clinical benefits and cost advantages. A large-scale study providing the benefits related to the use of IC to guide the prescription of nutrition support is needed.

5. Limitations

IC is the gold standard for measuring REE and for guiding nutrition support; however, several factors may limit the accuracy and/or the feasibility of the measurement (Table 3). During mechanical ventilation, air leakages in the respiratory circuit (particularly elevated in case of tracheostomy), high positive end expiratory pressure (PEEP > 10), fraction of inspired oxygen (FiO$_2$) > 80%, and presence of other gases than O$_2$, CO$_2$, and N$_2$ lead to unreliable results [1]. Thoracic drains are also a frequent cause of leakage in cardiothoracic units. Factors causing instability—such as agitation, fever, sedatives, and vasoactive adjustments during IC—limit the agreement between measured and real REE [54]. Likewise, organ support therapies such as continuous renal replacement therapy (CRRT) affect the respiratory pattern due to CO$_2$ removal, therefore measured REE does not reflect patient's real needs [54]. Similarly, to calculate real REE on extracorporeal membrane oxygenation (ECMO) patients requires gas exchange analysis by IC at both ventilator and ECMO sides [55,56].

Table 3. Factors limiting the reliability and feasibility of IC measurement.

Factors Limiting IC Measurement
• Agitation, fever, sedatives, and vasoactive adjustments during measurement
• Air leakages in respiratory circuit
• Dialysis or continuous renal replacement therapy
• ECMO
• Mechanical ventilation with PEEP > 10
• Mechanical ventilation with FiO$_2$ > 80%
• Noninvasive ventilation
• Other gases than O$_2$, CO$_2$, and N$_2$: helium
• Supplemental oxygen in spontaneous breathing patients

Moreover, not all subjects are good candidates to IC (i.e., spontaneous breathing patients who are claustrophobic, nauseous, vomiting, or do not tolerate a face mask or being under a canopy cannot undergo IC measurement). Patients who require supplemental oxygen or undergoing noninvasive ventilation are also difficult to test due to limitations of software and techniques. Other restraints for performing IC in clinical routine are related to the equipment and maintenance cost, poor health insurance reimbursement, lack of trained manpower, difficulties interpreting the results, and lack of time to carry out the measurements [13].

6. Current Developments

Many indirect calorimeters are commercially available, but most of them are bulky, expensive and poorly accurate compared to a reference device [57–60]. Some indirect calorimeters use the 'breath-by-breath' technology and generate rapid readings by measuring short intervals of gas samples, but this method is error-prone due to the response time of gas analyzers and software. Others are equipped with a mixing chamber and offer more stable measurements, because the gas is physically 'averaged' before being analyzed. However, the presence of the mixing chamber (3–5 L) results in a large dimension device, which requires prolonged measurements (>20 min) to allow gas concentrations stability. This limits the possibility of doing short-time reliable measurements [57–60].

In recent years, hand-held calorimeters such as the MedGem™ and BodyGem™ (Microlife, Dunedin, FL, USA) have also been developed. While traditional indirect calorimeters measure VO_2 and VCO_2, the hand-held devices measure only VO_2, while RQ is assumed to be 0.85. Advantages of these devices are portability, low degree of technical expertise required, and low cost. However, they cannot be used in ventilated patients, do not measure VCO_2, and are not validated in hospitalized patients [61].

Indeed, several comparison studies have been conducted both in adults and children comparing standard metabolic carts to determine whether the MedGem™ device is accurate and reliable. The hand-held calorimeter showed discrepant results compared to Deltatrac® in anorexia nervosa patients and healthy controls [62], overestimating REE by 8–11% [63] and agreeing only about 45% of the time in ambulatory adults [64]. MedGem® showed agreement only 21% of the time with Vmax measures in outpatients with cirrhosis [65] and tended to overestimate REE in obese individuals [66]. Similarly, it was found inaccurate in children and adolescents with and without obesity, overestimating REE by 7–10% [67,68] compared to other indirect calorimeters such as Parvomedics® and Deltatrac®, and underestimating by 8% [69] compared to Vmax®.

An international multicentric study (ICALIC), supported by two academic societies (ESPEN and ESICM), has recently led to the evaluation of a new generation calorimeter (Q-NRG®) developed to overcome the issue of inaccuracy, high cost, and lack of time [1]. It is equipped with a micro mixing chamber (2 mL) and features the technical characteristics required for measuring REE in both mechanically ventilated and spontaneous breathing subjects. In vitro evaluation showed gas analyzers' accuracy within 2% difference against a mass spectrometer (MS) for the measurements of predefined gas mixtures and within 5% in a mechanically ventilated setting at oxygen enrichment up to 70% for measurements of simulated VO_2 and VCO_2 [70]. Q-NRG® also showed very good accuracy and intra- and inter-unit precision in canopy mode both in vitro and in vivo compared to MS in healthy volunteers [71]. Studies to evaluate the ergonomics of the Q-NRG® in the ICU and hospitalized patients are ongoing within the frame of ICALIC study: they compare the currently used calorimeters. In addition to accuracy and precision, the innovation and performances of this new calorimeter are reactivity, portability, battery-powered, affordability, monthly gas calibration, and warm-up free operations. Current innovations also led to the development of original devices to facilitate the personal monitoring of REE. An example is the Breezing® device, a pocket-sized indirect calorimeter that measures oxygen consumption and carbon dioxide production rate in breath with a colorimetric technology. This device showed good agreement with the results from the Douglas Bag method for VO_2, VCO_2, EE, and RQ in healthy subjects but no tests were performed in clinical setting [72].

7. Alternative Methods to IC

So far, predictive equations remain the most common REE estimation method. They allow a rapid calculation of REE using anthropometric data (height, weight, sex, etc.) and have been validated among different group of hospitalized patients, but none is optimal (Table 4). Most of these equations have been developed in healthy subjects, resulting in large errors in case of critical illness and chronic diseases, despite the use of the correction factors [73]. Other methods for assessing REE have been explored and compared to IC in order to find a valid alternative.

Fick's principle uses cardiac output data, hemoglobin concentration, and arterial and mixed venous oxygen concentrations obtained from a pulmonary artery catheter to calculate REE. Comparison with IC in critically ill patients showed poor correlation with high variability between absolute values and variations of VO_2 measured, unacceptable for clinical use [74,75]. The error found may be mostly related to five factors: the accuracy of the blood gas analyzer used to calculate arterial and venous oxygen content, the mixed of venous and bronchial arterial blood sample, the hemoglobin levels, the cardiac output variation over the respiratory cycle and the assumption of a fixed RQ to calculate REE [74,76].

The calculation of EE based on CO_2 measurement collected from mechanical ventilators ($EEVCO_2$) has also been proposed. This technique considers a fixed value of RQ to calculate the oxygen consumption (VO_2) and REE through the Weir formula. Mainly due to the variability of RQ in critically ill patients, the accuracy of $EEVCO_2$ compared to the Deltatrac® metabolic monitor is poor [77–80].

The doubly labeled water method implies the oral administration of water with both hydrogen and oxygen atoms labeled with non-radioactive isotopes ($^2H/^1H$ and $^{18}O/^{16}O$) and uses their elimination rates in body liquids to calculate CO_2 production. By assuming a fixed RQ this method allows calculating TEE in any subjects and any environment, and can been used in complementation to IC to calculate Physical Activity Level [81,82]. However, this technique is expensive and requires long time to get the results, limiting its use in daily clinical practice [3].

Motion sensors devices initially developed for fitness settings may be useful in clinical practice to monitor activity induced energy expenditure (AEE), in particular for patients undergoing physiotherapy during rehabilitation programs, as well as for the management of daily activity and the dietary programs in patients with obesity and/or diabetes. These devices are wearable on the arm, wrist, or waist; user-friendly; relatively low-cost; and non-invasive. Energy expenditure is derived from acceleration data and individual parameters (sex, age, weight, heart rate) using manufacturer's confidential algorithms. However, the energy expenditure derived from these devices generally over- or underestimates the energy expenditure measured by IC by at least 10% [83]. Further studies are needed to validate their accuracy in clinical practice.

Measurements of body composition by bioelectrical impedance analysis (BIA) or dual energy X-ray absorptiometry (DXA) can be used to estimate REE. To this purpose predictive formula including FFM and FM values have been developed. This approach has been shown quite inaccurate in clinical populations compared to IC [73,84,85] and cannot be adopted in critically ill patients due to their abnormalities in hydration state and serum electrolyte concentrations that cause errors in the BIA-derived estimates of FFM and FM [86].

Table 4. Some predictive equations commonly used in clinical practice and tested among different hospitalized patients against IC.

Equations	Parameters Used for Calculation	Accuracy Rate *
General Hospitalized Population		
25 kcal/kg	25 × WT	43% [10] 23% [87]
Harris & Benedict (1919)	M: 13.75 × WT + 5.00 × HT − 6.75 × age + 66.47 F: 9.56 × WT + 1.85 × HT − 0.67 × age + 655.09	43% [10] 38% [87]
Ireton-Jones (1992)	1925 − 10 × age + 5 × WT + (281 if male) + (292 if trauma) + (851 if burn)	28% [10]
Mifflin-St Jeor (1990)	M: 10 × WT + 6.25 × HT − 5 × age + 5 F: 10 × WT + 6.25 × HT − 5 × age − 161	35% [10] 32% [87]
Schofield (1985)	8.4 × WT + 4.7 × HT + 200	42% [87]
Anorexic Patients (BMI < 16)		
Bernstein et al. (1983)	M: 11.02 × WT + 10.23 × HT − 5.8 × age − 1032 F: 7.48 × WT − 0.42 × HT − 3 × age + 844	40% [73]
Harris & Benedict (1919)	M: 13.75 × WT + 5.00 × HT − 6.75 × age + 66.47 F: 9.56 × WT + 1.85 × HT − 0.67 × age + 655.09	39% [73]
Huang et al. (2004)	10.16 × WT + 3.93 × HT − 1.44 × age + 273.82 × sex + 60.65	43% [73]
Lazzer et al. (2007)	M: 0.05 × WT + 4.65 × HT − 0.02 × age − 3.60 F: 0.04 × WT + 3.62 × HT − 2.68	39% [73]
Mifflin-St Jeor (1990)	M: 10 × WT + 6.25 × HT − 5 × age + 5 F: 10 × WT + 6.25 × HT − 5 × age − 161	40% [73]
Müller et al. (2004)	0.05 × WT + 1.01 × sex + 0.015 × age + 3.21	37% [73]
Owen (1987)	M: WT × 10.2 + 879 F: WT × 7.18 + 795	41% [73]
Obese Patients (BMI > 30)		
Bernstein et al. (1983)	M: 11.02 × WT + 10.23 × HT − 5.8 × age − 1032 F: 7.48 × WT − 0.42 × HT − 3 × age + 844	16% [88] 21% [89]
Harris & Benedict (1919)	M: 13.75 × WT + 5.00 × HT − 6.75 × age + 66.47 F: 9.56 × WT + 1.85 × HT − 0.67 × age + 655.09	64% [88]
Huang et al. (2004)	10.16 × WT + 3.93 × HT − 1.44 × age + 273.82 × sex + 60.65	66% [88] 53% [89] 54% [90]
Lazzer et al. (2007)	M: 0.05 × WT + 4.65 × HT − 0.02 × age − 3.60 F: 0.04 × WT + 3.62 × HT − 2.68	58% [88] 46% [90]
Mifflin-St Jeor (1990)	M: 10 × WT + 6.25 × HT − 5 × age + 5 F: 10 × WT + 6.25 × HT − 5 × age − 161	52% [89] 56% [90]
Müller et al. (2004)	0.05 × WT + 1.10 × sex + 0.016 × age + 2.92	60% [88] 58% [89] 47% [90]
Owen (1987)	M: WT × 10.2 + 879 F: WT × 7.18 + 795	38% [73] 40% [89]

Table 4. Cont.

Equations	Parameters Used for Calculation	Accuracy Rate *
Critically Ill Patients		
25 Kcal/Kg	25 × WT	12% [91]
Harris-Benedict (1919)	M: 13.75 × WT + 5.00 × HT − 6.75 × age + 66.47 F: 9.56 × WT + 1.85 × HT − 0.67 × age + 655.09	31% [91] 32% [92]
Ireton-Jones (1997)	1925 − 10 × age + 5 × WT + (281 if M) + (292 if trauma) + (851 if burn)	37% [93]
Mifflin-St Jeor (1990)	M: 10 × WT + 6.25 × HT − 5 × age + 5 F: 10 × WT + 6.25 × HT − 5 × age − 161	18% [91] 35% [10]
Owen (1987)	M: WT × 10.2 + 879 F: WT × 7.18 + 795	12% [91]
Penn State (2003)	0.85 × HB + 175 × Tmax + 33 × Ve − 6433	43% [10]
Swinamer (1990)	945 × BSA − 6.4 × age + 108 T + 24.2 × RR + 81.7 × VT − 4349	55% [93] 45% [10]

* % of patients where the predicted value (by equation) is within 10% of measured value (by IC). BSA, body surface area (m^2); HB, Harris–Benedict value; HT, height (cm); RR, respiratory rate (breath/min); sex: males (M) = 1, female (F); T, temperature (°C); Tmax, maximum temperature (°C) in previous 24 h; TV, tidal volume (L); Ve, expired minute ventilation at the time of collection (L/min); WT, weight (kg).

The agreement of predictive equations compared to IC results in critically ill patients was shown not to exceed 55%, especially in overweight or obese sarcopenic patients, and after prolonged physical immobilization [33,35,94]. Poor agreement is mainly due to the influence of body temperature, nutrition support, presence of sepsis, level of sedation, and therapies on REE [13]. The magnitude and the duration of the variations depend mostly on the severity of the disease with a considerable individual variability that cannot be assessed by equations [95]. Moreover, most of the equations base their calculations on anthropometric parameters, such as the body weight, which is often unknown and largely influenced by fluid retention or dehydration, leading to unreliable results [96].

Predictive equations tend to over (↑) or under (↓)—estimate REE in patients with chronic diseases such as:

- chronic obstructive pulmonary disease (↓) [97]
- chronic kidney disease (↑) [98]
- amyotrophic lateral sclerosis (↓) [85]
- fibro-calculous pancreatic diabetes and diabetes type 2 (↓) [99]
- cancer (↑) [100]
- cirrhosis (↓) [101]

Similarly, predictive equations are inaccurate in patients with extreme BMI (BMI < 16 kg/m^2 and BMI > 40 kg/m^2) [102]. Errors are mainly due to an excessive or deficient fat mass, which is less metabolically active than the lean body mass, and to the body weight considered for the calculation (current, ideal, adjusted, or estimated) [73]. Therefore, it seems clear that standard factors to estimate the energy needs of individual patients are inappropriate and should be discouraged to guide nutrition support. Pragmatically, the ESPEN guideline suggests to use the simplest equation in critically ill patients—i.e., 20 kcal/kg/day during the first days—and in absence of IC to increase to 25 kcal/kg/day after 7 days [34].

8. Conclusions

The optimization of nutrition therapy is crucial for global patient care. In order to prevent under- and over-feeding and their related complications, it is important to accurately assess REE in individual patients and to ensure adapted nutrition support. IC is considered as the gold standard to this purpose and ideally any patients in whom energy needs are uncertain should be measured. Recent developments should facilitate the widespread use of IC in medical routine and promote better clinical outcomes. Considering the ongoing debate, the widespread use of IC might finally enable the design of prospective studies which will be able to determine the optimal dose of energy to deliver during the different stages of disease, i.e., the ratio of the energy delivered to measured REE and timing of feeding.

Author Contributions: M.D.: conceptualization, writing—original draft preparation, visualization; N.A.: writing—review and editing; M.M.B.: writing—review and editing, supervision; C.P.: writing—review and editing, supervision.

Funding: Financial support came from the Public Foundation Nutrition 2000Plus.

Conflicts of Interest: CP received financial support as an unrestricted academic research grant from public institutions (Geneva University Hospital) and the Foundation Nutrition 2000 Plus. CP received financial support as research grants and an unrestricted academic research grant, as well as an unrestricted research grant and consulting fees, from Abbott, Baxter, B. Braun, Cosmed, Fresenius-Kabi, Nestle Medical Nutrition, Novartis, Nutricia-Numico, Pfizer, and Solvay, outside the submitted work. M.M.B. received research grants and public academic research grants, unrestricted research grand from Fresenius Kabi International, consulting fees from Fresenius Kabi International, and honoraria for lectures for Fresenius Kabi, Nestle. The other authors declare that they have no conflict of interest related to the current work. The funders had no role in the design of the study; in the collection, analyses, or interpretation of data; in the writing of the manuscript, or in the decision to publish the results.

References

1. Oshima, T.; Berger, M.M.; De Waele, E.; Guttormsen, A.B.; Heidegger, C.P.; Hiesmayr, M.; Singer, P.; Wernerman, J.; Pichard, C. Indirect calorimetry in nutritional therapy. A position paper by the ICALIC study group. *Clin. Nutr.* **2017**, *36*, 651–662. [CrossRef]
2. Gupta, R.D.; Ramachandran, R.; Venkatesan, P.; Anoop, S.; Joseph, M.; Thomas, N. Indirect Calorimetry: From Bench to Bedside. *Indian J. Endocrinol. Metab.* **2017**, *21*, 594–599. [CrossRef]
3. Fraipont, V.; Preiser, J.C. Energy Estimation and Measurement in Critically Ill Patients. *J. Parenter. Enter. Nutr.* **2013**, *37*, 705–713. [CrossRef]
4. Singer, P.; Anbar, R.; Cohen, J.; Shapiro, H.; Shalita-Chesner, M.; Lev, S.; Grozovski, E.; Theilla, M.; Frishman, S.; Madar, Z. The tight calorie control study (TICACOS), a prospective, randomized, controlled pilot study of nutritional support in critically ill patients. *Intensiv. Care Med.* **2011**, *37*, 601–609. [CrossRef]
5. Heidegger, C.P.; Berger, M.M.; Graf, S.; Zingg, W.; Darmon, P.; Costanza, M.C.; Thibault, R.; Pichard, C. Optimisation of energy provision with supplemental parenteral nutrition in critically ill patients: A randomised controlled clinical trial. *Lancet* **2013**, *381*, 385–393. [CrossRef]
6. Petros, S.; Horbach, M.; Seidel, F.; Weidhase, L. Hypocaloric vs Normocaloric Nutrition in Critically Ill Patients: A Prospective Randomized Pilot Trial. *J. Parenter. Enter. Nutr.* **2016**, *40*, 242–249. [CrossRef]
7. Allingstrup, M.J.; Kondrup, J.; Wiis, J.; Claudius, C.; Pedersen, U.G.; Hein-Rasmussen, R.; Bjerregaard, M.R.; Steensen, M.; Jensen, T.H.; Lange, T.; et al. Early goal-directed nutrition versus standard of care in adult intensive care patients: The single-centre, randomised, outcome assessor-blinded EAT-ICU trial. *Intensiv. Care Med.* **2017**, *43*, 1637–1647. [CrossRef]
8. Berger, M.M.; Pantet, O.; Jacquelin-Ravel, N.; Charriere, M.; Schmidt, S.; Becce, F.; Audran, R.; Spertini, F.; Tappy, L.; Pichard, C. Supplemental parenteral nutrition improves immunity with unchanged carbohydrate and protein metabolism in critically ill patients: The SPN2 randomized tracer study. *Clin. Nutr.* **2018**. [CrossRef]
9. Merritt, R. Use of indirect calorimetry in critically ill patients. In *The ASPEN Nutrition Support Practice Manual*, 2nd ed.; American Society for Parenteral and Enteral Nutrit: Silver Spring, MD, USA, 2006; pp. 277–280.
10. Boullata, J.; Williams, J.; Cottrell, F.; Hudson, L.; Compher, C. Accurate determination of energy needs in hospitalized patients. *J. Am. Diet. Assoc.* **2007**, *107*, 393–401. [CrossRef]
11. Wooley, J.A.; Sax, H.C. Indirect calorimetry: Applications to practice. *Nutr. Clin. Pract.* **2003**, *18*, 434–439. [CrossRef]

12. Berger, M.M.; Reintam-Blaser, A.; Calder, P.C.; Casaer, M.; Hiesmayr, M.J.; Mayer, K.; Montejo, J.C.; Pichard, C.; Preiser, J.C.; van Zanten, A.R.H.; et al. Monitoring nutrition in the ICU. *Clin. Nutr.* **2019**, *38*, 584–593. [CrossRef]
13. Singer, P.; Singer, J. Clinical Guide for the Use of Metabolic Carts: Indirect Calorimetry-No Longer the Orphan of Energy Estimation. *Nutr. Clin. Pract.* **2016**, *31*, 30–38. [CrossRef]
14. Weissman, C.; Kemper, M.; Hyman, A.I. Variation in the resting metabolic rate of mechanically ventilated critically ill patients. *Anesth. Analg.* **1989**, *68*, 457–461. [CrossRef]
15. Cuthbertson, D.P.; Angeles Valero Zanuy, M.A.; Leon Sanz, M.L. Post-shock metabolic response. 1942. *Nutr. Hosp.* **2001**, *16*, 176–182.
16. Rattanachaiwong, S.; Singer, P. Indirect Calorimetry as Point of Care Testing. *Clin. Nutr.* **2019**. [CrossRef]
17. Zusman, O.; Theilla, M.; Cohen, J.; Kagan, I.; Bendavid, I.; Singer, P. Resting energy expenditure, calorie and protein consumption in critically ill patients: A retrospective cohort study. *Crit. Care* **2016**, *20*, 367. [CrossRef]
18. Plank, L.D.; Hill, G.L. Sequential metabolic changes following induction of systemic inflammatory response in patients with severe sepsis or major blunt trauma. *World J. Surg.* **2000**, *24*, 630–638. [CrossRef]
19. Plank, L.D.; Connolly, A.B.; Hill, G.L. Sequential changes in the metabolic response in severely septic patients during the first 23 days after the onset of peritonitis. *Ann. Surg.* **1998**, *228*, 146–158. [CrossRef]
20. Brandi, L.S.; Oleggini, M.; Lachi, S.; Frediani, M.; Bevilacqua, S.; Mosca, F.; Ferrannini, E. Energy metabolism of surgical patients in the early postoperative period: A reappraisal. *Crit. Care Med.* **1988**, *16*, 18–22. [CrossRef]
21. Dickerson, R.N.; Vehe, K.L.; Mullen, J.L.; Feurer, I.D. Resting energy expenditure in patients with pancreatitis. *Crit. Care Med.* **1991**, *19*, 484–490. [CrossRef]
22. Schneeweiss, B.; Graninger, W.; Stockenhuber, F.; Druml, W.; Ferenci, P.; Eichinger, S.; Grimm, G.; Laggner, A.N.; Lenz, K. Energy metabolism in acute and chronic renal failure. *Am. J. Clin. Nutr.* **1990**, *52*, 596–601. [CrossRef]
23. Soncini Sanches, A.C.; de Góes, C.R.; Nogueira Berbel Bufarah, M.; Balbi, A.L.; Ponce, D. Does Acute Kidney Injury Alter Energy Metabolism of Septic Patients? *Arch. Ren. Dis. Manag.* **2016**, *2*, 19–23. [CrossRef]
24. Goes, C.R.; Balbi, A.L.; Ponce, D. Evaluation of Factors Associated with Hypermetabolism and Hypometabolism in Critically Ill AKI Patients. *Nutrients* **2018**, *10*, 505. [CrossRef]
25. Sabatino, A.; Theilla, M.; Hellerman, M.; Singer, P.; Maggiore, U.; Barbagallo, M.; Regolisti, G.; Fiaccadori, E. Energy and Protein in Critically Ill Patients with AKI: A Prospective, Multicenter Observational Study Using Indirect Calorimetry and Protein Catabolic Rate. *Nutrients* **2017**, *9*, 802. [CrossRef]
26. Kreymann, G.; Grosser, S.; Buggisch, P.; Gottschall, C.; Matthaei, S.; Greten, H. Oxygen consumption and resting metabolic rate in sepsis, sepsis syndrome, and septic shock. *Crit. Care Med.* **1993**, *21*, 1012–1019. [CrossRef]
27. Wu, C.; Wang, X.Y.; Yu, W.K.; Tian, F.; Liu, S.T.; Li, P.; Li, J.; Li, N. Hypermetabolism in the Initial Phase of Intensive Care Is Related to a Poor Outcome in Severe Sepsis Patients. *Ann. Nutr. Metab.* **2015**, *66*, 188–195. [CrossRef]
28. Puthucheary, Z.A.; Rawal, J.; McPhail, M.; Connolly, B.; Ratnayake, G.; Chan, P.; Hopkinson, N.S.; Phadke, R.; Dew, T.; Sidhu, P.S.; et al. Acute skeletal muscle wasting in critical illness. *JAMA* **2013**, *310*, 1591–1600. [CrossRef]
29. Jeon, J.; Kym, D.; Cho, Y.S.; Kim, Y.; Yoon, J.; Yim, H.; Hur, J.; Chun, W. Reliability of resting energy expenditure in major burns: Comparison between measured and predictive equations. *Clin. Nutr.* **2018**. [CrossRef]
30. McClave, S.A.; Martindale, R.G.; Kiraly, L. The use of indirect calorimetry in the intensive care unit. *Curr. Opin. Clin. Nutr. Metab. Care* **2013**, *16*, 202–208. [CrossRef]
31. Foley, N.; Marshall, S.; Pikul, J.; Salter, K.; Teasell, R. Hypermetabolism following moderate to severe traumatic acute brain injury: A systematic review. *J. Neurotrauma* **2008**, *25*, 1415–1431. [CrossRef]
32. Berger, M.M.; Pichard, C. Feeding should be individualized in the critically ill patients. *Curr. Opin. Crit. Care* **2019**, *25*, 307–313. [CrossRef]
33. Ndahimana, D.; Kim, E.K. Energy Requirements in Critically Ill Patients. *Clin. Nutr. Res.* **2018**, *7*, 81–90. [CrossRef]

34. Singer, P.; Blaser, A.R.; Berger, M.M.; Alhazzani, W.; Calder, P.C.; Casaer, M.P.; Hiesmayrh, M.; Mayeri, K.; Montejoj, J.C.; Pichard, C.; et al. ESPEN guideline on clinical nutrition in the intensive care unit. *Clin. Nutr.* **2019**, *38*, 48–79. [CrossRef]
35. Zusman, O.; Kagan, I.; Bendavid, I.; Theilla, M.; Cohen, J.; Singer, P. Predictive equations versus measured energy expenditure by indirect calorimetry: A retrospective validation. *Clin. Nutr.* **2018**. [CrossRef]
36. Wolfe, R.R. Sepsis as a modulator of adaptation to low and high carbohydrate and low and high fat intakes. *Eur. J. Clin. Nutr.* **1999**, *53*, S136–S142. [CrossRef]
37. Tappy, L.; Schwarz, J.M.; Schneiter, P.; Cayeux, C.; Revelly, J.P.; Fagerquist, C.K.; Jéquier, E.; Chioléro, R. Effects of isoenergetic glucose-based or lipid-based parenteral nutrition on glucose metabolism, de novo lipogenesis, and respiratory gas exchanges in critically ill patients. *Crit. Care Med.* **1998**, *26*, 860–867. [CrossRef]
38. Viana, M.V.; Pantet, O.; Bagnoud, G.; Martinez, A.; Favre, E.; Charriere, M.; Favre, D.; Eckert, P.; Berger, M.M. Metabolic and Nutritional Characteristics of Long-Stay Critically Ill Patients. *J. Clin. Med.* **2019**, *8*, 985. [CrossRef]
39. Reignier, J.; Boisrame-Helms, J.; Brisard, L.; Lascarrou, J.B.; Ait Hssain, A.; Anguel, N.; Argaud, L.; Asehnoune, K.; Asfar, P.; Bellec, F.; et al. Enteral versus parenteral early nutrition in ventilated adults with shock: A randomised, controlled, multicentre, open-label, parallel-group study (NUTRIREA-2). *Lancet* **2018**, *391*, 133–143. [CrossRef]
40. Avesani, C.M.; Draibe, S.A.; Kamimura, M.A.; Dalboni, M.A.; Colugnati, F.A.; Cuppari, L. Decreased resting energy expenditure in non-dialysed chronic kidney disease patients. *Nephrol. Dial. Transplant.* **2004**, *19*, 3091–3097. [CrossRef]
41. Neyra, R.; Chen, K.Y.; Sun, M.; Shyr, Y.; Hakim, R.M.; Ikizler, T.A. Increased resting energy expenditure in patients with end-stage renal disease. *J. Parenter. Enteral. Nutr.* **2003**, *27*, 36–42. [CrossRef]
42. Kamimura, M.A.; Draibe, S.A.; Avesani, C.M.; Canziani, M.E.; Colugnati, F.A.; Cuppari, L. Resting energy expenditure and its determinants in hemodialysis patients. *Eur. J. Clin. Nutr.* **2007**, *61*, 362–367. [CrossRef]
43. Ikizler, T.A.; Wingard, R.L.; Sun, M.; Harvell, J.; Parker, R.A.; Hakim, R.M. Increased energy expenditure in hemodialysis patients. *J. Am. Soc. Nephrol.* **1996**, *7*, 2646–2653.
44. Cekici, H.; Acar Tek, N. Determining energy requirement and evaluating energy expenditure in neurological diseases. *Nutr. Neurosci.* **2018**, 1–11. [CrossRef]
45. Huggett, R.J.; Scott, E.M.; Gilbey, S.G.; Stoker, J.B.; Mackintosh, A.F.; Mary, D.A. Impact of type 2 diabetes mellitus on sympathetic neural mechanisms in hypertension. *Circulation* **2003**, *108*, 3097–3101. [CrossRef]
46. Farooqi, N.; Carlsson, M.; Haglin, L.; Sandstrom, T.; Slinde, F. Energy expenditure in women and men with COPD. *Clin. Nutr. ESPEN* **2018**, *28*, 171–178. [CrossRef]
47. Carneiro, I.P.; Elliott, S.A.; Siervo, M.; Padwal, R.; Bertoli, S.; Battezzati, A.; Prado, C.M. Is Obesity Associated with Altered Energy Expenditure? *Adv. Nutr.* **2016**, *7*, 476–487. [CrossRef]
48. Cuerda, C.; Ruiz, A.; Velasco, C.; Breton, I.; Camblor, M.; Garcia-Peris, P. How accurate are predictive formulas calculating energy expenditure in adolescent patients with anorexia nervosa? *Clin. Nutr.* **2007**, *26*, 100–106. [CrossRef]
49. Yeh, D.D.; Fuentes, E.; Quraishi, S.A.; Cropano, C.; Kaafarani, H.; Lee, J.; King, D.R.; DeMoya, M.; Fagenholz, P.; Butler, K.; et al. Adequate Nutrition May Get You Home: Effect of Caloric/Protein Deficits on the Discharge Destination of Critically Ill Surgical Patients. *JPEN* **2016**, *40*, 37–44. [CrossRef]
50. Milte, R.K.; Ratcliffe, J.; Miller, M.D.; Crotty, M. Economic evaluation for protein and energy supplementation in adults: Opportunities to strengthen the evidence. *Eur. J. Clin. Nutr.* **2013**, *67*, 1243–1250. [CrossRef]
51. Correia, M.; Perman, M.I.; Pradelli, L.; Omaralsaleh, A.J.; Waitzberg, D.L. Economic burden of hospital malnutrition and the cost-benefit of supplemental parenteral nutrition in critically ill patients in Latin America. *J. Med. Econ.* **2018**, *21*, 1047–1056. [CrossRef]
52. Pradelli, L.; Graf, S.; Pichard, C.; Berger, M.M. Supplemental parenteral nutrition in intensive care patients: A cost saving strategy. *Clin. Nutr.* **2018**, *37*, 573–579. [CrossRef]
53. Berger, M.M.; Pichard, C. Parenteral nutrition in the ICU: Lessons learned over the past few years. *Nutrition* **2019**, *59*, 188–194. [CrossRef]
54. Haugen, H.A.; Chan, L.N.; Li, F. Indirect calorimetry: A practical guide for clinicians. *Nutr. Clin. Pract.* **2007**, *22*, 377–388. [CrossRef]

55. De Waele, E.; van Zwam, K.; Mattens, S.; Staessens, K.; Diltoer, M.; Honore, P.M.; Czapla, J.; Nijs, J.; La Meir, M.; Huyghens, L.; et al. Measuring resting energy expenditure during extracorporeal membrane oxygenation: Preliminary clinical experience with a proposed theoretical model. *Acta Anaesthesiol. Scand.* **2015**, *59*, 1296–1302. [CrossRef]
56. Wollersheim, T.; Frank, S.; Muller, M.C.; Skrypnikov, V.; Carbon, N.M.; Pickerodt, P.A.; Spies, C.; Mai, K.; Spranger, J.; Weber-Carstens, S. Measuring Energy Expenditure in extracorporeal lung support Patients (MEEP)-Protocol, feasibility and pilot trial. *Clin. Nutr.* **2018**, *37*, 301–307. [CrossRef]
57. Graf, S.; Karsegard, V.L.; Viatte, V.; Heidegger, C.P.; Fleury, Y.; Pichard, C.; Genton, L. Evaluation of three indirect calorimetry devices in mechanically ventilated patients: Which device compares best with the Deltatrac II(®)? A prospective observational study. *Clin. Nutr.* **2015**, *34*, 60–65. [CrossRef]
58. Graf, S.; Karsegard, V.L.; Viatte, V.; Maisonneuve, N.; Pichard, C.; Genton, L. Comparison of three indirect calorimetry devices and three methods of gas collection: A prospective observational study. *Clin. Nutr.* **2013**, *32*, 1067–1072. [CrossRef]
59. Sundstrom, M.; Tjader, I.; Rooyackers, O.; Wernerman, J. Indirect calorimetry in mechanically ventilated patients. A systematic comparison of three instruments. *Clin. Nutr.* **2013**, *32*, 118–121. [CrossRef]
60. Cooper, J.A.; Watras, A.C.; O'Brien, M.J.; Luke, A.; Dobratz, J.R.; Earthman, C.P.; Schoeller, D.A. Assessing validity and reliability of resting metabolic rate in six gas analysis systems. *J. Am. Diet. Assoc.* **2009**, *109*, 128–132. [CrossRef]
61. Hipskind, P.; Glass, C.; Charlton, D.; Nowak, D.; Dasarathy, S. Do handheld calorimeters have a role in assessment of nutrition needs in hospitalized patients? A systematic review of literature. *Nutr. Clin. Pract.* **2011**, *26*, 426–433. [CrossRef]
62. Hlynsky, J.; Birmingham, C.L.; Johnston, M.; Gritzner, S. The agreement between the MedGem indirect calorimeter and a standard indirect calorimeter in anorexia nervosa. *Eat. Weight Disord.* **2005**, *10*, e83–e87. [CrossRef]
63. Alam, D.S.; Hulshof, P.J.; Roordink, D.; Meltzer, M.; Yunus, M.; Salam, M.A.; van Raaij, J.M. Validity and reproducibility of resting metabolic rate measurements in rural Bangladeshi women: Comparison of measurements obtained by Medgem and by Deltatrac device. *Eur. J. Clin. Nutr.* **2005**, *59*, 651–657. [CrossRef]
64. Frankenfield, D.C.; Coleman, A. An evaluation of a handheld indirect calorimeter against a standard calorimeter in obese and nonobese adults. *JPEN* **2013**, *37*, 652–658. [CrossRef]
65. Schock, L.; Lam, L.; Tandon, P.; Taylor, L.; Raman, M. Indirect Calorimetry Performance Using a Handheld Device Compared to the Metabolic Cart in Outpatients with Cirrhosis. *Nutrients* **2019**, *11*, 1030. [CrossRef]
66. Anderson, E.J.; Sylvia, L.G.; Lynch, M.; Sonnenberg, L.; Lee, H.; Nathan, D.M. Comparison of energy assessment methods in overweight individuals. *J. Acad. Nutr. Diet.* **2014**, *114*, 273–278. [CrossRef]
67. White, D.A.; Staggs, V.S.; Williams, V.; Edwards, T.C.; Shook, R.; Shakhnovich, V. Handheld Indirect Calorimetry as a Clinical Tool for Measuring Resting Energy Expenditure in Children with and without Obesity. *Child. Obes.* **2019**, *15*, 280–287. [CrossRef]
68. Fields, D.A.; Kearney, J.T.; Copeland, K.C. MedGem hand-held indirect calorimeter is valid for resting energy expenditure measurement in healthy children. *Obesity (Silver Spring)* **2006**, *14*, 1755–1761. [CrossRef]
69. Woo, P.; Murthy, G.; Wong, C.; Hursh, B.; Chanoine, J.P.; Elango, R. Assessing resting energy expenditure in overweight and obese adolescents in a clinical setting: Validity of a handheld indirect calorimeter. *Pediatr Res.* **2017**, *81*, 51–56. [CrossRef]
70. Oshima, T.; Dupertuis, Y.M.; Delsoglio, M.; Graf, S.; Heidegger, C.P.; Pichard, C. In vitro validation of indirect calorimetry device developed for the ICALIC project against mass spectrometry. *Clin. Nutr. ESPEN.* **2019**, *32*, 50–55. [CrossRef]
71. Delsoglio, M.; Dupertuis, Y.M.; Oshima, T.; van der Plas, M.; Pichard, C. Evaluation of the accuracy and precision of a new generation indirect calorimeter in canopy dilution mode. *Clin. Nutr.* **2019**, in press.
72. Xiaojun, X.; Quach, A.; Bridgeman, D.; Tsow, F.; Forzani, E.; Tao, N. Personalized Indirect Calorimeter for Energy Expenditure (EE) Measurement. *Glob. J. Obes. Diabetes Metab. Syndr.* **2015**. [CrossRef]
73. Jesus, P.; Achamrah, N.; Grigioni, S.; Charles, J.; Rimbert, A.; Folope, V.; Petit, A.; Déchelotte, P.; Coëffier, M. Validity of predictive equations for resting energy expenditure according to the body mass index in a population of 1726 patients followed in a Nutrition Unit. *Clin. Nutr.* **2015**, *34*, 529–535. [CrossRef]

74. Soussi, S.; Vallee, F.; Roquet, F.; Bevilacqua, V.; Benyamina, M.; Ferry, A.; Cupaciu, A.; Chaussard, M.; De Tymowski, C.; Boccara, D.; et al. Measurement of Oxygen Consumption Variations in Critically Ill Burns Patients: Are the Fick Method and Indirect Calorimetry Interchangeable? *Shock* **2017**, *48*, 532–538. [CrossRef]
75. Inadomi, C.; Terao, Y.; Yamashita, K.; Fukusaki, M.; Takada, M.; Sumikawa, K. Comparison of oxygen consumption calculated by Fick's principle (using a central venous catheter) and measured by indirect calorimetry. *J. Anesth.* **2008**, *22*, 163–166. [CrossRef]
76. Ogawa, A.M.; Shikora, S.A.; Burke, L.M.; Heetderks-Cox, J.E.; Bergren, C.T.; Muskat, P.C. The thermodilution technique for measuring resting energy expenditure does not agree with indirect calorimetry for the critically ill patient. *J. Parenter. Enter. Nutr.* **1998**, *22*, 347–351. [CrossRef]
77. Oshima, T.; Graf, S.; Heidegger, C.P.; Genton, L.; Pugin, J.; Pichard, C. Can calculation of energy expenditure based on CO2 measurements replace indirect calorimetry? *Crit. Care* **2017**, *21*, 13. [CrossRef]
78. Stapel, S.N.; de Grooth, H.J.S.; Alimohamad, H.; Elbers, P.W.G.; Girbes, A.R.J.; Weijs, P.J.M.; Oudemans-van Straaten, H.M. Ventilator-derived carbon dioxide production to assess energy expenditure in critically ill patients: Proof of concept. *Crit. Care* **2015**, *19*, 370. [CrossRef]
79. Rousing, M.L.; Hahn-Pedersen, M.H.; Andreassen, S.; Pielmeier, U.; Preiser, J.C. Energy expenditure in critically ill patients estimated by population-based equations, indirect calorimetry and CO2-based indirect calorimetry. *Ann. Intensiv. Care* **2016**, *6*, 16. [CrossRef]
80. Kagan, I.; Zusman, O.; Bendavid, I.; Theilla, M.; Cohen, J.; Singer, P. Validation of carbon dioxide production (VCO2) as a tool to calculate resting energy expenditure (REE) in mechanically ventilated critically ill patients: A retrospective observational study. *Crit. Care* **2018**, *22*, 186. [CrossRef]
81. de Carvalho Bastone, A.; Ferriolli, E.; Pfrimer, K.; de Souza Moreira, B.; Diz, J.B.M.; Dias, J.M.D.; Dias, R.C. Energy Expenditure in Older Adults Who Are Frail: A Doubly Labeled Water Study. *J. Geriatr. Phys. Ther.* **2017**. [CrossRef]
82. Schutz, Y. Respiration chamber calorimetry and doubly labeled water: Two complementary aspects of energy expenditure? *Eur. J. Clin. Nutr.* **2018**, *72*, 1310–1313. [CrossRef]
83. Wahl, Y.; Duking, P.; Droszez, A.; Wahl, P.; Mester, J. Criterion-Validity of Commercially Available Physical Activity Tracker to Estimate Step Count, Covered Distance and Energy Expenditure during Sports Conditions. *Front. Physiol.* **2017**, *8*, 725. [CrossRef]
84. Hashizume, N.; Tanaka, Y.; Yoshida, M.; Fukahori, S.; Ishii, S.; Saikusa, N.; Masui, D.; Higashidate, N.; Sakamoto, S.; Tsuruhisa, S.; et al. Resting energy expenditure prediction using bioelectrical impedance analysis in patients with severe motor and intellectual disabilities. *Brain Dev. Jpn.* **2019**, *41*, 352–358. [CrossRef]
85. Jesus, P.; Marin, B.; Fayemendy, P.; Nicol, M.; Lautrette, G.; Sourisseau, H.; Preux, P.M.; Couratier, P.; Desport, J.C. Resting energy expenditure equations in amyotrophic lateral sclerosis, creation of an ALS-specific equation. *Clin. Nutr.* **2019**, *38*, 1657–1665. [CrossRef]
86. Barak, N.; Wall-Alonso, E.; Cheng, A.; Sitrin, M.D. Use of bioelectrical impedance analysis to predict energy expenditure of hospitalized patients receiving nutrition support. *JPEN* **2003**, *27*, 43–46. [CrossRef]
87. Kruizenga, H.M.; Hofsteenge, G.H.; Weijs, P.J. Predicting resting energy expenditure in underweight, normal weight, overweight, and obese adult hospital patients. *Nutr. Metab. (Lond.)* **2016**, *13*, 85. [CrossRef]
88. Achamrah, N.; Jesus, P.; Grigioni, S.; Rimbert, A.; Petit, A.; Dechelotte, P.; Folope, V.; Coëffier, M. Validity of Predictive Equations for Resting Energy Expenditure Developed for Obese Patients: Impact of Body Composition Method. *Nutrients* **2018**, *10*, 63. [CrossRef]
89. Orozco-Ruiz, X.; Pichardo-Ontiveros, E.; Tovar, A.R.; Torres, N.; Medina-Vera, I.; Prinelli, F.; Lafortuna, C.L.; Guevara-Cruz, M. Development and validation of new predictive equation for resting energy expenditure in adults with overweight and obesity. *Clin. Nutr.* **2018**, *37 Pt A*, 2198–2205. [CrossRef]
90. Cancello, R.; Soranna, D.; Brunani, A.; Scacchi, M.; Tagliaferri, A.; Mai, S.; Marzullo, P.; Zambon, A.; Invitti, C. Analysis of Predictive Equations for Estimating Resting Energy Expenditure in a Large Cohort of Morbidly Obese Patients. *Front. Endocrinol. (Lausanne)* **2018**, *9*, 367. [CrossRef]
91. Kross, E.K.; Sena, M.; Schmidt, K.; Stapleton, R.D. A comparison of predictive equations of energy expenditure and measured energy expenditure in critically ill patients. *J. Crit. Care* **2012**, *27*, 321.e5. [CrossRef]
92. Costa, N.A.; Marinho, A.D.; Cancado, L.R. Nutritional requirements of the critically ill patient. *Rev. Bras. Ter. Intensiv.* **2012**, *24*, 270–277. [CrossRef]

93. MacDonald, A.; Hildebrandt, L. Comparison of formulaic equations to determine energy expenditure in the critically ill patient. *Nutrition* **2003**, *19*, 233–239. [CrossRef]
94. Pichard, C.; Oshima, T.; Berger, M.M. Energy deficit is clinically relevant for critically ill patients: Yes. *Intensiv. Care Med.* **2015**, *41*, 335–338. [CrossRef]
95. Frankenfield, D.C.; Ashcraft, C.M. Estimating energy needs in nutrition support patients. *J. Parenter. Enter. Nutr.* **2011**, *35*, 563–570. [CrossRef]
96. Graf, S.; Pichard, C.; Genton, L.; Oshima, T.; Heidegger, C.P. Energy expenditure in mechanically ventilated patients: The weight of body weight! *Clin. Nutr.* **2017**, *36*, 224–228. [CrossRef]
97. Ramos, F.M.; Rossato, L.T.; Ramires, B.R.; Pimentel, G.D.; Venancio, L.S.; Orsatti, F.L.; de Oliveira, E.P. Comparison of predictive equations of resting energy expenditure in older adults with chronic obstructive pulmonary disease. *Rev. Port. Pneumol. (2006)* **2017**, *23*, 40–42. [CrossRef]
98. Kamimura, M.A.; Avesani, C.M.; Bazanelli, A.P.; Baria, F.; Draibe, S.A.; Cuppari, L. Are prediction equations reliable for estimating resting energy expenditure in chronic kidney disease patients? *Nephrol. Dial. Transplant.* **2011**, *26*, 544–550. [CrossRef]
99. Behera, K.K.; Joseph, M.; Shetty, S.K.; Chacko, A.; Sahoo, M.K.; Mahendri, N.V.; Nair, V.; Nadig, S.; Thomas, N. Resting energy expenditure in subjects with fibro-calculous pancreatic diabetes. *J. Diabetes* **2014**, *6*, 158–163. [CrossRef]
100. Khor, S.M.; Mohd, B.B. Assessing the resting energy expenditure of cancer patients in the Penang General Hospital. *Malays. J. Nutr.* **2011**, *17*, 43–53.
101. Eslamparast, T.; Vandermeer, B.; Raman, M.; Gramlich, L.; Den Heyer, V.; Belland, D.; Ma, M.; Tandon, P. Are Predictive Energy Expenditure Equations Accurate in Cirrhosis? *Nutrients* **2019**, *11*, 334. [CrossRef]
102. Frankenfield, D.C. Bias and accuracy of resting metabolic rate equations in non-obese and obese adults. *Clin. Nutr.* **2013**, *32*, 976–982. [CrossRef]

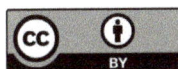

© 2019 by the authors. Licensee MDPI, Basel, Switzerland. This article is an open access article distributed under the terms and conditions of the Creative Commons Attribution (CC BY) license (http://creativecommons.org/licenses/by/4.0/).

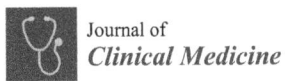

Review

Nutritional Challenges in Metabolic Syndrome

Irene Hoyas [1] and Miguel Leon-Sanz [2,*]

[1] Department of Endocrinology and Nutrition, University Hospital Doce de Octubre, 28041 Madrid, Spain
[2] Medical School, University Complutense, 28040 Madrid, Spain
* Correspondence: miguelle@ucm.es or Mlshdoc@gmail.com; Tel.: +34-91-779-2892

Received: 22 July 2019; Accepted: 19 August 2019; Published: 24 August 2019

Abstract: Metabolic Syndrome (MetS) is a combination of risk factors for the development of cardiovascular disease (CVD) and type 2 diabetes. Different diagnostic criteria were proposed, but a consensus was reached in 2009 based on values of waist circumference, blood pressure, fasting glycemia, triglycerides, and high-density lipoprotein (HDL)-cholesterol levels. The main underlying etiologic factor is insulin resistance. The quality and quantity of individual macronutrients have an influence on the development and resolution of this syndrome. However, the main treatment goal is weight loss and a decrease in insulin resistance. A controlled energy dietary recommendation, together with moderate levels of physical activity, may positively change the parameters of MetS. However, there is no single dietary or exercise prescription that works for all patients. Dietary patterns such as Mediterranean-style, dietary approaches to stop hypertension (DASH), low-carbohydrate, and low-fat diets can ameliorate insulin resistance and MetS. Long-term adherence to a healthy lifestyle is key in assuring that individuals significantly reduce the risk of CVD and diabetes mellitus.

Keywords: metabolic syndrome; insulin resistance; dietary pattern; carbohydrates; fat

1. Introduction

Metabolic Syndrome (MetS) is a combination of risk factors for the development of cardiovascular disease (CVD) and type 2 diabetes (T2DM). It is very common and occurs in all regions of the world in populations with reduced physical activity and excessive energy intake. Age, sex, socioeconomic status, and ethnic background may change the prevalence, but it is estimated that 25–35% of adults may have MetS. The grouping of risk factors for CVD was firstly proposed 100 years ago but was progressively developed over many decades and received different names, such as syndrome X, insulin resistance syndrome, and the deadly quartet [1].

MetS was also defined in various ways over time by different organizations and expert groups. There are four common components present in the different definitions: obesity, abdominal adiposity or indicators of insulin resistance, impaired glucose metabolism, hypertension, and atherogenic dyslipidemia. The differences among the diverse definitions depend on the cut-off points needed to fulfil the diagnostic criteria and the requirement of the obligatory presence of specific features to meet the definition of MetS [2].

In 2009, six organizations, the International Diabetes Federation, the American Heart Association, the National Heart, Liver, and Blood Institute, the World Heart Federation, the International Atherosclerosis Society, and the International Association for the Study of Obesity, reached a consensus for the definition of MetS [3]. According to the consensus, MetS can be diagnosed if the patient has any three of the following:

- Elevated waist circumference: population- and country-specific cut-off points;
- Blood pressure: systolic > 130 and/or diastolic > 85 mmHg or drug treatment;
- Fasting glucose: >100 mg/dL (5.6 mmol/L) or drug treatment;

- Triglycerides: >150 mg/dL (1.7 mmol/L) or drug treatment;
- High-density lipoprotein (HDL)-cholesterol: <40 mg/dL (1 mmol/L) (male) or <50 mg/dL (1.3 mmol/L) (female) or drug treatment.

MetS is not a disease but a cluster of individual risk factors, whose main purpose is to identify individuals with increased risk of developing CVD and diabetes mellitus. MetS facilitates the early identification of patients with excessive adipose tissue and insulin resistance, despite the fact that not every person at risk who fulfils the criteria for MetS has insulin resistance and, on the contrary, not all persons with insulin resistance have MetS [4]. The diagnosis of MetS may be helpful in convincing patients about the importance of adopting therapeutic measures to correct the different components of this syndrome. Patients who fulfil the criteria of MetS have a two-fold increased risk of CVD, 1.5-fold increased risk of all-cause mortality, and three-fold increased risk of diabetes [5,6]. These estimates may differ slightly depending on the MetS criteria set used and the population where they are applied.

However, the definition of this syndrome does not include some relevant CVD risk factors, such as family history, smoking habit, age, gender, or low-density lipoprotein (LDL)-cholesterol. That may explain why MetS is a good prognostic estimation in the long term, but other risk calculators may be more precise for prognosis at less than 10 years. MetS could also indicate risks not accounted for in other CVD risk calculators. In certain instances, it can move the CVD risk of a patient upward, from low to intermediate risk, according to traditional risk calculators, such as ATP-III, SCORE, or Framingham risk score [7].

2. Therapeutic Approach to Metabolic Syndrome

Among other reasons, sedentary life and the easy access to inexpensive foods contribute to the explanation of why MetS is currently so prevalent. Its treatment aims to decrease the risks of CVD and T2DM. The first and most important step is the implementation of a new lifestyle with changes in diet and physical activity, as well as the acquisition of healthier habits. Weight loss and lifestyle changes may improve individual MetS components. Behavioral interventions make it easier for individuals to incorporate and maintain these changes in their daily routines.

Weight reduction was the main goal of most intervention studies. It is associated with significant improvements in all parameters of MetS. Even moderate weight loss (around 7%) resulted in substantial reductions in blood pressure, and glucose, triglyceride, and total cholesterol concentrations [8,9]. In addition, weight reduction improves adipokines and inflammation markers, such as adiponectin and tumor necrosis factor alpha concentrations [10].

A reasonable first goal for obese patients is to aim for weight loss of approximately 10% of baseline weight in six months. If they achieve this objective, insulin resistance will improve along with risk reduction of MetS and CVD. Even a lower weight loss, between 5% and 10%, improves the sensitivity to insulin between 30 and 60%, an effect greater than that seen with insulin-sensitizing drugs [11].

Considering all the therapeutic options, caloric restriction is a very effective intervention because most persons with this syndrome are obese and sedentary. Changes in physical activity are always part of lifestyle interventions for MetS, and current scientific evidence supports the role of exercise as an effective treatment strategy for the syndrome. Along with dietary changes, a program of regular physical activity also leads to a reduction in insulin resistance and CVD risk [12].

In this review, we focus on the nutritional component of MetS therapy. We analyze the contributions of the three macronutrients to the development and treatment of MetS. We do not cover issues related to micronutrients, sweeteners, or alcohol consumption.

3. Influence of Dietary Macronutrients in MetS

The role of each macronutrient present in the diet in the development and treatment of MetS was extensively studied and we review the current state of knowledge of their contributions to this syndrome.

3.1. Carbohydrates

After oral administration, absorption, gastrointestinal and pancreatic hormone secretion, liver metabolism, and visceral and muscular uptake, carbohydrates are responsible for blood glucose and insulin levels. They should not be regarded as a homogeneous component of foods. Overall, there are three types: starch or complex carbohydrates, sugars or simple carbohydrates, and fiber, with different repercussions on the glycemic response. The metabolic effects of foods containing carbohydrates can be partially predicted by their glycemic index (GI), which ranks foods containing carbohydrates according to how they change blood glucose levels, usually by comparing 50 g of any given food with a reference food such as white bread. When the GI is low (55 or less) that particular food causes a lower and slower increase in blood glucose and, therefore, insulin levels. Related to this index is the concept of glycemic load (GL), which combines both the quantity and quality of carbohydrates. If the carbohydrate content of 100 g of potato is 14 g and the GI is 85, the GL will be 85 × 14/100 = 12, more than double the GL of 100 g of an apple, which is 5. The GL concept allows comparison of blood glucose response to different types and amounts of foods [13,14]. The GI depends not only on the carbohydrate composition but also on other factors (the physical form of the food, amylose or amylopectin content, complete composition of the food, presence of fiber, cooking process, etc.) [15]. Despite its conceptual appeal, the utility of GI and GL in clinical practice is not widely recognized because of lack of impact on glycemic control [16].

It is accepted that an elevated intake of carbohydrates of high GI causes insulin resistance directly and contributes to the development of T2DM in persons with MetS [17,18]. Generally, foods with low GI are also more abundant in fiber. A diet rich in fiber showed a reduction in insulinemia by 10% and insulin resistance (by HOMA index) by 13% [19]. Fiber intake increases satiety and also reduces the risk of developing T2DM, and, in patients already diagnosed with this disease, viscous fiber supplements improve conventional markers of glycemic control beyond usual care and should be considered in its management [20]. However, fiber intake through foods that are naturally high in dietary fiber is better than fiber supplements, because natural foods also provide other substances such as micronutrients and phytochemicals.

Carbohydrate and lipid contents of diets have a mutual influence on their metabolism. Diets with low GI produce lower concentrations of fasting triglycerides and LDL-cholesterol [21]. It is interesting to emphasize that, when simple carbohydrates are consumed in a proportion lower than 20–25%, they do not modify the levels of plasma triglycerides. However, in obese patients with insulin resistance, the intake of simple carbohydrates stimulates the synthesis of fatty acids and inhibits endothelial and hepatic lipoprotein lipase, and in this way promotes hypertriglyceridemia and lowers HDL-cholesterol levels [22]. In a more positive manner, the effect of carbohydrates on the increase in plasma triglyceride levels is lower if fiber intake is high. Low-glycemic-index diets are, thus, recommended for patients with MetS [23,24], contributing to decreased CVD risk, and reduced levels of glycosylated hemoglobin in type 1 and 2 DM patients [25,26].

In the last two decades, we saw a growing interest in diets with low carbohydrate content or ketogenic diets. Initially, they were discredited because it was thought that the elevated lipid content would increase the risk of CVD. However, several landmark studies showed greater weight loss during the first six months of follow-up compared to conventional low-fat hypocaloric diets [27,28]. No statistically significant differences in weight loss were seen after 12 months of follow-up. Interestingly, with these ketogenic diets, triglyceride concentrations decrease, HDL-cholesterol levels increase markedly, and insulin sensitivity and glycosylated hemoglobin (HbA1c) improve. In those cases of high HbA1c, there is a greater reduction in HbA1c levels after carbohydrate restriction rather than after protein or lipid restriction [29].

Fructose is a simple carbohydrate that deserves particular comment. When absorbed, it does not stimulate the secretion of insulin or leptin. Long-term daily consumption leads to an increase in weight and a decrease in insulin sensitivity, favoring the development of MetS and type 2 diabetes [30], both in children and in adults [31]. Soft drinks contain large amounts of high-fructose corn syrup (HFCS) and sucrose and add greater amounts of simple carbohydrates to the daily diet. It was stated that moderate fructose consumption of ≤50 g/day or 10% of energy has no deleterious effect on lipid and glucose control, and ≤100 g/day does not influence body weight. Nevertheless, a higher intake is not recommended, and the intake of sugar-sweetened beverages should be limited or avoided [32].

3.2. Lipids

In humans, energy intake is made up of carbohydrates and lipids. However, lipids also have functional features and play an important role in the pathogenesis of atherosclerosis. The accepted range of lipid calories in the diet is very broad and is the opposite of carbohydrates. Therefore, low-lipid or low-carbohydrate diets contain very different total amounts of lipids. For all adults, the acceptable macronutrient distribution of total fat is to be 20–35% of total calorie intake [33].

The amount of fat can influence insulin sensitivity and the risk of developing type 2 diabetes only with intakes greater than 35–40% of total energy intake [34]. A diet that contains 20–40% fat does not change insulin sensitivity, regardless of its effect on weight [35].

However, lipids in the diet are a heterogeneous group, and quality is as important as quantity. Generally, we classify lipids as saturated, monounsaturated, and polyunsaturated fats (SFAs, MUFAs, and PUFAs, respectively). The consumption of high amounts of saturated fats and *trans* fatty acids is associated with an alteration in the action of insulin, while the intake of monounsaturated fats has the opposite effect. Therefore, the ratio of monounsaturated fatty acids/saturated fat is related to insulin sensitivity (Table 1). Along with these effects on insulin, diets enriched with MUFAs improve the lipid profile, because they reduce LDL-cholesterol and triglycerides, and elevate HDL-cholesterol levels [36–38]. Polyunsaturated fats are associated with a lower relative risk of 40% for developing type 2 diabetes. In studies that included patients with type 2 diabetes, substitution of SFAs by PUFAs and carbohydrates by MUFAs caused a decrease in insulin resistance. Moreover, ω-3 PUFAs can reduce triglyceride levels, improve hypertension, reduce inflammation, and diminish cardiovascular risk in diabetic patients [39–42]. It was recently reported that the intake of 2 g of icosapent ethyl twice daily with statin therapy is associated with less CVD morbidity and mortality but with slightly higher rates of hospitalization for atrial fibrillation and serious bleeding [43].

Table 1. Influence of diet on insulin sensitivity.

Diet Component	Insulin Sensitivity
Total fatty acids (>40%)	(−)
Polyunsaturated fatty acids	(−)
trans Fatty acids	(−)
Monounsaturated fatty acids	(+)
Fiber cereal	(+)
Low glycemic index	(+)
Alcohol	(+)
Salt	(−)
Simple sugars (>20% energy)	(−)
Conjugated linoleic acid	(−)

(+): Increases insulin sensitivity. (−): Decreases insulin sensitivity.

A diet low in fat and rich in simple carbohydrates, as was used in the CARMEN study, may increase insulin resistance (measured by HOMA) and is associated with a significant increase in triglyceride levels [44]. For some time, the American Diabetic Association (ADA) recommended that the sum of carbohydrates and monounsaturated fatty acids should represent 60–70% of the total energy in the diet. Nevertheless, since the ADA 2014 position statement, there is no "first-line" approach with respect to the optimal carbohydrate quantity in the diet plan, because evidence remains inconclusive [45]. On the other hand, in overweight or obese individuals, low-fat diets are equal to but no better than other weight-reducing diets when the goal is weight reduction [46].

A healthy pattern limits saturated and *trans* fats, added sugars, and sodium. The recommendation for the general population is to consume less than 10% of calories per day as added sugars and less than 10% of calories per day as saturated fats. In the Dietary Guidelines for Americans, it is advised that individuals eat as little dietary cholesterol as possible while consuming a healthy eating pattern. The cholesterol intake in a healthy United States (US)-style diet contains approximately 100 to 300 mg of cholesterol across the 12 calorie levels [47]. European guidelines recommend that foods rich in *trans* or saturated fats (hard margarines, tropical oils, fatty or processed meat, sweets, cream, butter, and regular cheese) should be replaced with monounsaturated fats (extra virgin olive oil) and polyunsaturated fats (non-tropical vegetable oils). In this way, it is assumed that *trans* fats will be <1.0% of total energy and saturated fat <10% (<7% in the presence of high plasma cholesterol values) [48].

3.3. Proteins

Proteins are associated with increased satiety and the preservation of lean body mass during weight loss, but their role in the dietary recommendations for patients with MetS is less clear.

Guidelines recommend a wide range of 10–35% of energy intake as digestible protein for adults, or a minimum of 0.8 g/kg body weight per day. Within this range, ADA position statements suggest that patients with diabetes and normal renal function should consume 15–20% of their energy intake as protein. However, they recognize that there is no definitive evidence for recommending an ideal amount of protein in relation either to glycemic control or for improving CVD risk factors [49].

Protein may have an incretin role. Its consumption is associated with higher insulin secretion, equivalent to that caused by eating the same amount of glucose. Some amino acids, such as leucine, lysine, or alanine, stimulate insulin secretion. In contrast, homocysteine can inhibit it [50,51].

There are several studies that propose hyperproteic diets in the management of MetS due to the satiating effect of proteins [52–54]. These diets also contribute to the preservation of lean mass. However, these diets may favor an increase in urinary calcium excretion and bone remodeling, and their use is not totally accepted [55]. Overall, these concerns seem a little overstated. High-protein diets do not seem to lead to calcium bone loss, and have no damaging effect on the kidney unless there is a pre-existing metabolic renal dysfunction.

4. Dietary Patterns

The most effective intervention for metabolic intervention is caloric restriction. Nutrition change to support a 7–10% weight loss is an appropriate goal for people with prediabetes, unless additional weight loss is desired for other purposes. The contributions of different nutrients to success in the reduction have to be seen in the context of the general eating plan of the patient. There is no perfect combination of macronutrients useful for all individuals. Compliance with a healthier lifestyle and dietary intake are more important than a particular dietary pattern. This represents an advantage for patients confronting MetS. As there is no "one-size-fits-all" pattern, individuals can advance with any healthy plan that is easy for them to follow. It also opens the door to adaptations of dietary recommendations based on metabolic goals, socioeconomic factors, food availability, and personal and cultural preferences. Irrespective of the macronutrient balance in the diet, total energy intake should be appropriate to accomplish the weight management goals.

Several nutrition patterns are effective in improving diabetes control, but the optimal macronutrient composition in meal planning in persons with MetS is less well defined. As previously seen, the main concern with regard to MetS is the development of diabetes and the associated cardiovascular risk. Patients with MetS have a similar benefit to overweight/obese patients with diabetes from the adoption of several dietary patterns. As already stated, the goal in both conditions is achieving weight loss. A short description of the characteristics of the different dietary patterns and their potential benefits was recently published [49]. Multiple studies analyzed the effectiveness of different patterns and confirmed the emphasis on compliance. Table 2 summarizes the main benefits of different dietary patterns regarding weight, glucose and lipid metabolism, and blood pressure.

Table 2. Metabolic syndrome improvement observed with different dietary patterns. DASH—Dietary approaches to stop hypertension; CVD—Cardiovascular disease; LDL-C—Low-density lipoprotein cholesterol; HDL-C—High-density lipoprotein cholesterol.

Dietary Patterns	↓ Risk of Diabetes	↓ A1c	↓ Triglycerides	↓ CVD	Weight Loss	↓ LDL-C or HDL-C	↓ Blood Pressure
Low fat [1]	X				X		
Very low fat [2]					X		X
Low carbohydrate [3]		X			X	X	X
Very low carbohydrate [4]		X	X		X	X	X
Mediterranean-style	X	X	X	X			
DASH	X				X		X
Vegetarian or vegan	X	X			X	X	
Paleo diet			Lack of evidence				
Zone diet (40–30–30 diet)		Lack of evidence			x	Lack of evidence	
Healthy Nordic diet	x			x	x		

The content of the table is derived from References [56–59]. X means there is proven evidence of the benefit; x indicates hypothetical evidence. "↓" represents a decrease and improvement in risk factor. [1] Low fat = fat intake < 30% of total calories; [2] very low fat = fat intake <10% of total calories; [3] low carbohydrate = carbohydrate intake 26–45% of total calories; [4] very low carbohydrate = carbohydrate intake < 26% of total calories.

With the exception of low-carbohydrate diets, common to many of these patterns is the emphasis on no starchy vegetables, the reduction of added sugars and refined grains, and the exclusion of processed foods to favor whole foods instead. Adoption of a Mediterranean-style diet rich in whole grain cereals, fruits, vegetables, nuts, and olive oil, compared to a prudent dietary pattern (50–60% of energy as carbohydrate and <30% as fat), was associated with improvements in endothelial function and significant reductions in the markers of systemic vascular inflammation in MetS patients after two years of follow-up [60,61]. The DASH (dietary approaches to stop hypertension) diet, rich in fruits, vegetables, and low-fat dairy food and low in saturated and total fat intake, demonstrated weight reduction and a significant reduction in blood pressure [62–64]. Mediterranean-style, vegetarian, and DASH eating patterns have a lower risk of developing type 2 diabetes [59]. Overall, the lower the provision of carbohydrates is, the lower the value of A1c hemoglobin is [65]. Weight loss or A1c reductions may be statistically significant but with small differences, with, for example, vegetarian diets, of 2 kg and 0.3%, respectively [66].

Low-fat diets are used as the control or default intervention vs. other dietary patterns. Their benefits seem to derive from weight loss rather than the eating pattern itself [67]. Interestingly, when low-carbohydrate diets are used, the specific distribution of fats and, particularly, the amount of saturated fat must be taken into account because, otherwise, it may be higher than that recommended for healthy individuals [68].

If we can call intermittent fasting a dietary pattern, different forms of intermittent fasting can lead to improved beta cell responsiveness, insulin sensitivity, and blood pressure control [69].

5. Conclusions

MetS is a cluster of risk factors that identifies patients at risk of developing diabetes mellitus and CVD. Nutrition therapy, as part of a comprehensive lifestyle intervention, may improve obesity and insulin resistance, which play key roles in its pathogenesis.

Macronutrients may contribute to worsening or improving MetS. An elevated intake of carbohydrates of high GI causes insulin resistance directly and has an impact on the development of T2DM in persons with MetS. In contrast, low-GI diets, more abundant in fiber, increase satiety and decrease insulin resistance and the risk of developing T2DM. Low-GI diets are, thus, recommended for patients with MetS. Diets enriched with MUFAs also improve the lipid profile and increase insulin sensitivity compared with SFAs. A healthy pattern limits saturated and *trans* fats, added sugars, and sodium. Specifically, the recommendation for the general population is to consume less than 10% of calories per day as added sugars and less than 10% of calories per day as saturated fats. Proteins in the diet are associated with increased satiety, insulin secretion, and preservation of lean body mass during weight loss, and hyperproteic diets are suggested for the management of MetS.

The effects of macronutrients are important; however, we consume them combined in eating patterns. Several dietary patterns may be helpful in reversing MetS, such as Mediterranean-style, vegetarian, DASH, low-carbohydrate, or even low-fat diets. The different patterns have variable effects on each risk factor, but all of them must be compatible with caloric restriction, which is the most effective intervention for metabolic intervention.

Author Contributions: Both authors contributed to the literature search, summarized the information, and wrote the review.

Conflicts of Interest: The authors declare no conflicts of interest.

References

1. Eckel, R.H.; Grundy, S.M.; Zimmet, P. The metabolic syndrome. *Lancet* **2005**, *365*, 1415–1428. [CrossRef]
2. Samson, S.L.; Garber, A.J. Metabolic Syndrome. *Endocrinol. Metab. Clin. N. Am.* **2014**, *43*, 1–23. [CrossRef] [PubMed]
3. Alberti, K.G.; Eckel, R.H.; Grundy, S.M.; Zimmet, P.Z.; Cleeman, J.I.; Donato, K.A.; Fruchart, J.C.; James, W.P.; Loria, C.M.; Smith, S.C., Jr.; et al. Harmonizing the metabolic syndrome: A joint interim statement of the International Diabetes Federation Task Force on Epidemiology and Prevention; National Heart, Lung, and Blood Institute; American Heart Association; World Heart Federation; International Atherosclerosis Society; and International Association for the Study of Obesity. *Circulation* **2009**, *120*, 1642–1645.
4. Kahn, R. Metabolic syndrome: Is it a syndrome? Does it matter? *Circulation* **2007**, *115*, 1806–1810. [CrossRef] [PubMed]
5. Ford, E.S. Risk for All-Cause Mortality, Cardiovascular Disease, and Diabetes Associated with the Metabolic Syndrome. A summary of the evidence. *Diabetes Care* **2005**, *28*, 1769–1778. [CrossRef] [PubMed]
6. Mottillo, S.; Filiion, K.B.; Genest, J.; Joseph, L.; Pilote, L.; Poirier, P.; Rinfret, S.; Schiffrin, E.L.; Eisenberg, M.J. The Metabolic Syndrome and Cardiovascular Risk. A systematic review and meta-analysis. *J. Am. Coll. Cardiol.* **2010**, *56*, 1113–1132. [CrossRef] [PubMed]
7. Blaha, M.J.; Bausal, S.; Rouf, R.; Golden, S.H.; Blumenthal, R.S.; Defilippis, A.P. A practical "ABCDE" approach of the metabolic syndrome. *Mayo Clin. Proc.* **2008**, *83*, 932–941. [CrossRef]
8. Case, C.C.; Jones, P.H.; Nelson, K.; Smith, E.O.; Ballantyne, C.M. Impact of weight loss on the metabolic syndrome. *Diabetes Obes. Metab.* **2002**, *4*, 407–414. [CrossRef]
9. Phelan, S.; A Wadden, T.; I Berkowitz, R.; Sarwer, D.B.; Womble, L.G.; Cato, R.K.; Rothman, R. Impact of weight loss on the metabolic syndrome. *Int. J. Obes.* **2007**, *31*, 1442–1448. [CrossRef]
10. Xydakis, A.M.; Case, C.C.; Jones, P.H.; Hoogeveen, R.C.; Liu, M.-Y.; Smith, E.O.; Nelson, K.W.; Ballantyne, C.M. Adiponectin, Inflammation, and the Expression of the Metabolic Syndrome in Obese Individuals: The Impact of Rapid Weight Loss through Caloric Restriction. *J. Clin. Endocrinol. Metab.* **2004**, *89*, 2697–2703. [CrossRef]
11. Nestel, P. Nutritional aspects in the causation and management of the metabolic syndrome. *Endocrinol. Metab. Clin. N. Am.* **2004**, *33*, 483–492. [CrossRef] [PubMed]
12. Katzmarzyk, P.T.; Leon, A.S.; Wilmore, J.H.; Skinner, J.S.; Rao, D.C.; Rankinen, T.; Bouchard, C. Targeting the Metabolic Syndrome with Exercise: Evidence from the HERITAGE Family Study. *Med. Sci. Sports Exerc.* **2003**, *35*, 1703–1709. [CrossRef] [PubMed]
13. Liu, S.; Willett, W.C.; Stampfer, M.J.; Hu, F.B.; Franz, M.; Sampson, L.; Hennekens, C.H.; E Manson, J. A prospective study of dietary glycemic load, carbohydrate intake, and risk of coronary heart disease in US women. *Am. J. Clin. Nutr.* **2000**, *71*, 1455–1461. [CrossRef] [PubMed]
14. Burger, K.N.; Beulens, J.W.; Boer, J.M.; Spijkerman, A.M. Dietary glycemic load and glycemic index and risk of coronary heart disease and stroke in Dutch men and women: The EPIC-MORGEN study. *PLoS ONE* **2011**, *6*, e25955. [CrossRef] [PubMed]

15. Sichieri, R.; Moura, A.S.; Genelhu, V.; Hu, F.; Willett, W.C. An 18-month randomized trial of a low-glycemic-index diet and weight change in Brazilian women. *Am. J. Clin. Nutr.* **2007**, *86*, 707–713. [CrossRef] [PubMed]
16. Wheeler, M.L.; Dunbar, S.A.; Jaacks, L.M.; Karmally, W.; Mayer-Davis, E.J.; Wylie-Rosett, J.; Yancy, W.S.J. Macronutrients, food groups, and eating patterns in the management of diabetes: A systematic review of the literature, 2010. *Diabetes Care* **2012**, *35*, 434–445. [CrossRef] [PubMed]
17. Jenkins, D.J.; Jenkins, A.L.; Wolever, T.M. Low glycemic index: Lente carbohydrates and physiological effects of altered food frequency. *Am. J. Clin. Nutr.* **1994**, *59*, 706–709. [CrossRef]
18. Schulze, M.B.; Liu, S.; Rimm, E.B.; Manson, J.E.; Willett, W.C.; Hu, F.B. Glycemic index, glycemic load, and dietary fiber intake and incidence of type 2 diabetes in younger and middle-aged women. *Am. J. Clin. Nutr.* **2004**, *80*, 348–356. [CrossRef] [PubMed]
19. Pereira, M.A.; Jacobs, D.R.; Pins, J.J.; Raatz, S.K.; Gross, M.D.; Slavin, J.L.; Seaquist, E.R. Effect of whole grains on insulin sensitivity in overweight hyperinsulinemic adults. *Am. J. Clin. Nutr.* **2002**, *75*, 848–855. [CrossRef]
20. Jovanovski, E.; Khayyat, R.; Zurbau, A.; Komishon, A.; Mazhar, N.; Sievenpiper, J.L.; Mejia, S.B.; Ho, H.V.T.; Li, D.; Jenkins, A.L.; et al. Should Viscous Fiber Supplements Be Considered in Diabetes Control? Results from a Systematic Review and Meta-analysis of Randomized Controlled Trials. *Diabetes Care* **2019**, *42*, 755–766. [CrossRef]
21. Jarvi, A.E.; Karlstrom, B.E.; Granfeldt, Y.E.; Bjorck, I.E.; Asp, N.G.; Vessby, B.O. Improved glycemic control and lipid profile and normalized fibrinolytic activity on a low-glycemic index diet in type 2 diabetic patients. *Diabetes Care* **1999**, *22*, 10–18. [CrossRef] [PubMed]
22. Fried, S.K.; Rao, S.P. Sugars, hypertryglyceridemia, and cardiovascular disease. *Am. J. Clin. Nutr.* **2003**, *78*, 873–880. [CrossRef] [PubMed]
23. McMillan-Price, J.; Petocz, P.; Atkinson, F.; O'Neill, K.; Samman, S.; Caterson, I.; Brand-Miller, J. Comparison of 4 diets of varying glycemic load on weight loss and cardiovascular risk reduction in overweight and obese young adults: A randomized controlled trial. *Arch. Intern. Med.* **2006**, *166*, 1466–1475. [CrossRef] [PubMed]
24. Horton, E.S. Effects of lifestyle changes to reduce risks of diabetes and associated cardiovascular risks: Results from large-scale efficacy trials. *Obesity* **2009**, *17*, S43–S48. [CrossRef] [PubMed]
25. Buyken, A.E.; Toeller, M.; Heitkamp, G.; Karamanos, B.; Rottiers, R.; Muggeo, M.; The Eurodiab Iddm Complications Study Group. Glycemic index in the diet of European outpatients with type 1 diabetes: Relations to glycated hemoglobin and serum lipids. *Am. J. Clin. Nutr.* **2001**, *73*, 574–581. [CrossRef] [PubMed]
26. Brand-Miller, J.; Hayne, S.; Petocz, P.; Colagiuri, S. Low-glycemic index diets in the management of diabetes. A meta-analysis of randomized controlled trials. *Diabetes Care* **2003**, *26*, 2261–2267. [CrossRef] [PubMed]
27. Samaha, F.F.; Iqbal, N.; Seshadri, P.; Chicano, K.L.; Daily, D.A.; McGrory, J.; Williams, T.; Williams, M.; Gracely, E.J.; Stern, L. A Low-Carbohydrate as Compared with a Low-Fat Diet in Severe Obesity. *New Engl. J. Med.* **2003**, *348*, 2074–2081. [CrossRef]
28. Stem, L.; Iqbal, N.; Seshadri, P.; Chicano, K. The effects of low-carbohydrate versus conventional weight loss diets in severely obese adults: One-year follow-up of a randomized trial. *ACC Curr. J. Rev.* **2004**, *13*, 18. [CrossRef]
29. Saslow, L.R.; Kim, S.; Daubenmier, J.J.; Moskowitz, J.T.; Phinney, S.D.; Goldman, V.; Murphy, E.J.; Cox, R.M.; Morán, P.; Hecht, F.M. A Randomized Pilot Trial of a Moderate Carbohydrate Diet Compared to a Very Low Carbohydrate Diet in Overweight or Obese Individuals with Type 2 Diabetes Mellitus or Prediabetes. *PLoS ONE* **2014**, *9*, e91027. [CrossRef]
30. Bray, G.A.; Nielsen, S.J.; Popkin, B.M. Consumption of high-fructose corn syrup in beverages may play a role in the epidemic of obesity. *Am. J. Clin. Nutr.* **2004**, *79*, 537–543. [CrossRef]
31. Dekker, M.J.; Su, Q.; Baker, C.; Rutledge, A.C.; Adeli, K. Fructose: A highly lipogenic nutrient implicated in insulin resistance, hepatic steatosis, and the metabolic syndrome. *Am. J. Physiol. Endocrinol. Metab.* **2010**, *299*, E685–E694. [CrossRef] [PubMed]
32. Rizkalla, S.W. Health implications of fructose consumption: A review of recent data. *Nutr. Metab.* **2010**, *7*, 82. [CrossRef] [PubMed]
33. Institute of Medicine. *Dietary Reference Intakes for Energy, Carbohydrate, Fiber, Fat, Fatty Acids, Cholesterol, Protein, and Amino Acids*; The National Academies Press: Washington, DC, USA, 2005.

34. Vessby, B.; Uusitupa, M.; Hermansen, K. Substituting dietary saturated fat for monounsaturated fat impairs insulin sensitivity in healthy men and women. *Diabetologia* **2001**, *44*, 312–319. [CrossRef] [PubMed]
35. Riccardi, G.; Giaccob, R.; Rivellese, A.A. Dietary fat, insulin sensitivity and the metabolic syndrome. *Clin. Nutr.* **2004**, *23*, 447–456. [CrossRef] [PubMed]
36. Rivellese, A.; Maffettone, A.; Vessby, B.; Uusitupa, M.; Hermansen, K.; Berglund, L.; Louheranta, A.; Meyer, B.J.; Riccardi, G. Effects of dietary saturated, monounsaturated and n-3 fatty acids on fasting lipoproteins, LDL size and post-prandial lipid metabolism in healthy subjects. *Atherosclerosis* **2003**, *167*, 149–158. [CrossRef]
37. Thomsen, C.; Rasmussen, O.; Lousen, T.; Holst, J.J.; Fenselau, S.; Schrezenmeir, J.; Hermansen, K. Differential effects of saturated and monounsaturated fatty acids on postprandial lipemia and incretin responses in healthy subjects. *Am. J. Clin. Nutr.* **1999**, *69*, 1135–1143. [CrossRef] [PubMed]
38. Rasmussen, B.M.; Vessby, B.; Uusitupa, M.; Berglund, L.; Pedersen, E.; Riccardi, G.; A Rivellese, A.; Tapsell, L.; Hermansen, K.; KANWU Study Group. Effects of dietary saturated, monounsaturated, and n-3 fatty acids on blood pressure in healthy subjects. *Am. J. Clin. Nutr.* **2006**, *83*, 221–226. [PubMed]
39. Meyer, B.J.; Lane, A.E.; Mann, N.J. Comparison of Seal Oil to Tuna Oil on Plasma Lipid Levels and Blood Pressure in Hypertriglyceridaemic Subjects. *Lipids* **2009**, *44*, 827–835. [CrossRef] [PubMed]
40. Dangardt, F.; Osika, W.; Chen, Y.; Nilsson, U.; Gan, L.-M.; Gronowitz, E.; Strandvik, B.; Friberg, P. Omega-3 fatty acid supplementation improves vascular function and reduces inflammation in obese adolescents. *Atherosclerosis* **2010**, *212*, 580–585. [CrossRef]
41. McEwen, B.; Morel-Kopp, M.C.; Tofler, G.; Ward, C. Effect of omega-3 fish oil on cardiovascular risk in diabetes. *Diabetes Educ.* **2010**, *36*, 565–584. [CrossRef]
42. Summers, L.K.; Fielding, B.A.; Bradshaw, H.A.; Ilic, V.; Beysen, C.; Clark, M.L.; Moore, N.R.; Frayn, K.N. Substituting dietary saturated fat with polyunsaturated fat changes abdominal fat distribution and improves insulin sensitivity. *Diabetologia* **2002**, *45*, 369–377. [CrossRef] [PubMed]
43. Bhatt, D.L.; Steg, P.G.; Miller, M.; Brinton, E.A.; Jacobson, T.A.; Ketchum, S.B.; Doyle, R.T., Jr.; Juliano, R.A.; Jiao, L.; Granowitz, C.; et al. REDUCEIT Investigators. Cardiovascular risk reduction with icosapent ethyl for hypertriglyceridemia. *N. Engl. J. Med.* **2019**, *380*, 11–22. [CrossRef] [PubMed]
44. Saris, W.H.M.; Astrup, A.; Prentice, A.M.; Zunft, H.J.F.; Formiguera, X.; De Venne, W.P.H.G.V.-V.; Raben, A.; Poppitt, S.D.; Seppelt, B.; Johnston, S.; et al. Randomized controlled trial of changes in dietary carbohydrate/fat ratio and simple vs complex carbohydrates on body weight and blood lipids: The CARMEN study. *Int. J. Obes.* **2000**, *24*, 1310–1318. [CrossRef]
45. Evert, A.B.; Boucher, J.L.; Cypress, M.; Dunbar, S.A.; Franz, M.J.; Mayer-Davis, E.J.; Neumiller, J.J.; Nwankwo, R.; Verdi, C.L.; Urbanski, P.; et al. Nutrition therapy recommendations for the management of adults with diabetes. *Diabetes Care* **2013**, *36*, 3821–3842. [CrossRef] [PubMed]
46. Pirozzo, S.; Summerbell, C.; Cameron, C.; Glasziou, P. Should we recommend low-fat diets for obesity? *Obes. Rev.* **2003**, *4*, 83–90. [CrossRef] [PubMed]
47. U.S. Department of Health and Human Service; U.S. Department of Agriculture. 2015–2020 Dietary Guidelines for Americans, 8th ed. Available online: https://health.gov/dietaryguidelines/2015/guidelines/ (accessed on 28 June 2019).
48. Catapano, A.L.; Graham, I.; De Backer, G.; Wiklund, O.; Chapman, M.J.; Drexel, H.; Hoes, A.W.; Jennings, C.S.; Landmesser, U.; Pedersen, T.R.; et al. 2016 ESC/EAS Guidelines for the Management of Dyslipidaemias: The Task Force for the Management of Dyslipidaemias of the European Society of Cardiology (ESC) and European Atherosclerosis Society (EAS). Developed with the special contribution of the European Association for Cardiovascular Prevention & Rehabilitation (EACPR). *Eur. Heart J.* **2016**, *37*, 2999–3058. [PubMed]
49. Evert, A.B.; Dennison, M.; Gardner, C.D.; Garvey, W.T.; Lau, K.H.K.; MacLeod, J.; Mitri, J.; Pereira, R.F.; Rawlings, K.; Robinson, S.; et al. Nutrition Therapy for Adults With Diabetes or Prediabetes: A Consensus Report. *Diabetes Care* **2019**, *42*, 731–754. [CrossRef] [PubMed]
50. Gannon, M.C. Effect of Protein Ingestion on the Glucose Appearance Rate in People with Type 2 Diabetes. *J. Clin. Endocrinol. Metab.* **2001**, *86*, 1040–1047. [CrossRef] [PubMed]
51. Patterson, S.; Flatt, P.; Brennan, L.; Newsholme, P.; McClenaghan, N. Detrimental actions of metabolic syndrome risk factor, homocysteine, on pancreatic β-cell glucose metabolism and insulin secretion. *J. Endocrinol.* **2006**, *189*, 301–310. [CrossRef] [PubMed]

52. Stentz, F.B.; Brewer, A.; Wan, J.; Garber, C.; Daniels, B.; Sands, C.; Kitabchi, A.E. Remission of pre-diabetes to normal glucose tolerance in obese adults with high protein versus high carbohydrate diet: Randomized control trial. *BMJ Open Diabetes Res. Care* **2016**, *4*, e000258. [CrossRef] [PubMed]
53. Leidy, H.J.; Clifton, P.M.; Astrup, A.; Wycherley, T.P.; Westerterp-Plantenga, M.S.; Luscombe-Marsh, N.D.; Woods, S.C.; Mattes, R.D. The role of protein in weight loss and maintenance. *Am. J. Clin. Nutr.* **2015**, *101*, 1320–1329. [CrossRef] [PubMed]
54. Sluik, D.; Brouwer-Brolsma, E.M.; Berendsen, A.A.M.; Mikkilä, V.; Poppitt, S.D.; Silvestre, M.P.; Tremblay, A.; Pérusse, L.; Bouchard, C.; Raben, A.; et al. Protein intake and the incidence of pre-diabetes and diabetes in 4 population-based studies: The PREVIEW project. *Am. J. Clin. Nutr.* **2019**, *109*, 1310–1318. [CrossRef] [PubMed]
55. Calvez, J.; Poupin, N.; Chesneau, C.; Lassale, C.; Tomé, D. Protein intake, calcium balance and health consequences. *Eur. J. Clin. Nutr.* **2012**, *66*, 281–295. [CrossRef] [PubMed]
56. Mithril, C.; Dragsted, L.; Meyer, C.; Blauert, E.; Holt, M.; Astrup, A. Guidelines for the New Nordic Diet. *Public Health Nutr.* **2012**, *15*, 1941–1947. [CrossRef] [PubMed]
57. Cheuvront, S.N. The Zone Diet phenomenon: A closer look at the science behind the claims. *J. Am. Coll. Nutr.* **2003**, *22*, 9–17. [CrossRef] [PubMed]
58. Fenton, T.R.; Fenton, C.J. Paleo diet still lacks evidence. *Am. J. Clin. Nutr.* **2016**, *104*, 844. [CrossRef]
59. Uusitupa, M.; Hermansen, K.; Savolainen, M.J.; Schwab, U.; Kolehmainen, M.; Brader, L.; Mortensen, L.S.; Cloetens, L.; Johansson-Persson, A.; Onning, G.; et al. Effects of an isocaloric healthy Nordic diet on insulin sensitivity, lipid profile and inflammation markers in metabolic syndrome—A randomized study (SYSDIET). *J. Intern. Med.* **2013**, *274*, 52–66. [CrossRef]
60. Esposito, K.; Marfella, R.; Ciotola, M.; Di Palo, C.; Giugliano, F.; Giugliano, G.; D'Armiento, M.; D'Andrea, F.; Giugliano, D. Effect of a Mediterranean-Style Diet on Endothelial Dysfunction and Markers of Vascular Inflammation in the Metabolic Syndrome. *JAMA* **2004**, *292*, 1440. [CrossRef]
61. Paniagua, J.A.; De La Sacristana, A.G.; Sánchez, E.; Romero, I.; Vidal-Puig, A.; Berral, F.J.; Escribano, A.; Moyano, M.J.; Peréz-Martinez, P.; López-Miranda, J.; et al. A MUFA-rich diet improves posprandial glucose, lipid and GLP-1 responses in insulin-resistant subjects. *J. Am. Coll. Nutr.* **2007**, *26*, 434–444. [CrossRef]
62. Lien, L.F.; Brown, A.J.; Ard, J.D.; Loria, C.; Erlinger, T.P.; Feldstein, A.C.; Lin, P.-H.; Champagne, C.M.; King, A.C.; McGuire, H.L.; et al. Effects of PREMIER Lifestyle Modifications on Participants with and without the Metabolic Syndrome. *Hypertension* **2007**, *50*, 609–616. [CrossRef]
63. Sacks, F.M.; Obarzanek, E.; Windhauser, M.M.; Svetkey, L.P.; Vollmer, W.M.; McCullough, M.; Karanja, N.; Lin, P.H.; Steele, P.; Proschan, M.A. Rationale and design of the Dietary Approaches to Stop Hypertension trial (DASH). A multicenter controlled-feeding study of dietary patterns to lower blood pressure. *Ann. Epidemiology* **1995**, *5*, 108–118. [CrossRef]
64. Obarzanek, E.; Sacks, F.M.; Vollmer, W.M.; Bray, G.A.; Miller, E.R.; Lin, P.-H.; Karanja, N.M.; Most-Windhauser, M.M.; Moore, T.J.; Swain, J.F.; et al. Effects on blood lipids of a blood pressureÂ–lowering diet: The Dietary Approaches to Stop hypertension (DASH) Trial. *Am. J. Clin. Nutr.* **2001**, *74*, 80–89.
65. Sainsbury, E.; Kizirian, N.V.; Partridge, S.R.; Gill, T.; Colagiuri, S.; Gibson, A.A. Effect of dietary carbohydrate restriction on glycemic control in adults with diabetes: A systematic review and metaanalysis. *Diabetes Res. Clin. Pract.* **2018**, *139*, 239–252. [CrossRef]
66. Viguiliouk, E.; Kendall, C.W.; Kahleov'a, H.; Rahelić, D.; Salas-Salvadó, J.; Choo, V.L.; Mejia, S.B.; Stewartm, S.E.; Leiter, L.A.; Jenkins, D.J.; et al. Effect of vegetarian dietary patterns on cardiometabolic risk factors in diabetes: A systematic review and meta-analysis of randomized controlled trials. *Clin. Nutr.* **2018**, *38*, 1133–1145. [CrossRef]
67. Wing, R.R.; Bolin, P.; Brancati, F.L.; Bray, G.A.; Clark, J.M.; Coday, M.; Evans, M.; Look AHEAD Research Group. Cardiovascular effects of intensive lifestyle intervention in type 2 diabetes. *N. Engl. J. Med.* **2013**, *369*, 145–154.

68. Tay, J.; Thompson, C.H.; Luscombe-Marsh, N.D.; Thompson, C.H.; Luscombe-Marsh, N.D.; Wycherley, T.P.; Noakes, M.; Buckley, J.D.; Wittert, G.A.; Yancy, W.S., Jr.; et al. Effects of an energy-restricted low-carbohydrate, high unsaturated fat/low saturated fat diet versus a high-carbohydrate, low-fat diet in type 2 diabetes: A 2-year randomized clinical trial. *Diabetes Obes. Metab.* **2018**, *20*, 858–871. [CrossRef]
69. Sutton, E.F.; Beyl, R.; Early, K.S.; Cefalu, W.T.; Ravussin, E.; Peterson, C.M. Early time-restricted feeding improves insulin sensitivity, blood pressure, and oxidative stress even without weight loss in men with prediabetes. *Cell Metab.* **2018**, *27*, 1212–1221. [CrossRef]

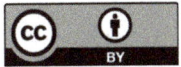

© 2019 by the authors. Licensee MDPI, Basel, Switzerland. This article is an open access article distributed under the terms and conditions of the Creative Commons Attribution (CC BY) license (http://creativecommons.org/licenses/by/4.0/).

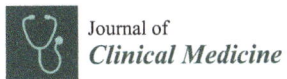

Review

Efficacy and Efficiency of Nutritional Support Teams

Emilie Reber [1,*], Rachel Strahm [1], Lia Bally [1], Philipp Schuetz [2,3] and Zeno Stanga [1]

[1] Department of Diabetes, Endocrinology, Nutritional Medicine and Metabolism, Bern University Hospital, and University of Bern, Freiburgstrasse 15, 3010 Bern, Switzerland
[2] Department of Medical University, Division of General Internal and Emergency Medicine, Kantonsspital Aarau, Tellstrasse 25, 5000 Aarau, Switzerland
[3] Department for Clinical Research, Medical Faculty, University of Basel, 4001 Basel, Switzerland
* Correspondence: emilie.reber@insel.ch

Received: 31 July 2019; Accepted: 20 August 2019; Published: 22 August 2019

Abstract: Malnutrition is frequent in patients during a hospital admission and may further worsen during the hospital stay without appropriate nutritional support. Malnutrition causes greater complication rates, morbidity, and mortality rates, which increases the length of hospital stay and prolongs rehabilitation. Early recognition of individual nutritional risk and timely initiation of a tailored nutritional therapy are crucial. Recent evidence from large-scale trials suggests that efficient nutritional management not only improves the nutritional status, but also prevents negative clinical outcomes and increases patients' quality of life. Multifaceted clinical knowledge is required to ensure optimal nutritional support, according to a patient's individual situation and to avoid potential complications. Furthermore, clear definition of responsibilities and structuring of patient, and work processes are indispensable. Interdisciplinary and multiprofessional nutritional support teams have been built up to ensure and improve the quality and safety of nutritional treatments. These teams continuously check and optimize the quality of procedures in the core areas of nutritional management by implementing nutritional screening processes using a validated tool, nutritional status assessment, an adequate nutritional care plan development, prompt and targeted nutritional treatment delivery, and provision of accurate monitoring to oversee all aspects of care, from catering to artificial nutrition. The foundation of any nutritional care plan is the identification of patients at risk. The aim of this narrative review is to provide an overview about composition, tasks, and challenges of nutritional support teams, and to discuss the current evidence regarding their efficiency and efficacy in terms of clinical outcome and cost effectiveness.

Keywords: nutritional support team; nutritional management; malnutrition; efficacy

---

1. Introduction

Malnutrition, which is defined as a state resulting from the lack of intake or uptake of nutrition leading to altered body composition, decreased mental and physical function, and impaired clinical outcome, is a lurking threat at hospitals in developing countries as well as in industrialized countries [1–5]. Up to 50% of admitted patients are malnourished or at high risk for malnutrition. Acutely ill patients frequently suffer from inflammation and subsequent anorexia, which leads to inadequate food intake and, therefore, to a catabolic state. Under these circumstances, the nutritional status further deteriorates, which may cause rapid weight loss [6].

The association between malnutrition and adverse clinical outcome is well described in the literature [7–32]. Nutritional treatment is urgently needed in malnourished patients to counteract negative metabolic and clinical consequences, to speed up recovery processes, and to enable better quality of life and patient autonomy [2,28,33–35].

The term "food chain" (Figure 1) has been adopted to emphasize that all stages in nutritional care must be adequate, from screening of patients and planning of menus to the distribution and serving of the food [36,37]. Because of the risks, and need for nutritional support, it is desirable for hospitals to appoint a multidisciplinary and multiprofessional nutrition steering group, including the clinical nutrition team, to oversee all aspects of nutritional care, from catering to artificial nutrition [36].

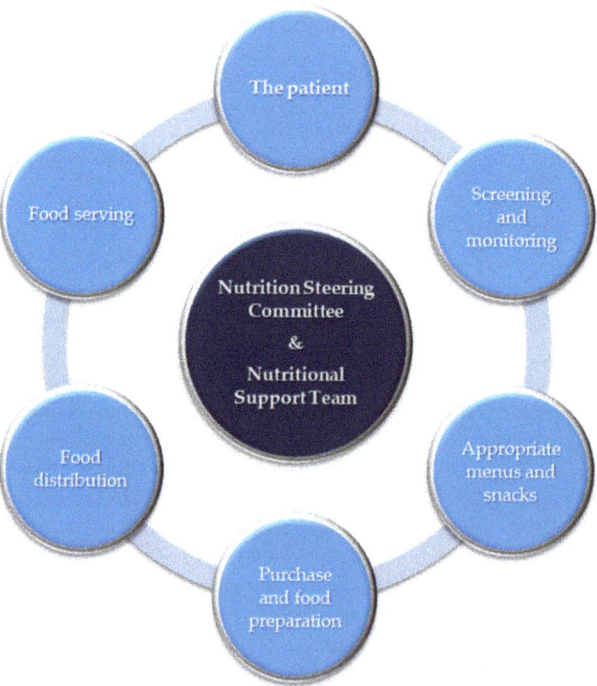

Figure 1. The food chain [36]. The food chain has been adopted to emphasize that all stages in the provision of food must be adequate, from screening of patients and planning of menus to the distribution and serving of the food.

Appropriate, high-quality hospital food is part of a multimodal therapy that includes a wide selection of meals, snacks between meals, and the option of fortified food. The majority of hospitals in industrialized countries should be able to provide such meals, which enable patients to meet their nutritional needs. The problem is that the number of hospitals have now outsourced the hospital kitchen, e.g., to catering companies, which may make it difficult to offer best quality food to patients. Meals may, for example, be frozen and unfrozen or heated twice, which causes an important loss of quality, e.g., regarding micronutrients. Remarkably, more than 40% of meals are left on the patient's plate and wasted, which means a patients' food consumption meets less than 80% of their nutritional needs, and causes additional costs for the hospital [38,39].

The high prevalence of malnutrition implies a close monitoring of food intake, on the one hand, by means of adequate meal-ordering systems and, on the other hand, by sensitizing hospital medical staff to nutritional issues. The keys to better manage nutritional support in hospitals are: (1) enhanced awareness and (2) profound knowledge of this complex matter. Attention to the organization is needed from the medical staff on the ward such as to prevent interruption of meals due to procedures or rounds, and to provide support for disabled patients who need assistance with eating. Such essential tasks have been shown to improve clinical outcomes and reduce healthcare costs in several studies [40–42].

In hospitals, competent nutritional management should rely on two structures: nutritional steering committees and multiprofessional nutritional support teams (NSTs) (Figure 2). The nutrition steering committee is the legislative body with direct access to hospital management (staff function). This committee consists of representative nurses, physicians, pharmacists, dieticians, cooks, managers, controllers, NST members, etc. [43]. It is responsible for promoting good nutrition as a policy, with explicit written nutritional standards, protocols, and guidelines. Further responsibilities are meant to guarantee choice of a wide range of meals and to support continuous improvement and monitoring of the nutritional therapy in terms of quality, safety, and medical efficacy [44]. This committee is also responsible for education, teaching, training, and research coordination. The nutrition steering committee and the NST should also collaborate closely with other hospitals and, in case of tertiary urban hospitals with the University as well as national and international nutritional societies, for clinical research and teaching purposes. NST exercises an executive function throughout the hospital (Figure 3). An optimal functioning institutionalized NST as described above is possible in an urban setting due to the high personal and financial resources allocated. In suburban or rural regions, it is also possible to build an NST but in a reduced format. Our long-lasting clinical experience shows that a single dietician with a physician with special interest in clinical nutrition can overtake the most important clinical tasks of an NST. There is a great opportunity to perform high standing qualitative nutritional care in any setting even if a dietician is available only once a week.

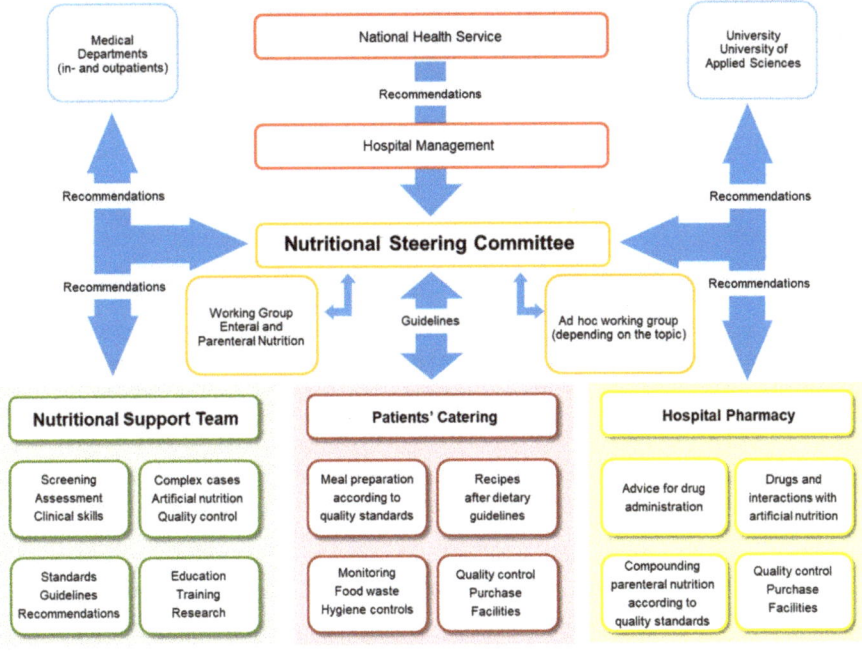

Figure 2. Nutritional management structure, with the Bern University Hospital, as an example.

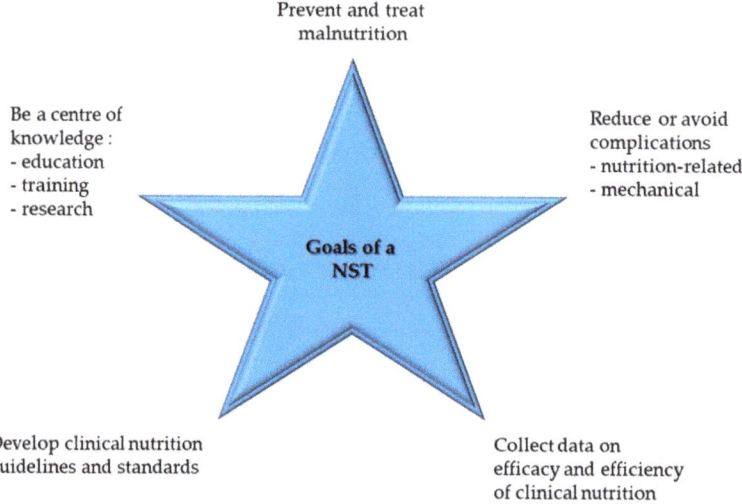

Figure 3. Goals of an NST, modified after [43].

Even though there has been considerable interest in NST to improve nutritional care and, thereby, patient outcomes, there is still a lack of strong scientific evidence mainly due to only a few randomized controlled studies with small heterogeneous study populations, different treatments, and non-standardized outcomes. The aim of this narrative review is to provide an overview about composition, tasks, and challenges of nutritional support teams and discuss the current evidence regarding their efficiency and efficacy in terms of clinical outcome and cost effectiveness.

2. Development of NSTs

While tube feeding (enteral nutrition) has been used since the Renaissance, parenteral nutrition was first successfully used in 1968 [45,46]. At that point, nutritional therapy was established in the clinical setting. Years later, case reports on negative outcomes caused by inadequate nutritional therapies were published. Several studies showed that medical staff often overlooks the clinical signs of malnutrition, which leads to longer hospital stays and higher mortality rates [47].

NSTs were developed to counteract these concerns. At the same time, international societies such as the American Society for Clinical Nutrition (ASPEN, 1976) and the European Society for Clinical Nutrition and Metabolism (ESPEN, 1979) were created. Their primary objective was to study metabolic problems associated with acute diseases and their nutritional implications, and to provide each patient with timely and appropriate nutritional care. A study in 2005 found that NST were present in 2.8% of the hospitals in Germany, 7.9% in Austria, and 2.4% in Switzerland [48]. Ten years later, a Swiss survey indicated that 62% of the country's hospitals had an NST composed of at least one physician and one dietician [49]. Currently, data from the "Nutrition Day Worldwide" shows that most hospitals (mostly urban hospitals) in Europe (approximately 66%) and in the USA (approximately 60%) have such NSTs. This shows the rising importance of clinical nutrition in the industrialized countries [50].

3. NST Composition and Collaboration

Simon Allison (Nottingham, UK) defines an NST as a multiprofessional team including professionals from different disciplines who are good communicators and possess knowledge of the optimal delivery of nutritional therapy [51,52]. An NST improves and ensures the therapy quality and reduces health care costs by preventing needless interventions (e.g., ensuring the appropriateness of indication, stopping unnecessary long fluid therapies, preventing unnecessary catheter removals) and optimizing current treatments (e.g., combining nutritional and drug therapies) [7,23,29]. Smooth multiprofessional and interdisciplinary cooperation as well as impeccable communication are key for the success of an NST. Such a team is traditionally composed of physicians, dieticians, and nurses specialized in clinical nutrition, and pharmacists, with the dieticians primarily assuming the lead in coordinating nutritional care during a hospital stay and, thereafter, in the outpatient clinic [17,53–56].

The composition of the team may vary according to the local needs and options in terms of human resources. Additionally, intensive collaboration with hospital departments responsible for infectious diseases and hospital hygiene is advisable, particularly in the area of parenteral nutrition. This cooperation allows the NST to share knowledge and competence in catheter handling, which is important for preventing, diagnosing, and possibly treating catheter-related bloodstream infections [17]. Other specialists may also collaborate with the NST, such as physiotherapists, occupational therapists, psychotherapists, or social workers [54,56]. Multiprofessional collaboration has to be perceived as an opportunity to integrate the personal and professional expertise of each individual.

4. Tasks and Challenges of NSTs

While the nutritional steering committee has a legislative role, an NST has an executive function throughout the hospital in terms of implementing standards, protocols, and guidelines in daily clinical practice. The core task of an NST is to ensure and promote high-level, evidence-based management of nutrition and to transfer this theoretical knowledge into clinical practice. The foundation of any nutritional care plan (Figure 4) is assessment of nutritional risk and early adequate provision of nutritional support to patients at risk of or suffering from malnutrition. Nutritional support is considered an essential part of the multimodal medical therapy concept, which has demonstrated good therapeutic outcomes. The individual tasks of the members of an NST are shown in Table 1.

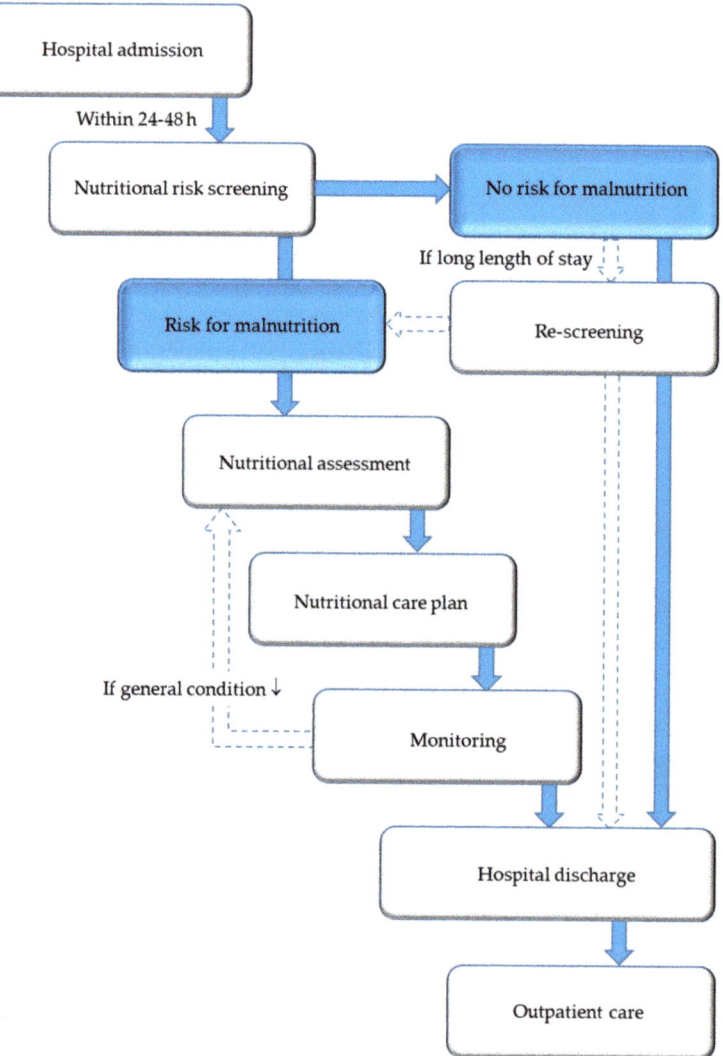

Figure 4. Nutritional care algorithm.

Table 1. Individual tasks of NST members [43].

Professional Function	Nutritional Care Tasks
Nurse	• Gives advice on routes, methods, and systems for delivery of enteral/parenteral nutrition; • Assesses adequacy of access to nutrition therapy; • Advises on use of tubes, feeding pumps, and enteral/parenteral equipment; • Implements and adapts protocols on methods of delivering enteral/parenteral nutrition to establish uniformity, save costs, and prevent mechanical complications; • Educates on enteral/parenteral nutrition and highly complex nutritional therapy; • Conducts research on complex nutritional therapy.
Physician	• Prescribes and manages enteral/parenteral therapy; • Promotes the established nutrition therapy within the host specialty; • Provides professional input for highly complex nutritional therapy; • Supports ongoing research and projects on complex nutritional therapy; • Informs colleagues, physicians in training, and members on the board of directors of the importance of good nutrition therapy on the ward.
Dietician	• Gives advice on enteral/parenteral nutrition (indications, choice of feeding solution, nutritional goals); • Advises about options for enteral/parenteral nutrition and other nutrients (e.g., immuno-nutrition, vitamins, trace elements); • Edits, implements, and adapts protocols on enteral/parenteral nutrition and complex nutritional therapy; • Develops and interprets screening tools; initiates and performs nutritional assessment; • Contributes to education and conducts research on complex nutritional solutions.
Pharmacist	• Provides logistical support for parenteral nutrition; • Oversees and provides information about possible chemical/pharmaceutical interactions between parenteral nutrition components; • Provides professional input on the composition of parenteral nutrition, on stability and compatibility of parenteral admixtures, and on drug/medication interactions with enteral/parenteral nutrition; • Supports ongoing research projects on complex nutritional therapy, develops and implements parenteral nutrition protocols.

4.1. Screening and Assessment

One of the most important missions of a, NST is to educate, to teach, and to train professionals in the skills related to clinical nutrition [51,53,56]. Sharing knowledge and experience with medical staff, health care providers, and students is part of effective nutritional management [55]. Awareness for malnutrition (sensitization), education, and training are, however, lacking [57]. It is a core task of the NST to implement nutritional standards, protocols, and guidelines in daily clinical practice, by establishing proper protocols for screening, assessment, and action [53,58]. The consequences of malnutrition are frequently underestimated and malnutrition is, unfortunately, rarely documented as a distinct diagnosis in medical reports and nurses' charts despite being of central medical and economic importance in hospitals [57].

The first step of nutritional care is the identification of patients at nutritional risk using simple, quick, and validated screening tools. Nutritional screening should be performed in all inpatients (and, preferably, also outpatients) within 24–48 h after hospital admission, respectively, as well as admission on the ward/intermediate care unit/intensive care unit. Nutritional screening should be performed by trained medical staff, at best, multi-professionally from nurses and physicians in charge of the patients, but, alternatively, from nurses, dietitians, or physicians only [59,60]. The Nutritional Risk Screening 2002 (NRS 2002) (Figure 5) is a widely used and well-validated screening tool used in hospitals to determine whether the patient is at nutritional risk [61]. If confirmed, a care plan has to be developed, based on more detailed nutritional assessment to determine the degree/severity of malnutrition. Patients with special metabolic, functional, or clinical problems that cannot be cared for by standard means should be referred to nutrition experts for more detailed nutritional assessment and design of a care plan.

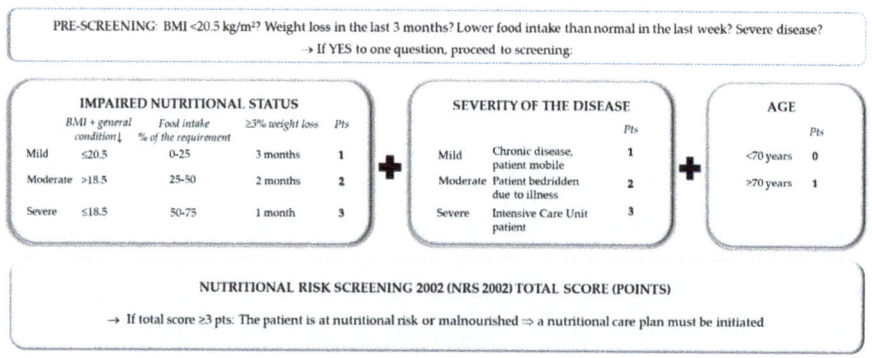

Figure 5. Nutritional risk screening 2002 [61].

Formal quantification of food intake may be helpful. Nutritional assessment can be carried out for at least two days using food diaries or food intake charts (e.g., semi-quantitative plate diagram) that are kept by nursing staff [62]. These can be used by dietitians to calculate energy and protein intake. Anthropometric measurements such as body weight, height, body mass index (BMI = weight ÷ (height in meters)^2), and, if applicable, mid-upper arm circumference or triceps skin fold tests may also be included [62,63]. In addition, according to the local circumstances and standards of care, the following additional measurements may complete the nutritional assessment: body composition (bioelectrical impedance analysis), muscle function (handgrip strength), activities of daily living (Barthel index), quality of life (mainly questionnaires such as SF-36 [64]), and calculation of energy requirements (e.g., Harris and Benedict formula, indirect calorimetry) [63]. Routine laboratory parameters (e.g., complete blood count, lipid profile, electrolytes, and liver parameters) may give information on the patient's nutritional state (proof of nutrient deficiency, information about the etiology of malnutrition, and follow-up of nutritional therapy), the disease severity and activity, and body composition changes to identify patients at nutritional risk [65]. However, none of these markers is very specific for nutritional deficiencies, and their medical interpretation is only possible in the context of the patient's clinical status and history. Thus, nutrition-related factors are hardly ever the sole cause of conspicuous laboratory findings, and there is no such thing as an optimal surrogate marker for malnutrition [65].

Laboratory values must, therefore, always be interpreted in a clinical context [66]. Nitrogen balance, albumin, prealbumin, transferrin, retinol binding protein, insulin growth factor-1, creatinine-height index, and total lymphocyte count are among the few parameters that may be used to quantify malnutrition in malnourished patients [65]. Concerning micronutrients, several potential deficiencies have been associated with malnutrition, including vitamins (i.e., vitamin B12, folic acid, fat-soluble vitamins A, D, E, K) and trace elements (especially zinc, iron, and selenium). The goal of nutritional assessment is to gain an understanding of the patient's nutritional status in order to develop a nutritional care plan containing an accurate calculation of the individual energy and protein requirements and choice of the most appropriate form of feeding (normal food, special consistency, fortified meals, snacks, oral nutritional supplements, or artificial nutrition support).

To call attention to the daily work of an NST (screening, assessment, and nutritional therapy) and, for the reimbursement of this procedure by insurance companies, it is crucial to record, document, and use the code for malnutrition in the Diagnosis Related Groups (DRG) tariff system. It is, therefore, important that the additional revenues arising from use of the DRG code for malnutrition and its therapy are reinvested to cover costs and promote NSTs.

4.2. Nutritional Therapy

NST offers a hospital-wide service with the aim to improve the quality of nutritional therapies targeting complex multimorbid patients, and, in general, to "fight against malnutrition." From a clinical and therapeutic standpoint, nutritional management starts with the identification of patients at nutritional risk—a status that will subsequently guide clinical decision-making—and focuses on those patients likely to benefit from nutritional therapy [67]. Using clinically important endpoints, there is now a substantial body of evidence showing that nutrition support improves outcome when it is implemented appropriately [28]. Thus, after an assessment has been completed and the severity of malnutrition has been determined, the attending medical staff—in cooperation with the NST—sets the individual nutritional plan and the strategy to achieve these goals (Figure 6). While the objective is always to fully meet the individual energy and protein requirements, one should strive for a nutritional intake of at least 75% of those needs [3,68]. Achievement of the goals set and adherence to therapy should be re-evaluated every 24–48 h. If necessary, the nutritional intervention should be adapted. Escalation of the support strategy—i.e., from oral to enteral or from enteral to parenteral nutrition—should be considered within five days [28].

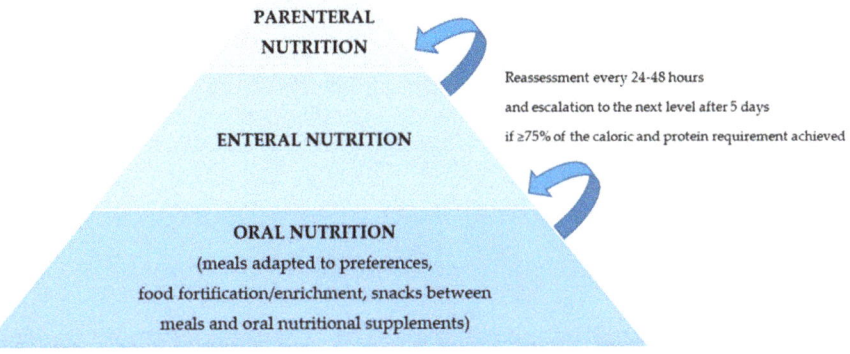

Figure 6. Strategy for nutritional therapy. The nutritional therapy is designed by an NST based on the patient's needs and current situation. The most physiologic route of nutrition delivery is preferable. Nutritional therapy should be regularly re-evaluated and escalated if needed.

4.3. Monitoring and Safety

An NST ensures the correct handling of the artificial nutrition, and reviews the appropriateness of the therapies and related prescriptions [51]. The initiation of a nutritional therapy in complex clinical situations and its proper documentation are also tasks of an NST [69]. An NST ensures the quality and safety of nutritional interventions, especially artificial nutrition, which helps to reduce potential mechanical and metabolic complications (e.g., blood glucose issues and refeeding syndrome) as well as infections [70]. The NST has a consultative role for the treating medical staff in the hospital and takes over the management of the nutritional therapy in outpatients.

4.4. Outpatient Management

Nutritional therapy is normally initialized during the hospital stay, and continued after discharge under close monitoring. The NST plays a key role in management of the therapy during the transition from the inpatient to the outpatient setting (Figure 7). The NST carries out regular visits on the wards, and, subsequently, plans and organizes the hospital discharge from a medical as well as a therapeutic point of view. It monitors the patients, when possible, in regular consultations in the outpatient' clinic. If artificial nutrition is needed at home, the multiprofessional NST instructs and educates patients as well as relatives and caregivers in close cooperation with the treating medical staff. After discharge, the NST remains the core contact for patients, their relatives, their general practitioners, and home care services regarding problems with nutritional therapy (intricate nutrition-related questions, complications, problems with devices, etc.). The NST also plays a central role in the outpatient setting, embedded in the complex interdisciplinary and multiprofessional therapeutic-medical network.

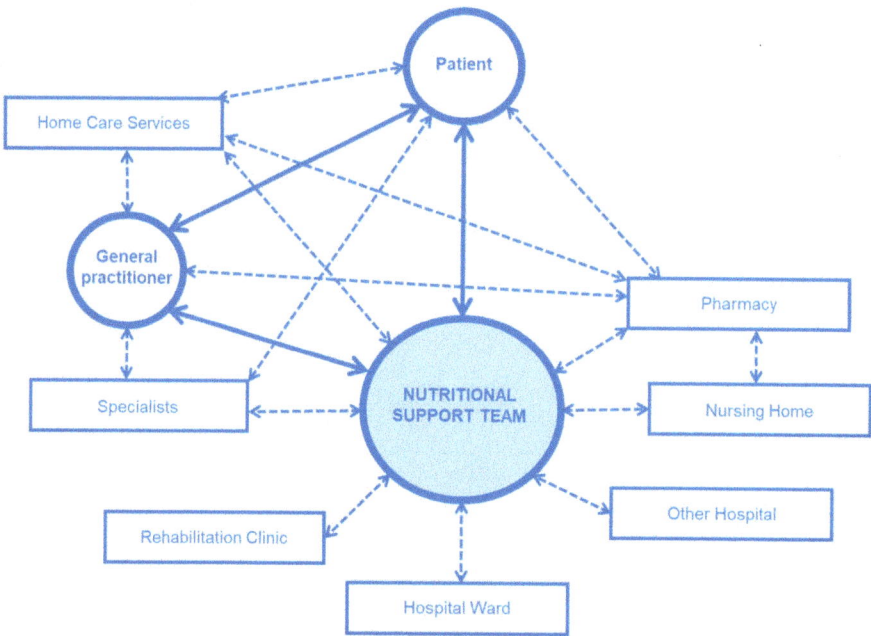

Figure 7. Network of an NST. NST has a central role in the management of patients with complex nutritional therapy in the inpatient and outpatient setting, during the hospital stay and beyond.

4.5. Standards and Processes

An NST monitors the clinical outcomes of the patients and regulates/optimizes processes of the nutritional intervention accordingly. Furthermore, NST periodically checks operating procedures as well as patient procedures, and proposes changes to optimize nutritional care. A good example is the transition from parenteral to enteral nutrition, or from enteral to oral therapy [58]. Since this is the platform of evidence-based practice, operational tasks of an NST include guaranteeing a wide range of meal choices, applying standards of care, implementing medical guidelines, developing standards for consultations, implementing evidence-based nutritional treatment, and maintaining high standards for the quality of hospital food (recipe management) in close collaboration with the catering department [36].

4.6. Education, Training, and Research

An NST also oversees and coordinates education and training in the field of nutritional management, according to the local possibilities and settings. This includes the dissemination of experience, expertise, and skills to trainees, students, and residents as well as other medical and para-medical staff. Multiprofessional work, connected thinking, and effective interdisciplinary communication are mandatory [54–56,71,72]. NST can ensure optimal treatment quality only when all professions and disciplines cooperate smoothly and the patient is given a place.

A respectful and strength-based team culture is the goal. Nutritional interventions and counseling should be scientifically-based whenever possible, and should correspond to the latest knowledge (evidence-based practice). The level of evidence that informs the daily clinical practice of an NST is not always satisfactory and is often based on long-term experience and expertise.

Beyond teaching, knowledge transfer, and skill development, NST should be able to perform clinical translational research and run clinical studies. A trial hypothesis may be generated in response to the concerns and challenges of everyday practice. Exchange of ideas, networking, and cooperation with other hospitals, universities, institutes, and societies is essential in this context, depending on the hospital setting [56].

5. Efficacy, Efficiency, and Positive Outcomes

An NST is often involved in defining the indications for and implementing artificial nutrition [73]. Through the involvement of an NST, there are significantly more correct indications for parenteral nutrition, and, as a result, many labor-intensive interventions can be avoided [53]. In the study of Sriram et al., the number of indicated parenteral therapies increased from 71.3% to 83.4% between 2003 and 2006 due to the intervention of NST [29]. At the same time, non-indicated interventions decreased from 16.5% to 8.9%, which is a sign of higher treatment quality [29]. Boitano et al. investigated compliance with the ASPEN guidelines for parenteral nutrition, which were implemented between 2007 and 2010 [7]. Through changes in the prescription forms, implementation of NST visits on the wards, and the education of physicians, the number of non-indicated therapies could be reduced. The percentage of indicated parenteral therapies increased from 60% to 97%, and around 85% of the patients were able to meet their energy and protein needs, versus 54% before [7]. The close monitoring of nutritional therapy showed an increase in correctly documented laboratory values from 53% to 83%. Additionally, the percentage of patients with hyperglycemia, which is the most frequent complication of parenteral nutrition, could be reduced from 47% to 3% [7]. Besides the obvious increase in treatment quality, the hospital was able to save a total of $5.3 million USD. In the study of Trujillo et al., including consecutive patients treated with parenteral nutrition, 15% of the nutritional interventions were non-indicated and 23% could have been avoided, for a total cost savings of $183,309 per year [32]. Through the interventions of an NST, metabolic complications could also be significantly reduced, from 66% to 34%, which represents $510,746 USD yearly. During 1997, in a Swiss university hospital, 69% of the parenteral nutrition prescriptions were done without involvement of an NST, and 28% of these were non-indicated [23]. Of these non-indicated therapies, 58% were inadequate. In 62% of the patients, energy intake was too low. In 20% of the patients, it was too high, and an additional 17% of patients received no vitamins or trace elements. After an NST was involved, the percentage of patients receiving parenteral nutrition decreased to 35% (2765 bags in 1995 vs 1812 bags in 1998), which leads to more enteral tube feeding. Furthermore, the number of catheter-related infections decreased from 25 (1995) to 3 (1998). Through the direct involvement of an NST, a total of 245,000 Euros per year could be saved [23]. In England, savings of over 50,715 British Pounds were achieved yearly, through the NST monitoring among medical and surgical patients [20]. Through the involvement of an NST, Chris Anderson et al. demonstrated a reduction of the yearly parenteral nutrition costs from $2107 to $1784 USD (mean total per day on parenteral nutrition) [8].

Already in the 1970s and 1980s, studies showed the efficacy (drop in severe catheter-related infections) and the associated cost-effectiveness of involving an NST [9,11,13,17,18,25,26]. Later on, further studies revealed that NST optimizes nutritional therapy and decreases metabolic complications. Moreover, through its interventions, NST is able to reduce the occurrence of electrolyte imbalance, especially in patients on home parenteral nutrition [44–47,57,74]. The recent study of Park et al. showed that the early intervention of an NST in critically ill patients with gastrointestinal diseases positively influences survival [22]. A significant reduction in 90-day mortality under oral nutritional therapy was reported in the study of Deutz et al. [10]. Benefits of NST interventions (oral, enteral, or parenteral) on patients' clinical outcomes could be demonstrated in many other randomized controlled trials over the last two decades, including improved energy and protein intake, shorter length of hospital stay, fewer complications, a lower elective rehospitalization rate, less weight loss, improved muscle function, and an improvement in quality of life [12,14–16,19,21,24,27,28,30,51]. In the study of Johansen et al., NST was responsible for the nutritional management only in the intervention group [19]. The primary endpoint was a composite of nutrition-related factors, which may influence the length of the hospital stay (mobilization, signs of infection, complications). Energy and protein intake of ≥75% of the requirements could be achieved in 62% of the patients in the intervention group versus 36% in the control group [19]. The hospital length of stay of patients who developed complications was significantly shorter in the intervention group [19]. Nutritional therapy may be carried out easily at home with the support of home care services, which results in substantial cost savings [31].

More recently, the efficacy and efficiency of an NST (counseling, therapy, and patient procedures, according to a protocol) were confirmed in the multicenter randomized, controlled Effect of early nutritional support on Frailty, Functional Outcomes, and Recovery of malnourished medical inpatients Trial (EFFORT) of Schuetz et al. [28]. In this study, more than 2000 polymorbid medical inpatients at nutritional risk (NRS 2002 total score ≥3) were randomly assigned to either receive a standard hospital diet versus individualized nutritional support, according to a nutritional protocol [75]. After 30 days, the positive effect of the individualized nutritional management through an NST could be shown. A total of 79% of the intervention group reached their energy and protein requirements, with 76% even within three days (high compliance rate). In the control group, 54% of the patients reached their energy requirements, and 55% reached the protein requirements. Quality of life, functional status, and clinical outcome were also significantly improved. Improved outcome can be translated into a need to treat 25 patients to prevent one adverse clinical outcome and 37 to prevent one death [28]. Notably, there was no increase in side-effects or complications, such as refeeding syndrome, associated with nutritional support [76,77]. These results show that malnutrition is a mostly modifiable risk factor and that a global strategy aimed at meeting the needs of individual patients is of decisive importance. Cachexia may not be fully reversed with nutritional support but remains essential until refractory cachexia occurs [78,79] (Table 2).

Table 2. Clinical studies showing efficacy and efficiency of NST.

Outcome	Correct Indication	Cost Savings	Decreased Complication Rates	Reduced Mortality	Improved Monitoring	Increased Dietary Intake	Positive Influence of Individualized Nutritional Support
Studies	Boitano et al. [7] Piquet et al. [23] Trujilo et al. [32] Sriram et al. [29]	Boitano et al. [7] ChrisAnderson et al. [8] Curry et al. [9] Faubion et al. [11] Goldmann et al. [13] Jacobs et al. [18] Kennedy et al. [20] Piquet et al. [23] Ryan et al. [25] Sanders et al. [26] Trujilo et al. [32]	Boitano et al. [7] Curry et al. [9] Faubion et al. [11] Gariballa et al. [12] Goldmann et al. [13] Ha et al. [14] Hegerova et al. [15] Hickson et al. [16] Jacobs et al. [18] Johansen et al. [19] Norman et al. [21,41] Piquet et al. [23] Ruefenacht et al. [24] Ryan et al. [25] Sanders et al. [26] Somanchi et al. [27] Schuetz et al. [28] Starke et al. [30] Stratton et al. [31] Trujilo et al. [32] ten Dam et al. [43] Dudrick et al. [45] Fürst et al. [46] Butterworth [47] Allison [51] Council of Europe [57]	Park et al. [22] Schuetz et al. [28] Deutz et al. [10]	Boitano et al. [7] Kennedy et al. [20]	Boitano et al. [7] Gariballa et al. [12] Ha et al. [14] Hegerova et al. [15] Hickson et al. [16] Johansen et al. [19] Norman et al. [21,41] Ruefenacht et al. [24] Somanchi et al. [27] Schuetz et al. [28] Starke et al. [30] Stratton et al. [31] ten Dam et al. [43] Dudrick et al. [45] Fürst et al. [46] Allison [51] Council of Europe [57]	Johansen et al. [19] Ruefenacht et al. [24] Schuetz et al. [28]

6. Strength of Evidence Regarding Nutritional Support Teams

Evidence-based medicine is intended to optimize the decision-making of physicians and patients by emphasizing the use of evidence from well-designed and well-conducted research including typically randomized trials and meta-analyses summarizing effects of such single trials. For many fields of clinical nutrition, including NSTs, there has been an important lack of large-scale interventional studies providing such high-quality evidence, and much of today's knowledge is based on observational research and experience of physician and dieticians. As a consequence, current clinical practice guidelines, often give weak recommendations regarding nutritional topics. However, as outlined above, there are some new and important clinical trials in the field, which provide strong evidence in favor of nutritional support and thus also in favor of NSTs [10,28]. However, there is clearly room for further improvements in our understanding on how to best use nutrition in individual patients.

7. Conclusions and Outlook

Malnutrition is a mostly modifiable condition with potentially deleterious consequences, if left untreated. Malnourished patients can be detected early and treated in a timely fashion through comprehensive nutritional care management. This contributes to improvements in the patient's clinical outcome, as recently shown in the EFFORT trial [28]. An interdisciplinary approach and nutritional therapies are effective in cost containment (improving quality of treatment, avoiding unnecessary interventions, and simplifying management), which is especially relevant for the modern healthcare policy. These results show that NSTs should be widely propagated and implemented in a hospital. There is growing evidence from clinical trials demonstrating the efficacy and efficiency of NSTs. The success of nutritional medicine strongly depends on their institutionalization and visibility of the field and the role of the NSTs in modern multimodal medical care. The key task of NSTs is to implement a comprehensive nutritional care system, so that every patient who could potentially benefit from nutritional support receives it rapidly, adequately, and with the highest standards of quality.

Author Contributions: Conceptualization, E.R. and Z.S. Writing—original draft preparation, E.R. Writing—review and editing, E.R., R.S., L.B., and P.S. Supervision, Z.S.

Funding: The Research Found of the Department of Diabetes, Endocrinology, Nutritional medicine and Metabolism and in parts by Nestlé Health Science (grant to the institution: Grant J. Clin. Med. Special Issue 2019_ZS17.12.2018) funded the APC.

Conflicts of Interest: The authors declare no conflicts of interest.

References

1. Aeberhard, C.; Birrenbach, T.; Joray, M.; Muhlebach, S.; Perrig, M.; Stanga, Z. Simple training tool is insufficient for appropriate diagnosis and treatment of malnutrition: A pre-post intervention study in a tertiary center. *Nutrition* **2016**, *32*, 355–361. [CrossRef] [PubMed]
2. Felder, S.; Lechtenboehmer, C.; Bally, M.; Fehr, R.; Deiss, M.; Faessler, L.; Kutz, A.; Steiner, D.; Rast, A.C.; Laukemann, S.; et al. Association of nutritional risk and adverse medical outcomes across different medical inpatient populations. *Nutrition* **2015**, *31*, 1385–1393. [CrossRef] [PubMed]
3. McWhirter, J.P.; Pennington, C.R. Incidence and recognition of malnutrition in hospital. *BMJ* **1994**, *308*, 945–948. [CrossRef] [PubMed]
4. Pirlich, M.; Schutz, T.; Norman, K.; Gastell, S.; Lubke, H.J.; Bischoff, S.C.; Bolder, U.; Frieling, T.; Güldenzoph, H.; Hahn, K.; et al. The German hospital malnutrition study. *Clin. Nutr.* **2006**, *25*, 563–572. [CrossRef] [PubMed]
5. Sorensen, J.; Kondrup, J.; Prokopowicz, J.; Schiesser, M.; Krahenbuhl, L.; Meier, R.; Liberda, M. EuroOOPS: An international, multicentre study to implement nutritional risk screening and evaluate clinical outcome. *Clin. Nutr.* **2008**, *27*, 340–349. [CrossRef] [PubMed]
6. Rinninella, E.; Cintoni, M.; De Lorenzo, A.; Anselmi, G.; Gagliardi, L.; Addolorato, G.; Miggiano, G.A.; Gasbarrini, A.; Mele, M.C. May nutritional status worsen during hospital stay? A sub-group analysis from a cross-sectional study. *Intern. Emerg. Med.* **2019**, *14*, 51–57. [CrossRef] [PubMed]

7. Boitano, M.; Bojak, S.; McCloskey, S.; McCaul, D.S.; McDonough, M. Improving the safety and effectiveness of parenteral nutrition: Results of a quality improvement collaboration. *Nutr. Clin. Pract.* **2010**, *25*, 663–671. [CrossRef]
8. ChrisAnderson, D.; Heimburger, D.C.; Morgan, S.L.; Geels, W.J.; Henry, K.L.; Conner, W.; Hensrud, D.D.; Thompson, G.; Weinsier, R.L. Metabolic complications of total parenteral nutrition: Effects of a nutrition support service. *JPEN J. Parenter. Enteral. Nutr.* **1996**, *20*, 206–210. [CrossRef]
9. Curry, C.R.; Quie, P.G. Fungal septicemia in patients receiving parenteral hyperalimentation. *N. Engl. J. Med.* **1971**, *285*, 1221–1225. [CrossRef]
10. Deutz, N.E.; Matheson, E.M.; Matarese, L.E.; Luo, M.; Baggs, G.E.; Nelson, J.L.; Hegazi, R.A.; Tappenden, K.A.; Ziegler, T.R. NOURISH Study Group. Readmission and mortality in malnourished, older, hospitalized adults treated with a specialized oral nutritional supplement: A randomized clinical trial. *Clin. Nutr.* **2016**, *35*, 18–26. [CrossRef]
11. Faubion, W.C.; Wesley, J.R.; Khalidi, N.; Silva, J. Total parenteral nutrition catheter sepsis: Impact of the team approach. *JPEN J. Parenter. Enteral. Nutr.* **1986**, *10*, 642–645. [CrossRef]
12. Gariballa, S.; Forster, S.; Walters, S.; Powers, H. A randomized, double-blind, placebo-controlled trial of nutritional supplementation during acute illness. *Am. J. Med.* **2006**, *119*, 693–699. [CrossRef]
13. Goldmann, D.A.; Maki, D.G. Infection control in total parenteral nutrition. *JAMA* **1973**, *223*, 1360–1364. [CrossRef]
14. Ha, L.; Hauge, T.; Spenning, A.B.; Iversen, P.O. Individual, nutritional support prevents undernutrition, increases muscle strength and improves QoL among elderly at nutritional risk hospitalized for acute stroke: A randomized, controlled trial. *Clin. Nutr.* **2010**, *29*, 567–573. [CrossRef]
15. Hegerova, P.; Dedkova, Z.; Sobotka, L. Early nutritional support and physiotherapy improved long-term self-sufficiency in acutely ill older patients. *Nutrition* **2015**, *31*, 166–170. [CrossRef]
16. Hickson, M.; Bulpitt, C.; Nunes, M.; Peters, R.; Cooke, J.; Nicholl, C.; Frost, G. Does additional feeding support provided by health care assistants improve nutritional status and outcome in acutely ill older in-patients?—A randomised control trial. *Clin. Nutr.* **2004**, *23*, 69–77. [CrossRef]
17. National Institute for Health and Clinical Excellence. Nutrition Support for Adults: Oral Nutrition Support, Enteral Tube Feeding and Parenteral Nutrition (clinical guideline 32). Available online: https://www.nice.org.uk/Guidance/CG32 (accessed on 20 August 2019).
18. Jacobs, D.O.; Melnik, G.; Forlaw, L.; Gebhardt, C.; Settle, R.G.; DiSipio, M.; Rombeau, J.L. Impact of a nutritional support service on VA surgical patients. *J. Am. Coll. Nutr.* **1984**, *3*, 311–315. [CrossRef]
19. Johansen, N.; Kondrup, J.; Plum, L.M.; Bak, L.; Norregaard, P.; Bunch, E.; Bærnthsen, H.; Andersen, J.R.; Larsen, I.H.; Martinsen, A. Effect of nutritional support on clinical outcome in patients at nutritional risk. *Clin. Nutr.* **2004**, *23*, 539–550. [CrossRef]
20. Kennedy, J.F.; Nightingale, J.M. Cost savings of an adult hospital nutrition support team. *Nutrition* **2005**, *21*, 1127–1133. [CrossRef]
21. Norman, K.; Kirchner, H.; Freudenreich, M.; Ockenga, J.; Lochs, H.; Pirlich, M. Three month intervention with protein and energy rich supplements improve muscle function and quality of life in malnourished patients with non-neoplastic gastrointestinal disease–a randomized controlled trial. *Clin. Nutr.* **2008**, *27*, 48–56. [CrossRef]
22. Park, Y.E.; Park, S.J.; Park, Y.; Cheon, J.H.; Kim, T.I.; Kim, W.H. Impact and outcomes of nutritional support team intervention in patients with gastrointestinal disease in the intensive care unit. *Medicine* **2017**, *96*, e8776. [CrossRef]
23. Piquet, M.A.; Bertrand, P.C.; Roulet, M. Role of a nutrition support team in reducing the inappropriate use of parenteral nutrition. *Clin. Nutr.* **2004**, *23*, 437; author reply 8. [CrossRef]
24. Rufenacht, U.; Ruhlin, M.; Wegmann, M.; Imoberdorf, R.; Ballmer, P.E. Nutritional counseling improves quality of life and nutrient intake in hospitalized undernourished patients. *Nutrition* **2010**, *26*, 53–60. [CrossRef]
25. Ryan, J.A., Jr.; Abel, R.M.; Abbott, W.M.; Hopkins, C.C.; Chesney, T.M.; Colley, R.; Phillips, K.; Fischer, J.E. Catheter complications in total parenteral nutrition: A prospective study of 200 consecutive patients. *N. Engl. J. Med.* **1974**, *290*, 757–761. [CrossRef]
26. Sanders, R.A.; Sheldon, G.F. Septic complications of total parenteral nutrition: A five year experience. *Am. J. Surg.* **1976**, *132*, 214–220. [CrossRef]

27. Somanchi, M.; Tao, X.; Mullin, G.E. The facilitated early enteral and dietary management effectiveness trial in hospitalized patients with malnutrition. *JPEN J. Parenter. Enteral. Nutr.* **2011**, *35*, 209–216. [CrossRef]
28. Schuetz, P.; Fehr, R.; Baechli, V.; Geiser, M.; Gomes, F.; Kutz, A.; Tribolet, P.; Bregenzer, T.; Braun, N.; Hoess, C. Individualized nutritional support in medical inpatients at nutritional risk: A randomized clinical trial. *Lancet* **2019**, *393*, 2312–2321. [CrossRef]
29. Sriram, K.; Cyriac, T.; Fogg, L.F. Effect of nutritional support team restructuring on the use of parenteral nutrition. *Nutrition* **2010**, *26*, 735–739. [CrossRef]
30. Starke, J.; Schneider, H.; Alteheld, B.; Stehle, P.; Meier, R. Short-term individual nutritional care as part of routine clinical setting improves outcome and quality of life in malnourished medical patients. *Clin. Nutr.* **2011**, *30*, 194–201. [CrossRef]
31. Stratton, R.J.; Green, C.J.; Elia, M. *Disease-Related Malnutrition: An Evidence-Based Approach to Treatment*; CABI Publishing: Wallingford, UK, 2003.
32. Trujillo, E.B.; Young, L.S.; Chertow, G.M.; Randall, S.; Clemons, T.; Jacobs, D.O.; Robinson, M.K. Metabolic and monetary costs of avoidable parenteral nutrition use. *JPEN J. Parenter. Enteral. Nutr.* **1999**, *23*, 109–113. [CrossRef]
33. Casaer, M.P.; Hermans, G.; Wilmer, A.; Van den Berghe, G. Impact of early parenteral nutrition completing enteral nutrition in adult critically ill patients (EPaNIC trial): A study protocol and statistical analysis plan for a randomized controlled trial. *Trials* **2011**, *12*, 21. [CrossRef]
34. Kubrak, C.; Jensen, L. Malnutrition in acute care patients: A narrative review. *Int. J. Nurs. Stud.* **2007**, *44*, 1036–1054. [CrossRef]
35. Villet, S.; Chiolero, R.L.; Bollmann, M.D.; Revelly, J.P.; Cayeux, R.N.M.; Delarue, J.; Berger, M.M. Negative impact of hypocaloric feeding and energy balance on clinical outcome in ICU patients. *Clin. Nutr.* **2005**, *24*, 502–509. [CrossRef]
36. Iff, S.; Leuenberger, M.; Rosch, S.; Knecht, G.; Tanner, B.; Stanga, Z. Meeting the nutritional requirements of hospitalized patients: An interdisciplinary approach to hospital catering. *Clin. Nutr.* **2008**, *27*, 800–805. [CrossRef]
37. Allison, S.; Stanga, Z.G.; Odlund Olin, A. Organization of nutritional care. In *Basics in Clinical Nutrition*, 3rd ed.; Sobotka, L., Ed.; Galen: Prague, Czechia, 2011; pp. 135–139.
38. Barton, A.D.; Beigg, C.L.; Macdonald, I.A.; Allison, S.P. High food wastage and low nutritional intakes in hospital patients. *Clin. Nutr.* **2000**, *19*, 445–449. [CrossRef]
39. Dias-Ferreira, C.; Santos, T.; Oliveira, V. Hospital food waste and environmental and economic indicators—A Portuguese case study. *Waste Manag.* **2015**, *46*, 146–154. [CrossRef]
40. Elia, M.; Parsons, E.L.; Cawood, A.L.; Smith, T.R.; Stratton, R.J. Cost-effectiveness of oral nutritional supplements in older malnourished care home residents. *Clin. Nutr.* **2018**, *37*, 651–658. [CrossRef]
41. Norman, K.; Pirlich, M.; Smoliner, C.; Kilbert, A.; Schulzke, J.D.; Ockenga, J.; Lochs, H.; Reinhold, T. Cost-effectiveness of a 3-month intervention with oral nutritional supplements in disease-related malnutrition: A randomised controlled pilot study. *Eur. J. Clin. Nutr.* **2011**, *65*, 735–742. [CrossRef]
42. Zhong, Y.; Cohen, J.T.; Goates, S.; Luo, M.; Nelson, J.; Neumann, P.J. The Cost-Effectiveness of Oral Nutrition Supplementation for Malnourished Older Hospital Patients. *Appl. Health Econ. Health Policy* **2017**, *15*, 75–83. [CrossRef]
43. ten Dam, S.; Droop, A.; Arjaans, W.; de Groot, S.; van Bokhorst-de van der Schueren, M. Organisation of Nutritional Care Ethical and Legal Aspects. Module 11.1 Organisation of a nutritional support team, 2012. Available online: https://lllnutrition.com/mod/page/view.php?id=3422 (accessed on 20 August 2019).
44. Ockenga, J.; Valentini, L. Organisationsstruktur der ernährungsmedizinischen Kompetenz, Ernährungsteams und Ernährungskommissionen. In *Ernährungsmedizin*, 5th ed.; Biesalski, H.K., Bischoff, S.C., Pirlich, M., Weimann, A., Eds.; Georg Thieme Verlag KG: Stuttgart, Germany, 2017; pp. 469–476.
45. Dudrick, S.J.; Wilmore, D.W.; Vars, H.M.; Rhoads, J.E. Long-term total parenteral nutrition with growth, development, and positive nitrogen balance. *Surgery* **1968**, *64*, 134–142.
46. Fürst, P.; Stehle, P. Künstliche Ernährung–gestern, heute, morgen. *Transfus. Med. Hemother.* **1990**, *17*, 237–244. [CrossRef]
47. Butterworth, C.E. The skeleton in the hospital closet. 1974. *Nutrition* **1994**, *10*, 435–441.

48. Shang, E.; Hasenberg, T.; Schlegel, B.; Sterchi, A.B.; Schindler, K.; Druml, W.; Koletzko, B.; Meier, R. An European survey of structure and organisation of nutrition support teams in Germany, Austria and Switzerland. *Clin. Nutr.* **2005**, *24*, 1005–1013. [CrossRef]
49. Aubry, E.; Mareschal, J.; Gschweitl, M.; Zvingelis, M.; Schuetz, P.; Stanga, Z. Facts zum Management der Klinischen Ernährung—Eine Online-Befragung. *Aktuel. Ernaehrungsmed.* **2018**, *42*, 452–460. [CrossRef]
50. NutritionDay Worldwide 2018. Available online: https://www.nutritionday.org/en/about-nday/national-reports/index.html (accessed on 20 August 2019).
51. Allison, S.P. Nutritional support—Who needs it and who does it? *Clin. Nutr.* **1992**, *11*, 165–166. [CrossRef]
52. Allison, S. Hospital food as treatment. In *A Report by a Working Party of BAPEN*; BAPEN: Maidenhead, UK, 1999.
53. Delegge, M.; Wooley, J.A.; Guenter, P.; Wright, S.; Brill, J.; Andris, D.; Wagner, P.; Filibeck, D. ASPEN Board of Directors. The state of nutrition support teams and update on current models for providing nutrition support therapy to patients. *Nutr. Clin. Pract.* **2010**, *25*, 76–84.
54. Nightingale, J. Nutrition support teams: How they work, are set up and maintained. *Frontline Gastroenterol.* **2010**, *1*, 171–177. [CrossRef]
55. Payne-James, J. Cost-effectiveness of nutrition support teams. Are they necessary? *Nutrition* **1997**, *13*, 928–930. [CrossRef]
56. Suchner, U.; Dormann, A.; Hund-Wissner, E.; Shang, E.; Senkal, M. Anforderungen an Struktur und Funktion eines Ernährungsteams. *Anaesthesist* **2000**, *49*, 675–684. [CrossRef]
57. Council of Europe, Committee of Ministers. Resolution ResAP (2003) on Food and Nutritional Care in Hospitals. 2004. Available online: https://search.coe.int/cm/Pages/result_details.aspx?ObjectID=09000016805de855 (accessed on 20 August 2019).
58. Schneider, P.J. Nutrition support teams: An evidence-based practice. *Nutr. Clin. Pract.* **2006**, *21*, 62–67. [CrossRef]
59. Reber, E.; Gomes, F.; Bally, L.; Schuetz, P.; Stanga, Z. Nutritional Management of Medical Inpatients. *J. Clin. Med.* **2019**, *8*, 1130. [CrossRef]
60. Reber, E.; Gomes, F.; Vasiloglou, M.F.; Schuetz, P.; Stanga, Z. Nutritional Risk Screening and Assessment. *J. Clin. Med.* **2019**, *8*, 1065. [CrossRef]
61. Kondrup, J.; Rasmussen, H.H.; Hamberg, O.; Stanga, Z. Nutritional risk screening (NRS 2002): A new method based on an analysis of controlled clinical trials. *Clin. Nutr.* **2003**, *22*, 321–336. [CrossRef]
62. Soeters, P.B.; Reijven, P.L.; van Bokhorst-de van der Schueren, M.A.; Schols, J.M.; Halfens, R.J.; Meijers, J.M.; van Gemerta, W.G. A rational approach to nutritional assessment. *Clin. Nutr.* **2008**, *27*, 706–716. [CrossRef]
63. Barbosa-Silva, M.C. Subjective and objective nutritional assessment methods: What do they really assess? *Curr. Opin. Clin. Nutr. Metab. Care* **2008**, *11*, 248–254. [CrossRef]
64. Ware, J.E., Jr.; Sherbourne, C.D. The MOS 36-item short-form health survey (SF-36). I. Conceptual framework and item selection. *Med. Care* **1992**, *30*, 473–483. [CrossRef]
65. Keller, U. Nutritional Laboratory Markers in Malnutrition. *J. Clin. Med.* **2019**, *8*, 775. [CrossRef]
66. Leuenberger, M.; Nuoffer, J.-M.; Stanga, Z. Sinnvolle laborchemische Diagnostik in der Mangelernährung. *Pipette* **2007**, *2*, 15–19.
67. Allison, S.P. Malnutrition, disease, and outcome. *Nutrition* **2000**, *16*, 590–593. [CrossRef]
68. Kondrup, J.; Bak, L.; Hansen, B.S.; Ipsen, B.; Ronneby, H. Outcome from nutritional support using hospital food. *Nutrition* **1998**, *14*, 319–321. [CrossRef]
69. Valentini, L.; Jadma, K. Zehn Jahre Ernährungsteam in Österreich: Definitionen, Aufgaben und Perspektiven. *J. Ernährungsmed.* **2004**, *6*, 17–23.
70. Laesser, C.; Cumming, P.; Reber, E.; Stanga, Z.; Muka, T.; Bally, L. Management of Glucose Control in Noncritically Ill, Hospitalized Patients Receiving Parenteral and/or Enteral Nutrition: A Systematic Review. *JCM* **2019**, *8*, 935. [CrossRef]
71. Burch, N.E.; Stewart, J.; Smith, N. Are nutrition support teams useful? Results from the NCEPOD study into parenteral nutrition. *Gut* **2011**, *60* (Suppl. 1), A2. [CrossRef]
72. Rasmussen, N.M.L.; Belqaid, K.; Lugnet, K.; Nielsen, A.L.; Rasmussen, H.H.; Beck, A.M. Effectiveness of multidisciplinary nutritional support in older hospitalised patients: A systematic review and meta-analyses. *Clin. Nutr. ESPEN* **2018**, *27*, 44–52. [CrossRef]

73. Riley, K.; Sulo, S.; Dabbous, F.; Partridge, J.; Kozmic, S.; Landow, W.; VanDerBosch, G.; Falson, M.K.; Sriram, K. Reducing Hospitalizations and Costs: A Home Health Nutrition-Focused Quality Improvement Program. *JPEN J. Parenter. Enteral. Nutr.* **2019**. [CrossRef]
74. Valentini, L.; Volkert, D.; Schütz, T.; Ockenga, J.; Pirlich, M.; Druml, W.; Schindler, K.; Ballmer, P.E.; Bischoff, S.C.; Weimann, A.; et al. Leitlinie der Deutschen Gesellschaft für Ernährungsmedizin (DGEM). *Aktuelle Ernährungsmedizin* **2013**, *38*, 97–111. [CrossRef]
75. Bounoure, L.; Gomes, F.; Stanga, Z.; Keller, U.; Meier, R.; Ballmer, P.; Fehr, R.; Mueller, B.; Genton, L.; Bertrand, P.C.; et al. Detection and treatment of medical inpatients with or at-risk of malnutrition: Suggested procedures based on validated guidelines. *Nutrition* **2016**, *32*, 790–798. [CrossRef]
76. Friedli, N.; Stanga, Z.; Sobotka, L.; Culkin, A.; Kondrup, J.; Laviano, A.; Mueller, B.; Schuetz, P. Revisiting the refeeding syndrome: Results of a systematic review. *Nutrition* **2017**, *35*, 151–160. [CrossRef]
77. Friedli, N.; Stanga, Z.; Culkin, A.; Crook, M.; Laviano, A.; Sobotka, L.; Kressig, R.W.; Kondrup, J.; Mueller, B.; Schuetz, P. Management and prevention of refeeding syndrome in medical inpatients: An evidence-based and consensus-supported algorithm. *Nutrition* **2018**, *47*, 13–20. [CrossRef]
78. Arends, J.; Baracos, V.; Bertz, H.; Bozzetti, F.; Calder, P.C.; Deutz, N.E.P.; Erickson, N.; Laviano, A.; Lisanti, M.P.; Lobo, D.N.; et al. ESPEN expert group recommendations for action against cancer-related malnutrition. *Clin. Nutr.* **2017**, *36*, 1187–1196. [CrossRef]
79. Fearon, K.; Strasser, F.; Anker, S.D.; Bosaeus, I.; Bruera, E.; Fainsinger, R.L.; Jatoi, A.; Loprinzi, C.; MacDonald, N.; Mantovani, G.; et al. Definition and classification of cancer cachexia: An international consensus. *Lancet Oncol.* **2011**, *12*, 489–495. [CrossRef]

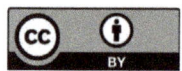

© 2019 by the authors. Licensee MDPI, Basel, Switzerland. This article is an open access article distributed under the terms and conditions of the Creative Commons Attribution (CC BY) license (http://creativecommons.org/licenses/by/4.0/).

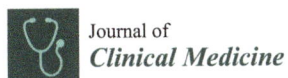

Review

Nutrition in Cancer Patients

Paula Ravasco [1,2,3]

1. University Hospital of Santa Maria, 1649-035 Lisbon, Portugal; p.ravasco@medicina.ulisboa.pt
2. University of Lisbon, 1649-028 Lisbon, Portugal
3. Centre for Interdisciplinary Research in Health (CIIS) of the Portuguese Catholic University, 1649-023 Lisbon, Portugal

Received: 3 July 2019; Accepted: 4 August 2019; Published: 14 August 2019

Abstract: Background: Despite being recognised that nutritional intervention is essential, nutritional support is not widely accessible to all patients. Given the incidence of nutritional risk and nutrition wasting, and because cachexia management remains a challenge in clinical practice, a multidisciplinary approach with targeted nutrition is vital to improve the quality of care in oncology. **Methods:** A literature search in PubMed and Cochrane Library was performed from inception until 26 March. The search consisted of terms on: cancer, nutrition, nutritional therapy, malnutrition, cachexia, sarcopenia, survival, nutrients and guidelines. Key words were linked using "OR" as a Boolean function and the results of the four components were combined by utilizing the "AND" Boolean function. Guidelines, clinical trials and observational studies written in English, were selected. Seminal papers were referenced in this article as appropriate. Relevant articles are discussed in this article. **Results:** Recent literature supports integration of nutrition screening/assessment in cancer care. Body composition assessment is suggested to be determinant for interventions, treatments and outcomes. Nutritional intervention is mandatory as adjuvant to any treatment, as it improves nutrition parameters, body composition, symptoms, quality of life and ultimately survival. Nutrition counselling is the first choice, with/without oral nutritional supplements (ONS). Criteria for escalating nutrition measures include: (1) 50% of intake vs. requirements for more than 1–2 weeks; (2) if it is anticipated that undernourished patients will not eat and/or absorb nutrients for a long period; (3) if the tumour itself impairs oral intake. N-3 fatty acids are promising nutrients, yet clinically they lack trials with homogeneous populations to clarify the identified clinical benefits. Insufficient protein intake is a key feature in cancer; recent guidelines suggest a higher range of protein because of the likely beneficial effects for treatment tolerance and efficacy. Amino acids for counteracting muscle wasting need further research. Vitamins/minerals are recommended in doses close to the recommended dietary allowances and avoid higher doses. Vitamin D deficiency might be relevant in cancer and has been suggested to be needed to optimise protein supplements effectiveness. **Conclusions:** A proactive assessment of the clinical alterations that occur in cancer is essential for selecting the adequate nutritional intervention with the best possible impact on nutritional status, body composition, treatment efficacy and ultimately reducing complications and improving survival and quality of life.

Keywords: cancer; nutrition; nutritional therapy; nutritional support; malnutrition; cachexia; sarcopenia; survival

---

1. Introduction

Cancer is a complex disease that results from multiple interactions between genes and the environment, and is regarded as one of the current leading causes of mortality worldwide [1,2]. Metabolic and nutritional alterations can influence survival and recovery of cancer patients: malnutrition, sarcopenia and cachexia [3,4]. Malnutrition ensues from an inflammatory state that promotes anorexia and consequently, weight loss. It is highly prevalent in cancer patients [5] as 15 to 40% of patients report weight loss at diagnosis [6]. It is estimated that 40 to 80% of all cancer patients will be malnourished during the course of the disease. Furthermore, malnutrition can influence treatment outcomes, delay wound healing, worsen muscle function and increase the risk of post-operative complications. It can also impair tolerance and response to antineoplastic treatments, which can in turn lead to extended hospital stay, increase the risk for treatment interruptions, and possible reduced survival [7,8]. Sarcopenia is characterised by a decrease in lean body mass with an impact both on strength and physical function that may decrease the quality of life [9]. As cancer-related weight loss in obese patients cannot be identified by a low body mass index (BMI), sarcopenic obesity, defined as low lean body mass in obese patients, is frequently overlooked [10]. In these patients, changes in body composition result in an increased metabolic risk, and it seems to be a significant predictor of treatment related adverse events [11,12]. Cancer cachexia is a complex multifactorial syndrome that results from a combination of metabolic alterations, systemic inflammation and decreased appetite. It is characterised by an involuntary sustained weight loss and loss of skeletal muscle mass, with or without loss of fat mass that are irreversible by conventional nutritional support [13].

In addition to the disease, antineoplastic treatments and/or surgery have a significant impact on patients' nutritional status [14–16]. During chemotherapy (CT), more than 50% of patients experience dysgeusia, nausea, vomiting and mucositis, and radiotherapy (RT) related complications are also common. It is also established that poor nutritional status increases surgical morbidity and post-surgical complications [17]. Nutritional intervention in cancer patients aim to identify, prevent and treat malnutrition through nutritional counselling with or without oral nutritional supplements (ONS) or via artificial nutrition, i.e., enteral or parenteral nutrition [18–20], as well as to address metabolic and nutritional alterations that influence patients' recovery and survival [19,20]. Despite the fact that nutritional intervention is a key component, nutritional support is not widely accessible to all patients at nutritional risk [21–23]. Additionally, given the incidence of nutritional risk in cancer and the fact that the management of cachexia remains a challenge in clinical practice [24], a multidisciplinary approach is vital to define efficient strategies that can improve quality of care in cancer patients. According to the reviewed data and guidelines, nutritional intervention should be central and adjuvant to any treatment and should be included in the multidisciplinary approach mandatory in oncology. This will allow for more adequate and efficient results in these patients. Multidisciplinary follow-up, with early and regular nutritional intervention, is of major importance in oncology, thus being a key factor for successful treatment and recovery. The present article aims to provide insights and an overview of the most recent literature regarding key nutritional aspects in cancer patients.

Based on this framework, a literature search in PubMed and Cochrane Library was performed from inception until 26 March. The search consisted of terms: cancer, nutrition, nutritional therapy, malnutrition, cachexia, sarcopenia, survival, nutrients, guidelines. Key words were linked using "OR" as a Boolean function and the results of the four components were combined by utilizing the "AND" Boolean function. Guidelines, clinical trials and observational studies written in English, were selected. Seminal papers in the area, even if dated outside the search timeline, were referenced in this article as appropriate.

2. Results

2.1. Nutritional Screening and Assessment

Screening for nutritional risk as early as possible allows for the identification of patients at risk of becoming malnourished [25]. Screening should be done as early as possible, and recent literature suggests that it should be done at diagnosis or at hospital admission; screening should be repeated in the course of treatment for referral for evaluation if needed [19,21,23,25–27]. Evidence supports the integration of malnutrition screening in cancer patients care. The adequate tool for screening undernutrition should be brief and easy to fill, inexpensive, highly sensitive and have good specificity [25]. MUST (Malnutrition Universal Screening Tool) and NRS-2002 (Nutritional Risk Screening-2002) are considered suitable [28–30]; the MNA (Mini Nutritional Assessment) is a suitable tool for nutritional assessment in the senior population [19,23].

When nutritional risk is present, screening should be followed by comprehensive nutritional assessment to better determine the course of nutritional intervention. It seems there is no consensus on the best method to perform this assessment, but SGA (Subjective Global Assessment) and PG-SGA (Patient Generated-Subjective Global Assessment) have been validated for nutritional assessment of adult oncology patients [25,26,31].

When used isolated, weight loss is ineffective to detect malnutrition, as it has low sensitivity for metabolic changes that occur in cancer patients. Yet, its early and regular assessment, combined with the evaluation of nutritional intake, BMI and inflammatory status is a standard clinical recommendation [19,26]. As for BMI, it has low sensitivity to detect changes in the nutritional status, especially in obese patients, thus it should only be used combined with other assessment tools [26,32].

Body composition provides valuable information in the management of cancer patients, as imaging methods detect loss of muscle mass as well as fatty muscle infiltration [2]. In cancer patients at risk for malnutrition, sarcopenia and cachexia, muscle mass should be assessed [19,21]. Methods available are dual X-ray absorptiometry (DEXA), computed tomography scans at the level of the 3rd vertebra or bioimpedance analysis (BIA). Additionally, it has been recommended that nutritional assessment should be performed for the stages of cancer cachexia, as nutritional intervention is most effective in the stages of precachexia and cachexia [13].

2.2. Nutritional Intervention

In order to tackle nutritional deterioration, gathering objective data on nutritional status and its evolution throughout the disease course is of prime concern. Different cancer types or locations display different nutritional patterns that require tailored nutritional therapy. Nutritional deterioration is a multifactorial end-result determined by cancer-related and nutrition- and/or metabolic-related factors. Proper nutrition can alleviate symptom burden, improve health across the cancer continuum, support cancer survivorship [33–36] and is a hallmark of successful cancer treatment.

Nutritional interventions will vary according to patients' medical history, type and stage of cancer, as well as to the response to treatment. If the patient can eat and has a functional gastrointestinal tract, nutritional counselling, with or without ONS should be the elected intervention to address altered nutritional demands due to treatment or disease [19,21,26]. ONS may be necessary, as a means to compensate for lower food intake and to try to prevent nutritional deterioration during the course of treatments. Monitoring compliance with the selected nutritional intervention is essential.

2.2.1. Individualised Nutritional Counselling

In clinical practice, oral nutrition is always the priority. Oral nutrition is the preferred route of feeding as it is a significant part of the patient's daily routine and does contribute substantially to the patients' autonomy [19]. It represents a privileged time to spend with family and friends, avoiding the tendency for isolation. The acknowledgement that the prescribed diet is individualized, adapted and adequate to individual needs, empowers the patient with a feeling of control, thus it is also a highly effective approach for psychological modulation. All these factors may potentially contribute to improve the patients' quality of life, and may modulate acute and late treatment morbidity. The referral for a nutrition professional responsible for the individualised dietary counselling should always be based on decision-making plans (Figure 1).

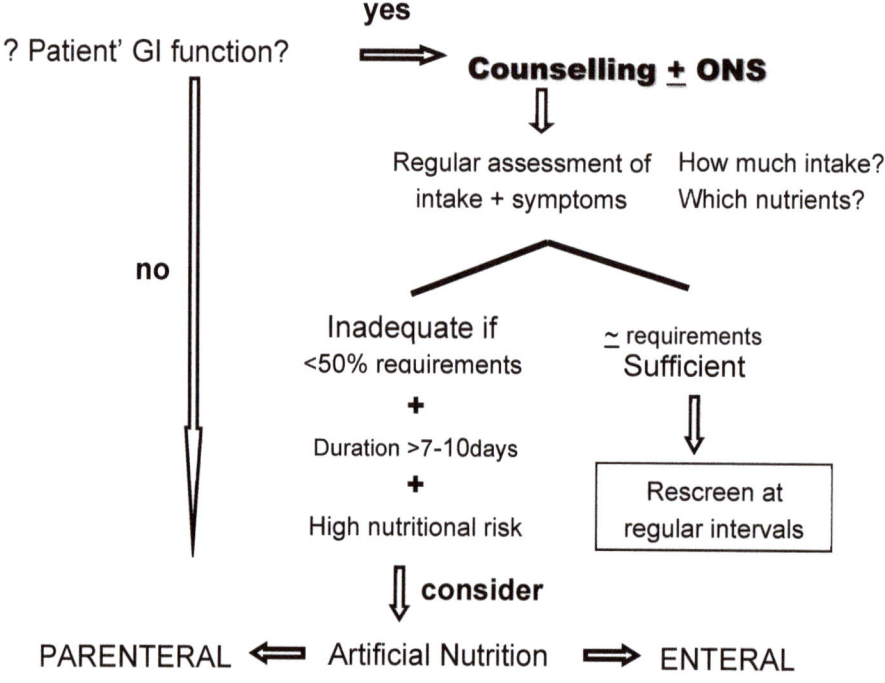

Figure 1. Evidence based decision making plan.

As clinicians we have to recognise the dimensions that are determinant for the patients. Indeed, the diet is the only factor that the patient feels he/she can control during the whole course of treatments and interventions. Also, an adequate food intake is recognised by the patient as well as by the family and caregivers, as essential to maintain the daily activity, energy, functional capacity and to overcome treatments more successfully. Notably, nutritional wasting is common regardless of the cancer stage (curative, adjuvant, to palliative) and is an independent predictor of poor physical function, lower quality of life, surgical complications, and reduced survival [3,10,13,37]. Cancer wasting is characterised by muscle mass deterioration that occurs in more than 50% of newly diagnosed cancer patients, in comparison with 15% prevalence in healthy individuals of similar age [38]. Since both muscle mass and adipose tissue play a role in oncological outcomes, strategies to optimize body composition are an important part of successful cancer therapy. Hence, a major goal of nutrition intervention is to favourably influence body composition, with the potential to improve cancer therapy outcomes, morbidities and ultimately, prognosis.

To be effective, individualised counselling has to be based on a thorough assessment of various nutritional and clinical parameters: nutritional status and dietary intake, usual dietary pattern, intolerances or food aversions, patients' psychological status, autonomy, cooperation, need for help or support of others in the act of eating. A thorough symptom assessment is also mandatory (Table 1).

Table 1. Common causes for a poor nutrient intake in cancer patients.

- Deterioration in taste, smell and appetite, as a consequence of the tumour and/or therapy
- Altered food preferences/food avoidance/food aversion
- Eating problems (teeth, chewing)
- Dysphagia, odynophagia or partial/total gastrointestinal obstruction
- Early satiety, nausea and vomiting
- Soreness, xerostomia, sticky saliva, painful throat, trismus
- Oral lesions and oesophagitis
- Radiotherapy/chemotherapy induced mucositis
- Acute or chronic radiation enteritis during and after radiotherapy
- Depression, anxiety
- Pain

Individualised nutritional counselling taking into consideration patients' clinical condition and symptoms, was the most effective nutrition intervention, assuring a sustained and adequate diet, which was able to overcome the predictable deterioration subsequent to RT [35,36,39–42]. Positive effects were experienced in the long term with a possible impact of patients' prognosis [43] as recently showed in a randomized trial, the preliminary results of which were presented in the ESPEN Congress in 2018. Another randomised trial of nutritional therapy showed that intervention had an impact in maintaining patients' nutritional status and function [39]. In this study, individualised intensive nutrition counselling was compared with individualised on-demand nutrition counselling by a dietician prior to and during oncologic treatment. On-demand nutrition counselling requested by physician/nurse referral, seemed not inferior to intensive counselling; thus, these results do emphasise the importance of establishing multimodal nutrition teams to effectively and timely screen and orient patients for adequate nutrition [39]. Several guidelines to date do include nutritional counselling as their standard of care for malnourished patients or at risk of malnutrition [19–21,23,26,27] or during anti-neoplastic treatments in head-neck (HNC), oesophageal and colorectal cancers as these patients are in particular risk of malnutrition due to tumour location and irradiated area [14].

If/when oral nutrition is inadequate/insufficient, artificial nutrition should be considered [19–21,23,26,27]. Criteria for the escalation in nutritional measures are: (1) inadequate food intake (<50% of requirements) is anticipated for more than 10 days due to surgery or chemotherapy (CT)/radiotherapy (RT); (2) if food intake is less than 50% of the requirements for more than one to two weeks; (3) if it is anticipated that undernourished patients will not be able to eat and/or absorb the adequate amount of nutrients for a long period time, due to antineoplastic treatments; (4) if the tumour mass itself impairs oral intake and food progression through the upper GI tract. The decision between enteral nutrition (EN) and parenteral nutrition (PN) must take into account the site of the tumour, its extent, complications, treatment plan and intent, prognosis, patients' overall physical status and the duration of the nutritional support [19–21,23,26,27,44].

2.2.2. Artificial Nutrition

If the intestinal functions are preserved, EN should be preferred in order to maintain gut integrity and reduce bacterial translocation [45], as well as to reduce infectious complications [19–21,23,26]. A standard polymeric feeding formula should be preferred. EN is recommended in undernourished or at-risk patients during CT if undernutrition is present or if inadequate food intake is present or anticipated [19,22,23,27,46]. Systematic artificial nutrition during CT treatment is not recommended [19–21,23,26]. In radiation-induced severe mucositis or in obstructive tumours of the head-neck or thorax, either PEG or nasogastric tube are recommended [19,20]. EN is contraindicated in: intestinal obstruction or ileus, severe shock, intestinal ischaemia, high output fistula, severe intestinal haemorrhage, intestinal insufficiency due to radiation enteritis, short bowel syndrome, peritoneal carcinomatosis chylothorax [19,21,23,26]. In these situations, or whenever EN is insufficient, a combination of EN and PN or PN alone should be considered [19,21,23,26].

As for PN, it should be initiated early [19,21,23,26] whenever indicated. PN is the first option of nutritional support in cases of intestinal failure; whenever macro and micronutrient' requirements can only be fulfilled via the parenteral route, long term artificial nutrition as home parenteral nutrition (HPN) is standard recommendation [19,44,47,48].

As for the macronutrients in PN, amino acids (AA) requirement of cancer patients relies on: negative balance between whole body protein synthesis and breakdown, doses of AA closer to 2 g/kg/day may be required to control catabolism and stimulate synthesis vs. 0.8 g/kg/day as recommended for healthy subjects [49], and for older subjects and chronic disease, most recent clinical guidelines recommend >1.0 g/kg/day of protein. Hence, to support protein balance, up to 1.5 g/kg/day or more of protein is the consensual recommendation. In the nutritive PN admixtures, essential AA should be present in approximately 50% of AA and branched chain AA should account for the remainder 50% of total AA [50]. In what concerns fat as an energy substrate, the most consensual regimens have fat accounting for $\approx$50% of non-protein calories [51,52].

Recently, PN as a supplemental route of nutrient administration (SHPN) emerged as a possible resource to optimise nutrient delivery. Prospective studies [53–57] on SHPN suggest a possible benefit in energy balance, increased body fat, greater maximum exercise capacity and QoL. A recent randomised trial showed that SHPN may prevent loss of MM in patients with incurable gastrointestinal cancer [57]. Hence, there is yet insufficient evidence to recommend SHPN in cancer patients to improve QoL and nutrition parameters. Additionally, practice of HPN differs between countries; most do not consider the use of PN if there is a functional gastrointestinal tract, while others may consider its use if it is according to the will of the patient [58–60].

Refeeding syndrome can occur when severe shifts in fluids and electrolytes happen in severely malnourished patients receiving EN or PN, and it may cause hypophosphatemia, hypokalaemia, hypomagnesaemia, thiamine deficiency, changes in sodium, glucose and fluid balance and also in protein and lipid metabolism [19,21]. Its prevention is recommended when BMI < 16 kg/m^2 or in the presence of unintentional weight loss >15% within the last three to six months or whenever there is little or no nutritional intake for more than 10 days or if there are decreased levels of potassium, phosphate or magnesium prior to feeding. If a severe decrease in food intake occurs for at least five days, it is recommended a gradual increase in nutrition over several days, and no more than 50% of the calculated energy requirements should be supplied during the first two days of feeding [19,25]. The identified fluid and electrolytes imbalances should be corrected, and the circulatory volume, fluid balance, heart rate and rhythm, as well as clinical status, should be monitored closely. Attention to the refeeding syndrome risk is currently contemplated in guidelines for cancer management [19–23,26,27].

2.2.3. Surgery

In order to minimise the metabolic stress response and catabolism associated with surgery in undernourished patients, the enhanced recovery after surgery program (ERAS) is recommended for all cancer patients undergoing curative or palliative surgery [18,22,61]. Within ERAS protocol the following principles should be followed: Screening for malnutrition and give additional nutritional support if necessary [18,22]; avoid preoperative fasting; preoperative carbohydrate treatment should be considered as well as the reestablishment of oral feeding on the first postoperative day; and early mobilisation [18,22]. To avoid preoperative fasting, patients with no risk of aspiration, are allowed to eat solid food until six hours and drink clear fluids until two hours before anaesthesia [18].

In oncologic surgical patients, with moderate to severe nutritional risk, nutritional support is recommended before and after surgery [18,25]. If severe malnutrition is present, delaying surgery may be necessary [18,25]. When submitted to major surgery, nutritional support should be provided routinely, with particular attention to elderly sarcopenic patients.

Besides the ERAS protocol, an early start of nutritional supplementation can significantly diminish the degree of weight loss and incidence of complications [22,25]. If it is anticipated that after surgery, the patient will be unable to eat for more than seven days, it is advised to start nutrition therapy even in well-nourished patients [18,22,25]. After surgery, oral nutrition should also be preferred to EN and the latter should be preferred to PN. If oral intake is possible, it should start after surgery without interruption, after assessing individual tolerance. If oral nutrition is not possible, EN should be initiated within 24 h, preferring standard polymeric enteral formulae if adequate [25].

2.2.4. Radiotherapy and Chemotherapy

Oral mucositis, dysphagia and diarrhoea are common complications of RT and/or CT treatments [12–22]. During RT, nutritional counselling is also recommended, especially in HNC, thorax and gastrointestinal (GI) tract cancers [12–23]. When deemed necessary, ONS should be provided [62], and when severe mucositis is present, artificial nutrition should be considered [23]. When dietary counselling and ONS are insufficient to reduce weight loss or if in the presence of severe mucositis or obstructive tumours of the head or neck or thorax, artificial nutrition should be considered [19,20,23]. In patients treated with RT or chemoradiotherapy, PN is not recommended [19], and it should only be considered when adequate nutrition cannot be assured with oral or EN [19].

2.3. Specific Nutrients

Nutritional strategies that potentially allow better management of cancer have been widely investigated, but few have reached conclusive results.

2.3.1. Protein

Many patients with cancer do not meet the recommended intake (1.2–1.5 g/kg/day), and not even the one for healthy individuals (0.8 g/kg/day) [63]. Limited protein intake ensues mainly from nutrition impact symptoms that affect dietary intake [64]. Recent guidelines do suggest a higher range of protein intake (1.2–1.5 g/kg/day), because of the positive results of higher protein intake in protein balancing and in maintaining muscle mass. Of additional interest is a recent study showing an inverse association between red meat consumption and seven-year mortality among 992 individuals with stage III colon cancer [65], suggesting that higher protein intake may actually be beneficial in cancer.

Interventions with amino acids have been tested in cancer, aiming to optimise nutritional status and counteract muscle mass wasting. They include supplementation with branched chain amino acids (leucine, isoleucine and valine) [63], β-hydroxy β-methyl butyrate, carnitine and creatine. Yet further research is needed to clarify potential benefits.

As for glutamine, its supplementation in cases of oral mucositis or to prevent/treat diarrhoea during pelvic RT, is not recommended [19,22,26]. As for its use when PN is required for patients undergoing haematopoietic stem cell transplant, guidelines are not identical: there is a fair graded recommendation for eventual use of 0.2–0.5 g/kg/day [26], and the indication that there is not enough evidence to recommend for or against glutamine to reduce anticancer therapy side effects, especially in high dose protocols [19]. In what concerns its potential to improve muscle mass, there is not enough data to support it.

2.3.2. Eicosapentaenoic Acid and Fish Oil

Eicosapentaenoic acid (EPA) has been identified as a promising nutrient with appointed clinical benefits. Several mechanisms have been proposed to explain the potential benefits of EPA on the body composition: inhibition of catabolic stimuli by modulating the production of pro-inflammatory cytokines and enhancing insulin sensitivity that induces protein synthesis. Intervention studies showed that EPA may attenuate deterioration of nutritional status and may aid in improving calorie and protein intake. Recent systematic reviews found that EPA can reduce inflammation and has a potential to modulate the nutritional status/body composition [66,67]. Furthermore, some studies suggest that n−3 fatty acids inhibit proliferation of cancer cells [68] and might decrease CT toxicity [69]. Given the large number of studies reporting a positive impact of n−3 fatty acids on the muscle mass, it is likely that this would be a practical and effective intervention for preventing loss of muscle without significant side effects [19]. It is noteworthy that the strength of recommendation somewhat differs for the use of n−3 fatty acids supplementation in weight losing cancer patients not responding to standard nutritional therapy. This recommendation has been rated as strong [26] and weak [19]. Nevertheless, both guidelines are inclined to consider supplementation with long chain fatty acids and fish oil to decrease systemic inflammation and improve appetite, food intake and body weight.

Trials with homogeneous patient populations regarding cancer type, stage, anti-neoplastic regimens, supplement dosage and modality of administration are needed to clarify clinical benefits. Indeed, it is noteworthy that in view of the modest survival benefits of CT/RT in some cancers, important issues for physicians are to optimize well-being, quality of life via nutritional status and adequate body composition [70].

2.3.3. Micronutrients

Because of the adverse effects of therapy and restricted diet of many patients, the American Institute for Cancer Research [71], American Cancer Society [72] and the European Society for Clinical Nutrition and Metabolism—ESPEN [19] support the use of a multivitamin-multimineral supplement in doses close to the recommended dietary allowance. High doses of vitamins and minerals are discouraged in the absence of specific deficiencies [19,20]. Vitamin D deficiency might be relevant in cancer [19]; also, an association has been reported between low vitamin D and muscle wasting. As a consequence, vitamin D may be needed to optimise protein supplements effectiveness. In light of the recent literature, vitamin D supplementation with 600–800 international units (RDA) in cancer patients can be beneficial in the context of preventing muscle wasting, but further research is needed.

3. Discussion

In cancer, deterioration and muscle wasting result from the combination of reduced nutrient absorption, alterations in appetite, taste and/or dietary intake, hormone-induced metabolic changes and cancer-related immune activation with cytokine release. Regardless of the underlying mechanisms, cancer-related weight loss is a multidimensional manifestation that worsens patients' well-being, tolerance to antineoplastic therapies and prognosis. Clinically speaking, weight loss is frequent in cancer patients, and depending on the location of the tumour, it is present in 15 to 40% of cancer patients at diagnosis. Weight loss is frequently the first sign of the nutritional alterations that occur in the course of the disease and is associated with poor prognosis, reduced quality of life and morbidity [62]. Cancer cachexia can be defined as *'a multi-factorial syndrome defined by an ongoing loss of skeletal muscle mass (with or without loss of fat mass) that cannot be fully reversed by conventional nutritional support. It leads to progressive functional impairment. Its pathophysiology is characterized by a negative protein and energy balance driven by a variable combination of reduced food intake and abnormal metabolism'*. The agreed diagnostic criterion for cachexia was weight loss >5%, or weight loss >2% in individuals already showing depletion of body weight (BMI < 20 kg/m^2) or of skeletal muscle (sarcopenia). Assessment for classification and clinical management should also include the following domains: 'anorexia/reduced food intake, catabolic drive, muscle mass and strength, functional and psychosocial impairment' [13].

The main nutritional problem in cancer is wasting of muscle mass, acknowledged to be a predictor of lower quality of life, impaired functionality, surgical complications and shortened survival [10,63,73,74]. Of note that sarcopenia occurs independently of loss of weight or of fat mass. Thus, a clinically relevant phenotype that also emerged in cancer is characterised by sarcopenia with excessive fat mass. Additionally, to the previous studies demonstrating the major impact of muscle mass depletion on survival and treatment toxicity [73,74], a recent study in a cohort of head-neck cancer patients, showed that patients with cachexia had a worse disease-free survival compared with non-cachectic patients [12,39].

Bearing this in mind, the clinical efforts and priority given to improve treatment outcomes, will logically have to include nutritional intervention and adequacy of body composition. The search for an effective nutritional intervention that improves body composition (preservation of muscle mass and muscle quality) is of utmost importance for clinicians and patients, given the implications for prognosis. Early detection of malnutrition and cachexia should be part of a multimodal approach to improve both patient-centred and oncology outcomes [47].

4. Conclusions

In the present article, the most recent guidelines for the management of cancer patients, as well as original studies in nutrition and cancer, were included. Nutrition is a central factor in oncology, influencing the development of the disease, tumour inherent symptoms, response to, and recovery after anti-neoplastic treatment(s), thus having a strong impact on the quality of life and prognosis of the disease. A main nutritional feature is wasting of muscle mass, strongly associated with decreased functional capacity, higher incidence of chemotherapy toxicity, increased hospitalization and complication rate, as well as mortality. Nutritional risk screening and assessment in cancer patients allows for the early detection of malnourished patients and also for a prompt nutritional intervention aiming to prevent nutritional deterioration and muscle wasting. A proactive assessment of the clinical alterations that occur during treatments and during the disease course, is essential for selecting the adequate nutritional intervention, aiming for the best impact on patients' outcomes. Early tailored intervention has the potential to improve body composition and treatment' efficacy, and as evidence stands, it is an obligatory adjuvant intervention, with the likelihood of improving prognosis of the disease itself.

Conflicts of Interest: The authors declare no conflict of interest.

References

1. Fearon, K.; Barber, M. Moses A: The cancer cachexia syndrome. *Surg. Oncol. Clin. N. Am.* **2001**, *10*, 109–126. [CrossRef]
2. Mattox, T.W. Cancer Cachexia: Cause, Diagnosis, and Treatment. *Nutr. Clin. Pract.* **2017**, *32*, 599–606. [CrossRef] [PubMed]
3. Brown, J.C.; Caan, B.J.; Meyerhardt, J.A.; Weltzien, E.; Xiao, J.; Feliciano, E.M.C.; Kroenke, C.H.; Castillo, A.; Kwan, M.L.; Prado, C.M. The deterioration of muscle mass and radiodensity is prognostic of poor survival in stage I–III colorectal cancer: A population-based cohort study (C-SCANS). *J. Cachex Sarcopenia Muscle* **2018**, *9*, 664–672. [CrossRef] [PubMed]
4. Demark-Wahnefried, W.; Peterson, B.L.; Winer, E.P.; Marks, L.; Aziz, N.; Marcom, P.K.; Blackwell, K.; Rimer, B.K. Changes in Weight, Body Composition, and Factors Influencing Energy Balance Among Premenopausal Breast Cancer Patients Receiving Adjuvant Chemotherapy. *J. Clin. Oncol.* **2001**, *19*, 2381–2389. [CrossRef] [PubMed]
5. De Wys, W.D.; Begg, C.; Lavin, P.T.; Band, P.R.; Bennett, J.M.; Bertino, J.R.; Cohen, M.H.; Douglass, H.O., Jr.; Engstrom, P.F.; Ezdinli, E.Z.; et al. Prognostic effect of weight loss prior to chemotherapy in cancer patients. *Am. J. Med.* **1980**, *69*, 491–497. [CrossRef]
6. Wigmore, S.J.; Plester, C.E.; Ross, J.A.; Fearon, K.C.H.; Wigmore, S. Contribution of anorexia and hypermetabolism to weight loss in anicteric patients with pancreatic cancer. *BJS* **1997**, *84*, 196–197. [CrossRef]
7. Belghiti, J.; Langonnet, F.; Bourstyn, E.; Fekete, F. Surgical implications of malnutrition and immunodeficiency in patients with carcinoma of the esophagus. *Br. J. Surg.* **1983**, *70*, 339–341. [CrossRef]
8. Mantzorou, M.; Koutelidakis, A.; Theocharis, S.; Giaginis, C. Clinical Value of Nutritional Status in Cancer: What is its Impact and how it Affects Disease Progression and Prognosis? *Nutr. Cancer* **2017**, *69*, 1–26. [CrossRef]
9. Ravasco, P.; Grillo, I.M.; Vidal, P.; Camilo, M. Nutritional Deterioration in Cancer: The Role of Disease and Diet. *Clin. Oncol.* **2003**, *15*, 443–450. [CrossRef]
10. Prado, C.M.; Cushen, S.J.; Orsso, C.E.; Ryan, A.M. Sarcopenia and cachexia in the era of obesity: Clinical and nutritional impact. *Proc. Nutr. Soc.* **2016**, *75*, 188–198. [CrossRef]
11. Bazzan, A.J.; Newberg, A.B.; Cho, W.C.; Monti, D.A. Diet and nutrition in cancersurvivorship and palliative care. *Evid. Based Complement. Alternat. Med.* **2013**, *2013*, 917647. [CrossRef] [PubMed]

12. Orell-Kotikangas, H.; Österlund, P.; Mäkitie, O.; Saarilahti, K.; Ravasco, P.; Schwab, U.; Mäkitie, A.A. Cachexia at diagnosis is associated with poor survival in head and neck cancer patients. *Acta Oto-Laryngol.* **2017**, *137*, 778–785. [CrossRef] [PubMed]
13. Fearon, K.; Strasser, F.; Anker, S.D.; Bosaeus, I.; Bruera, E.; Fainsinger, R.L.; Jatoi, A.; Loprinzi, C.; MacDonald, N.; Mantovani, G.; et al. Definition and classification of cancer cachexia: An international consensus statement. *Lancet Oncol.* **2011**, *12*, 489–495. [CrossRef]
14. Donaldson, S. Nutritional consequences of radiotherapy. *Cancer Res.* **1997**, *37*, 2407–2413.
15. Chao, K.S.C.; Perez, C.A.; Brady, L.W. (Eds.) Fundamentals of patient management. In *Radiation Oncology: Management Decisions*; Lippincot-Raven: Philadelphia, PA, USA, 2014; pp. 1–13.
16. Blauwhoff-Buskermolen, S.; Versteeg, K.S.; De Van Der Schueren, M.A.; Braver, N.R.D.; Berkhof, J.; Langius, J.A.; Verheul, H.M. Loss of Muscle Mass During Chemotherapy Is Predictive for Poor Survival of Patients with Metastatic Colorectal Cancer. *J. Clin. Oncol.* **2016**, *34*, 1339–1344. [CrossRef]
17. Van der Schueren, M.A.; Van Leeuwen, P.A.; Sauerwein, H.P.; Kuik, D.J.; Snow, G.B.; Quak, J.J. Assessment of malnutrition parameters in head and neck cancer patients and their relation to postoperative complications. *Head Neck* **1997**, *19*, 419–425. [CrossRef]
18. Weimann, A.; Braga, M.; Carli, F.; Higashiguchi, T.; Hübner, M.; Klek, S.; Laviano, A.; Ljungqvist, O.; Lobo, D.N.; Martindale, R.; et al. ESPEN guideline: Clinical nutrition in surgery. *Clin. Nutr.* **2017**, *36*, 623–650. [CrossRef]
19. Arends, J.; Bachmann, P.; Baracos, V.; Barthelemy, N.; Bertz, H.; Bozzetti, F.; Fearon, K.; Hütterer, E.; Isenring, E.; Kaasa, S.; et al. ESPEN guidelines on nutrition in cancer patients. *Clin. Nutr.* **2017**, *36*, 11–48. [CrossRef]
20. Arends, J.; Baracos, V.; Bertz, H.; Bozzetti, F.; Calder, P.; Deutz, N.; Erickson, N.; Laviano, A.; Lisanti, M.; Lobo, D.; et al. ESPEN expert group recommendations for action against cancer-related malnutrition. *Clin. Nutr.* **2017**, *36*, 1187–1196. [CrossRef]
21. De Las Peñas, R.; Majem, M.; Perez-Altozano, J.; Virizuela, J.A.; Cancer, E.; Diz, P.; Donnay, O.; Hurtado, A.; Jimenez-Fonseca, P.; Ocon, M.J. SEOM clinical guidelines on nutrition in cancer patients (2018). *Clin. Transl. Oncol.* **2019**, *21*, 87–93. [CrossRef]
22. Raspé, C.; Flöther, L.; Schneider, R.; Bucher, M.; Piso, P. Best practice for perioperative management of patients with cytoreductive surgery and HIPEC. *Eur. J. Surg. Oncol.* **2017**, *43*, 1013–1027. [CrossRef]
23. French Speaking Society of Clinical Nutrition and Metabolism (SFNEP). Clinical nutrition guidelines of the French Speaking Society of Clinical Nutrition and Metabolism (SFNEP): Summary of recommendations for adults undergoing non-surgical anticancer treatment. *Dig. Liver Dis.* **2014**, *46*, 667–674. [CrossRef]
24. Prado, C.M.; Sawyer, M.B.; Ghosh, S.; Lieffers, J.R.; Esfandiari, N.; Antoun, S.; Baracos, V. Central tenet of cancer cachexia therapy: Do patients with advanced cancer have exploitable anabolic potential? *Am. J. Clin. Nutr.* **2013**, *98*, 1012–1019. [CrossRef]
25. Benoist, S.; Brouquet, A. Nutritional assessment and screening for malnutrition. *J. Visc. Surg.* **2015**, *152* (Suppl. 1), S3–S7. [CrossRef]
26. Thompson, K.L.; Elliott, L.; Fuchs-Tarlovsky, V.; Levin, R.M.; Voss, A.C.; Piemonte, T. Rd Oncology Evidence-Based Nutrition Practice Guideline for Adults. *J. Acad. Nutr. Diet.* **2017**, *117*, 297–310. [CrossRef]
27. Talwar, B.; Donnelly, R.; Skelly, R.; Donaldson, M. Nutritional management in head and neck cancer: United Kingdom National Multidisciplinary Guidelines. *J. Laryngol. Otol.* **2016**, *130*, S32–S40. [CrossRef]
28. Orell-Kotikangas, H.; Österlund, P.; Saarilahti, K.; Ravasco, P.; Schwab, U.; Mäkitie, A.A. NRS-2002 for pre-treatment nutritional risk screening and nutritional status assessment in head and neck cancer patients. *J. Support. Care Cancer* **2015**, *23*, 1495–1502. [CrossRef]
29. Boléo-Tomé, C.; Monteiro Grillo, I.; Camilo, M.E.; Ravasco, P. Validation of the Malnutrition Universal Screening Tool (MUST) in cancer. *Br. J. Nutr.* **2012**, *108*, 343–348. [CrossRef]
30. Boléo-Tomé, C.; Chaves, M.; Monteiro-Grillo, I.; Camilo, M.; Ravasco, P. Teaching Nutrition Integration: MUST Screening in Cancer. *Oncologist* **2011**, *16*, 239–245. [CrossRef]
31. Ottery, F. Definition of standardised nutritional assessment and interventional pathways in oncology. *Nutrition* **1996**, *12*, s15–s19. [CrossRef]
32. Ortiz, C. Analysis of clinical guidelines in oncology. *Nutr. Hosp.* **2016**, *33* (Suppl. 1), 40–49.
33. Ravasco, P.; Monteiro-Grillo, I.; Camilo, M.E. Does nutrition influence quality of life in cancer patients undergoing radiotherapy? *Radiother. Oncol.* **2003**, *67*, 213–220. [CrossRef]

34. Monteiro-Grillo, I.; Vidal, P.M.; Camilo, M.E.; Ravasco, P. Cancer: Disease and nutrition are key determinants of patients' quality of life. *Support. Care Cancer* **2004**, *12*, 246–252. [CrossRef]
35. Ravasco, P.; Monteiro Grillo, I.; Marques Vidal, P.; Camilo, M.E. Dietary conseling improves patient outcomes: A prospective, randomized, controlled trial in colorectal cancer patients undergoing radiotherapy. *J. Clin. Oncol.* **2005**, *23*, 1431–1438. [CrossRef]
36. Ravasco, P.; Vidal, P.M.; Camilo, M.E.; Monteiro-Grillo, I.; Monteiro-Grillo, I. Impact of nutrition on outcome: A prospective randomized controlled trial in patients with head and neck cancer undergoing radiotherapy. *Head Neck* **2005**, *27*, 659–668. [CrossRef]
37. Martin, L.; Senesse, P.; Gioulbasanis, I.; Antoun, S.; Bozzetti, F.; Deans, C.; Strasser, F.; Thoresen, L.; Jagoe, R.T.; Chasen, M.; et al. Diagnostic criteria for the classification of cancer-associated weight loss. *J. Clin. Oncol.* **2015**, *33*, 90–99. [CrossRef]
38. Von Haehling, S.; Morley, J.E.; Anker, S.D. An overview of sarcopenia: Facts and numbers on prevalence and clinical impact. *J. Cachexia Sarcopenia Muscle* **2010**, *1*, 129–133. [CrossRef]
39. Orell-Kotikangas, H.; Österlund, P.; Saarilahti, K.; Ravasco, P.; Schwab, U.; Mäkitie, A.A. Nutritional Counseling for Head and Neck Cancer Patients Undergoing (Chemo) Radiotherapy-A Prospective Randomized Trial. *Front. Nutr.* **2019**, *18*, 22. [CrossRef]
40. Van Bokhorst-de van der Schueren, M.A. Nutritional support strategies for malnourished cancer patients. *Eur. J. Oncol. Nurs.* **2005**, *9* (Suppl. 2), S74–S83. [CrossRef]
41. Bauer, J.; Isenring, E.; Ferguson, M. Dietary counseling: Evidence in chemotherapy patients. *Support. Oncol.* **2008**, *6*, 354–355.
42. Isenring, E.A.; Bauer, J.D.; Capra, S. Nutrition Support Using the American Dietetic Association Medical Nutrition Therapy Protocol for Radiation Oncology Patients Improves Dietary Intake Compared with Standard Practice. *J. Am. Diet. Assoc.* **2007**, *107*, 404–412. [CrossRef]
43. Ravasco, P.; Monteiro Grillo, I.; Camilo, M. Dietary individualized counseling benefits in colorectal cancer: The long term follow-up of a randomized controlled trial of nutritional therapy. *Am. J. Clin. Nutr.* **2012**, *96*, 1346–1353. [CrossRef]
44. Staun, M.; Pironi, L.; Bozzetti, F.; Baxter, J.; Forbes, A.; Joly, F.; Jeppesena, P.; Morenog, J.; Hebuterne, X.; Pertkiewicz, M.; et al. ESPEN Guidelines on Parenteral Nutrition: Home Parenteral Nutrition (HPN) in Adult Patients. Available online: http://espen.info/documents/0909/HomeParenteralNutritioninadults.pdf (accessed on 17 July 2019).
45. Souza, N.C.S.; Simões, B.P.; Júnior, A.A.J.; Chiarello, P.G. Changes in Intestinal Permeability and Nutritional Status after Cytotoxic Therapy in Patients with Cancer. *Nutr. Cancer* **2014**, *66*, 576–582. [CrossRef]
46. O'Reilly, D.; Fou, L.; Hasler, E.; Hawkins, J.; O'Connell, S.; Pelone, F.; Callaway, M.; Campbell, F.; Capel, M.; Charnley, R.; et al. Diagnosis and management of pancreatic cancer in adults: A summary of guidelines from the UK National Institute for Health and Care Excellence. *Pancreatology* **2018**, *18*, 962–970. [CrossRef]
47. Lis, C.G.; Gupta, D.; Lammersfeld, C.A.; Markman, M.; Vashi, P.G. Role of nutritional status in predicting quality of life outcomes in cancer—A systematic review of the epidemiological literature. *Nutr. J.* **2012**, *11*, 27. [CrossRef]
48. Nightingale, J.; Young, A.; Hawthorne, B.; McKee, R.; McKinlay, A.; Rafferty, G.; Protheroe, S.; Culkin, A.; Eastwood, J.; Farrer, K.; et al. Position Statement from BIFA Committee. Available online: https://www.bapen.org.uk/nutrition-support/parenteral-nutrition/position-statement-from-bifa-committee (accessed on 17 July 2019).
49. Bozzetti, F.; Bozzetti, V. Is the intravenous supplementation of amino acid to cancer patients adequate? A critical appraisal of literature. *Clin. Nutr.* **2013**, *32*, 142–146. [CrossRef]
50. Wolfe, R.R. The 2017 Sir David P Cuthbertson lecture. Amino acids and muscle protein metabolism in critical care. *Clin. Nutr.* **2018**, *37*, 1093–1100. [CrossRef]
51. Körber, J.; Pricelius, S.; Heidrich, M.; Muller, M.J. Increased lipid utilization in weight losing and weight stable cancer patients with normal body weight. *Eur. J. Clin. Nutr.* **1999**, *53*, 740–745. [CrossRef]
52. Cao, D.-X.; Wu, G.-H.; Zhang, B.; Quan, Y.-J.; Wei, J.; Jin, H.; Jiang, Y.; Yang, Z.-A. Resting energy expenditure and body composition in patients with newly detected cancer. *Clin. Nutr.* **2010**, *29*, 72–77. [CrossRef]
53. Finocchiaro, C.; Gervasio, S.; Agnello, E.; Appiano, S.; Bertetto, O.; Ciuffreda, L.; Montrucchio, G.; Luisa, A.M.; D'andrea, F.; Domeniconi, D.; et al. Multicentric study on home parenteral nutrition in advanced cancer patients. *Riv. Ital. Nutr. Parenter. Enter.* **2002**, *20*, 98–107.

54. Seys, P.; Tadmouri, A.; Senesse, P.; Radji, A.; Rotarski, M.; Balian, A.; Culine, S.; Dufour, P.; Chambrier, C. Home parenteral nutrition in elderly patients with cancer: An observational prospective study. *Bull. Cancer* **2014**, *101*, 243–249. [CrossRef]

55. Culine, S.; Chambrier, C.; Tadmouri, A.; Senesse, P.; Seys, P.; Radji, A.; Rotarski, M.; Balian, A.; Dufour, P. Home parenteral nutrition improves quality of life and nutritional status in patients with cancer: A French observational multicentre study. *Support. Care Cancer* **2014**, *22*, 1867–1874. [CrossRef]

56. Vashi, P.G.; Dahlk, S.; Popiel, B.; Lammersfeld, C.A.; Ireton-Jones, C.; Gupta, D. A longitudinal study investigating quality of life and nutritional outcomes in advanced cancer patients receiving home parenteral nutrition. *BMC Cancer* **2014**, *14*, 593. [CrossRef]

57. Girke, J.; Seipt, C.; Markowski, A.; Luettig, B.; Schettler, A.; Momma, M.; Schneider, A.S. Quality of Life and Nutrition Condition of Patients Improve Under Home Parenteral Nutrition: An Exploratory Study. *Nutr. Clin. Pract.* **2016**, *31*, 659–665. [CrossRef]

58. Keane, N.; Fragkos, K.C.; Patel, P.S.; Bertsch, F.; Mehta, S.J.; Di Caro, S.; Rahman, F. Performance status, prognostic scoring, and parenteral nutrition requirements predict survival in patients with advanced cancer receiving home parenteral nutrition. *Nutr. Cancer* **2018**, *70*, 73–82. [CrossRef]

59. Bozzetti, F.; Arends, J.; Lundholm, K.; Micklewright, A.; Zürcher, G.; Muscaritoli, M. ESPEN Guidelines on Parenteral Nutrition: Non-surgical oncology. *Clin. Nutr.* **2009**, *28*, 445–454. [CrossRef]

60. Scolapio, J.; Picco, M.; Tarrosa, V. Enteral versus parenteral nutrition: The patient's preference. *J. Parenter. Enter. Nutr.* **2002**, *26*, 248–250. [CrossRef]

61. Obermair, A.; Simunovic, M.; Isenring, L.; Janda, M. Nutrition interventions in patients with gynecological cancers requiring surgery. *Gynecol. Oncol.* **2017**, *145*, 192–199. [CrossRef]

62. Baldwin, C.; Weekes, C.E. Dietary counselling with or without oral nutritional supplements in the management of malnourished patients: A systematic review and meta-analysis of randomised controlled trials. *J. Hum. Nutr. Diet.* **2012**, *25*, 411–426. [CrossRef]

63. Deutz, N.E.; Safar, A.; Schutzler, S.; Memelink, R.; Ferrando, A.; Spencer, H.; Van Helvoort, A.; Wolfe, R.R. Muscle protein synthesis in cancer patients can be stimulated with a specially formulated medical food. *Clin. Nutr.* **2011**, *30*, 759–768. [CrossRef]

64. Omlin, A.; Blum, D.; Wierecky, J.; Haile, S.R.; Ottery, F.D.; Strasser, F. Nutrition impact symptoms in advanced cancer patients: Frequency and specific interventions, a case–control study. *J. Cachex Sarcopenia Muscle* **2013**, *4*, 55–61. [CrossRef]

65. Van Blarigan, E.L.; Fuchs, C.S.; Niedzwiecki, D.; Zhang, S.; Saltz, L.B.; Mayer, R.J.; Mowat, R.B.; Whittom, R.; Hantel, A.; Benson, A.; et al. Association of Survival with Adherence to the American Cancer Society Nutrition and Physical Activity Guidelines for Cancer Survivors After Colon Cancer Diagnosis: The CALGB 89803/Alliance Trial. *JAMA Oncol.* **2018**, *4*, 783–790. [CrossRef]

66. Papallardo, G.; Almeida, A.; Ravasco, P. Eicosapentaenoic acid in cancer: Does it improve body composition and modulate metabolism? *Nutrition* **2015**, *31*, 549–555. [CrossRef]

67. Ravasco, P.; Lavriv, D.; Neves, P. Should omega-3 be used in cancer cachexia? *Clin. Nutr. ESPEN* **2018**, *25*, 18–25.

68. Hering, J.; Garrean, S.; Dekoj, T.R.; Razzak, A.; Saied, A.; Trevino, J.; Babcock, T.A.; Espat, N.J. Inhibition of Proliferation by Omega-3 Fatty Acids in Chemoresistant Pancreatic Cancer Cells. *Ann. Surg. Oncol.* **2007**, *14*, 3620–3628. [CrossRef]

69. Murphy, R.A.; Mourtzakis, M.; Mazurak, V.C. n-3 polyunsaturated fatty acids: The potential role for supplementation in cancer. *Curr. Opin. Clin. Nutr. Metab. Care* **2012**, *15*, 246–251. [CrossRef]

70. Geisler, C.; Prado, C.; Müller, M. Inadequacy of Body Weight-Based Recommendations for Individual Protein Intake—Lessons from Body Composition Analysis. *Nutrients* **2017**, *9*, 23. [CrossRef]

71. Norman, H.A.; Butrum, R.R.; Feldman, E.; Picciano, M.F.; Rivlin, R.; Simopoulos, A.; Wargovich, M.J.; Weisburger, E.K.; Zeisel, S.H.; Heber, D.; et al. The Role of Dietary Supplements during Cancer Therapy. *J. Nutr.* **2003**, *133*, 3794S–3799S. [CrossRef]

72. Rock, C.L.; Doyle, C.; Demark-Wahnefried, W.; Meyerhardt, J.; Courneya, K.S.; Schwartz, A.L.; Bandera, E.V.; Hamilton, K.K.; Grant, B.; McCullough, M.; et al. Nutrition and physical activity guidelines for cancer survivors. *CA Cancer J. Clin.* **2012**, *62*, 242–274. [CrossRef]

73. Stene, G.B.; Helbostad, J.L.; Amundsen, T.; Sørhaug, S.; Hjelde, H.; Kaasa, S.; Grønberg, B.H. Changes in skeletal muscle mass during palliative chemotherapy in patients with advanced lung cancer. *Acta Oncol.* **2015**, *54*, 340–348. [CrossRef]
74. Lieffers, J.R.; Bathe, O.F.; Fassbender, K.; Winget, M.; Baracos, V.E. Sarcopenia is associated with postoperative infection and delayed recovery from colorectal cancer resection surgery. *Br. J. Cancer* **2012**, *107*, 931–936. [CrossRef]

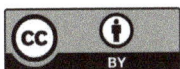

© 2019 by the author. Licensee MDPI, Basel, Switzerland. This article is an open access article distributed under the terms and conditions of the Creative Commons Attribution (CC BY) license (http://creativecommons.org/licenses/by/4.0/).

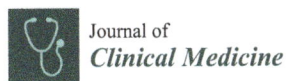

Review

Nutritional Management of Medical Inpatients

Emilie Reber [1,*,†], **Filomena Gomes** [2,†], **Lia Bally** [1], **Philipp Schuetz** [3,4] **and Zeno Stanga** [1]

1. Department of Diabetes, Endocrinology, Nutritional Medicine and Metabolism, Bern University Hospital, and University of Bern, 3010 Bern, Switzerland
2. The New York Academy of Sciences, New York, NY 10007, USA
3. Department of Medical University, Division of General Internal and Emergency Medicine, Kantonsspital Aarau, 5000 Aarau, Switzerland
4. Department for Clinical Research, Medical Faculty, University of Basel, 4001 Basel, Switzerland
* Correspondence: emilie.reber@insel.ch
† These authors contributed equally to the manuscript.

Received: 27 June 2019; Accepted: 26 July 2019; Published: 30 July 2019

Abstract: Malnutrition is a common condition in hospitalized patients that is often underdiagnosed and undertreated. Hospital malnutrition has multifactorial causes and is associated with negative clinical and economic outcomes. There is now growing evidence from clinical trials for the efficiency and efficacy of nutritional support in the medical inpatient population. Since many medical inpatients at nutritional risk or malnourished are polymorbid (i.e., suffer from multiple comorbidities), this makes the provision of adequate nutritional support a challenging task, given that most of the clinical nutrition guidelines are dedicated to single diseases. This review summarizes the current level of evidence for nutritional support in not critically ill polymorbid medical inpatients.

Keywords: malnutrition; nutritional management; nutritional therapy

1. Introduction

Hippocrates of Kos, one of the most outstanding figures in the history of medicine in the fourth to fifth century BCE stated that "The patient ought likewise to be consider'd, whether he is able to hold out with the prescribed diet, even in the height of the disease; for if the diet is not sufficient, the patient will grow too faint, and be overcome by the disease." [1]. He considered nutritional interventions to cure diseases as reflected in his well-known statement "Let food be thy medicine and medicine be thy food".

Around 80 years ago, Studley described weight loss of >20% of body weight as a factor increasing mortality (+33%) in chronic peptic ulcer patients undergoing non-emergency surgery, "regardless of the appearance of the individual" [2]. Some years later, more than 30 years ago, concerns regarding prevalence and adverse effects of disease-related malnutrition (malnutrition triggered by illness or disease) and in hospitalized patients were first reported [3–5]. Nowadays, the link between malnutrition and clinical negative outcomes, e.g., muscle wasting, higher infection rates, longer length of hospital stay, morbidity and mortality rates, is clearly established [6–10]. In high-income countries, where access to food should not be limited, every third patient is at risk for malnutrition or already malnourished at hospital admission [11]. Most patients further lose weight during their hospital stay, and, as consequence, their nutritional status deteriorates. A study of Barton et al. showed that 40% of the hospital food served to patients is left on the plates and returned, thus resulting in patients eating less than 80% of their individual energy and protein requirements [12]. There are several factors leading to progressive unintentional weight loss, such as gastrointestinal symptoms, inactivity, depression or low mood, advanced age, effects of illness on protein and energy homeostasis, protein catabolism, inflammation, hormonal function and loss of appetite [13]. Loss of appetite may develop during hospital stays either as a consequence of an underlying disease or treatment or preexist as a primary condition. This loss of appetite arises as a physiological response to acute illness and predisposes inpatients to serious caloric and protein deficits [14]. In combination with immobilization and a pronounced inflammatory and endocrine stress response, these nutritional deficits contribute to muscle wasting and progressive deterioration of metabolic and functional status, particularly in medical inpatients with multiple morbidities [9,15]. An initial loss of appetite does, however, not confer a risk to fail achievement of nutritional targets since this improves quite rapidly after the initiation of nutritional support [16].

There is some evidence from high-quality trials in critical care settings reporting harmful effects of hypercaloric replacement nutrition strategies [14]. These negative effects might be explained by suppression of autophagy with inadequate clearance of acute cell damage associated with illness [17]. Autophagy is a body mechanism to get rid of damaged cells organelles and toxic products. Loss of appetite may therefore be a protective mechanism in an acute disease with the goals to accelerate recovery from disease by improving autophagy. Importantly, in patients suffering from chronic diseases, this protective physiological response may have been exaggerated thereby causing malnutrition. Thus, in patients with multiple chronic diseases, who have milder disease severities, lost weight and muscle mass over time, use of an adequate eucaloric nutritional support has a potentially positive effect. They might have better metabolism and nutrients use due to decreased insulin resistance and decreased risk that nutrition would interfere with autophagy [7,18]. Thus, since critically ill patients have different nutritional needs from the patients on the medical wards, this review focuses on the nutritional support of non-critically ill medical inpatients; as such, the critically ill population is the focus of another publication in this special issue ("Kopp-Lugli et al. Nutrition therapy in critically ill patients treated on intensive and intermediate care units: a literature review").

Understanding the optimal use of nutritional support is highly complex because timing, route of delivery, and the amount and type of nutrients may all have important roles and potentially affect patient's outcomes. Furthermore, it has been questioned whether nutritional support in polymorbid medical inpatients differs from the ones suffering from a single disease. Polymorbidity (or multimorbidity) is mostly defined as the co-occurrence of at least two chronic medical conditions in one patient. Polymorbidity is frequent in hospitals and, despite being common in older people, is not necessarily associated with higher age. Nevertheless, older adult patients require special attention, as they tend to be more polymorbid than younger patients are. In addition to the disease burden, older patients often experience malnutrition by multifactor, such as anorexia of aging, presbyphagia and dysphagia due to sarcopenia [19–21]. While there are plenty of clinical nutrition guidelines available focusing on individual diseases, [22–26] Gomes et al. recently published new guidelines for the nutritional support in polymorbid medical inpatients [13].

2. Today's Clinical Evidence Level

Recent meta-analyses, which investigated the effects of nutritional support on clinical outcomes concluded that nutritional support leads to an increase in energy and protein intake, an increase in body weight but there were no significant effects on clinical outcomes such as mortality and morbidity, and only little effect on non-elective hospital readmissions [27,28]. The results showed no benefit in critical ill patients, possibly due to a suppression of autophagy and increased risk of refeeding syndrome [28]. In fact, these systematic reviews found (from the included heterogeneous trials and with high risk for bias) an important lack of evidence in this area, as high quality randomized, interventional trials, needed to establish causal relationships, were missing. Thus, the lack of significant results regarding mortality and morbidity may be rather due to methodological issues and low statistical power, and not lack of effectiveness per se.

In fact, other recent studies showed results that are more promising. The multicenter randomized placebo controlled double-blind "NOURISH-trial", conducted by Deutz and his colleagues, evaluated the effect of specialized, energy-dense ONS on postdischarge outcomes including nonelective readmission and mortality in initially hospitalized, malnourished, older adults. Patients were randomly allocated to receive during hospitalization and after discharge either a specialized, energy-dense ONS or a carbohydrate-only ONS. Results showed that energy-dense, specialized ONS extending beyond discharge improved body weight but could not reduce readmission rate. A significant reduction in 90-day mortality in the intervention group compared to the placebo group (4.8% vs. 9.7%) resulting in a number needed to treat (NNT) of 20 [29]. However, it remains unclear whether this beneficial effect is attributable to the specific formula (containing a leucine metabolite) used in this study or the high protein and energy amount provided by the oral nutritional supplement, given that control patients received a low protein and calorie placebo product. The very recently published open-label, non-blinded, multicenter, randomized-controlled trial, the "EFFORT trial", conducted by Schuetz and colleagues, assessed the effect of a protocol-guided individualized nutritional support to reach nutritional needs (determined either with the Harris-Benedict formula or with indirect calorimetry) of medical inpatients. Protocol-guided nutritional support reduced the primary outcome (all-cause mortality, admission to intensive care, non-elective hospital readmission, major complications, and decline in functional status) by 4% (22.9% vs. 26.9%) by 30 days when compared to usual care, translating into a NNT of 25 to prevent one severe complication [30]. Additionally, mortality rate was significantly lower in the intervention group compared to the control group (7.2% vs. 9.9%, NNT of 37) and notable improvements in functional outcomes and in quality of life measures were observed. Notably, in the nutrition support group, 91% received oral nutrition, and, perhaps most importantly, an individualized nutritional care plan from a specialist dietitian. Conversely, enteral or parenteral nutrition was used in eight and 12 participants respectively [30]. The effect of nutritional support on the risk for the primary endpoint was consistent across predefined subgroups. Thus, these results provide strong evidence for the concept of systematically screening medical inpatients on hospital admission in terms of nutritional risk, independent of the medical condition, followed by a nutritional assessment and initiation of individualized nutritional support in at-risk patients. The results also contradict the hypothesis that provision of nutritional support during the acute phase of illness would have harmful effects—at least in the non-critically ill setting [30]. Unlike the NOURISH trial that investigated the effect of a specific formula of an oral nutritional supplement, within EFFORT a variety of nutritional support strategies were used by trained dieticians to reach the individual nutritional goals of each patient. Thus, EFFORT does not provide evidence regarding single nutritional components or types of foods, but rather proves that the overall strategy of providing tailored nutritional support to reach the nutritional requirements during the acute phase of illness is beneficial for medical inpatients [30].

3. Nutritional Therapy

Since there is growing evidence for the positive effect of nutritional therapy (Figure 1), proper definition and thus diagnosis are lacking. The Global Leadership Initiative on Malnutrition (GLIM) working group recently published an umbrella approach to diagnose malnutrition in various clinical settings [31]. This aims to early identify nutritional risk in polymorbid patients to individually treat them and improve their clinical outcome [31]. The GLIM working group supports a two-step process with screening and assessment, targeting a standardization of nutritional support [31].

There are differences of prognosis of nutritional status and nutritional strategy among the etiology of malnutrition; malnutrition with severe inflammation (e.g., severe infection, multiple trauma), with persistent inflammation due to chronic disease (e.g., cancer, congestive heart failure), malnutrition with minimum or no inflammation in chronic disease patients (e.g., short bowel syndrome, dysphagia after stroke and anorexia nervosa) and malnutrition due to simple starvation (e.g., poverty, dementia, lack of appropriate nutrition care in the hospital/facilities). Patients with severe inflammation are often difficult to recover their nutritional status by only nutritional support, so the goal of nutrition support is to minimize deterioration of nutritional status. On the other hand, nutritional status of the patients with no or minimum inflammation, or those after simple starvation, can be improved if appropriate nutrition support provided by the nutrition specialists.

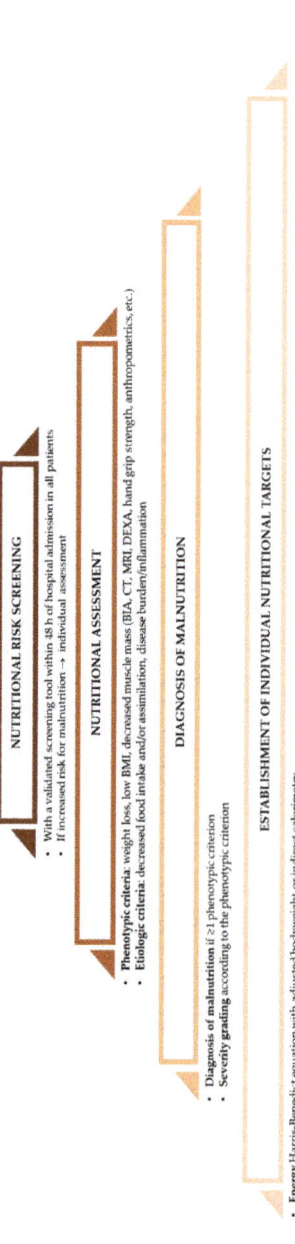

Figure 1. Nutritional algorithm, after [30].

3.1. Organization of Nutritional Support

Nutritional support in hospitals ideally relies on two main structures: A hospital nutrition steering committee and multidisciplinary nutritional support teams. The nutrition steering committee is working within the clinical governance framework (sets nutritional standards, protocols and guidelines) and has a direct access to hospital management. Members of the nutrition steering committee should be drawn from the management, and include senior representation from medical staff, catering, nursing, dietetics, pharmacy and other healthcare professionals [32,33]. A nutritional support team has an executive function within the hospital, implementing standards, protocols and guidelines in daily clinical practice. Such a team consisting of physicians, dieticians, nurses, and pharmacists, ensures and improves nutritional treatments quality and safety, and is continuously checking and optimizing procedures of nutritional management (see dedicated manuscript in this special issue). Interdisciplinary cooperation and good communication between healthcare professionals is important and mandatory to provide an individualized nutritional support to all patients who need it.

3.2. Screening and Assessment

The identification of malnutrition has been typically based on anthropometric, biochemical and physical parameters, among others. There is no universally accepted gold standard (best method) for the assessment of nutritional status [34,35]. Commonly used criteria include unintentional weight loss (percentage of body weight) in the past 3–6 months, low BMI, reduced muscle mass, reduced dietary intake in the past week, reduced absorptive capacity, and disease burden/inflammation [31].

Standardized procedures are needed in order to initiate a timely and adequate nutritional therapy [36]. Systematic screening for nutritional risk, followed by a comprehensive nutritional assessment should be implemented and lead to the development of a personalized nutritional care plan (see dedicated manuscript in this special issue: Reber et al., Nutritional screening and assessment) [13,33,37]. Nutrition screening is the first step in determining nutritional problems. Screening should rapidly and accurately identify individuals who should be referred to the nutrition specialist (e.g., dietitian, expert clinician) for a further assessment, where it would be possible to gather more information and determine if there truly is a nutrition problem, to understand the cause of the problem and to determine its severity. Nutritional screening should be done with validated screening tools, such as malnutrition universal screening (MUST), mini nutritional assessment short form (MNA-SF) and nutritional risk screening 2002 (NRS-2002), each of them having strength and limitations and may not be sufficiently validated in specific populations like polymorbid patients (see dedicated manuscript in this special issue: Reber et al., Nutritional screening and assessment) [38,39]. In general, nutritional assessment continues the data gathering process initiated in the screen. The types of data collected in nutritional assessment are often similar to data collected in the screening process but in more depth [40]. In summary, nutritional support should be initiated with a detailed nutritional care plan (appropriate monitoring procedures and clear guidelines for action e.g., food record charts or dietetic referral) in people who are at risk of malnutrition or manifestly malnourished according to the result of the nutritional risk screening and assessment results [41].

3.3. Nutritional Targets

Meeting the nutritional requirement is important to maintain or gain weight, muscle mass and function, to improve clinical outcomes, and reduce complications and rehospitalization rates.

Dietitians and medical staff trained in nutrition support should ensure that the patients' dietary intake meets the individual energy, protein, fluid, electrolyte, mineral, micronutrients and fiber needs [33]. The activity levels and the underlying clinical condition (e.g., catabolism, pyrexia, gastrointestinal tolerance, potential metabolic instability), as well as the likely duration of nutrition support, should also be taken into account.

3.3.1. Energy

Determining the patients' energy requirements is a central point of nutritional assessment. The total energy expenditure consists of the resting energy expenditure, diet-induced thermogenesis and the energy expended during physical activity [13]. The gold standard to measure energy requirements is the indirect calorimetry, but when not possible, these may be calculated with published prediction equations adjusted for age sex, and weight (e.g., Harris-Benedict formula) in addition to activity and stress factors, or roughly estimated weight-based formulae (it has been suggested 27 kcal/kg/day for polymorbid older patients) [13]. In individuals with very low BMI, the higher value of 30 kcal/kg/d should slowly be targeted [13]. Reaching the energy targets too quickly and/or feeding at too high rates potentially lead to complications such as the refeeding syndrome or overfeeding [42].

3.3.2. Proteins

The general protein requirement is 1 g/kg/d for the polymorbid medical inpatient population. In case of acute or chronic kidney failure, protein requirements may have to be reduced to 0.8–1 g/kg/d unless dialysis, but there are no specific recommendations for polymorbid patients suffering from kidney failure [13]. In case of dialysis, the protein requirements are the same as normal and there is a need for 20 g of proteins after the dialysis (dialytic loss). For older patients suffering acute or chronic disease, recommendations are 1.2–15. g/kg/d [43,44]. An individual target has to be defined for each patient, since other factors such as hypermetabolism can change protein requirements (e.g., major trauma and burns). Patients undergoing paracentesis need 10 g proteins per liter ascites.

3.3.3. Micronutrients

In malnourished polymorbid inpatients, micronutrients requirements may be higher due to reduced food intake or due to higher needs (disease-depending). Micronutrients should be supplemented according to the recommended daily intake, and/or substituted if deficiencies are occurring [13]. The daily micronutrients requirements are considered to be covered in case of the amount of enteral nutrition is ≥1500 mL per day. Vitamins and trace elements should be provided to patients receiving parenteral nutrition since there are none in the nutritional solutions.

3.4. Nutritional Route

Oral nutrition should be the first-line choice of nutritional support, including meals adapted to the individual patient preferences, additional energy dense snacks (e.g., "homemade" milkshakes), food fortification with powdered carbohydrate and protein supplements, and the commercial oral nutritional supplements [13]. The use of the convenient commercial oral nutritional supplements have been shown to maintain the muscle mass, to lower the complication rate and hospital readmission rate after six months [13,45–48], but a combination of oral nutritional support strategies (using both traditional and commercially available products) also results in the improvement of important clinical outcomes [30].

If oral nutrition is not possible, safe or sufficient, enteral and eventually parenteral nutrition should be considered, whereas the enteral nutrition should be the preferred route due to lower risk of infectious and non-infectious complications [13]. The energy and protein intake should be assessed every 24–48 h and escalated after 5 days if the patient does not meet at least 75% of his/her requirements [49].

3.5. Nutrition for Specific Medical Conditions

Patients with renal failure need restrictions in potassium and phosphate. Patients with congestive heart failure may benefit from sodium and water restrictions in given cases.

There is weak evidence to support the use of specialized oral nutritional supplements or enteral nutrition formulas in polymorbid medical inpatients. Arginine, glutamine, and beta-hydroxy-beta-metylbuturate (HMB) may be used in patients suffering from pressure ulcers [13,50].

Arginine (semi-essential amino acid) is required for promotion of nitrogen balance, cell proliferation, T lymphocyte function and collagen accumulation. It also changes into nitric oxide, which is known for its vasodilatory and angiogenic properties. Glutamine (conditionally essential amino acid) plays a key role in the immune system, and its deficiency may significantly slow the healing process. HMB (metabolite of leucine, an essential amino acid) supplementation was associated with increased muscle mass accretion by inhibiting muscle proteolysis and modulating protein turnover. A mixture of soluble and insoluble fibers can be used in older polymorbid patients receiving enteral nutrition and suffering from diarrhea or constipation, which are frequent complications of enteral nutrition [13]. Special attention should then be paid to the hydration state as it may cause obstipation [51].

3.6. Timing

An early start of nutritional support (within 48 h after hospital admission) is recommended to maintain or improve patient's nutritional and functional status, and prevent sarcopenia [13]. Even though the optimal length of the nutritional support is still unclear, it is usually recommended to treat beyond hospital discharge, as this continued nutritional intervention is known to increase patients' quality of life and nutritional and functional status, and in the older (>65 years) polymorbid patients it results in lower mortality rates [13,52,53].

3.7. Monitoring

Experienced clinical teams with the relevant skills and training in nutritional monitoring should review the indications, route, risks, benefits and goals of nutrition support at regular intervals. This interval depends on the patient and the parameter that is being monitored (e.g., nutritional, anthropometric, biochemical, clinical condition), and may increase when the patient's condition is stable under nutritional treatment. For example, nutrient intake from oral, enteral or parenteral nutrition (including any change in conditions that are affecting food intake) is recommended to be monitored daily initially, reducing to twice weekly when stable [33]. Similarly, laboratory parameters (e.g., sodium, potassium, urea, creatinine) should be monitored more frequently initially, i.e., at baseline and daily until stable, and then reduced to 1 or 2 times a week. In addition to the nutritional parameters used to monitor responses to nutritional support, functional indices (e.g., handgrip strength) should be used regularly to asses other clinical outcomes (i.e., survival, quality of life) in polymorbid medical inpatients.

4. Barriers to the Adequate Provision of Nutritional Support

The awareness about malnutrition must be raised primarily among hospital medical staff, where nutritional support is not seen as being part of the medical treatment. Malnutrition is often unrecognized as a diagnosis and is, subsequently, being under-reported and not being treated. Clearly defined protocols and responsibilities are needed to address this hidden problem, starting with a systematic nutritional risk screening and nutritional assessment for all patients on admission to hospital. Malnutrition should become a topic in the education and training of medical staff. At the same time, because the causes of malnutrition are often multifactorial (from depression and lack of appetite to inability to self-feed), communication and collaboration should be improved between the different members of the multidisciplinary team and between the team and the patient, in order to efficiently address those causes [16]. A recently published study showed that 78% of the hospitals and 22% of the nursing homes in Switzerland have a nutritional steering committee, and 92% and 14%, respectively, have dieticians available. Around 80% of the hospitals and nursing homes did not implement a systematic nutritional risk screening procedure, resulting in around 60% of the patients being screened at least at one time point (in hospitals and nursing homes); 25% of the hospital do screen the patients as they feel a problem [54]. Further, 56% of the institutions monitor the food intake of their patients and 50% monitor and document the nutritional status [54]. The nutritionDay survey 2018, a survey on nutritional care conducted worldwide (https://www.nutritionday.org/en/network/imprint/index.html;

Table 1) showed that 76.4% of the participating centers had NST available on site, and that 61.6% of the participating centers use a specific screening tool to screen the patients at hospital admission.

Table 1. National reports from the nutritionDay 2018, available from https://www.nutritionday.org/en/about-nday/national-reports/index.html.

Country	Number of Participating Centers	Percentage of Hospitals with NST Present on Site	Percentage of Screening at Hospital Admission
Australia	1	100	100
Austria	4	100	45.5
Belgium	52	88	77.3
Brazil	12	100	80.0
Bulgaria	1	66.7	0
China	9	100	56.5
Colombia	35	69.1	56.6
Croatia	3	55.6	20.0
Germany	36	60.9	49.5
Greece	3	100	0
India	13	7.7	50.1
Japan	9	100	50
Netherlands	1	100	0
Poland	4	0	60
Portugal	4	100	66.7
Singapore	1	0	82.6
Spain	5	100	50.0
Sweden	2	100	100
Switzerland	1	66.7	16.7
Thailand	1	100	66.7
United States of America	16	62.5	96.0

Individual factors such as patients' symptoms, disease severity (e.g., causing dysphagia and loss of appetite), mood and orientation, impaired functional and cognitive status, social environment (e.g., isolation, loneliness, lack of family support) may all significantly reduce the food (and nutrient) intake of hospitalized patients and contribute for the deterioration of their nutritional status. Polypharmacy, especially in polymorbid patients, may further influence their nutritional status, causing drug–drug and drug–nutrients interactions as well as gastrointestinal symptoms. This calls for the need of frequent monitoring of the nutritional status of the hospitalized patient (e.g., weekly monitoring of the body weight). For those patients receiving nutritional support, regular visits by the dietitian allow the patient to receive the encouragement to comply with the nutritional care plan, and the adaptation of this plan to the changing needs of the patient [55].

5. Conclusions and Outlook

Nutritional support has been shown to be a highly effective treatment option to prevent and/or treat malnutrition, decreasing morbidity and mortality rates. Nutritional interventions deserve as much attention as any other therapeutic interventions, and clinicians should aim to maximize their efficacy and minimize side effects. Further studies should also investigate the cost-effectiveness of nutritional interventions in medically ill patients. It will be equally important to determine which medical inpatients have the most benefit from nutritional support interventions through metabolomics and microbiome research, walking towards an evidence-based personalized nutrition approach.

Author Contributions: Conceptualization, E.R. and Z.S.; writing—original draft preparation, E.R.; writing—review and editing, F.G. and L.B. and P.S. and Z.S.; supervision, Z.S.

Funding: The APC was funded by the Research Found of the Department of Diabetes, Endocrinology, Nutritional medicine and Metabolism and in part by Nestlé Health Science (grant to the institution).

Conflicts of Interest: The authors declare no conflict of interest. The funders had no role in the design of the study; in the collection, analyses, or interpretation of data; in the writing of the manuscript, or in the decision to publish the results.

References

1. Sprengell, C. *Hippocrates: The Aphorisms of Hippocrates, and The Sentences of Celsus; with Explanations and References to the Most Considerable Writers*, 2nd ed.; Wilkin, F., Bonwick, F., Eds.; Gale Ecco: London, UK, 1735.
2. Studley, H.O. Percentage of weight loss: A basic indicator of surgical risk in patients with chronic peptic ulcer. *J. Am. Med. Assoc.* **1936**, *106*, 458–460. [CrossRef]
3. McWhirter, J.P.; Pennington, C.P. Incidence and recognition of malnutrition in hospital. *Br. Med. J.* **1994**, *308*, 945–948. [CrossRef] [PubMed]
4. Hill, G.L.; Pickford, I.; Young, G.A.; Schorah, C.J.; Blackett, R.L.; Burkinshaw, L.; Warren, J.V.; Morgan, D.B. Malnutrition in surgical patients: An unrecognised problem. *Lancet* **1977**, *309*, 689–692. [CrossRef]
5. Bistrian, B.R.; Blackburn, G.L.; Vitale, J.; Cochran, D.; Naylor, J. Prevalence of malnutrition in general medical patients. *JAMA* **1976**, *235*, 1567–1570. [CrossRef] [PubMed]
6. Kubrak, C.; Jensen, L. Malnutrition in acute care patients: A narrative review. *Int. J. Nurs. Stud.* **2007**, *44*, 1036–1054. [CrossRef]
7. Schutz, P.; Bally, M.; Stanga, Z.; Keller, U. Loss of appetite in acutely ill medical inpatients: Physiological response or therapeutic target? *Swiss Med. Wkly.* **2014**, *144*, w13957. [CrossRef]
8. Casaer, M.P.; Hermans, G.; Wilmer, A.; Van den Berghe, G. Impact of early parenteral nutrition completing enteral nutrition in adult critically ill patients (EPaNIC trial): A study protocol and statistical analysis plan for a randomized controlled trial. *Trials* **2011**, *12*, 21. [CrossRef]
9. Felder, S.; Lechtenboehmer, C.; Bally, M.; Fehr, R.; Deiss, M.; Faessler, L.; Kutz, A.; Steiner, D.; Rast, A.C.; Laukemann, S.; et al. Association of nutritional risk and adverse medical outcomes across different medical inpatient populations. *Nutrition* **2015**, *31*, 1385–1393. [CrossRef]
10. Villet, S.; Chiolero, R.L.; Bollmann, M.D.; Revelly, J.P.; Cayeux, M.C.; Delarue, J.; Berger, M.M. Negative impact of hypocaloric feeding and energy balance on clinical outcome in ICU patients. *Clin. Nutr.* **2005**, *24*, 502–509. [CrossRef]
11. Sorensen, J.; Kondrup, J.; Prokopowicz, J.; Schiesser, M.; Krahenbuhl, L.; Meier, R.; Liberda, M. EuroOOPS: An international, multicentre study to implement nutritional risk screening and evaluate clinical outcome. *Clin. Nutr.* **2008**, *27*, 340–349. [CrossRef]
12. Barton, A.D.; Beigg, C.L.; Macdonald, I.A.; Allison, S.P. High food wastage and low nutritional intakes in hospital patients. *Clin. Nutr.* **2000**, *19*, 445–449. [CrossRef] [PubMed]
13. Gomes, F.; Schuetz, P.; Bounoure, L.; Austin, P.; Ballesteros-Pomar, M.; Cederholm, T.; Fletcher, J.; Laviano, A.; Norman, K.; Poulia, K.A.; et al. ESPEN guidelines on nutritional support for polymorbid internal medicine patients. *Clin. Nutr.* **2018**, *37*, 336–353. [CrossRef] [PubMed]
14. Casaer, M.P.; Van den Berghe, G. Nutrition in the acute phase of critical illness. *N. Engl. J. Med.* **2014**, *370*, 1227–1236. [CrossRef] [PubMed]
15. Felder, S.; Braun, N.; Stanga, Z.; Kulkarni, P.; Faessler, L.; Kutz, A.; Steiner, D.; Laukemann, S.; Haubitz, S.; Huber, A.; et al. Unraveling the Link between Malnutrition and Adverse Clinical Outcomes: Association of Acute and Chronic Malnutrition Measures with Blood Biomarkers from Different Pathophysiological States. *Ann. Nutr. Metab.* **2016**, *68*, 164–172. [CrossRef] [PubMed]
16. Tribolet, P.; Fehr, R.; Bächli, V.; Geiser, M.; Toplak, H.; Stanga, Z.; Schuetz, P. What are Barriers of Nutritional Therapy in Malnourished Medical Inpatients? An Observational Study. *Aktuel Ernahr.* **2017**, *42*, 167–179.
17. Schetz, M.; Casaer, M.P.; Van den Berghe, G. Does artificial nutrition improve outcome of critical illness? *Crit. Care* **2013**, *17*, 302. [CrossRef]
18. Russell, R.C.; Yuan, H.X.; Guan, K.L. Autophagy regulation by nutrient signaling. *Cell Res.* **2014**, *24*, 42–57. [CrossRef] [PubMed]
19. Fujishima, I.; Fujiu-Kurachi, M.; Arai, H.; Hyodo, M.; Kagaya, H.; Maeda, K.; Mori, T.; Nishioka, S.; Oshima, F.; Ogawa, S.; et al. Sarcopenia and dysphagia: Position paper by four professional organizations. *Geriatr. Gerontol. Int.* **2019**, *19*, 91–97. [CrossRef]

20. Morley, J.E. Defining Undernutrition (Malnutrition) in Older Persons. *J. Nutr. Health Aging* **2018**, *22*, 308–310. [CrossRef]
21. Ortega, O.; Martin, A.; Clave, P. Diagnosis and Management of Oropharyngeal Dysphagia Among Older Persons, State of the Art. *J. Am. Med. Direct. Assoc.* **2017**, *18*, 576–582. [CrossRef]
22. Arends, J.; Bachmann, P.; Baracos, V.; Barthelemy, N.; Bertz, H.; Bozzetti, F.; Fearon, K.; Hutterer, E.; Isenring, E.; Kaasa, S.; et al. ESPEN guidelines on nutrition in cancer patients. *Clin. Nutr.* **2017**, *36*, 11–48. [CrossRef] [PubMed]
23. Forbes, A.; Escher, J.; Hebuterne, X.; Klek, S.; Krznaric, Z.; Schneider, S.; Shamir, R.; Stardelova, K.; Wierdsma, N.; Wiskin, A.E.; et al. ESPEN guideline: Clinical nutrition in inflammatory bowel disease. *Clin. Nutr.* **2017**, *36*, 321–347. [CrossRef] [PubMed]
24. Meier, R.; Beglinger, C.; Layer, P.; Gullo, L.; Keim, V.; Laugier, R.; Friess, H.; Schweitzer, M.; Macfie, J. ESPEN guidelines on nutrition in acute pancreatitis. European Society of Parenteral and Enteral Nutrition. *Clin. Nutr.* **2002**, *21*, 173–183. [CrossRef] [PubMed]
25. Plauth, M.; Bernal, W.; Dasarathy, S.; Merli, M.; Plank, L.D.; Schutz, T.; Bischoff, S.C. ESPEN guideline on clinical nutrition in liver disease. *Clin. Nutr.* **2019**, *38*, 485–521. [CrossRef] [PubMed]
26. Turck, D.; Braegger, C.P.; Colombo, C.; Declercq, D.; Morton, A.; Pancheva, R.; Robberecht, E.; Stern, M.; Strandvik, B.; Wolfe, S.; et al. ESPEN-ESPGHAN-ECFS guidelines on nutrition care for infants, children, and adults with cystic fibrosis. *Clin. Nutr.* **2016**, *35*, 557–577. [CrossRef] [PubMed]
27. Bally, M.R.; Blaser Yildirim, P.Z.; Bounoure, L.; Gloy, V.L.; Mueller, B.; Briel, M.; Schuetz, P. Nutritional Support and Outcomes in Malnourished Medical Inpatients: A Systematic Review and Meta-analysis. *JAMA Intern. Med.* **2016**, *176*, 43–53. [CrossRef] [PubMed]
28. Feinberg, J.; Nielsen, E.E.; Korang, S.K.; Halberg Engell, K.; Nielsen, M.S.; Zhang, K.; Didriksen, M.; Lund, L.; Lindahl, N.; Hallum, S.; et al. Nutrition support in hospitalised adults at nutritional risk. *Cochrane Database Syst. Rev.* **2017**, *5*, Cd011598. [CrossRef]
29. Deutz, N.E.; Matheson, E.M.; Matarese, L.E.; Luo, M.; Baggs, G.E.; Nelson, J.L.; Hegazi, R.A.; Tappenden, K.A.; Ziegler, T.R. Readmission and mortality in malnourished, older, hospitalized adults treated with a specialized oral nutritional supplement: A randomized clinical trial. *Clin. Nutr.* **2016**, *35*, 18–26. [CrossRef]
30. Schuetz, P.; Fehr, R.; Baechli, V.; Geiser, M.; Gomes, F.; Kutz, A.; Tribolet, P.; Bregenzer, T.; Hoess, C.; Pavlicek, V.; et al. Individualised nutritional support in medical inpatients at nutritional risk: A randomized clinical trial. *Lancet* **2019**, *393*, 2312–2321. [CrossRef]
31. Cederholm, T.; Jensen, G.L.; Correia, M.; Gonzalez, M.C.; Fukushima, R.; Higashiguchi, T.; Baptista, G.; Barazzoni, R.; Blaauw, R.; Coats, A.J.S.; et al. GLIM criteria for the diagnosis of malnutrition—A consensus report from the global clinical nutrition community. *J. Cachexia Sarcopenia Muscle* **2019**, *10*, 207–217. [CrossRef]
32. Ten Dam, S.; Droop, A.; Arjaans, W.; de Groot, S.; van Bokhorst-de van der Schueren, M. Module 11.1 Organisation of a Nutritional Support Team. In *ESPEN LLL, Organisation of Nutritional Care Ethical and Legal Aspects: ESPEN*; 2012; Available online: https://lllnutrition.com/mod/page/view.php?id=3422, (accessed on 29 July 2019).
33. National Institute for Health and Clinical Excellence. *Nutrition Support for Adults: Oral Nutrition Support, Enteral Tube Feeding and Parenteral Nutrition (Clinical Guidance 32) London: National Collaborating Centre for Acute Care (UK)*; National Institute for Health and Clinical Excellence: London, UK, 2006.
34. Donini, L.M.; Savina, C.; Rosano, A.; Cannella, C. Systematic review of nutritional status evaluation and screening tools in the elderly. *J. Nutr. Health Aging* **2007**, *11*, 421–432. [PubMed]
35. Foley, N.C.; Salter, K.L.; Robertson, J.; Teasell, R.W.; Woodbury, M.G. Which Reported Estimate of the Prevalence of Malnutrition After Stroke Is Valid? *Stroke* **2009**, *40*, E66–E74. [CrossRef] [PubMed]
36. Bauer, J.M.; Kaiser, M.J.; Sieber, C.C. Evaluation of nutritional status in older persons: Nutritional screening and assessment. *Curr. Opin. Clin. Nutr. Metab. Care* **2010**, *13*, 8–13. [CrossRef] [PubMed]
37. Weekes, C.E.; Elia, M.; Emery, P.W. The development, validation and reliability of a nutrition screening tool based on the recommendations of the British Association for Parenteral and Enteral Nutrition (BAPEN). *Clin. Nutr.* **2004**, *23*, 1104–1112. [PubMed]
38. Power, L.; Mullally, D.; Gibney, E.R.; Clarke, M.; Visser, M.; Volkert, D.; Bardon, L.; de van der Schueren, M.A.E.; Corish, C.A. A review of the validity of malnutrition screening tools used in older adults in community and healthcare settings—A MaNuEL study. *Clin. Nutr. ESPEN* **2018**, *24*, 1–13. [CrossRef] [PubMed]

39. Van Bokhorst-de van der Schueren, M.A.; Guaitoli, P.R.; Jansma, E.P.; de Vet, H.C. Nutrition screening tools: Does one size fit all? A systematic review of screening tools for the hospital setting. *Clin. Nutr.* **2014**, *33*, 39–58. [CrossRef] [PubMed]
40. Charney, P. Nutrition screening vs. nutrition assessment: How do they differ? *Nutr. Clin. Pract.* **2008**, *23*, 366–372. [CrossRef] [PubMed]
41. Elia, M. *Guidelines for Detection and Management of Malnutrition*; British Association for Parenteral and Enteral Nutrition: Redditch, UK, 2000.
42. Friedli, N.; Stanga, Z.; Culkin, A.; Crook, M.; Laviano, A.; Sobotka, L.; Kressig, R.W.; Kondrup, J.; Mueller, B.; Schuetz, P. Management and prevention of refeeding syndrome in medical inpatients: An evidence-based and consensus-supported algorithm. *Nutrition* **2018**, *47*, 13–20. [CrossRef] [PubMed]
43. Deutz, N.E.; Bauer, J.M.; Barazzoni, R.; Biolo, G.; Boirie, Y.; Bosy-Westphal, A.; Cederholm, T.; Cruz-Jentoft, A.; Krznaric, Z.; Nair, K.S.; et al. Protein intake and exercise for optimal muscle function with aging: Recommendations from the ESPEN Expert Group. *Clin. Nutr.* **2014**, *33*, 929–936. [CrossRef] [PubMed]
44. Volkert, D.; Beck, A.M.; Cederholm, T.; Cruz-Jentoft, A.; Goisser, S.; Hooper, L.; Kiesswetter, E.; Maggio, M.; Raynaud-Simon, A.; Sieber, C.C.; et al. ESPEN guideline on clinical nutrition and hydration in geriatrics. *Clin. Nutr.* **2019**, *38*, 10–47. [CrossRef] [PubMed]
45. Gariballa, S.; Forster, S.; Walters, S.; Powers, H. A randomized, double-blind, placebo-controlled trial of nutritional supplementation during acute illness. *Am. J. Med.* **2006**, *119*, 693–699. [CrossRef] [PubMed]
46. Hegerova, P.; Dedkova, Z.; Sobotka, L. Early nutritional support and physiotherapy improved long-term self-sufficiency in acutely ill older patients. *Nutrition* **2015**, *31*, 166–170. [CrossRef] [PubMed]
47. Starke, J.; Schneider, H.; Alteheld, B.; Stehle, P.; Meier, R. Short-term individual nutritional care as part of routine clinical setting improves outcome and quality of life in malnourished medical patients. *Clin. Nutr.* **2011**, *30*, 194–201. [CrossRef] [PubMed]
48. Volkert, D.; Hubsch, S.; Oster, P.; Schlierf, G. Nutritional support and functional status in undernourished geriatric patients during hospitalization and 6-month follow-up. *Aging Clin. Exp. Res.* **1996**, *8*, 386–395. [CrossRef]
49. Bounoure, L.; Gomes, F.; Stanga, Z.; Keller, U.; Meier, R.; Ballmer, P.; Fehr, R.; Mueller, B.; Genton, L.; Bertrand, P.C.; et al. Detection and treatment of medical inpatients with or at-risk of malnutrition: Suggested procedures based on validated guidelines. *Nutrition* **2016**, *32*, 790–798. [CrossRef] [PubMed]
50. Wong, A.; Chew, A.; Wang, C.M.; Ong, L.; Zhang, S.H.; Young, S. The use of a specialised amino acid mixture for pressure ulcers: A placebo-controlled trial. *J. Wound Care* **2014**, *23*, 259–260. [CrossRef] [PubMed]
51. Vandewoude, M.F.; Paridaens, K.M.; Suy, R.A.; Boone, M.A.; Strobbe, H. Fibre-supplemented tube feeding in the hospitalised elderly. *Age Ageing* **2005**, *34*, 120–124. [CrossRef] [PubMed]
52. Beck, A.M.; Holst, M.; Rasmussen, H.H. Oral nutritional support of older (65 years+) medical and surgical patients after discharge from hospital: Systematic review and meta-analysis of randomized controlled trials. *Clin. Rehabil.* **2013**, *27*, 19–27. [CrossRef] [PubMed]
53. Munk, T.; Tolstrup, U.; Beck, A.M.; Holst, M.; Rasmussen, H.H.; Hovhannisyan, K.; Thomsen, T. Individualised dietary counselling for nutritionally at-risk older patients following discharge from acute hospital to home: A systematic review and meta-analysis. *J. Hum. Nutr. Diet.* **2016**, *29*, 196–208. [CrossRef] [PubMed]
54. Aubry, E.; Mareschal, J.; Gschweitl, M.; Zvingelis, M.; Schuetz, P.; Stanga, Z. Facts zum Management der Klinischen Ernährung—Eine Online-Befragung. *Aktuel Ernahr.* **2018**, *42*, 452–460. [CrossRef]
55. Lobo, D.N. Improving outcomes with a little EFFORT. *Lancet* **2019**, *393*, 2278–2280. [CrossRef]

© 2019 by the authors. Licensee MDPI, Basel, Switzerland. This article is an open access article distributed under the terms and conditions of the Creative Commons Attribution (CC BY) license (http://creativecommons.org/licenses/by/4.0/).

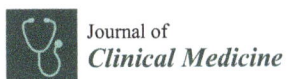

Review

Gastroparesis and Dumping Syndrome: Current Concepts and Management

Stephan R. Vavricka [1,2,*] and Thomas Greuter [2]

1   Center of Gastroenterology and Hepatology, CH-8048 Zurich, Switzerland
2   Department of Gastroenterology and Hepatology, University Hospital Zurich, CH-8091 Zurich, Switzerland
*   Correspondence: stephan.vavricka@hin.ch

Received: 21 June 2019; Accepted: 23 July 2019; Published: 29 July 2019

Abstract: Gastroparesis and dumping syndrome both evolve from a disturbed gastric emptying mechanism. Although gastroparesis results from delayed gastric emptying and dumping syndrome from accelerated emptying of the stomach, the two entities share several similarities among which are an underestimated prevalence, considerable impairment of quality of life, the need for a multidisciplinary team setting, and a step-up treatment approach. In the following review, we will present an overview of the most important clinical aspects of gastroparesis and dumping syndrome including epidemiology, pathophysiology, presentation, and diagnostics. Finally, we highlight promising therapeutic options that might be available in the future.

Keywords: gastroparesis; dumping syndrome; pathophysiology; clinical presentation; treatment

1. Introduction

Gastroparesis and dumping syndrome both evolve from a disturbed gastric emptying mechanism. While gastroparesis results from significantly delayed gastric emptying, dumping syndrome is a consequence of increased flux of food into the small bowel [1,2]. The two entities share several important similarities: (i) gastroparesis and dumping syndrome are frequent, but also frequently overlooked; (ii) they affect patient's quality of life considerably due to possibly debilitating symptoms; (iii) patients should be taken care of within a multidisciplinary team setting; and (iv) treatment should follow a step-up approach from dietary modifications and patient education to pharmacological interventions and, finally, surgical procedures and/or enteral feeding. Most importantly, the two diagnoses have to be considered by one of the treating specialists, regardless of whether this is the endocrinologist, nutritional specialist or gastroenterologist, when symptoms are present. Pre-test probability based on comorbidities (such as diabetes in case of gastroparesis or surgical history for dumping syndrome) together with the presence of typical symptoms should lead to a high degree of clinical suspicion. However, for both disorders, diagnostic evaluations should follow in order to confirm the diagnosis before initiation of treatment. Firstly, because treatment options might be invasive and require proper diagnostic evaluations beforehand. Secondly, several differential diagnoses might show a similar presentation. Such diagnoses are peptic ulcer disease, gastric cancer, celiac disease, abdominal angina for gastroparesis, anastomotic ulcers, internal herniation and gallbladder disease for early dumping syndrome and insulinoma, surreptitious use of glucose-lowering medication for late dumping [2–5]. In the following review, we will present an overview of the most important clinical aspects of gastroparesis and dumping syndrome including epidemiology, pathophysiology, presentation, diagnostics and treatment. Finally, we highlight promising therapeutic options that might be available in the future.

2. Definitions and Epidemiology

Gastroparesis and dumping syndrome are frequent, but their prevalence and incidence vary depending on definitions and studied populations. Therefore, heterogenous results have been reported in the literature.

2.1. Gastroparesis

Gastroparesis is a syndrome characterized by an objectively delayed gastric emptying in the absence of a mechanical gastric outlet obstruction and the presence of cardinal symptoms such as early satiety, postprandial fullness and nausea-vomiting [6]. The prevalence of gastroparesis in the general population is uncertain. A wide range in different at-risk populations has been reported. In addition, gastroparesis is likely significantly under diagnosed. While an epidemiological study from Olmsted county revealed a prevalence of 24.2/100,000 for definite gastroparesis and 50.5/100,000 for definite, probable or possible gastroparesis [7], prevalence might be as high as 1.8% [8]. Patients with type 1 diabetes are at particular risk. Here, 10-year incidence rates of 5.2% have been reported (in contrast to a rate of 1% for type 2 diabetes and 0.2% for non-diabetic patients [9]. Other studies demonstrate even higher rates for diabetics with 58% for type 1 and 30% for type 2 [10,11]. However, most of the performed studies have a considerable selection bias with inclusion of patients from tertiary referral centers only. Still, there might be a large proportion of undetected gastroparesis patients, because either the patient does not seek medical attention or the treating doctors are reluctant to evaluate symptoms and/or further diagnostics. The incidence of postsurgical gastroparesis after gastrectomy is approximately 0.4% to 5.0% [12]. Overall, the incidence of gastroparesis after surgery depends on the surgical procedure and the surgical site. In the early postoperative period after pylorus-preserving pancreatoduodenectomy, postsurgical gastroparesis occurs in up to 20% to 50% of patients [12]. In one study, 67% of patients who underwent pancreatic cancer cryoablation were found to suffer from gastroparesis [13]. There seems to be a gender-specific differences with women accounting for up to 70% of the affected population. Interestingly, elderly patients (>65 years old) are at particular risk [14].

2.2. Dumping Syndrome

Dumping syndrome is a frequently encountered postsurgical complication that can be divided into an early and late subtype [2]. Alterations in gastric anatomy after esophageal, gastric and bariatric surgery result in rapid passage of food into the small intestine, which leads to early gastrointestinal and vasomotor symptoms (within 1 h) and late hypoglycemia (1 to 3 h after meal ingestion) [15,16]. Reliable population-based prevalence data for dumping syndrome are still lacking. As of yet, the frequency of postsurgical dumping syndrome is estimated at 25%–50% with 5 to 10% of patients experiencing a severe disabling form [17]. These rates vary depending on type of surgery prodecure [2]. While 20% of patients suffer from symptoms of dumping syndrome after vagotomy and pyloroplasty, these rates rise to 40% after Roux-en-Y bypass and sleeve gastrectomy, and peak at 50% after esophagectomy [18–22]. The incidence and prevalence of dumping syndrome has been increasing due to the current obesity epidemics and the consecutive climb in gastric bypass surgeries [23]. Early dumping represents the most common type, while isolated late dumping is observed in only 25% [2,22]. Due to considerable overlap in clinical presentation it is, however, sometimes difficult to differentiate between the two and co-occurrence is frequently encountered.

3. Pathophysiology and Clinical Presentation

The occurrence of cardinal symptoms after ingestion of a meal in a patient with high pre-test probability should rise suspicion for the presence of gastroparesis or dumping syndrome. The symptoms per se are rather non-specific and might occur with many other diseases. However, the existence of risk factors such as diabetes for gastroparesis or bariatric surgery for dumping makes the diagnoses more likely (Tables 1 and 2).

3.1. Gastroparesis

Several aspects contribute to a delayed gastric emptying in gastroparesis patients. Among these are extrinsic denervation of the stomach, impaired inhibitory input to smooth muscles due to loss of nitric oxide in enteric nerves, loss of interstitial cells of Cajal (ICC, "pacemaker cells), smooth muscle atrophy and altered function of immune cells [1]. ICC generate electrical slow waves in the stomach, and disrupted ICC networks and gastric dysrhythmias have been associated with gastroparesis [24]. For details see Figure 1. The most frequent etiologies are diabetes and surgery [25]. In a high proportion of patients, the underlying cause remains unknown (so called idiopathic gastroparesis) [25]. This form is found in particular in younger women and appears to be associated with viral infection (in up to 20%) [26–28]. Less frequent etiologic factors are Parkinson's disease, amyloid, tumors (paraneoplastic gastroparesis), scleroderma, or mesenteric ischemia [29]. Importantly, medication-induced gastroparesis has to be considered in all patients. Typically here are opioids, ciclosporine, anticholinergics and glucagon-like peptide 1 (GLP1)-agonists [30–32]. The latter should be particularly suspected in diabetic patients before considering the gastroparesis to be caused by diabetes and poor control of blood glucose. From a clinical perspective, the simplest classification of gastroparesis is into the two categories diabetic vs. non-diabetic. Delayed gastric emptying can be observed in 28% to 65% of unselected patients with diabetes [33,34]. Patients with type 1 diabetes have a higher incidence of gastroparesis as compared with type 2 (5.25 vs. 1%) and an earlier age at onset [7,9,29]. Type 2 diabetics, however, have more serious symptoms. Gastroparesis in diabetic patients usually occurs 10 years after the onset of diabetes and it parallels other forms of diabetic microvascular disease, including neuropathy and retinopathy. Severe symptoms of diabetic gastroparesis cause poor glycemic control and poor nutritional status, and increase the risk of hypoglycaemia [35].

Gastroparesis is often a debilitating disease associated with significant morbidity and mortality [36,37]. The most frequently reported symptoms are: early satiety, postprandial fullness, nausea-vomiting, bloating and upper abdominal pain [38]. The latter is somewhat neglected by physicians, but appear to occur in up to 72%–90% of patients. Pain is often experienced after meals (72%), but can also occur during night time (74%) [29,39]. The presence of non-prandial abdominal pain can, therefore, not be used to rule out the diagnosis. It rather appears to be another piece in the wide presentation of the disease. Weight loss is not a typical feature of gastroparesis patients. Symptoms can vary depending on the specific etiology. Nausea, at least, is similar in all patients with gastroparesis, irrespectively of the underlying cause. Both nausea and vomiting significantly correlate with a reduced quality of life [40]. It should be kept in mind that the presence of symptoms is a sine qua non for the diagnosis of gastroparesis.

3.2. Dumping Syndrome

In early dumping syndrome, rapid transition of food into the small intestine results in a fluid shift (due to hyperosmolarity) and release of gastrointestinal hormones such as vasoactive substances (neurostatin, vasoactive intestinal peptide (VIP), incretins (gastric inhibitory polypeptide (GIP), GLP1) and glucose-modulators (insulin, glucagon) [2,15,41–43]. This results in gastrointestinal and vasomotor symptoms; the latter is characterized by hypotension (due to the above mentioned fluid shift) and a consecutive sympathetic nerve system response [15,16]. In late dumping, rapid absorption of glucose (due to the presence of undigested carbohydrates in the small intestine) increases incretin release (GLP1), which exaggerates insulin response [2,44–46]. This ultimately leads to hypoglycaemia within 1 to 3 h after meal intake (so called incretin-driven hyperinsulinemic response) [15,16]. Although these mechanisms are typically and frequently seen as a postsurgical complication, dumping can also occur in the absence of previous surgery [47]. While in these cases, there is no alteration in gastric anatomy, gastric emptying is accelerated due to a disturbed intrinsic gastric innervation [2]. Diabetes is the main contributor [47,48]. Thus, diabetes can be associated with both delayed (see gastroparesis) and increased gastric emptying. The latter is particularly seen in early diabetes and more so in type 2 than 1. Due to overlapping symptoms, it might be difficult to distinguish gastroparesis from dumping syndrome in diabetic patients. Vomiting makes gastroparesis more probable, while dumping should be considered in particular in the presence of diarrhea [49]. Idiopathic forms of dumping have been described also. Similarly to gastroparesis, viral infections are a possible cause [50]. About 50% of patients with idiopathic dumping syndrome report a history of gastroenteritis symptoms [50].

Symptoms of early and late dumping are quite different. Early dumping includes the following symptoms that occur within 1 h, typically 30 min after a meal ingestion [15]: abdominal pain, bloating, borborygmi, nausea, diarrhea (gastrointestinal symptoms); and fatigue, desire to lie down, flushing, palpitations/perspiration, tachycardia, hypotension and rarely syncope (vasomotor symptoms). For late dumping, typical symptoms can be divided into neuroglycopenia and autonomic reactivity [17]. While the first group comprises fatigue, weakness, confusion, hunger and syncope, the latter includes perspiration, palpitations, tremor and irritability. Dumping syndrome can result in significant weight loss (30%) and considerably affects quality of life [51]. It may lead to hospitalizations due to hypoglycemia, episodes of confusion, seizures and even epilepsy [52].

Table 1. Symptoms and causes of gastroparesis.

Symptoms and Causes of Gastroparesis
Symptoms:
Postprandial fullness, early satiety, bloating, abdominal distension, nausea, and vomiting, abdominal pain, and dysphagia
Causes:
Diabetes
Non-diabetic causes
Surgery (such as gastrectomy with vagotomy, vagal nerve injury, Roux-en-Y, pancreatectomy, anti-reflux operations, lung transplant)
Gastrointestinal disorders: gastroesophageal reflux, gastric ulcer disease, gastritis, atrophic gastritis, pancreatitis
Diseases of the nervous system (such as parkinsonism)
Connective tissue diseases (such as scleroderma)
Unknown ("idiopathic gastroparesis")
Paraneoplastic
Mesenteric ischemia
Viral infections: e.g., CMV
Side effect of medications
Metabolic and endocrine disorders: hypothyroidism, pregnancy, uremia

Table 2. Symptoms and causes of dumping syndrome.

Symptoms and Causes of Dumping Syndrome
Symptoms:
Early dumping syndrome (within 1 h after meal ingestion)
Gastrointestinal symptoms: Abdominal pain, epigastric fullness, diarrhea, nausea, vomiting, borborygmi, and bloating
Vasomotor symptoms: desire to lie down, palpitations and tachycardia, fatigue, faintness, syncope, perspiration, headache, light-headedness, hypotension, flushing, and pallor
Late dumping syndrome (1–3 h after meal ingestion)
Neuroglycopenia: fatigue, weakness, confusion, hunger and syncope
Autonomic reactivity: perspiration, palpitations, tremor and irritability
Causes:
Surgery: gastrojejunostomy, antrectomy, pylorectomy, pyloroplasty, esophagectomy, vagotomy, Roux-en Y bypass, Nissen fundoplication
Not-surgery related: diabetes mellitus, viral illness, unkown ("idiopathic")

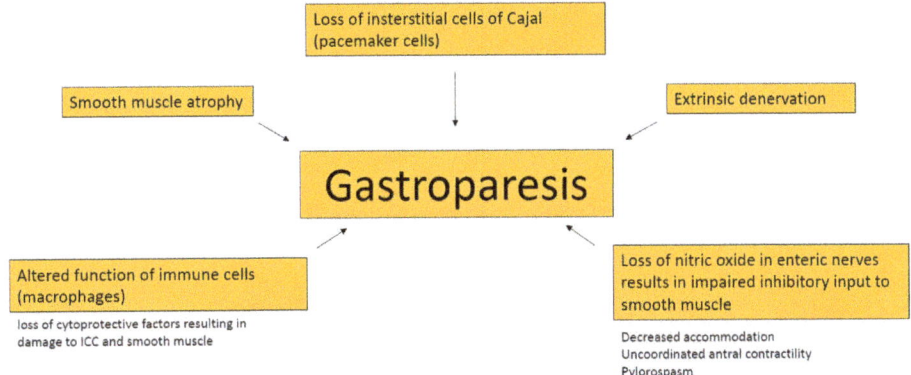

Figure 1. Pathophysiology of gastroparesis. ICC, interstitial cells of Cajal.

4. Diagnostic Evaluations

Gastroparesis and dumping syndrome have to be distinguished from several organic and functional diseases. Distinction between irritable bowel syndrome, functional dyspepsia and gastroparesis, dumping syndrome might be particularly difficult [29,53]. Many cardinal symptoms are shared between these entities. Diagnostic evaluations are therefore key to clearly establish the diagnosis of gastroparesis and dumping syndrome [54].

4.1. Gastroparesis

Gastroparesis is diagnosed by a thorough history and physical examination, which help to identify the presence of characteristic symptoms of gastroparesis and exclude alternative diagnoses. Once the syndrome is suspected, an upper endoscopy is necessary to rule out mechanical gastric obstruction. Although an upper gastrointestinal series may suggest the diagnosis, there is a limited role for imaging in the workup for gastroparesis and delayed emptying should be confirmed by gastric transit testing such as gastric scintigraphy, breath testing, and wireless motility capsule [55,56]. Gastroparesis is diagnosed if typical symptoms are present, a delayed gastric emptying is documented and a correlation of symptoms with food intake is observed [29]. This definition of gastroparesis highlights two key points: (1) objective measures of delayed gastric emptying are needed to establish the diagnosis; and (2) symptoms are a sine-qua-non [29]. A test that is positive for delayed gastric emptying does not make the diagnosis if a patient is asymptomatic. Scintigraphy is the gold-standard to establish decreased gastric emptying and the most widely used technique. However, there are regional differences. Some European centers use breath tests more often because there are simply to handle and have been shown to correlate nicely with scintigraphy results [57]: A test meal (usually white bread, butter, water and an egg omelette with 13C octanoic acid) is ingested and 13C measured using expired breath gas analysis [58]. Magnetic resonance imaging (MRI) assesses gastric physiology by simultaneously measuring gastric emptying and motility without the need of ionizing radiation [59]. There is increasing evidence that MRI is a reliable non-invasive tool in the diagnostic evaluation of gastroparesis [59]. Given the importance of disrupted ICC networks in the pathophysiology of gastroparesis, slow wave measurements are another potential diagnostic test. In fact, a combination of electrogastrogram and magnetogastrogram is able to distinguish gastroparesis patients from controls [60].

4.2. Dumping Syndrome

Increased pre-test probability such as a past surgical history and the presence of typical symptoms result in a high clinical suspicion for the presence of dumping syndrome. Two questionnaires have been established for the identification of clinically relevant symptoms of dumping syndrome, the Sigstad's score and the Arts' dumping questionnaire [2,51]. A simple visual analogue scale might also be used [61]. Objective measurements are less established compared to gastroparesis. Measuring glucose has a low diagnostic yield, but might be considered when symptoms of late dumping syndrome are present [2]. Importantly, glucose should be measured in the plasma and not in the capillary blood, since low glucose levels are less reliable in the latter. Suggested cut-offs are 2.8 and 3.3 mmol/L [62]. Provocation tests might have higher predictive values. Two options are available, oral glucose tolerance test (OGTT) and the mixed meal tolerance test [2,63]. For OGTT, 50 or 75 g sugar is ingested and blood glucose, haematocrit, pulse and blood pressure are measured every 30 min for 3 h [15]. An increase in the haematocrit by 3% and/or pulse acceleration by 10 min suggest early dumping syndrome, while development of hypoglycemia suggests late dumping syndrome [15]. In the mixed meal tolerance test, carbohydrates, fats and proteins are ingested, and glucose, insulin are checked every 30 min [44,64]. The ordering physician should keep in mind that even healthy individuals can show a drop in their blood sugar levels after meal intake and that therefore the test has a high false positive rate [65]. Gastric emptying studies are potential alternatives, but their specificity and sensitivity is rather low [2].

5. Treatment of Gastroparesis

Treatment strategies are quite similar in gastroparesis and dumping syndrome. In a multidisciplinary setting, a step-wise approach should be followed, where dietary modifications and patient education represent the first step, pharmacological interventions the second, and surgical interventions the last option (Figure 2). In the acute setting of gastroparesis, dehydration and electrolyte abnormalities should be corrected by oral or intravenous routes, as appropriate [66]. In severe cases, gastric decompression by insertion of a nasogastric tube might be necessary [29]. In a more chronic setting, the first step in the management of gastroparesis are nutritional counselling and dietary modifications. The patient should be educated to eat small, low-fat, low-fibre meals [29]. Counselling by a nutritional expert is of paramount importance, because gastroparesis can lead to considerable malnutrition due to inadequate oral intake and vomiting [67,68]. In case of underlying diabetes, controlling blood glucose levels should be aimed for [29]. Epidemiological studies have linked poor diabetes control with gastroparesis [69]. As of yet, there are no randomized controlled trials proving that lowering HbA1c indeed improves gastroparesis symptoms. Nonetheless, controlling diabetes makes sense for numerous reasons. When these initial steps do not lead to clinical improvement, pharmacological interventions are needed. The armamentarium is limited, but at least a few drugs are available [70]. Among those are the prokinetics metoclopramide and domperidone that act as dopamine 2 receptor antagonists. Their efficacy has been demonstrated in several randomized trials [71,72]. However, their efficacy appears to be independent of their potential for accelerating gastric emptying, since gastric emptying has been shown to poorly correlate with symptomatic response [73]. Other mechanisms such as affecting gastric hypersensitivity or gastric accommodation may be responsible for their effect [74]. Data about their long-term effects are sparse, and several potentially deleterious side-effects limit their use in clinical practice. Metoclopramide imposes a risk for tardive dyskinesia in 1% of patients, while domperidone has been linked to serious cardiac side-effects. Use of metoclopramide should, therefore, be restricted to a maximum of 3 months, at the lowest possible dose [75]. Erythromycin, a macrolide antibiotic, improves gastric emptying through stimulating the motilin receptor and represents an option for short-term treatment, when metoclopramide and domperidone have failed [76]. Nausea, a frequent and bothersome symptom in gastroparesis, can be treated with antiemetics such as prochlorperazine, diphenhydramine, or a 5-HT3 antagonist [66]. Aprepitant can also be considered given its effects on nausea, vomiting and overall symptoms in gastroparesis patients [77]. Iberogast, an over-the-counter herbal preparation is frequently used in functional dyspepsia. Despite having no effect on gastric emptying, iberogast has been shown to positively affect gastroparesis symptoms in a placebo-controlled crossover trial [78]. Several interventional approaches have been developed and hyped in the past with different outcomes.

The injection of botulinum toxin during upper endoscopy into the pyloric muscle might be effective, albeit only in the short term [79–82]. However, the two only randomized controlled trials failed to show efficacy of pyloric botox [83,84]. Whether this was due to small sample size and consecutive lack of power has yet to be determined. Another therapy option is gastric electrical stimulation (GES), where electric current is delivered to gastric smooth muscles via implanted electrodes with a positive impact on gastroparesis symptoms and gastric emptying [85]. GES has been proposed as an alternative for patients with intractable gastroparesis, but a double-blind controlled trial showed only minor improvement with a significant complication rate [86]. A meta-analysis, including 10 studies, suggested that diabetic gastroparesis patients seem to benefit the most, whereas idiopathic gastroparesis patients and postsurgical patients are less responsive and need further research [87]. Another technique, the gastric peroral endoscopic pyloromyotomy (G-POEM) showed some efficacy in gastroparesis patients but further studies are needed [88–93]. Esoflip is currently the newest kid on the block. It is a balloon catheter that was developed for dilations in the gastrointestinal tract. Non-controlled studies revealed high rates of technical success with increased distensibility and symptomatic improvement after pyloric dialation [94]. Esoflip might have its role in difficult to treat patients before considering surgical interventions, but more data, particularly randomized controlled trials are needed first. Surgery should be seen as treatment of last resort and should be discussed individually in a multidisciplinary team setting due to the sparse clinical data. At least, a recent case series including 28 patients suggested improvement of symptoms, gastric emptying and a consecutive reduction in the need for prokinetic treatment 3 months after surgery [95]. However, surgery clearly has its role when oral nutritional intake is compromised. In these cases, jejunostomy feeding should be considered. A percutaneous or surgical placement of a gastrostomy-jejunostomy tube enables decompression of the stomach and permits enteral feeding [96].

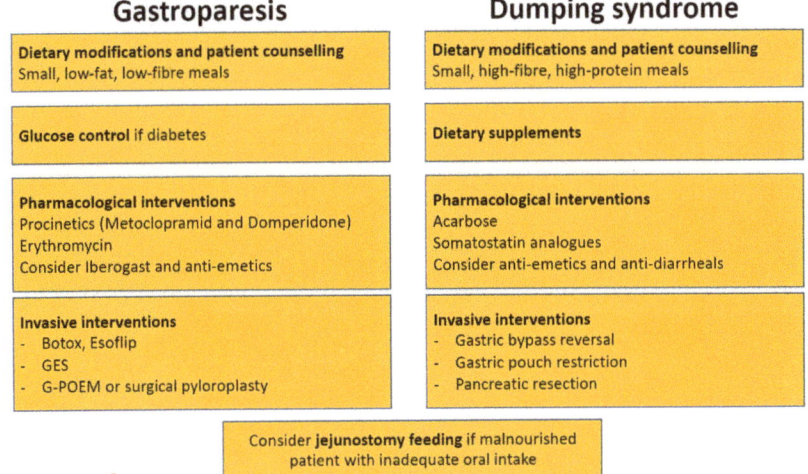

Figure 2. Treatment algorithm for gastroparesis and dumping syndrome. GES, gastric electrical stimulation; G-POEM, gastric peroral endoscopic pyloromyotomy.

6. Treatment of Dumping Syndrome

Similarly to gastroparesis, dietary modifications and patient education by a nutritional expert are the first steps in the treatment of dumping syndrome [2,97–100]. Smaller and more frequent meals (around six per day) are recommended [2]. Intake of fluids should be delayed by at least 30 min. Rapidly absorbable carbohydrates and alcoholic beverages should be avoided, while intake of high-fibre, high-protein food is recommended [2]. The rationale behind is that liquids further accelerate gastric emptying. Lying down after a meal for 30 min may further delay emptying of the stomach [15,101]. As a second step, dietary supplements such as guar gum, pectin or glucomannan can be added to enhance food viscosity [102–104]. However, most patients do not tolerate these agents due to frequent side-effects such as gas formation and bloating [2]. Pharmacological interventions are the third step in the therapeutic ladder. However, it should be kept in mind that as of yet no treatment has been approved for dumping syndrome. The currently available options are (1) acarbose and (2) for severe cases somatostatin analogues. Acarbose is an alpha-glucosidase inhibitor that decreases intraluminal digestion of carbohydrates in the duodenum. Therefore, it is used to treat postprandial hypoglycemia in late dumping syndrome [105–108]. However, as seen for the dietary supplements, acarbose is associated with side-effects such as flatulence occurring in a high proportion of patients [109]. Somatostatin analogues can improve dumping syndrome by affecting several disease mechanisms: (i) delaying gastric emptying; (ii) slowering small intestine transit; (iii) decreasing release of gastrointestinal hormones including insulin secretion; and (iv) inhibition of postprandial vasodilation [2,51]. Somatostatin analogues such as octreotide can be applied either subcutaneously three times a day or intramuscularly every 2 to 4 weeks [51,110–112]. The latter is probably preferred by the majority of patients. Most important side-effects are steatorrhea, diarrhea, nausea, gallstone formation, pain at injection site and weight gain. Due to these side-effects daily applied doses should start as low as 25 mcg and then titrated up to a maximum of 100 mcg. Treatment should be stopped after 2 weeks (subcutaneous application) or 2 months (intramuscular application) if no improvement is observed [2]. Non-specific symptoms such as nausea and diarrhea may be symptomatically treated with antiemetics (meclizine, promethazine) and antidiarrheals (tincture of opium, loperamide). Anticholinergics like dicyclomine, hyoscyamine, and propantheline slow gastric emptying and are antispasmotic. Diazoxide is a potassium channel activator, which influences hypoglycaemia and is used in late dumping [113]. However, these drugs have been studied in only few patients with dumping syndrome. As for gastroparesis, surgical interventions (revision surgery) should be discussed on a case to case basis, since data for their efficacy are limited [2].

7. Conclusions

Gastroparesis and dumping syndrome are frequent disorders, particularly in diabetic and postsurgical patients. Since symptoms are non-specific, these two entities have to be distinguished from several differential diagnoses and require objective measures that document delayed or accelerated gastric emptying. A multidisciplinary team approach including nutritional experts, endocrinologists and gastroenterologists is key to success. Within this setting, optimal treatment strategies can be discussed and individually tailored to each patient. This is particularly important in cases that are difficult to treat, where possible treatment options are limited and data for their efficacy conflicting.

Author Contributions: Conceptualization, S.R.V. and T.G.; methodology, S.R.V. and T.G.; writing—original draft preparation, S.R.V. and T.G.; writing—review and editing, S.R.V. and T.G.; visualization, T.G.; supervision, S.R.V. and T.G.; project administration, S.R.V.

Conflicts of Interest: T.G. has a consulting contract with Sanofi-Aventis, received a travel grant from Falk Pharma GmbH and Vifor, and an unrestricted research grant from Novartis. S.R.V. received consultant fees and unrestricted research grants from Abbott, Ferring, MSD, Pfizer, Takeda, Tillots, UCB, Vifor and Falk Pharma GmbH.

References

1. Camilleri, M.; Bharucha, A.E.; Farrugia, G. Epidemiology, mechanisms, and management of diabetic gastroparesis. *Clin. Gastroenterol. Hepatol.* **2011**, *9*, 5–12. [CrossRef] [PubMed]
2. van Beek, A.P.; Emous, M.; Laville, M.; Tack, J. Dumping syndrome after esophageal, gastric or bariatric surgery: Pathophysiology, diagnosis, and management. *Obes. Rev.* **2017**, *18*, 68–85. [CrossRef] [PubMed]
3. Talley, N.J.; Vakil, N.B.; Moayyedi, P. American gastroenterological association technical review on the evaluation of dyspepsia. *Gastroenterology* **2005**, *129*, 1756–1780. [CrossRef] [PubMed]

4. Mulla, C.M.; Storino, A.; Yee, E.U.; Lautz, D.; Sawnhey, M.S.; Moser, A.J.; Patti, M.E. Insulinoma After Bariatric Surgery: Diagnostic Dilemma and Therapeutic Approaches. *Obes. Surg.* **2016**, *26*, 874–881. [CrossRef] [PubMed]
5. Mathur, A.; Gorden, P.; Libutti, S.K. Insulinoma. *Surg. Clin. N. Am.* **2009**, *89*, 1105–1121. [CrossRef] [PubMed]
6. Bharucha, A.E. Epidemiology and natural history of gastroparesis. *Gastroenterol. Clin. N. Am.* **2015**, *44*, 9–19. [CrossRef] [PubMed]
7. Jung, H.K.; Choung, R.S.; Locke, G.R.; Schleck, C.D.; Zinsmeister, A.R.; Szarka, L.A.; Mullan, B.; Talley, N.J. The incidence, prevalence, and outcomes of patients with gastroparesis in Olmsted County, Minnesota, from 1996 to 2006. *Gastroenterology* **2009**, *136*, 1225–1233. [CrossRef] [PubMed]
8. Rey, E.; Choung, R.S.; Schleck, C.D.; Zinsmeister, A.R.; Talley, N.J.; Locke, G.R. Prevalence of hidden gastroparesis in the community: The gastroparesis "iceberg". *J. Neurogastroenterol. Motil.* **2012**, *18*, 34–42. [CrossRef]
9. Choung, R.S.; Locke, G.R.; Schleck, C.D.; Zinsmeister, A.R.; Melton, L.J.; Talley, N.J. Risk of gastroparesis in subjects with type 1 and 2 diabetes in the general population. *Am. J. Gastroenterol.* **2012**, *107*, 82–88. [CrossRef]
10. Horowitz, M.; Harding, P.E.; Maddox, A.F.; Wishart, J.M.; Akkermans, L.M.; Chatterton, B.E.; Shearman, D.J. Gastric and oesophageal emptying in patients with type 2 (non-insulin-dependent) diabetes mellitus. *Diabetologia* **1989**, *32*, 151–159. [CrossRef]
11. Horowitz, M.; Maddox, A.F.; Wishart, J.M.; Harding, P.E.; Chatterton, B.E.; Shearman, D.J. Relationships between oesophageal transit and solid and liquid gastric emptying in diabetes mellitus. *Eur. J. Nucl. Med.* **1991**, *18*, 229–234. [CrossRef] [PubMed]
12. Dong, K.; Yu, X.J.; Li, B.; Wen, E.G.; Xiong, W.; Guan, Q.L. Advances in mechanisms of postsurgical gastroparesis syndrome and its diagnosis and treatment. *Chin. J. Dig. Dis.* **2006**, *7*, 76–82. [CrossRef] [PubMed]
13. Dong, K.; Li, B.; Guan, Q.L.; Huang, T. Analysis of multiple factors of postsurgical gastroparesis syndrome after pancreaticoduodenectomy and cryotherapy for pancreatic cancer. *World J. Gastroenterol.* **2004**, *10*, 2434–2438. [CrossRef] [PubMed]
14. Nusrat, S.; Bielefeldt, K. Gastroparesis on the rise: Incidence vs awareness? *Neurogastroenterol. Motil.* **2013**, *25*, 16–22. [CrossRef] [PubMed]
15. Tack, J.; Arts, J.; Caenepeel, P.; De Wulf, D.; Bisschops, R. Pathophysiology, diagnosis and management of postoperative dumping syndrome. *Nat. Rev. Gastroenterol. Hepatol.* **2009**, *6*, 583–590. [CrossRef]
16. Tack, J.; Deloose, E. Complications of bariatric surgery: Dumping syndrome, reflux and vitamin deficiencies. *Best Pract. Res. Clin. Gastroenterol.* **2014**, *28*, 741–749. [CrossRef] [PubMed]
17. Eagon, J.C.; Miedema, B.W.; Kelly, K.A. Postgastrectomy syndromes. *Surg. Clin. N. Am.* **1992**, *72*, 445–465. [CrossRef]
18. Vecht, J.; Masclee, A.A.; Lamers, C.B. The dumping syndrome. Current insights into pathophysiology, diagnosis and treatment. *Scand. J. Gastroenterol. Suppl.* **1997**, *223*, 21–27.
19. McLarty, A.J.; Deschamps, C.; Trastek, V.F.; Allen, M.S.; Pairolero, P.C.; Harmsen, W.S. Esophageal resection for cancer of the esophagus: Long-term function and quality of life. *Ann. Thorac. Surg.* **1997**, *63*, 1568–1572. [CrossRef]
20. Banerjee, A.; Ding, Y.; Mikami, D.J.; Needleman, B.J. The role of dumping syndrome in weight loss after gastric bypass surgery. *Surg. Endosc.* **2013**, *27*, 1573–1578. [CrossRef]
21. Papamargaritis, D.; Koukoulis, G.; Sioka, E.; Zachari, E.; Bargiota, A.; Zacharoulis, D.; Tzovaras, G. Dumping symptoms and incidence of hypoglycaemia after provocation test at 6 and 12 months after laparoscopic sleeve gastrectomy. *Obes. Surg.* **2012**, *22*, 1600–1606. [CrossRef] [PubMed]
22. Tzovaras, G.; Papamargaritis, D.; Sioka, E.; Zachari, E.; Baloyiannis, I.; Zacharoulis, D.; Koukoulis, G. Symptoms suggestive of dumping syndrome after provocation in patients after laparoscopic sleeve gastrectomy. *Obes. Surg.* **2012**, *22*, 23–28. [CrossRef] [PubMed]
23. Berg, P.; McCallum, R. Dumping Syndrome: A Review of the Current Concepts of Pathophysiology, Diagnosis, and Treatment. *Dig. Dis. Sci.* **2016**, *61*, 11–18. [CrossRef]
24. O'Grady, G.; Angeli, T.R.; Du, P.; Lahr, C.; Lammers, W.J.E.P.; Windsor, J.A.; Abell, T.L.; Farrugia, G.; Pullan, A.J.; Cheng, L.K. Abnormal initiation and conduction of slow-wave activity in gastroparesis, defined by high-resolution electrical mapping. *Gastroenterology* **2012**, *143*, 589–598.e583. [CrossRef] [PubMed]

25. Hyett, B.; Martinez, F.J.; Gill, B.M.; Mehra, S.; Lembo, A.; Kelly, C.P.; Leffler, D.A. Delayed radionucleotide gastric emptying studies predict morbidity in diabetics with symptoms of gastroparesis. *Gastroenterology* **2009**, *137*, 445–452. [CrossRef] [PubMed]
26. Chen, J.D.; Lin, Z.; Pan, J.; McCallum, R.W. Abnormal gastric myoelectrical activity and delayed gastric emptying in patients with symptoms suggestive of gastroparesis. *Dig. Dis. Sci.* **1996**, *41*, 1538–1545. [CrossRef] [PubMed]
27. Oh, J.J.; Kim, C.H. Gastroparesis after a presumed viral illness: Clinical and laboratory features and natural history. *Mayo Clin. Proc.* **1990**, *65*, 636–642. [CrossRef]
28. Bityutskiy, L.P.; Soykan, I.; McCallum, R.W. Viral gastroparesis: A subgroup of idiopathic gastroparesis–clinical characteristics and long-term outcomes. *Am. J. Gastroenterol.* **1997**, *92*, 1501–1504.
29. Camilleri, M.; Parkman, H.P.; Shafi, M.A.; Abell, T.L.; Gerson, L. Clinical guideline: Management of gastroparesis. *Am. J. Gastroenterol.* **2013**, *108*, 18–37. [CrossRef]
30. Mittal, R.K.; Frank, E.B.; Lange, R.C.; McCallum, R.W. Effects of morphine and naloxone on esophageal motility and gastric emptying in man. *Dig. Dis. Sci.* **1986**, *31*, 936–942. [CrossRef]
31. Salehi, M.; Aulinger, B.A.; D'Alessio, D.A. Targeting beta-cell mass in type 2 diabetes: Promise and limitations of new drugs based on incretins. *Endocr. Rev.* **2008**, *29*, 367–379. [CrossRef] [PubMed]
32. Maes, B.D.; Vanwalleghem, J.; Kuypers, D.; Ghoos, Y.; Rutgeerts, P.J.; Vanrentergham, Y.F. Differences in gastric motor activity in renal transplant recipients treated with FK-506 versus cyclosporine. *Transplantation* **1999**, *68*, 1482–1485. [CrossRef] [PubMed]
33. Samsom, M.; Vermeijden, J.R.; Smout, A.J.; Van Doorn, E.; Roelofs, J.; Van Dam, P.S.; Martens, E.P.; Eelkman-Rooda, S.J.; Van Berge-Henegouwen, G.P. Prevalence of delayed gastric emptying in diabetic patients and relationship to dyspeptic symptoms: A prospective study in unselected diabetic patients. *Diabetes Care* **2003**, *26*, 3116–3122. [CrossRef]
34. Jones, K.L.; Russo, A.; Stevens, J.E.; Wishart, J.M.; Berry, M.K.; Horowitz, M. Predictors of delayed gastric emptying in diabetes. *Diabetes Care* **2001**, *24*, 1264–1269. [CrossRef] [PubMed]
35. Horváth, V.J.; Izbéki, F.; Lengyel, C.; Kempler, P.; Várkonyi, T. Diabetic gastroparesis: Functional/morphologic background, diagnosis, and treatment options. *Curr. Diabetes Rep.* **2014**, *14*, 527. [CrossRef] [PubMed]
36. Woodhouse, S.; Hebbard, G.; Knowles, S.R. Psychological controversies in gastroparesis: A systematic review. *World J. Gastroenterol.* **2017**, *23*, 1298–1309. [CrossRef] [PubMed]
37. Bielefeldt, K. Gastroparesis: Concepts, controversies, and challenges. *Scientifica (Cairo)* **2012**, *2012*, 424802. [CrossRef]
38. Liu, N.; Abell, T. Gastroparesis Updates on Pathogenesis and Management. *Gut Liver* **2017**, *11*, 579–589. [CrossRef]
39. Cherian, D.; Sachdeva, P.; Fisher, R.S.; Parkman, H.P. Abdominal pain is a frequent symptom of gastroparesis. *Clin. Gastroenterol. Hepatol.* **2010**, *8*, 676–681. [CrossRef]
40. Cherian, D.; Parkman, H.P. Nausea and vomiting in diabetic and idiopathic gastroparesis. *Neurogastroenterol. Motil.* **2012**, *24*, 217–222. [CrossRef]
41. Tack, J. Gastric motor disorders. *Best Pract. Res. Clin. Gastroenterol.* **2007**, *21*, 633–644. [CrossRef] [PubMed]
42. Mayer, E.A.; Thompson, J.B.; Jehn, D.; Reedy, T.; Elashoff, J.; Meyer, J.H. Gastric emptying and sieving of solid food and pancreatic and biliary secretion after solid meals in patients with truncal vagotomy and antrectomy. *Gastroenterology* **1982**, *83 Pt 2*, 184–192.
43. Lawaetz, O.; Blackburn, A.M.; Bloom, S.R.; Aritas, Y.; Ralphs, D.N. Gut hormone profile and gastric emptying in the dumping syndrome. A hypothesis concerning the pathogenesis. *Scand. J. Gastroenterol.* **1983**, *18*, 73–80. [CrossRef] [PubMed]
44. Salehi, M.; Gastaldelli, A.; D'Alessio, D.A. Blockade of glucagon-like peptide 1 receptor corrects postprandial hypoglycemia after gastric bypass. *Gastroenterology* **2014**, *146*, 669–680. [CrossRef] [PubMed]
45. Toft-Nielsen, M.; Madsbad, S.; Holst, J.J. Exaggerated secretion of glucagon-like peptide-1 (GLP-1) could cause reactive hypoglycaemia. *Diabetologia* **1998**, *41*, 1180–1186. [CrossRef] [PubMed]
46. Eloy, R.; Garaud, J.C.; Moody, A.; Jaeck, D.; Grenier, J.F. Jejunal factor stimulating insulin release in the isolated perfused canine pancreas and jejunum. *Horm. Metab. Res.* **1975**, *7*, 461–467. [CrossRef]
47. Mehagnoul-Schipper, D.J.; Lenders, J.W.; Willemsen, J.J.; Hopman, W.P. Sympathoadrenal activation and the dumping syndrome after gastric surgery. *Clin. Auton. Res.* **2000**, *10*, 301–308. [CrossRef]

48. Holdsworth, C.D.; Turner, D.; McIntyre, N. Pathophysiology of post-gastrectomy hypoglycaemia. *Br. Med. J.* **1969**, *4*, 257–259. [CrossRef]
49. Hejazi, R.A.; Patil, H.; McCallum, R.W. Dumping syndrome: Establishing criteria for diagnosis and identifying new etiologies. *Dig. Dis. Sci.* **2010**, *55*, 117–123. [CrossRef]
50. Berg, P.; McCallum, R.; Hall, M.; Sarosiek, I. Dumping Syndrome: Updated Perspectives on Etiologies and Diagnosis. *Pract. Gastroenterol.* **2014**, *38*, 30–38.
51. Arts, J.; Caenepeel, P.; Bisschops, R.; Dewulf, D.; Holvoet, L.; Piessevaux, H.; Bourgeois, S.; Sifrim, D.; Janssens, J.; Tack, J. Efficacy of the long-acting repeatable formulation of the somatostatin analogue octreotide in postoperative dumping. *Clin. Gastroenterol. Hepatol.* **2009**, *7*, 432–437. [CrossRef] [PubMed]
52. Marsk, R.; Jonas, E.; Rasmussen, F.; Näslund, E. Nationwide cohort study of post-gastric bypass hypoglycaemia including 5,040 patients undergoing surgery for obesity in 1986–2006 in Sweden. *Diabetologia* **2010**, *53*, 2307–2311. [CrossRef] [PubMed]
53. Tack, J.; Bisschops, R.; Sarnelli, G. Pathophysiology and treatment of functional dyspepsia. *Gastroenterology* **2004**, *127*, 1239–1255. [CrossRef] [PubMed]
54. Bredenoord, A.J.; Chial, H.J.; Camilleri, M.; Mullan, B.P.; Murray, J.A. Gastric accommodation and emptying in evaluation of patients with upper gastrointestinal symptoms. *Clin. Gastroenterol. Hepatol.* **2003**, *1*, 264–272. [CrossRef]
55. Abell, T.L.; Camilleri, M.; Donohoe, K.; Hasler, W.L.; Lin, H.C.; Maurer, A.H.; McCallum, R.W.; Nowak, T.; Nusynowitz, M.L.; Parman, H.P.; et al. Consensus recommendations for gastric emptying scintigraphy: A joint report of the American Neurogastroenterology and Motility Society and the Society of Nuclear Medicine. *Am. J. Gastroenterol.* **2008**, *103*, 753–763. [CrossRef] [PubMed]
56. Tougas, G.; Eaker, E.Y.; Abell, T.L.; Abrahamsson, H.; Boivin, M.; Chen, J.; Hocking, M.P.; Quigley, E.M.; Koch, K.L.; Tokayer, A.Z.; et al. Assessment of gastric emptying using a low fat meal: Establishment of international control values. *Am. J. Gastroenterol.* **2000**, *95*, 1456–1462. [CrossRef] [PubMed]
57. Keller, J.; Bassotti, G.; Clarke, J.; Dinning, P.; Fox, M.; Grover, M.; Hellström, P.M.; Ke, M.; Layer, P.; Malagelada, C.; et al. Expert consensus document: Advances in the diagnosis and classification of gastric and intestinal motility disorders. *Nat. Rev. Gastroenterol. Hepatol.* **2018**, *15*, 291–308. [CrossRef]
58. Camilleri, M. Clinical practice. Diabetic gastroparesis. *N. Engl. J. Med.* **2007**, *356*, 820–829. [CrossRef]
59. de Zwart, I.M.; de Roos, A. MRI for the evaluation of gastric physiology. *Eur. Radiol.* **2010**, *20*, 2609–2616. [CrossRef]
60. Bradshaw, L.A.; Cheng, L.K.; Chung, E.; Obioha, C.B.; Erickson, J.C.; Gorman, B.L.; Somarajan, S.; Richars, W.O. Diabetic gastroparesis alters the biomagnetic signature of the gastric slow wave. *Neurogastroenterol. Motil.* **2016**, *28*, 837–848. [CrossRef]
61. Mine, S.; Sano, T.; Tsutsumi, K.; Murakami, Y.; Ehara, K.; Saka, M.; Hara, K.; Fukagawa, T.; Udagawa, H.; Katai, H. Large-scale investigation into dumping syndrome after gastrectomy for gastric cancer. *J. Am. Coll. Surg.* **2010**, *211*, 628–636. [CrossRef] [PubMed]
62. Ritz, P.; Hanaire, H. Post-bypass hypoglycaemia: A review of current findings. *Diabetes Metab.* **2011**, *37*, 274–281. [CrossRef] [PubMed]
63. van der Kleij, F.G.; Vecht, J.; Lamers, C.B.; Masclee, A.A. Diagnostic value of dumping provocation in patients after gastric surgery. *Scand. J. Gastroenterol.* **1996**, *31*, 1162–1166. [CrossRef] [PubMed]
64. Khoo, C.M.; Muehlbauer, M.J.; Stevens, R.D.; Pamuklar, Z.; Chen, J.; Newgard, C.B.; Torquati, A. Postprandial metabolite profiles reveal differential nutrient handling after bariatric surgery compared with matched caloric restriction. *Ann. Surg.* **2014**, *259*, 687–693. [CrossRef] [PubMed]
65. Emous, M.; Ubels, F.L.; van Beek, A.P. Diagnostic tools for post-gastric bypass hypoglycaemia. *Obes. Rev.* **2015**, *16*, 843–856. [CrossRef] [PubMed]
66. Waseem, S.; Moshiree, B.; Draganov, P.V. Gastroparesis: Current diagnostic challenges and management considerations. *World J. Gastroenterol.* **2009**, *15*, 25–37. [CrossRef]
67. Ogorek, C.P.; Davidson, L.; Fisher, R.S.; Krevsky, B. Idiopathic gastroparesis is associated with a multiplicity of severe dietary deficiencies. *Am. J. Gastroenterol.* **1991**, *86*, 423–428.
68. Parkman, H.P.; Yates, K.P.; Hasler, W.L.; Nguyan, L.; Pasricha, P.J.; Snape, W.J.; Farrugia, G.; Calles, J.; Koch, K.L.; Abell, T.L.; et al. Dietary intake and nutritional deficiencies in patients with diabetic or idiopathic gastroparesis. *Gastroenterology* **2011**, *141*, 486–498. [CrossRef]

69. Bytzer, P.; Talley, N.J.; Hammer, J.; Young, L.J.; Jones, M.P.; Horowitz, M. GI symptoms in diabetes mellitus are associated with both poor glycemic control and diabetic complications. *Am. J. Gastroenterol.* **2002**, *97*, 604–611. [CrossRef]
70. Quigley, E.M. Pharmacotherapy of gastroparesis. *Expert Opin. Pharmacother.* **2000**, *1*, 881–887. [CrossRef]
71. Patterson, D.; Abell, T.; Rothstein, R.; Koch, K.; Barnett, J. A double-blind multicenter comparison of domperidone and metoclopramide in the treatment of diabetic patients with symptoms of gastroparesis. *Am. J. Gastroenterol.* **1999**, *94*, 1230–1234. [PubMed]
72. McCallum, R.W.; Ricci, D.A.; Rakatansky, H.; Behar, J.; Rhodes, J.B.; Salen, G.; Deren, J.; Ippoliti, A.; Olsen, H.W.; Falchuk, K.; et al. A multicenter placebo-controlled clinical trial of oral metoclopramide in diabetic gastroparesis. *Diabetes Care* **1983**, *6*, 463–467. [CrossRef] [PubMed]
73. Janssen, P.; Harris, M.S.; Jones, M.; Masaoka, T.; Farre, R.; Törnblom, H.; Van Oudenhove, L.; Simren, M.; Tack, J. The relation between symptom improvement and gastric emptying in the treatment of diabetic and idiopathic gastroparesis. *Am. J. Gastroenterol.* **2013**, *108*, 1382–1391. [CrossRef] [PubMed]
74. Stanghellini, V.; Tack, J. Gastroparesis: Separate entity or just a part of dyspepsia? *Gut* **2014**, *63*, 1972–1978. [CrossRef] [PubMed]
75. Rao, A.S.; Camilleri, M. Review article: Metoclopramide and tardive dyskinesia. *Aliment. Pharmacol. Ther.* **2010**, *31*, 11–19. [CrossRef] [PubMed]
76. Richards, R.D.; Davenport, K.; McCallum, R.W. The treatment of idiopathic and diabetic gastroparesis with acute intravenous and chronic oral erythromycin. *Am. J. Gastroenterol.* **1993**, *88*, 203–207. [PubMed]
77. Pasricha, P.J.; Yates, K.P.; Sarosiek, I.; McCallum, R.W.; Abell, T.L.; Koch, K.L.; Nguyen, L.A.B.; Snape, W.J.; Hasler, W.L.; Clarke, J.O.; et al. Aprepitant Has Mixed Effects on Nausea and Reduces Other Symptoms in Patients With Gastroparesis and Related Disorders. *Gastroenterology* **2018**, *154*, 65–76. [CrossRef] [PubMed]
78. Braden, B.; Caspary, W.; Börner, N.; Vinson, B.; Schneider, A.R. Clinical effects of STW 5 (Iberogast) are not based on acceleration of gastric emptying in patients with functional dyspepsia and gastroparesis. *Neurogastroenterol. Motil.* **2009**, *21*, 632–638. [CrossRef] [PubMed]
79. Friedenberg, F.; Gollamudi, S.; Parkman, H.P. The use of botulinum toxin for the treatment of gastrointestinal motility disorders. *Dig. Dis. Sci.* **2004**, *49*, 165–175. [CrossRef] [PubMed]
80. Ezzeddine, D.; Jit, R.; Katz, N.; Gopalswamy, N.; Bhutani, M.S. Pyloric injection of botulinum toxin for treatment of diabetic gastroparesis. *Gastrointest. Endosc.* **2002**, *55*, 920–923. [CrossRef] [PubMed]
81. Lacy, B.E.; Zayat, E.N.; Crowell, M.D.; Schuster, M.M. Botulinum toxin for the treatment of gastroparesis: A preliminary report. *Am. J. Gastroenterol.* **2002**, *97*, 1548–1552. [CrossRef] [PubMed]
82. Miller, L.S.; Szych, G.A.; Kantor, S.B.; Bromer, M.Q.; Knight, L.C.; Maurer, A.H.; Fisher, R.S.; Parkman, H.P. Treatment of idiopathic gastroparesis with injection of botulinum toxin into the pyloric sphincter muscle. *Am. J. Gastroenterol.* **2002**, *97*, 1653–1660. [CrossRef] [PubMed]
83. Arts, J.; Holvoet, L.; Caenepeel, P.; Bisschops, R.; Sifrim, D.; Verbeke, K.; Janssens, J.; Tack, J. Clinical trial: A randomized-controlled crossover study of intrapyloric injection of botulinum toxin in gastroparesis. *Aliment. Pharmacol. Ther.* **2007**, *26*, 1251–1258. [CrossRef] [PubMed]
84. Friedenberg, F.K.; Palit, A.; Parkman, H.P.; Hanlon, A.; Nelson, D.B. Botulinum toxin A for the treatment of delayed gastric emptying. *Am. J. Gastroenterol.* **2008**, *103*, 416–423. [CrossRef] [PubMed]
85. Angeli, T.R.; Du, P.; Midgley, D.; Paskaranandavadivel, N.; Sathar, S.; Lahr, C.; Abell, T.L.; Cheng, L.K.; O'Grady, G. Acute Slow Wave Responses to High-Frequency Gastric Electrical Stimulation in Patients With Gastroparesis Defined by High-Resolution Mapping. *Neuromodulation* **2016**, *19*, 864–871. [CrossRef] [PubMed]
86. Abell, T.; McCallum, R.; Hocking, M.; Koch, K.; Abrahamsson, H.; Leblanc, I.; Lindberg, G.; Konturek, J.; Nowak, T.; Quigley, E.M.; et al. Gastric electrical stimulation for medically refractory gastroparesis. *Gastroenterology* **2003**, *125*, 421–428. [CrossRef]
87. Chu, H.; Lin, Z.; Zhong, L.; McCallum, R.W.; Hou, X. Treatment of high-frequency gastric electrical stimulation for gastroparesis. *J. Gastroenterol. Hepatol.* **2012**, *27*, 1017–1026. [CrossRef]
88. Khashab, M.A.; Ngamruengphong, S.; Carr-Locke, D.; Bapaye, A.; Benias, P.C.; Serouya, S.; Dorwat, S.; Chaves, D.M.; Artifon, E.; de Moura, E.G.; et al. Gastric per-oral endoscopic myotomy for refractory gastroparesis: Results from the first multicenter study on endoscopic pyloromyotomy (with video). *Gastrointest. Endosc.* **2017**, *85*, 123–128. [CrossRef]

89. Khashab, M.A.; Stein, E.; Clarke, J.O.; Saxena, P.; Kumbhari, V.; Chander Roland, B.; Kalloo, A.N.; Stavropoulos, S.; Pasricha, P.; Inoue, H. Gastric peroral endoscopic myotomy for refractory gastroparesis: First human endoscopic pyloromyotomy (with video). *Gastrointest. Endosc.* **2013**, *78*, 764–768. [CrossRef]
90. Dacha, S.; Mekaroonkamol, P.; Li, L.; Shahnavaz, N.; Sakaria, S.; Keilin, S.; Willingham, F.; Christie, J.; Cai, Q. Outcomes and quality-of-life assessment after gastric per-oral endoscopic pyloromyotomy (with video). *Gastrointest. Endosc.* **2017**, *86*, 282–289. [CrossRef]
91. Gonzalez, J.M.; Benezech, A.; Vitton, V.; Barthet, M. G-POEM with antro-pyloromyotomy for the treatment of refractory gastroparesis: Mid-term follow-up and factors predicting outcome. *Aliment. Pharmacol. Ther.* **2017**, *46*, 364–370. [CrossRef] [PubMed]
92. Gonzalez, J.M.; Lestelle, V.; Benezech, A.; Cohen, J.; Vitton, V.; Grimaud, J.C.; Barthet, M. Gastric per-oral endoscopic myotomy with antropyloromyotomy in the treatment of refractory gastroparesis: Clinical experience with follow-up and scintigraphic evaluation (with video). *Gastrointest. Endosc.* **2017**, *85*, 132–139. [CrossRef] [PubMed]
93. Rodriguez, J.H.; Haskins, I.N.; Strong, A.T.; Plescia, R.L.; Allemang, M.T.; Butler, R.S.; Cline, M.S.; El-Hayek, K.; Ponsky, J.L.; Kroh, M.D. Per oral endoscopic pyloromyotomy for refractory gastroparesis: Initial results from a single institution. *Surg. Endosc.* **2017**, *31*, 5381–5388. [CrossRef] [PubMed]
94. Gourcerol, G.; Tissier, F.; Melchior, C.; Touchais, J.Y.; Huet, E.; Prevost, G.; Leroi, A.M.; Ducrotte, P. Impaired fasting pyloric compliance in gastroparesis and the therapeutic response to pyloric dilatation. *Aliment. Pharmacol. Ther.* **2015**, *41*, 360–367. [CrossRef]
95. Hibbard, M.L.; Dunst, C.M.; Swanström, L.L. Laparoscopic and endoscopic pyloroplasty for gastroparesis results in sustained symptom improvement. *J. Gastrointest. Surg.* **2011**, *15*, 1513–1519. [CrossRef]
96. Felsher, J.; Chand, B.; Ponsky, J. Decompressive percutaneous endoscopic gastrostomy in nonmalignant disease. *Am. J. Surg.* **2004**, *187*, 254–256. [CrossRef]
97. Pittman, A.C.; Robinson, F.W. Dietary management of the "dumping" syndrome. Long-term follow-up. *J. Am. Diet. Assoc.* **1962**, *40*, 108–110.
98. Robinson, F.W.; Pittman, A.C. Dietary management of postgastrectomy dumping syndrome. *Surg. Gynecol. Obstet.* **1957**, *104*, 529–534.
99. Khoshoo, V.; Reifen, R.M.; Gold, B.D.; Sherman, P.M.; Pencharz, P.B. Nutritional manipulation in the management of dumping syndrome. *Arch. Dis. Child.* **1991**, *66*, 1447–1448. [CrossRef]
100. Kellogg, T.A.; Bantle, J.P.; Leslie, D.B.; Redmond, J.B.; Slusarek, B.; Swan, T.; Buchwald, H.; Ikramuddin, S. Postgastric bypass hyperinsulinemic hypoglycemia syndrome: Characterization and response to a modified diet. *Surg. Obes. Relat. Dis.* **2008**, *4*, 492–499. [CrossRef]
101. Ukleja, A. Dumping syndrome: Pathophysiology and treatment. *Nutr. Clin. Pract.* **2005**, *20*, 517–525. [CrossRef] [PubMed]
102. Jenkins, D.J.; Gassull, M.A.; Leeds, A.R.; Metz, G.; Dilawari, J.B.; Slavin, B.; Blendis, L.M. Effect of dietary fiber on complications of gastric surgery: Prevention of postprandial hypoglycemia by pectin. *Gastroenterology* **1977**, *73*, 215–217. [CrossRef]
103. Harju, E.; Larmi, T.K. Efficacy of guar gum in preventing the dumping syndrome. *JPEN J. Parenter. Enter. Nutr.* **1983**, *7*, 470–472. [CrossRef] [PubMed]
104. Kneepkens, C.M.; Fernandes, J.; Vonk, R.J. Dumping syndrome in children. Diagnosis and effect of glucomannan on glucose tolerance and absorption. *Acta Paediatr. Scand.* **1988**, *77*, 279–286. [CrossRef] [PubMed]
105. Ng, D.D.; Ferry, R.J.; Kelly, A.; Weinzimer, S.A.; Stanley, C.A.; Katz, L.E. Acarbose treatment of postprandial hypoglycemia in children after Nissen fundoplication. *J. Pediatr.* **2001**, *139*, 877–879. [CrossRef] [PubMed]
106. Ritz, P.; Vaurs, C.; Bertrand, M.; Anduze, Y.; Guillaume, E.; Hanaire, H. Usefulness of acarbose and dietary modifications to limit glycemic variability following Roux-en-Y gastric bypass as assessed by continuous glucose monitoring. *Diabetes Technol. Ther.* **2012**, *14*, 736–740. [CrossRef] [PubMed]
107. Speth, P.A.; Jansen, J.B.; Lamers, C.B. Effect of acarbose, pectin, a combination of acarbose with pectin, and placebo on postprandial reactive hypoglycaemia after gastric surgery. *Gut* **1983**, *24*, 798–802. [CrossRef] [PubMed]
108. McLoughlin, J.C.; Buchanan, K.D.; Alam, M.J. A glycoside-hydrolase inhibitor in treatment of dumping syndrome. *Lancet* **1979**, *2*, 603–605. [CrossRef]

109. Hasegawa, T.; Yoneda, M.; Nakamura, K.; Ohnishi, K.; Harada, H.; Kyouda, T.; Yoshida, Y.; Makino, I. Long-term effect of alpha-glucosidase inhibitor on late dumping syndrome. *J. Gastroenterol. Hepatol.* **1998**, *13*, 1201–1206. [CrossRef] [PubMed]
110. Didden, P.; Penning, C.; Masclee, A.A. Octreotide therapy in dumping syndrome: Analysis of long-term results. *Aliment. Pharmacol. Ther.* **2006**, *24*, 1367–1375. [CrossRef] [PubMed]
111. Penning, C.; Vecht, J.; Masclee, A.A. Efficacy of depot long-acting release octreotide therapy in severe dumping syndrome. *Aliment. Pharmacol. Ther.* **2005**, *22*, 963–969. [CrossRef] [PubMed]
112. Deloose, E.; Bisschops, R.; Holvoet, L.; Arts, J.; De Wulf, D.; Caenepeel, P.; Lannoo, M.; Vanuytsel, T.; Andrews, C.; Tack, J. A pilot study of the effects of the somatostatin analog pasireotide in postoperative dumping syndrome. *Neurogastroenterol. Motil.* **2014**, *26*, 803–809. [CrossRef] [PubMed]
113. Vilarrasa, N.; Goday, A.; Rubio, M.A.; Caixas, A.; Pellitero, S.; Ciudin, A.; Calanas, A.; Botella, J.I.; Breton, I.; Morales, M.J.; et al. Hyperinsulinemic Hypoglycemia after Bariatric Surgery: Diagnosis and Management Experience from a Spanish Multicenter Registry. *Obes. Facts* **2016**, *9*, 41–51. [CrossRef] [PubMed]

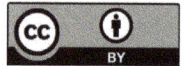

© 2019 by the authors. Licensee MDPI, Basel, Switzerland. This article is an open access article distributed under the terms and conditions of the Creative Commons Attribution (CC BY) license (http://creativecommons.org/licenses/by/4.0/).

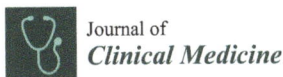

Review

Nutritional Risk Screening and Assessment

Emilie Reber [1,*,†], **Filomena Gomes** [2,†], **Maria F. Vasiloglou** [3], **Philipp Schuetz** [4,5] and **Zeno Stanga** [1]

1. Department of Diabetes, Endocrinology, Nutritional Medicine and Metabolism, Bern University Hospital, and University of Bern, Freiburgstrasse 15, 3010 Bern, Switzerland
2. The New York Academy of Sciences, 250 Greenwich Sweet, 40th floor, New York, NY 10007, USA
3. Diabetes Technology Research Group, ARTORG Center for Biomedical Engineering Research, University of Bern, Murtenstrasse 50, 3008 Bern, Switzerland
4. Medical University Department, Division of General Internal and Emergency Medicine, Kantonsspital Aarau, Tellstrasse 25, 5000 Aarau, Switzerland
5. Department for Clinical Research, Medical Faculty, University of Basel, 4001 Basel, Switzerland
* Correspondence: emilie.reber@insel.ch
† Contributed equally to this manuscript.

Received: 30 May 2019; Accepted: 9 July 2019; Published: 20 July 2019

Abstract: Malnutrition is an independent risk factor that negatively influences patients' clinical outcomes, quality of life, body function, and autonomy. Early identification of patients at risk of malnutrition or who are malnourished is crucial in order to start a timely and adequate nutritional support. Nutritional risk screening, a simple and rapid first-line tool to detect patients at risk of malnutrition, should be performed systematically in patients at hospital admission. Patients with nutritional risk should subsequently undergo a more detailed nutritional assessment to identify and quantify specific nutritional problems. Such an assessment includes subjective and objective parameters such as medical history, current and past dietary intake (including energy and protein balance), physical examination and anthropometric measurements, functional and mental assessment, quality of life, medications, and laboratory values. Nutritional care plans should be developed in a multidisciplinary approach, and implemented to maintain and improve patients' nutritional condition. Standardized nutritional management including systematic risk screening and assessment may also contribute to reduced healthcare costs. Adequate and timely implementation of nutritional support has been linked with favorable outcomes such as a decrease in length of hospital stay, reduced mortality, and reductions in the rate of severe complications, as well as improvements in quality of life and functional status. The aim of this review article is to provide a comprehensive overview of nutritional screening and assessment methods that can contribute to an effective and well-structured nutritional management (process cascade) of hospitalized patients.

Keywords: nutritional risk screening; nutritional assessment; malnutrition

1. Introduction

Nutrition is a basic need of life and thus plays an important role in health promotion and disease prevention. Nutritional intake and its controlling mechanisms (e.g., appetite, satiety) are highly complex physiological processes. These processes have a strong influence on nutritional status, which in turn depends on nutritional intake, its balanced supply of macro and micronutrients, and fluid intake. For various reasons, ill people may struggle to meet their nutritional and hydration requirements, and as a consequence, 20–50% of patients are malnourished or at high risk of malnutrition upon hospital admission [1]. One in five patients does not consume enough food to cover their energy or protein needs [2]. The underlying disease may directly impair nutritional intake and may induce metabolic and/or psychological disorders, which increase the nutritional needs or decrease food intake [3–5].

Frequent problems such as chewing and swallowing issues, immobility, and side effects of drugs and polypharmacy should not be underestimated in this regard [6,7]. A protracted decline in nutritional status results in a catabolic metabolism and chronic low-grade inflammation, potentially leading to several harmful consequences, such as loss of fat-free mass, immune dysfunction, higher complications and mortality rates, reduced quality of life, and prolonged hospital stays [8,9]. Malnutrition also influences the efficacy or tolerance of several treatments, such as antibiotic therapy, chemotherapy, radiotherapy, and surgery. The increased metabolism due to the stress of eventual surgical procedures further aggravates the nutritional metabolic risk, and is characterized by activation of the sympathetic nervous system, endocrine responses, and immunological and hematological changes—all leading to a hypermetabolic state, which may further increase patients' nutritional needs. In addition, the fasting periods before many examinations and interventions, as well as inappropriate meal services, inadequate quality and flexibility of hospital catering, and insufficient assistance provided by the health care staff to the most vulnerable patients, lead to further inadequate food intake and deterioration of patients' nutritional status.

Malnutrition should be considered and treated as an additional disease, as it has been shown to worsen clinical outcomes and to increase morbidity, mortality, and complication rates, thus causing additional costs [3,4,7,10–14]. However, malnutrition is preventable and mostly reversible with early adequate nutritional therapy. It often remains undetected due to lack of awareness, knowledge, and clinical protocols to identify and treat this problem within hospitals. The identification of malnutrition has typically been based on anthropometric, biochemical, and physical parameters, among others. However, there is currently no universally accepted gold standard (best method) for the assessment of nutritional status [15,16].

A systematic and standardized approach to identifying this condition is needed, and that is where nutritional screening tools play an important role [17]. When malnutrition is diagnosed, an individual nutritional care plan should be established by a nutrition specialist (e.g., dietitian, expert clinician) in consultation with a multidisciplinary team, and monitored regularly throughout the hospital stay. To improve the overall outcomes from nutritional treatment it is necessary to select patients with overt malnutrition, and those at most risk of developing nutritional deficiencies during their hospitalization. A systematic approach to addressing malnutrition in hospitals should start with the screening of all patients on admission, proceeding to a detailed assessment of nutritional status in those found to be at increased risk. In patients who are identified as malnourished or at nutritional risk, an appropriate nutritional intervention tailored to the individual patient's needs should follow. Unfortunately, although the need for this process is well-recognized and forms part of several national and international guidelines, it is not carried out everywhere. In the well-known cross-sectional "NutriDay" survey conducted in 2007–2008, 21,007 patients from 325 hospitals in 25 European countries were included. Results showed that a screening routine existed in only half (53%) of the hospitals in the different regions, mostly performed with locally developed methods. While the routine screening of patients for malnutrition on hospital admission existed for 93% of units in the United Kingdom, less than 33% of units had this practice in Austria, Germany, and the South Eastern region. In addition, more than a quarter of all patients (27%) were considered to be at risk of malnutrition, and energy goals were not met in almost half (43%) of the surveyed population [18]. It remains necessary to raise awareness of malnutrition and to improve the outcomes of patients' nutritional treatments.

We aimed to provide an extensive and critical overview of the nutritional screening and nutritional assessment methods of hospitalized patients, complemented by the description of the most novel technological approaches developed to improve the accuracy of dietary assessment. We hope that this review will be helpful to update clinicians involved in the nutritional care of this patient population.

2. Screening

Nutritional risk screening tools are very helpful in the daily routine to detect potential or manifest malnutrition in a timely manner. Such tools should be easy to use, quick, economical, standardized, and validated. Screening tools should be both sensitive and specific, and if possible, predictors of the success of the nutritional therapy. Nutritional screening should be part of a defined clinical protocol that results in a plan of action if the screening result is positive.

Diverse scores and screening systems were established in past decades for use in various clinical settings and patient populations (inpatients, community, geriatrics, etc.). Screening should be performed within the first 24–48 h after hospital admission and at regular intervals thereafter (e.g., weekly), in order to rapidly and accurately identify individuals who should be referred to the nutrition specialist (e.g., dietitian, expert clinician) for further assessment. Nutritional screening should include dynamic parameters rather than static ones—for example, recent weight loss, current body mass index (BMI), recent food intake, and disease severity. According to the systematic review conducted by van Bokhorst-de van der Schueren et al., at least 33 different nutritional risk screening tools exist [19]. The present work will use three as examples. The present work will use three examples thereof, which the European Society for Clinical Nutrition and Metabolism (ESPEN) recommends: the Nutritional Risk Screening 2002 (NRS-2002) for the inpatient setting, the Malnutrition Universal Screening Tool (MUST) for the ambulatory setting and the Mini Nutritional Assessment (MNA) for institutionalized geriatric patients [20].

One of the nutritional risk screening tools used most often in hospitals worldwide is the NRS-2002 (Table 1). The NRS-2002 was developed by Kondrup et al., and is meant to be a generic tool in the hospital setting—that is, useful in detecting most of the patients who would benefit from nutritional therapy [21]. This was recently shown in a large multicenter randomized controlled study in a medical inpatient population, which demonstrated a reduction of important clinical outcomes, including mortality, in patients at risk of malnutrition as determined by the NRS-2002 [22]. The NRS-2002 is a simple and well-validated tool which incorporates pre-screening with four questions. If one of these is answered positively, a screening follows which includes surrogate measures of nutritional status, with static and dynamic parameters and data on the severity of the disease (stress metabolism). For each parameter, a score from 0 to 3 can result. Age over 70 years is considered as a risk factor, and is included in the screening tool as well, giving 1 point. A total score of ≥3 points means that the patient is at risk of malnutrition or already malnourished and therefore a nutritional therapy is indicated. The NRS-2002 has been assessed and validated in hundreds of studies, including randomized controlled trials, and has been shown to be very reliable if administered by trained staff.

The MUST (Table 2) was developed to identify malnourished individuals in all care settings (hospitals, nursing homes, home care, etc.) [23]. It was the basis for the NRS-2002 [21]. Recent food intake is not included, and calculations of the weight loss percentage may be a barrier for the busy healthcare staff on the wards.

The MNA is the screening tool most frequently used in institutionalized geriatric patients (Table 3). It combines screening and assessment features. Unlike the NRS-2002, the MNA includes diverse components (loss of appetite, altered sense of taste and smell, loss of thirst, frailty, depression) often relevant for the nutritional status of older people. It also includes anthropometric measurements, nutritional habits, general condition, and self-evaluation. Both the MNA (complete form) as well as a short-form MNA (MNA-SF) are available. The complete MNA includes eighteen items in four domains (Appendix A). The MNA-SF includes only six items, but is quicker and as effective as the long version. If the total score is 11 points or less, the patient is considered at risk of malnutrition or malnourished and the full version (assessment) should be performed.

It is important for clinicians to understand how the tools were validated and for which population and care setting they were developed in order to determine if the tool is appropriate for use in their institution [24]. For example, a study that aimed to identify the most appropriate nutritional screening tool for predicting unfavorable clinical outcomes in 705 patients admitted to a Brazilian hospital compared the performance of NRS-2002, MNA-SF, and MUST. The authors observed that the NRS-2002 and MNA-SF had similar performance in predicting complications, very long length of hospital stay, and mortality, but the NRS-2002 had the best yield, and therefore recommended the use of this tool in the Brazilian inpatient population [25].

Table 1. Nutritional Risk Screening 2002. APACHE: acute physiology and chronic health evaluation; BMI: body mass index; COPD: chronic obstructive pulmonary disease; ONS: oral nutritional supplement.

Pre-Screening	
Is the BMI of the patient < 20.5 kg/m²	Yes
Did the patient lose weight in the past 3 months?	Yes
Was the patient's food intake reduced in the past week?	Yes
Is the patient critically ill?	Yes

If yes to one of those questions, proceed to screening.
If no for all answers, the patient should be re-screened weekly.

Screening			
Nutritional status	score	Stress metabolism (severity of the disease)	score
None	0	None	0
Mild Weight loss >5% in 3 months OR 50–75% of the normal food intake in the last week	1	Mild stress metabolism Patient is mobile Increased protein requirement can be covered with oral nutrition *Hip fracture, chronic disease especially with complications e.g., liver cirrhosis, COPD, diabetes, cancer, chronic hemodialysis*	1
Moderate Weight loss >5% in 2 months OR BMI 18.5–20.5 kg/m² AND reduced general condition OR 25–50% of the normal food intake in the last week	2	Moderate stress metabolism Patient is bedridden due to illness Highly increased protein requirement, may be covered with ONS *Stroke, hematologic cancer, severe pneumonia, extended abdominal surgery*	2
Severe Weight loss >5% in 1 month OR BMI <18.5 kg/m² AND reduced general condition OR 0–25% of the normal food intake in the last week	3	Severe stress metabolism Patient is critically ill (intensive care unit) Very strongly increased protein requirement can only be achieved with (par)enteral nutrition *APACHE-II >10, bone marrow transplantation, head traumas*	3
Total (A)		Total (B)	
Age			
<70 years: 0 pt			
≥70 years: 1 pt			
TOTAL = (A) + (B) + Age			
≥3 points: patient is at nutritional risk. Nutritional care plan should be set up			
<3 points: repeat screening weekly			

Table 2. The Malnutrition Universal Screening Tool.

Malnutrition Universal Screening Tool (MUST)			
BMI (kg/m^2)		Unintentional weight loss in the past 3–6 months		Acute illness with reduced food intake (estimated) for ≥5 days
≥20	0	≤5%	0	No = 0
18.5–20.0	1	5–10%	1	Yes = 2
≤18.5	2	≥10%	2	
Overall Risk for Malnutrition			
Total	Risk	Procedure	Implementation
0	Low	Routine clinical care	Clinic: weekly Nursing home: monthly Outpatient: yearly in at-risk patient groups, e.g., age >75 years
1	Medium	Observe	Clinic, nursing home, and outpatient: Document dietary intake for 3 days. If adequate: little concern and repeat screening (hospital weekly, care home at least monthly, community at least every 2–3 months). If inadequate: clinical concern. Follow local policy, set goals, improve and increase overall nutritional intake, monitor and review care plan regularly.
≥2	High	Treat	Clinic, nursing home, and outpatient: Refer to dietitian, Nutritional Support Team, or implement local policy. Set goals, improve and increase overall nutritional intake. Monitor and review care plan (hospital weekly, care home monthly, community monthly).

Table 3. The Mini Nutritional Assessment Short-Form.

	Screening		
A	Has food intake declined over the past 3 months due to loss of appetite, digestive problems, or chewing or swallowing difficulties?		0 = severe decrease in food intake 1 = moderate decrease in food intake 2 = no decrease in food intake
B	Weight loss during the last 3 months		0 = weight loss greater than 3 kg 1 = does not know 2 = weight loss between 1 and 3 kg 3 = no weight loss
C	Mobility		0 = bedridden or chair bound 1 = able to get out of bed/chair but does not go out 2 = goes out
D	Has the patient suffered psychological stress or acute disease in the past 3 months?		0 = yes 2 = no
E	Neuropsychological problems		0 = severe dementia or depression 1 = mild dementia 2 = no psychological problems
F1	Body mass index (BMI)		0 = BMI less than 19 1 = BMI 19 to less than 21 2 = BMI 21 to less than 23 3 = BMI 23 or greater
If BMI is not available, replace question F1 with F2. Do not answer F2 if F1 is already completed.			
F2	Calf circumference (CC) in cm		0 = CC less than 31 3 = CC 31 or greater
Screening Score			
12–14 points	Normal nutritional status		
8–11 points	At risk of malnutrition		
0–7 points	Malnourished		

3. Assessment

Nutritional assessment should be performed in patients identified as at nutritional risk according to the first step (i.e., screening for risk of malnutrition). Assessment allows the clinician to gather more information and conduct a nutrition-focused physical examination in order to determine if there is truly a nutrition problem, to name the problem, and to determine the severity of the problem [26]. The data collected in a nutritional assessment are often similar to data collected in the screening process, but in more depth. Screening assesses risk whereas assessment actually determines nutritional status [26]. The observation and documentation of oral nutritional intake, including qualitative and quantitative aspects, and measurement of energy, protein, and micronutrient intake, is an important part of nutritional assessment.

There is a limited number of tools used for the assessment of nutritional status. The most-used tool is the Subjective Global Assessment (SGA), which includes information on a medical history (weight loss; dietary intake change; gastrointestinal and functional impairment) and physical examination (loss of subcutaneous fat; muscle wasting; ankle edema, sacral edema, and ascites). Each patient is classified as either well nourished (SGA A), moderately or suspected of being malnourished (SGA B), or severely malnourished (SGA C). A limitation of using SGA is that it only classifies subjects into three general groups, and it does not reflect subtle changes in nutritional status. Furthermore, it is subjective, does not account for biochemical values (e.g., visceral protein levels), and its sensitivity, precision, and reproducibility over time have not been extensively studied in some patient populations. Thus, here we describe the several components that should be part of the nutritional assessment process and interpreted by specialized clinical staff (e.g., dietitians) [27–29].

Most of these components have limited sensitivity and specificity when used individually; therefore, methods for identifying malnourished patients require the use of several parameters and the clinical judgment of experienced and specialized clinical staff. Detailed evaluation leads to an understanding of the nature and cause of the nutrition-related problem, and will inform the design of a personalized nutritional care plan [30].

3.1. Anthropometric Measurements

3.1.1. Body Weight and Body Mass Index

Body weight, height, and the resulting BMI are important parameters which are relatively easy to obtain from patients with acute as well as chronic diseases. If height cannot be assessed (e.g., in bedridden patients or patients that are unable to stand), knee height or demi-span (also recommended by the MNA) may be used to estimate height by means of standard formulas [31,32]. The body weight measurement should be standardized (e.g., measured at the same time of day and with the same amount of light clothing) to obtain a reliable weight trend. The BMI is an indicator of chronic malnutrition. Europeans are considered underweight when BMI is <18.5 kg/m^2. BMI values under this cutoff are associated with poor outcome and higher mortality rates, as are BMI values greater than 30 kg/m^2 (typically classified as obesity). In older adults the cut-off for the definition of underweight is higher, that is, <22 kg/m^2, as carrying some extra weight seems to be protective in this population. However, the BMI has some limitations. For example, it may be biased by fluid overload and edemas, and does not describe body composition (for example, a high BMI can be seen in fat individuals and also in very muscular athletes). Thus, the BMI does not reflect potentially pathological weight loss nor the patient's actual food intake. Unintentional weight loss is paramount for the assessment of nutritional status, as it points to a catabolic metabolic situation and is associated with higher morbidity and mortality rates.

3.1.2. Skinfold Measurements

One of the easiest and lowest-priced non-invasive methods is the measurement of the circumference of a limb (e.g., mid-arm, calf) and of skinfold thickness (SFT). The subcutaneous fat tissues normally account for half of the entire body fat mass, and the measurement of SFT gives information on the energy stores of the body, mainly fat stores (i.e., triglycerides). To estimate the total amount of body fat, four skinfolds need to be measured [33]:

- Biceps skinfold (front side of the middle upper arm);
- Triceps skinfold (back side of the middle upper arm);
- Subscapular skinfold (under the lowest point of the shoulder blade); and
- Suprailiac skinfold (above the upper bone of the hip).

The measurement of SFT requires trained staff and defined conditions. The high interindividual variability is a clear disadvantage of this method, as age, gender, and ethnicity influence the fat mass. The mid-upper-arm muscle circumference (MAMC) reflects the muscle mass, while the mid-arm muscle area (MAMA) gives information about the muscle protein stores, as half of the body's proteins are stored in the skeletal muscles. The MAMA is calculated from the MAMC and the triceps SFT (MAMA = MAMC − (0.314 × SFT)). The decrease in MAMA shows the loss of muscle mass, as a mobilization of the endogenous proteins. This method is not reliable in patients with fluid overload, however, nor does it represent short-term modifications of the nutritional status. The reliability of both the SFT and the MAMA strongly depend on the reference values. For these reasons, triceps skin fold and MAMA are mostly used for research purposes and not in daily clinical routine, as they give validated data—especially when measurements are performed by the same investigator and repeated in a given time period.

3.1.3. Body Composition

Body weight—including weight loss, calculation of the BMI, and measurement of the length, circumference, or thickness of various body parts—is useful for the assessment of nutritional status. Body composition describes the body compartments, such as fat mass, fat-free mass, muscle mass, and bone mineral mass, depending on the body composition model used (Figure 1). Body composition measurements may serve as an early diagnostic tool, as quantification, or as a follow-up method that helps to assess nutritional status [34]. Such measurements contribute to the diagnosis of sarcopenia and sarcopenic adiposity, and may establish reference values (energy expenditure/kg fat-free mass (FFM) or power/g muscle). Body composition may change due to disease, age, physical activity, and starvation. There are several methods available to determinate body composition, more or less invasively, as described in the following section (Table 4).

3.1.4. Bioelectrical Impedance Analysis (BIA)

Bioelectrical impedance analysis (BIA) is a simple, inexpensive, non-invasive method of estimating body composition. It is suitable for bedside measurements which depend on the body's proportions of fat, muscle, and water. BIA relies on the conduction of an alternating electrical current by the human body. The current passes easily through tissues containing a lot of water and electrolytes like blood and muscles, whereas fat tissues, air, and bone are harder to pass through. Therefore, the larger the fat-free mass, the greater the capacity of the body to conduct the current. BIA gives good information about total body water, body cell mass, and fat mass when correcting for age, sex, and ethnicity. However, BIA is not recommended in patients with fluid overload, in patients at extremes of BMI (<16 or >34 kg/m^2), in intensive care unit patients, or in the elderly [35,36]. The newly developed bioelectrical impedance vector analysis (BIVA) provides information about hydration status, body cell mass, and cell integrity through the vector length and position. Both malnutrition and obesity are clearly reflected by BIVA, making it attractive to assess and monitor patients' nutritional status.

3.1.5. Creatinine Height Index (CHI)

Creatine is metabolized to creatinine at a more or less stable rate, and reflects the amount of muscle mass [37]. Creatinine excretion correlates with lean body mass and body weight. The creatinine height index (CHI) [38] is a measure of lean body mass and is calculated as follows: CHI (%) = measured 24 h urinary creatinine × 100/normal 24 h urinary creatinine. Urinary creatinine excretion may be influenced by several factors, such as renal insufficiency, meat consumption, physical activity, fever, infections, and trauma. Additionally, the collection of 24-h urine is challenging in daily practice and further limits the use of this method.

3.1.6. Dual Energy X-ray Absorptiometry (DXA)

DXA is currently considered the gold standard of body composition measurement. It is increasingly used in clinical practice and in research, despite some exposure to radiation. DXA depends on radiological density analysis (usually in the hip and spine) and is a useful, indirect method of measuring fat mass, fat-free mass, and bone mineral mass.

3.1.7. Magnetic Resonance Tomography (MRT) and Computed Tomography (CT)

Magnetic resonance tomography (MRT) and computed tomography (CT) allow the quantification of fat mass and fat-free mass, giving information about the fat distribution and enabling an estimation of skeletal muscle mass. Unlike CT, MRT does not require ionizing radiation. These two methods are mainly used in research due to their restricted availability, their cost, and the time expended [39]. However, it is often possible to obtain nutritional information from scans taken for general diagnostic purposes.

3.1.8. Further Methods Used to Measure Body Composition

Several other methods are available, mainly for research purposes due to their complexity. These demanding and expensive methods include air displacement plethysmography (ADP), dilution methods, the measurement of total body potassium, and in vivo neutron activation analysis [40].

Air displacement plethysmography (ADP) is a method to determine the body density (body weight/body volume). It is based on the determination of the body volume by means of air displacement having regard to the residual air volume in the lungs and the gastrointestinal tract. Since the density of fat differs from the density of fat free mass, they can both be determined using a two-compartment model. ADP may also be used in ill patients, unlike other densitometry measurement using hydrodensitometry.

The dilution methods aim to determinate the total body water by means of dilution of non-radioactive isotopes (e.g., deuterium). Such tracers are given orally or parenterally, and their concentrations in urine and blood are measured after a defined time. Extracellular water can then be determined using bromide or sulfate, allowing the definition of intracellular water.

Since potassium is mostly found intracellularly and the natural isotope K^{40} is present in constant fraction, the measurement of the potassium allows the calculation of the body cell mass and thus enables the very accurate determination of the body cell mass.

With the in vivo neutron activation, the body is irradiated with neutron radiation, inducing the emission of a characteristic spectrum of gamma-radiations. This expensive method allows the quantification of single elements such as nitrogen, calcium, sodium, etc.

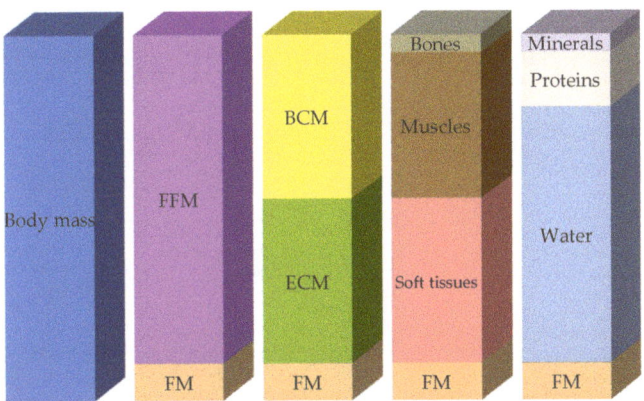

Figure 1. Compartment models of body composition. FFM: fat-free mass, FM: fat mass, BCM: body cell mass, ECM: extracellular cell mass. Modified after [40].

Table 4. Advantages and disadvantages of methods used to assess body composition.

Method	Target	Precision	Expenditure (Time/Apparatus)	Costs
Anthropometrics	FM, fat distribution, MM	↓	↓	↓↓
Bioelectrical impedance analysis	TBW, FM, FFM, BCM phase angle	↑	↓	↓
Creatinine height index	MM	↓	-	↓
Dual energy X-ray absorptiometry	FM, bone mineral content, soft tissues, bone density	↑	↑	↑
Magnetic resonance tomography	MM, FM, fat distribution	↑	↑	↑↑
Computed tomography	FM, fat distribution, MM	↑	↑	↑
Dilution method	TBW, FM, FFM (deuterium) ECW, ICW (bromide)	↑	↑	-
Potassium count	BCM, FFM, FM	↑	↑	↑↑
Neutron activation	Ca, Na, Cl, PO$_4$, N, H, O, C	↑	↑	↑↑

FM: fat mass; FFM: fat-free mass; MM: muscle mass; TBW: total body water; BCM: body cell mass; ECW: extracellular water; ICW: intracellular water; Ca: calcium; Na: sodium; Cl: chloride; PO$_4$: phosphate; N: nitrogen; H: hydrogen; O: oxygen; C: carbon.

3.2. Biochemical Analysis

There is no single parameter that can thoroughly assess nutritional status or monitor nutritional therapy. However, a set of laboratory parameters in the clinical routine (e.g., complete blood count, lipid profile, electrolytes, liver parameters) may provide valuable information about a patient's nutritional status (e.g., proof of nutrient deficiency, information about the etiology of malnutrition, follow-up nutritional therapy), about the severity and activity of the disease, and about changes in body composition (Table 5) [41]. Laboratory values—particularly in chronically malnourished patients—may help to detect deficiencies in vitamins (C, D, E, K, thiamine, B6, B12, and folic acid) and trace elements (zinc, selenium, and iron) and help to monitor current substitution therapies. In the early phase of refeeding, potassium, phosphate, and magnesium deficiencies may occur, potentially leading to severe complications (e.g., refeeding syndrome); hence, there is a need for close monitoring of these electrolytes.

Table 5. Laboratory values to detect malnutrition and monitor nutritional status [41].

Laboratory Value	Nutrition Independent Factors	Half-Life	Appropriateness to Detect Malnutrition	Appropriateness to Monitor Nutritional Therapy
Albumin	↑ dehydration ↓ inflammation, infections, trauma, heart failure, edema, liver dysfunction, nephrotic syndrome	20 d	+/++ Not appropriate in case of anorexia and acute illness	Not appropriate due to high suggestibility and long half-life
Transferrin	↑ renal failure, iron status, acute hepatitis, hypoxia ↓ inflammation, chronic infections hemochromatosis, nephrotic syndrome, liver dysfunction	10 d	+ Low sensitivity and specificity	+ Concentration is independent of the energy and protein intake
Prealbumin/Transthyretin (TTR)	↑ renal dysfunction, dehydration, corticosteroid therapy ↓ inflammation, hyperthyreosis, liver disease, overhydration	2 d	++ Not appropriate to detect anorexia Subnormal values within one week in case of fasting	++/+++ One of the most appropriate proteins
Retinol binding protein (RBP)	↑ kidney failure, alcohol abuse ↓ hyperthyreosis, chronic liver diseases, vitamin A deficiency, selenium deficiency	12 h	Idem prealbumin	Idem prealbumin
Insulin-like growth factor 1 (IGF-1)	↑ kidney failure ↓ liver diseases, severe catabolic status, age	24 h	++ Rapid decrease in fasting periods	+++ More specific than retinol-binding protein and prealbumin/transthyretin
Urinary creatinine	↑ collection time >24h, infection, trauma ↓ insufficient collection time, acute kidney failure	-	1 mmol of creatinine is derived from 1.9 kg of skeletal muscle mass	Not appropriate, very slow
Lymphocytes	↑ healing phase after infection, hematologic diseases ↓ sepsis, hematologic disease, immune suppressants, steroids	-	+ Very unspecific	Not appropriate, very slow

Laboratory values are mostly delayed and costly, and largely dependent on the analytic method and the analyzing laboratory. Additionally, numerous non-nutrition-related factors may influence the laboratory parameters (e.g., inflammatory markers such as CRP), leading to distorted values. Thus, laboratory values must always be interpreted within the clinical context.

3.3. Clinical Evaluation

3.3.1. Patient Clinical History

The patient's clinical history is a subjective and retrospective description of the patient's condition. It is the starting point of the nutritional assessment. Factors leading to malnutrition such as pain, gastrointestinal symptoms (e.g., diarrhea, vomiting, constipation), weight loss, loss of appetite, inability to chew or swallow, and poor dentition/oral health are discussed with the patient. The patient's clinical history should include previous medical condition (chronic or acute disease, symptoms of psychiatric illness, presence of conditions that may lead to metabolic stress (e.g., infection), as well as the actual functional capacity and physiological changes possibly influencing nutritional requirements or body composition (e.g., loss of muscle mass).

3.3.2. Physical Examination

Physical examination is an objective method of detecting clinical signs and symptoms of nutritional deficiencies of vitamins and minerals (e.g., poor muscle control, night vision impairment, vertical lip cracks, depression), and allows the assessment of tolerance to nutritional support (e.g., abdominal distention, vomiting, diarrhea) [42]. Some clinical signs are specific to a specific disease or nutrient deficiency. Others are non-specific and need further tests to elucidate their etiology (Table 6). Physical examination includes the control of vital parameters, the inspection and palpation for water retention (edema and ascites), and a rough assessment of muscle mass and subcutaneous fat stores.

Table 6. Clinical signs and symptoms of micronutrient deficiencies [40,42].

Body Region	Signs	Possible Deficiencies
Skin	Petechiae	Vitamins A, C
	Purpura	Vitamins C, K
	Pigmentation	Niacin
	Edema	Protein, vitamin B1
	Pallor	Folic acid, iron, biotin, vitamins B12, B6
	Decubitus	Protein, energy
	Seborrheic dermatitis	Vitamin B6, biotin, zinc, essential fatty acids
	Unhealed wounds	Vitamin C, protein, zinc
Nails	Pallor or white coloring	
	Clubbing, spoon-shape, or transverse ridging/banding; excessive dryness, darkness in nails, curved nail ends	Iron, protein, vitamin B12
Head/Hair	Dull/lackluster; banding/sparse; alopecia; depigmentation of hair; scaly/flaky scalp	Protein and energy, biotin, copper, essential fatty acid
Eyes	Pallor conjunctiva	Vitamin B12, folic acid, iron
	Night vision impairment	Vitamin A
	Photophobia	Zinc
Oral cavity	Glossitis	Vitamins B2, B6, B12, niacin, iron, folic acid
	Gingivitis	Vitamin C
	Fissures, stomatitis	Vitamin B2, iron, protein
	Cheilosis	Niacin, vitamins B2, B6, protein
	Pale tongue	Iron, vitamin B12
	Atrophied papillae	Vitamin B2, niacin, iron
Nervous system	Mental confusion	Vitamins B1, B2, B12, water
	Depression, lethargy	Biotin, folic acid, vitamin C
	Weakness, leg paralysis	Vitamins B1, B6, B12, pantothenic acid
	Peripheral neuropathy	Vitamins B2, B6, B12
	Ataxia	Vitamin B12
	Hyporeflexia	Vitamin B1
	Muscle cramps	Vitamin B6, calcium, magnesium
	Fatigue	Energy, biotin, magnesium, iron

3.3.3. Physical Function

Functional measurements are increasingly important in nutritional assessment. Indeed, muscle strength and cognitive functions all influence quality of life. Energy deficiency diminishes muscle strength and power, as well as overall physical condition. It is therefore very relevant to have information about muscle function and strength in the clinical setting. Muscle function tests are very sensitive to nutritional deficiencies, and therefore also to nutritional interventions. Changes can therefore be noticed much earlier than through body composition tests, for example. Hand dynamometry has been validated as a nutritional marker, correlates very well with the nutritional status, and is simultaneously a good predictor of surgical outcome, increased hospital length of stay, higher re-hospitalization rates, and decreased physical status. It is additionally a good predictor for short- and long-term mortality [43]. This test is easy, quick, and low-priced, but largely depends on the patient's cooperation. Other possible measurements are knee extension, hip flexion strength, or peak expiratory flow. Measurement of the distance walked in a given time (e.g., at a 4-m gait speed) may also provide good information on the global condition [44].

3.3.4. Medication

A patient's prescribed medications (including vitamin/mineral/botanical supplements) should be examined regarding potential drug–nutrient interactions and nutrition-related side effects (interactions with appetite, gastrointestinal function or symptoms).

3.4. Dietary History, Current Dietary Intake, and Innovative Dietary Assessment Methods

The dietary history includes the patient's dietary habits and preferences, including cultural and religious habits, special diets, as well as food allergies or intolerances. Fluid and alcohol intake should also be recorded.

The energy and protein balance and the comparison between food intake and energy expenditure reflect the current nutritional status—whether the patient's dietary intake is sufficient or not.

The quantification of food intake is one of the key approaches to assessing nutritional risk in individual patients. The assessment of macronutrients (fat, carbohydrates, and proteins) is as important as the assessment of micronutrients (vitamins, trace elements). There are numerous standardized methods of measuring food intake, such as 24 h food recall, food frequency questionnaires, and direct observation (food records are frequently used by nurses for institutionalized patients). These provide (semi-) quantitative information. The accurate assessment of food intake is difficult and error-prone. There is a growing need for more accurate dietary assessment methods. High-quality data are essential for research on the association between diet and health, for an understanding of dietary patterns, and for the identification of nutrition-related health problems [45].

Innovative technologies that improve dietary assessment have been proposed recently, and can be classified into four principal groups according to the technological features that each of them incorporate [46–50]:

- *Manual dietary assessment*—The user inserts all required data (e.g., portion size estimation, type of food) on a web page, smartphone app, etc. [50]. This method replaces the paper-based methods of dietary assessment into an electronic form by the use of pictures, video, text, or voice without the inclusion of automatic features.
- *Dietitian-supported assessment*—The user takes photos of the food and sends them to the dietitian. These data are then analyzed by nutrition experts who use standardized methods (e.g., nutritional software) to estimate the corresponding amount of nutrients [51]. No automation features are usually incorporated.
- *Wearable devices monitoring food intake*—Devices that directly measure eating behavior [52], such as detection systems which identify eating gestures (ear-based chewing and swallowing) in order to complement self-reporting of nutrient intake.
- *Computer-aided assessment*—this includes:

    (i) Systems that incorporate some degree of automation. These either use bar-code readers in order to automatically recognize packaged food labels [50], or utilize smartphone applications that integrate the automatic recognition of food items. In this case, the user takes photos of the food and the system recognizes the type of food. Typically, in this situation the user needs to manually insert or select the volume/portion of the food items in order for the system to be able to translate the information into macronutrients and energy [53].

    (ii) Systems that are completely based on artificial intelligence. In a typical scenario, the user takes photo(s) of the food and then the system automatically and in real-time identifies the different food items (identification), recognizes the type of each of them (labeling), and creates a 3D model of each of them (3D reconstruction) [54–58]. Supported by food composition databases, food images are translated into nutrient values such as grams of macronutrients or calories [54,56].

These new technologies have several advantages. They do not (fully) rely on a respondent's memory; they are based on a number of automatic data-processing steps, thus minimizing user-related variability [45]; there is minimal participant burden; and there are reduced research and administrative costs [50]. Additionally, these technologies offer portability and greater social acceptability than paper-based methods [59]. Some additional advantages of computer-aided methods include decreased workload and costs (excluding costs for software development) [48], minimization of researchers' transcription errors [60], reduced paper waste and postage costs, and the optimization of space, security, and organization required for paper file storage [61].

However, there are also some limitations for each group. The manual dietary assessment methods provide all the disadvantages of paper-based methods except for expenditures related to paper usage. Body sensor monitoring provides no input about the type or quality of the food that is captured [50]. What is more, dietician-supported assessment is labor-intense and expensive to analyze [50]. Moreover, with the AI-based systems, it is not possible to capture all the basic nutrient information (including cooking methods) with one single image [45], and the majority of the existing apps are manual or semi-automatic in terms of food logging, and non-automatic in portion size estimation. Individuals tend to estimate portion size inaccurately [62]; almost half of the errors found in food records are attributed to such faulty estimations [63]. Other possible disadvantages are under-reporting due to either poor image quality or user negligence in taking an adequate number of pictures before and after food and drink consumption [64]. In addition, some food types such as mixed foods or liquids are difficult to analyze with automated image analysis [58]. Tools that include only some AI components are usually non-validated; they include a limited number of food categories, and questions relating to the used nutrient databases arise [50]. The most important limitation of the majority of these technologies is the need for a tech-savvy user [45].

Several studies have compared dietary assessment by traditional methods versus innovative technologies. Some of them conclude that electronic records would be a useful tool, both for large-scale epidemiological studies and in the clinical context [61]. Others conclude that apps could replace the traditional 24-h recall and serve as feasible tools for dieticians investigating dietary intake at a population level [65]. The longer the app recording periods are, the better the correlation between the traditional and the innovative methods seems to be [66]. However, novel technologies for dietary assessment appear valid at the population level rather than for individualized support [67–69]. Even though there are an increasing number of studies in the domain of innovative technologies, sample sizes are relatively low, and duration is usually short. Therefore, there is a need for well-designed long-term studies to explore and analyze the combination of traditional methods and state-of-the-art technological tools which characterizes the new era of nutritional assessment.

Energy requirements are calculated from the basal energy requirement multiplied by an activity factor. They can be calculated with formulae (e.g., the Harris–Benedict formula [70]) or through a simplified general rule based on energy values between 25–35 kcal per kg of body weight per day, with adjustment for underweight and overweight patients (30 × body weight, +20% if BMI <20 kg/m^2 or −20% if BMI >30 kg/m^2) [71]. These formulae cannot be used in special situations (e.g., in ICU patients). The protein requirement may be estimated by using 1.2–1.5 g/kg body weight per day (0.8 g/kg/d in case of chronic kidney failure) [22]. The specific macronutrient requirements are described in Table 7. Indirect calorimetry remains the gold standard for the assessment of energy requirements, but in many clinical settings this option is not available, as indirect calorimeters may not be easy to operate and may not be portable or affordable.

Table 7. Macronutrient requirements for adults.

Macronutrient	Energy Content/g	Recommended Amount/kg Body Weight/d
Proteins	4 kcal	1.0–1.5 g
Carbohydrates	4 kcal	max. 3–5 g
Fats	9 kcal	0.8–1.5 g

Several conditions may impair food intake and should be taken into account as well. Among these are chewing and/or swallowing problems and functional limitations impairing independent eating. Additionally, cognitive changes affecting appetite and ability to feed oneself, and physiological changes that affect the desire to eat, may negatively impact the dietary intake.

3.5. Quality of Life

The assessment of quality of life is a more subjective parameter that is being increasingly included in nutritional assessment. It reflects the current health status, and may be used as an outcome parameter to monitor nutritional therapy. It is based on the perception of wellbeing in different domains—for example, symptoms (pain), physical (mobility, strength), psychological (anxiety, depression), and social (isolation), all potentially having an effect on eating. There are many questionnaires available, but there is no established consensus on which should optimally be used.

4. Conclusions and Outlook

Malnutrition is a frequent threat in hospitals, and is associated with negative outcomes. However, it remains a mostly treatable condition when there is adequate nutritional management. It is crucial to identify patients who are at nutritional risk or malnourished as early as possible, allowing the start of timely and effective nutritional support. Identifying patients at risk of malnutrition is the first step in the nutritional care process within a multimodal care system. Nutritional risk screening with simple and rapid tools should be performed systematically in each patient at hospital admission to detect patients who are nutritionally at risk or malnourished. Comprehensive detailed nutritional assessment should be performed thereafter in those patients identified as at risk of malnutrition or who are malnourished. This screening should be performed by a specialist (e.g., a dietician) using subjective and objective parameters such as clinical history, physical examination, body composition measurements, functional assessment, and laboratory values. New assessment methods may be very helpful, as they are accurate and quick. A nutritional care plan should be drawn up using an interdisciplinary approach and implemented to improve the patient's condition. Systematic nutritional risk screening and standardized nutritional management may also contribute to reduced healthcare costs.

Author Contributions: Conceptualization, E.R. and Z.S.; writing—original draft preparation E.R. and F.G.; writing—review and editing, M.V., P.S., and Z.S.; supervision, Z.S.

Funding: The APC was funded by the Research Fund of the Department of Diabetes, Endocrinology, Nutritional Medicine and Metabolism and in part by Nestlé Health Science (grant to the institution).

Conflicts of Interest: The authors declare no conflicts of interest.

Appendix A

Table A1. MNA full screening tool.

	Screening	
A	Has food intake declined over the past 3 months due to loss of appetite, digestive problems, chewing or swallowing difficulties?	0 = severe decrease in food intake 1 = moderate decrease in food intake 2 = no decrease in food intake
B	Weight loss during the past 3 months	0 = weight loss greater than 3 kg 1 = does not know 2 = weight loss between 1 and 3 kg 3 = no weight loss

Table A1. Cont.

C	Mobility	0 = bedridden or chair bound 1 = able to get out of bed/chair but does not go out 2 = goes out
D	Has suffered psychological stress or acute disease in the past 3 months?	0 = yes 2 = no
E	Neuropsychological problems	0 = severe dementia or depression 1 = mild dementia 2 = no psychological problems
F1	Body mass index (BMI)	0 = BMI less than 19 1 = BMI 19 to less than 21 2 = BMI 21 to less than 23 3 = BMI 23 or greater
	Screening Score (subtotal max. 14 points)	
12–14 points	Normal nutritional status	
8–11 points	At risk of malnutrition	
0–7 points	Malnourished	
For a more in-depth assessment, continue with questions G-R		
	Assessment	
G	Lives independently (not in nursing home or hospital)	0 = yes 1 = no
H	Takes more than 3 prescription drugs per day	0 = yes 1 = no
I	Pressure sores or skin ulcers	0 = yes 1 = no
J	How many full meals does the patient eat daily?	0 = 1 meal 1 = 2 meals 2 = 3 meals
K	Selected consumption markers for protein intake • Meat, fish or poultry every day • ≥1 serving of dairy products (milk, cheese, yoghurt) per day • ≥2 servings of legumes or eggs per week	0.0 = if 0 or 1 yes 0.5 = if 2 yes 1.0 = if 3 yes Yes/No Yes/No Yes/No
L	Consumes ≥2 servings of fruit or vegetables per day?	0 = yes 1 = no
M	How much fluid (water, juice, coffee, tea, milk…) is consumed per day?	0.0 = less than 3 cups 0.5 = 3 to 5 cups 1.0 = more than 5 cups
N	Mode of feeding	0 = unable to eat without assistance 1 = self-fed with some difficulty 2 = self-fed without any problem
O	Self view of nutritional status	0 = views self as being malnourished 1 = is uncertain of nutritional status 2 = views self as having no nutritional problem
P	In comparison with other people of the same age, how does the patient consider his/her health status?	0.0 = not as good 0.5 = does not know 1.0 = as good 2.0 = better
Q	Mid-arm circumference (MAC) in cm	0.0 = MAC less than 21 0.5 = MAC 21 to 22 1.0 = MAC greater than 22
R	Calf circumference (CC) in cm	0 = CC less than 31 1 = CC 31 or greater
	Malnutrition Indicator Score	
24–30 points	Normal nutritional status	
17–23.5 points	At risk of malnutrition	
<17 points	Malnourished	

References

1. Sorensen, J.; Kondrup, J.; Prokopowicz, J.; Schiesser, M.; Krahenbuhl, L.; Meier, R.; Liberda, M.; EuroOOPS Study Group. EuroOOPS: An international, multicentre study to implement nutritional risk screening and evaluate clinical outcome. *Clin. Nutr.* **2008**, *27*, 340–349. [CrossRef]
2. Dupertuis, Y.M.; Kossovsky, M.P.; Kyle, U.G.; Raguso, C.A.; Genton, L.; Pichard, C. Food intake in 1707 hospitalised patients: A prospective comprehensive hospital survey. *Clin. Nutr.* **2003**, *22*, 115–123. [CrossRef]
3. Schwegler, I.; von Holzen, A.; Gutzwiller, J.P.; Schlumpf, R.; Muhlebach, S.; Stanga, Z. Nutritional risk is a clinical predictor of postoperative mortality and morbidity in surgery for colorectal cancer. *Br. J. Surg.* **2010**, *97*, 92–97. [CrossRef]
4. Sun, Z.; Kong, X.J.; Jing, X.; Deng, R.J.; Tian, Z.B. Nutritional Risk Screening 2002 as a predictor of postoperative outcomes in patients undergoing abdominal surgery: A systematic review and meta-analysis of prospective cohort studies. *PLoS ONE* **2015**, *10*, e0132857. [CrossRef]
5. Imoberdorf, R.; Meier, R.; Krebs, P.; Hangartner, P.J.; Hess, B.; Staubli, M.; Wegmann, D.; Rühlin, M.; Ballmer, P.E. Prevalence of undernutrition on admission to Swiss hospitals. *Clin. Nutr.* **2010**, *29*, 38–41. [CrossRef]
6. Studley, H.O. Percentage of weight loss: A basic indicator of surgical risk in patients with chronic peptic ulcer. 1936. *Nutr Hosp.* **2001**, *16*, 141–143.
7. Meguid, M.M.; Debonis, D.; Meguid, V.; Hill, L.R.; Terz, J.J. Complications of abdominal operations for malignant disease. *Am. J. Surg.* **1988**, *156*, 341–345. [CrossRef]
8. Pikul, J.; Sharpe, M.D.; Lowndes, R.; Ghent, C.N. Degree of preoperative malnutrition is predictive of postoperative morbidity and mortality in liver transplant recipients. *Transplantation* **1994**, *57*, 469–472. [CrossRef]
9. Soeters, P.B.; Schols, A.M. Advances in understanding and assessing malnutrition. *Curr. Opin. Clin. Nutr. Metab. Care* **2009**, *12*, 487–494. [CrossRef]
10. Guo, W.; Ou, G.; Li, X.; Huang, J.; Liu, J.; Wei, H. Screening of the nutritional risk of patients with gastric carcinoma before operation by NRS 2002 and its relationship with postoperative results. *J. Gastroenterol. Hepatol.* **2010**, *25*, 800–803. [CrossRef]
11. Lieffers, J.R.; Bathe, O.F.; Fassbender, K.; Winget, M.; Baracos, V.E. Sarcopenia is associated with postoperative infection and delayed recovery from colorectal cancer resection surgery. *Br. J. Cancer* **2012**, *107*, 931–936. [CrossRef]
12. Schiesser, M.; Kirchhoff, P.; Muller, M.K.; Schafer, M.; Clavien, P.A. The correlation of nutrition risk index, nutrition risk score, and bioimpedance analysis with postoperative complications in patients undergoing gastrointestinal surgery. *Surgery* **2009**, *145*, 519–526. [CrossRef]
13. Schiesser, M.; Muller, S.; Kirchhoff, P.; Breitenstein, S.; Schafer, M.; Clavien, P.A. Assessment of a novel screening score for nutritional risk in predicting complications in gastro-intestinal surgery. *Clin. Nutr.* **2008**, *27*, 565–570. [CrossRef]
14. Sungurtekin, H.; Sungurtekin, U.; Balci, C.; Zencir, M.; Erdem, E. The influence of nutritional status on complications after major intraabdominal surgery. *J. Am. Coll. Nutr.* **2004**, *23*, 227–232. [CrossRef]
15. Donini, L.M.; Savina, C.; Rosano, A.; Cannella, C. Systematic review of nutritional status evaluation and screening tools in the elderly. *J. Nutr. Health. Aging* **2007**, *11*, 421–432.
16. Foley, N.C.; Salter, K.L.; Robertson, J.; Teasell, R.W.; Woodbury, M.G. Which reported estimate of the prevalence of malnutrition after stroke is valid? *Stroke* **2009**, *40*, E66–E74. [CrossRef]
17. Bauer, J.M.; Kaiser, M.J.; Sieber, C.C. Evaluation of nutritional status in older persons: Nutritional screening and assessment. *Curr. Opin. Clin. Nutr. Metab. Care* **2010**, *13*, 8–13. [CrossRef]
18. Schindler, K.; Pernicka, E.; Laviano, A.; Howard, P.; Schutz, T.; Bauer, P.; Grecu, I.; Jonkers, C.; Kondrup, J.; Ljungqvist, O.; et al. How nutritional risk is assessed and managed in European hospitals: A survey of 21,007 patients findings from the 2007–2008 cross-sectional nutritionDay survey. *Clin. Nutr.* **2010**, *29*, 552–559. [CrossRef]
19. Van Bokhorst-de van der Schueren, M.A.E.; Guaitoli, P.R.; Jansma, E.P.; de Vet, H.C.W. Nutrition screening tools: Does one size fit all? A systematic review of screening tools for the hospital setting. *Clin. Nutr.* **2014**, *33*, 39–58. [CrossRef]

20. Kondrup, J.; Allison, S.P.; Elia, M.; Vellas, B.; Plauth, M. ESPEN guidelines for nutrition screening 2002. *Clin. Nutr.* **2003**, *22*, 415–421. [CrossRef]
21. Kondrup, J.; Rasmussen, H.H.; Hamberg, O.; Stanga, Z. Nutritional risk screening (NRS 2002): A new method based on an analysis of controlled clinical trials. *Clin. Nutr.* **2003**, *22*, 321–336. [CrossRef]
22. Schuetz, P.; Fehr, R.; Baechli, V.; Geiser, M.; Gomes, F.; Kutz, A.; Tribolet, P.; Bregenzer, T.; Braun, N.; Hoess, C.; et al. Individualized nutritional support in medical inpatients at nutritional risk: A randomized clinical trial. *Lancet* **2019**, *393*, 2312–2321. [CrossRef]
23. Weekes, C.E.; Elia, M.; Emery, P.W. The development, validation and reliability of a nutrition screening tool based on the recommendations of the British, Association for Parenteral and Enteral Nutrition (BAPEN). *Clin. Nutr.* **2004**, *23*, 1104–1112.
24. Anthony, P.S. Nutrition screening tools for hospitalized patients. *Nutr. Clin. Pract.* **2008**, *23*, 373–382. [CrossRef]
25. Raslan, M.; Gonzalez, M.C.; Dias, M.C.; Nascimento, M.; Castro, M.; Marques, P.; Segatto, S.; Torrinhas, R.S.; Cecconello, I.; Waitzberg, D.L.; et al. Comparison of nutritional risk screening tools for predicting clinical outcomes in hospitalized patients. *Nutrition* **2010**, *26*, 721–726. [CrossRef]
26. Charney, P. Nutrition screening vs. nutrition assessment: How do they differ? *Nutr. Clin. Pract.* **2008**, *23*, 366–372. [CrossRef]
27. Detsky, A.S.; McLaughlin, J.R.; Baker, J.P.; Johnston, N.; Whittaker, S.; Mendelson, R.A.; Jeejeebhoy, K.N. What is subjective global assessment of nutritional status? 1987. Classical article. *Nutr. Hosp.* **2008**, *23*, 400–407.
28. Koom, W.S.; Ahn, S.D.; Song, S.Y.; Lee, C.G.; Moon, S.H.; Chie, E.K.; et al. Nutritional status of patients treated with radiotherapy as determined by subjective global assessment. *Radiat. Oncol. J.* **2012**, *30*, 132–139. [CrossRef]
29. National Kidney Foundation. KDOQI Clinical Practice Guidelines for Nutrition in Chronic Renal Failure 2000. Available online: https://kidneyfoundation.cachefly.net/professionals/KDOQI/guidelines_nutrition/nut_a09.html (accessed on 24 June 2019).
30. British Dietetic Association. *Parenteral and Enteral Nutrition Group. A Pocket Guide to Clinical Nutrition*, 4th ed.; Parenteral and Enteral Nutrition Group of the British Dietetic Association: Birmingham, UK, 2011.
31. Han, T.S.; Lean, M.E. Lower leg length as an index of stature in adults. *Int. J. Obes. Relat. Metab. Disord.* **1996**, *20*, 21–27.
32. Reeves, S.L.; Varakamin, C.; Henry, C.J. The relationship between arm-span measurement and height with special reference to gender and ethnicity. *Eur. J. Clin. Nutr.* **1996**, *50*, 398–400.
33. Maastricht UMC+. Nutritional Assessment Body Composition Skinfold Measurements 2019. Available online: https://nutritionalassessment.mumc.nl/en/skinfold-measurements (accessed on 12 July 2019).
34. Bosy-Westphal, A.; Kromeyer-Hausschild, K.; Pirlich, M.; Schlattmann, A.; Scholz, G. Body composition analysis—What can be measured with practical value? *Aktuel Ernahrungsmed.* **2004**, *1*, 189–195.
35. Kyle, U.; Bosaeus, I.; De Lorenzo, A.; Deurenberg, P.; Elia, M.; Gomez, J.; Heitmann, B.L.; Kent-Smith, L.; Melchior, J.C.; Pirlich, M.; et al. Bioelectrical impedance analysis—Part I: Review of principles and methods. *Clin. Nutr.* **2004**, *23*, 1226–1243. [CrossRef]
36. Kyle, U.; Bosaeus, I.; De Lorenzo, A.; Deurenberg, P.; Elia, M.; Manuel Gomez, J.; Lilienthal Heitmann, B.; Kent-Smith, L.; Melchior, J.C.; Pirlich, M.; et al. Bioelectrical impedance analysis—Part II: Utilization in clinical practice. *Clin. Nutr.* **2004**, *23*, 1430–1453. [CrossRef]
37. Forbes, G.B.; Bruining, G.J. Urinary creatinine excretion and lean body mass. *Am. J. Clin. Nutr.* **1976**, *29*, 1359–1366. [CrossRef]
38. Stratton, R.J.; Green, C.J.; Elia, M. *Disease-Related Malnutrition: An Evidence-Based Approach to Treatment*; CABI Publishing: Wallingford, UK, 2003.
39. MacDonald, A.J.; Greig, C.A.; Baracos, V. The advantages and limitations of cross-sectional body composition analysis. *Curr. Opin. Support Palliat. Care.* **2011**, *5*, 342–349. [CrossRef]
40. Pirlich, M.; Norman, K. *Bestimmung des Ernährungszustands (inkl. Bestimmung der Körperzusammensetzung und ernährungsmedizinisches Screening) in Biesalski, rnährungsmedizin*; Georg Thieme Verlag KG: Stuttgart, Germany, 2018.
41. Leuenberger, M.S.; Joray, M.L.; Kurmann, S.; Stanga, Z. How to assess the nutritional status of my patient. *Praxis (Bern 1994)* **2012**, *101*, 307–315. [CrossRef]

42. Esper, D.H. Utilization of nutrition-focused physical assessment in identifying micronutrient deficiencies. *Nutr. Clin. Pract.* **2015**, *30*, 194–202. [CrossRef]
43. Norman, K.; Stobaus, N.; Gonzalez, M.C.; Schulzke, J.D.; Pirlich, M. Hand grip strength: Outcome predictor and marker of nutritional status. *Clin. Nutr.* **2011**, *30*, 135–142. [CrossRef]
44. Studenski, S.; Perera, S.; Wallace, D.; Chandler, J.M.; Duncan, P.W.; Rooney, E.; Fox, M.; Guralnik, J.M. Physical performance measures in the clinical setting. *J. Am. Geriatr. Soc.* **2003**, *51*, 314–322. [CrossRef]
45. Food and Agriculture Organization of the United Nations. *Dietary Assessment: A Resource Guide to Method Selection and Application in Low Resource Settings*; Food and Agriculture Organization of the United Nations: Rome, Italy, 2018.
46. Forster, H.; Walsh, M.C.; Gibney, M.J.; Brennan, L.; Gibney, E.R. Personalised nutrition: The role of new dietary assessment methods. *Proc. Nutr. Soc.* **2016**, *75*, 96–105. [CrossRef]
47. Gemming, L.; Utter, J.; Ni Mhurchu, C. Image-assisted dietary assessment: A systematic review of the evidence. *J. Acad. Nutr. Diet.* **2015**, *115*, 64–77. [CrossRef]
48. Illner, A.K.; Freisling, H.; Boeing, H.; Huybrechts, I.; Crispim, S.P.; Slimani, N. Review and evaluation of innovative technologies for measuring diet in nutritional epidemiology. *Int. J. Epidemiol.* **2012**, *41*, 1187–1203. [CrossRef]
49. Stumbo, P.J. New technology in dietary assessment: A review of digital methods in improving food record accuracy. *Proc. Nutr. Soc.* **2013**, *72*, 70–76. [CrossRef]
50. Archundia Herrera, M.C.; Chan, C.B. Narrative Review of New Methods for Assessing Food and Energy Intake. *Nutrients* **2018**, *10*, 1064. [CrossRef]
51. Martin, C.K.; Correa, J.B.; Han, H.; Allen, H.R.; Rood, J.C.; Champagne, C.M.; Gunturk, B.K.; Bray, G.A. Validity of the Remote Food Photography Method (RFPM) for estimating energy and nutrient intake in near real-time. *Obesity (Silver Spring)* **2012**, *20*, 891–899. [CrossRef]
52. Dong, Y.; Hoover, A.; Scisco, J.; Muth, E. A new method for measuring meal intake in humans via automated wrist motion tracking. *Appl Psychophysiol. Biofeedback* **2012**, *37*, 205–215. [CrossRef]
53. Kawano, Y.; Yanai, K. FoodCam: A real-time food recognition system on a smartphone. *Multimed. Tool. Appl.* **2015**, *74*, 5263–5287. [CrossRef]
54. Anthimopoulos, M.; Dehais, J.; Shevchik, S.; Ransford, B.H.; Duke, D.; Diem, P.; Mougiakakou, S. Computer vision-based carbohydrate estimation for type 1 patients with diabetes using smartphones. *J. Diabetes Sci. Technol.* **2015**, *9*, 507–515. [CrossRef]
55. Bally, L.; Dehais, J.; Nakas, C.T.; Anthimopoulos, M.; Laimer, M.; Rhyner, D.; Rosenberg, G.; Zueger, T.; Diem, P.; Mougiakakou, S.; et al. Carbohydrate Estimation Supported by the GoCARB System in Individuals With Type 1 Diabetes: A Randomized Prospective Pilot Study. *Diabetes Care* **2017**, *40*, e6–e7. [CrossRef]
56. Dehais, J.; Anthimopoulos, M.; Shevchik, S.; Mougiakakou, S. Two-view 3D reconstruction for food volume estimation. *IEEE Trans. Multimed.* **2017**, *19*, 1090–1099. [CrossRef]
57. Rhyner, D.; Loher, H.; Dehais, J.; Anthimopoulos, M.; Shevchik, S.; Botwey, R.H.; Duke, D.; Stettler, C.; Diem, P.; Mougiakakou, S.; et al. Carbohydrate Estimation by a Mobile Phone-Based System Versus Self-Estimations of Individuals With Type 1 Diabetes Mellitus: A Comparative Study. *J. Med. Int. Res.* **2016**, *18*, e101. [CrossRef]
58. Vasiloglou, M.F.; Mougiakakou, S.; Aubry, E.; Bokelmann, A.; Fricker, R.; Gomes, F.; Guntermann, C.; Meyer, A.; Studerus, D.; Stanga, Z. A Comparative Study on Carbohydrate Estimation: GoCARB vs. Dietitians. *Nutrients* **2018**, *10*, 741. [CrossRef]
59. Ambrosini, G.L.; Hurworth, M.; Giglia, R.; Trapp, G.; Strauss, P. Feasibility of a commercial smartphone application for dietary assessment in epidemiological research and comparison with 24-h dietary recalls. *Nutr. J.* **2018**, *17*, 5. [CrossRef]
60. Bucher Della Torre, S.; Carrard, I.; Farina, E.; Danuser, B.; Kruseman, M. Development and Evaluation of e-CA, an Electronic Mobile-Based Food Record. *Nutrients* **2017**, *9*, 76.
61. Bejar, L.M.; Sharp, B.N.; Garcia-Perea, M.D. The e-EPIDEMIOLOGY Mobile Phone App for Dietary Intake Assessment: Comparison with a Food Frequency Questionnaire. *JMIR Res. Protoc.* **2016**, *5*, e208. [CrossRef]
62. Poslusna, K.; Ruprich, J.; de Vries, J.H.; Jakubikova, M.; van't Veer, P. Misreporting of energy and micronutrient intake estimated by food records and 24 hour recalls, control and adjustment methods in practice. *Br. J. Nutr.* **2009**, *101*, S73–85. [CrossRef]

63. Beasley, J.; Riley, W.T.; Jean-Mary, J. Accuracy of a PDA-based dietary assessment program. *Nutrition* **2005**, *21*, 672–677. [CrossRef]
64. Casperson, S.L.; Sieling, J.; Moon, J.; Johnson, L.; Roemmich, J.N.; Whigham, L. A mobile phone food record app to digitally capture dietary intake for adolescents in a free-living environment: Usability study. *JMIR Mhealth Uhealth* **2015**, *3*, e30. [CrossRef]
65. Ashman, A.M.; Collins, C.E.; Brown, L.J.; Rae, K.M.; Rollo, M.E. Validation of a Smartphone Image-Based Dietary Assessment Method for Pregnant Women. *Nutrients* **2017**, *9*, 73. [CrossRef]
66. Recio-Rodriguez, J.I.; Rodriguez-Martin, C.; Gonzalez-Sanchez, J.; Rodriguez-Sanchez, E.; Martin-Borras, C.; Martinez-Vizcaino, V.; Arietaleanizbeaskoa, M.S.; Magdalena-Gonzalez, O.; Fernandez-Alonso, C.; Maderuelo-Fernandez, J.A.; et al. EVIDENT Smartphone App, a New Method for the Dietary Record: Comparison With a Food Frequency Questionnaire. *JMIR Mhealth Uhealth* **2019**, *7*, e11463. [CrossRef]
67. Carter, M.C.; Burley, V.J.; Nykjaer, C.; Cade, J.E. 'My Meal Mate' (MMM): Validation of the diet measures captured on a smartphone application to facilitate weight loss. *Br. J. Nutr.* **2013**, *109*, 539–546. [CrossRef]
68. Conrad, J.; Nothlings, U. Innovative approaches to estimate individual usual dietary intake in large-scale epidemiological studies. *Proc. Nutr. Soc.* **2017**, *76*, 213–219. [CrossRef]
69. Lemacks, J.L.; Adams, K.; Lovetere, A. Dietary Intake Reporting Accuracy of the Bridge2U Mobile Application Food Log Compared to Control Meal and Dietary Recall Methods. *Nutrients* **2019**, *11*, 199. [CrossRef]
70. Harris, J.A.; Benedict, F.G. A Biometric Study of Human Basal Metabolism. *Proc. Natl. Acad. Sci. USA* **1918**, *4*, 370–373. [CrossRef]
71. Druml, W.; Jadrna, K. *Recommendations for Enteral and Parenteral Nutrition in Adults*; English Edition/Pocket Version; Austrian Society of Clinical Nutrition (AKE): Vienna, Austria, 2008.

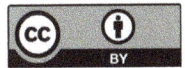

© 2019 by the authors. Licensee MDPI, Basel, Switzerland. This article is an open access article distributed under the terms and conditions of the Creative Commons Attribution (CC BY) license (http://creativecommons.org/licenses/by/4.0/).

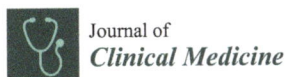

Review

Nutritional Management and Outcomes in Malnourished Medical Inpatients: Anorexia Nervosa

Cristina Cuerda [1,*], Maria F. Vasiloglou [2] and Loredana Arhip [1]

[1] Nutrition Unit, Instituto de Investigación Sanitaria Gregorio Marañón, Hospital General Universitario Gregorio Marañón, Calle del Dr. Esquerdo, 46, 28007 Madrid, Spain
[2] Diabetes Technology Research Group, ARTORG Center for Biomedical Engineering Research, University of Bern, Murtenstrasse 50, 3008 Bern, Switzerland
* Correspondence: cuerda.cristina@gmail.com

Received: 31 May 2019; Accepted: 15 July 2019; Published: 17 July 2019

Abstract: Background: Anorexia Nervosa (AN) is a psychiatric disorder characterised by a physical and psychosocial deterioration due to an altered pattern on the intake and weight control. The severity of the disease is based on the degree of malnutrition. The objective of this article is to review the scientific evidence of the refeeding process of malnourished inpatients with AN; focusing on the clinical outcome. Methods: We conducted an extensive search in Medline and Cochrane; on April 22; 2019; using different search terms. After screening all abstracts; we identified 19 papers that corresponded to our inclusion criteria. Results: The article focuses on evidence on the characteristics of malnutrition and changes in body composition; energy and protein requirements; nutritional treatment; physical activity programmes; models of organisation of the nutritional treatment and nutritional support related outcomes in AN patients. Conclusion: Evidence-based standards for clinical practice with clear outcomes are needed to improve the management of these patients and standardise the healthcare process.

Keywords: anorexia nervosa; refeeding syndrome; weight gain; mortality; length of stay

1. Introduction

AN is a psychiatric disorder characterised by a persistent restriction of energy intake leading to significantly low body weight, an intense fear of gaining weight or of becoming fat and a disturbance in the way one's body weight or shape is experienced.

The diagnostic criteria of AN according to the latest edition of the Diagnostic and Statistical Manual of Mental Disorders (DSM-5) is represented in Table 1 [1].

The prevalence of AN is estimated to be 1% [2], with a ratio between women and men of 9:1. The age of onset of AN is usually adolescence or youth, although some cases appear after 40 years or in childhood.

This disease has a great tendency to chronicity, it can produce serious medical complications, it can interfere with the individual's psychological and social development and it can even cause death. AN is associated with a high mortality rate (5%–10%) due to suicide, hydro-electrolyte alterations and arrhythmias, which places it at the head of psychiatric disorders [3].

Its aetiology is multifactorial and includes biological, psychological and cultural factors. Family and twin studies suggest a strong genetic component in AN. Within the biological factors are the neurochemical alterations [3,4]. The best known of these is the dysregulation of serotonin, which could also explain the high incidence of psychiatric comorbidities in these patients such as depression, anxiety and obsessive-compulsive disorders, which are associated with alterations in the serotonin system. Alterations have been found in these patients in some genes linked to different neurotransmitters (5HT2A receptor gene, MAOA monoamine oxidase gene, SERT serotonin transporter gene, NET noradrenaline transporter gene, among others) [4].

Table 1. Diagnostic criteria of anorexia nervosa according to DSM-5 classification.

Anorexia nervosa	A.	Restriction of energy intake relative to requirements leading to a significantly low body weight in the context of age, sex, developmental trajectory, and physical health. Significantly low weight is defined as a weight that is less than minimally normal or, for children and adolescents, less than that minimally expected.
	B.	Intense fear of gaining weight or becoming fat, or persistent behaviour that interferes with weight gain, even though at a significantly low weight.
	C.	Disturbance in the way in which one's body weight or shape is experienced, undue influence of body weight or shape on self-evaluation, or persistent lack of recognition of the seriousness of the current low body weight.

In addition, there are usually psychological problems and family dynamics. Patients with AN are described as anxious, depressive, perfectionists and with low self-esteem. Cultural influences are also important with the emphasis on thinness in our society, exacerbated by the media. All these factors can conclude in the appearance of AN in a vulnerable adolescent [5].

The treatment of AN requires a multidisciplinary team in which specialised professionals (physicians, nurses, dietitians, psychiatrists, psychologists, among others) work together. The treatment is based on the nutritional rehabilitation, management of complications, as well as on psychotherapy and psychotropic drugs [6].

The clinical manifestations of AN are multisystemic. A summary of them is presented in Table 2. The treatment of these alterations can be found in the literature [7,8].

Table 2. Clinical manifestations of anorexia nervosa.

Cardiovascular	Bradycardia and hypotension due to alterations in the autonomic nervous system. Electrocardiographic alterations: Atrial, ventricular arrhythmias and alterations in the QTc space. Myocardial alterations: decrease in cardiac mass, prolapse of the mitral valve and pericardial effusion.
Gastrointestinal	Delayed gastric emptying and constipation. Alterations of liver function tests. Parotid hypertrophy, loss of tooth enamel, gastroesophageal reflux, esophagitis, and oesophageal complications, Mallory–Weiss syndrome (especially in patients with purging habits, due to the chronicity of vomiting).
Neurological	Cortical atrophy and ventricular dilatation alterations. Alterations in psychological and cognitive tests.
Renal and Hydro electrolytic	Decrease in glomerular filtration rate. Hypokalaemia and hypochloremic metabolic alkalosis (vomit-induced) Metabolic acidosis (laxative abuse). Hyponatremia (diuretics abuse, potomania). Hypophosphatemia, hypokalaemia, and hypomagnesemia (refeeding syndrome, RS).
Bone	Osteopenia. Osteoporosis. Osteomalacia.
Endocrinological	Hypogonadotropic hypogonadism. Hypometabolism (resting energy expenditure, REE). Hypercortisolism, without the stigmas of Cushing's syndrome. Euthyroid sick syndrome (low-normal range of T4 and TSH, with low levels of T3 and an increase in rT3). Hypoglycaemia.Growth and developmental delay in children.
Haematological	Bone marrow hypoplasia with gelatinous transformation presenting variable degrees of anaemia, leukopenia, and thrombocytopenia.
Dermatological	Russell's sign. Xerosis. Lanugo. Hypercarotenaemia.

The objective of this article is to review the scientific evidence of the refeeding process of malnourished inpatients with AN, focusing on the clinical outcome.

2. Methods

We conducted an extensive search in Medline and Cochrane, on April 22nd 2019, using the following search terms: "Anorexia nervosa", "inpatients", "refeeding", "nutritional treatment", "tube-feeding", "energy expenditure", "physical activity", "exercise", "refeeding syndrome", "mortality", "weight gain", "rehospitalisation", "length of stay", in title and abstracts. We repeated the search using MeSH terms. We identified 259 papers. After screening all abstracts, we identified 19 papers that corresponded to our inclusion criteria. These were: (1) papers in English and Spanish in the last 15 years; (2) were performed in AN inpatients; (3) reported results on weight or body mass index (BMI) at admission and at discharge, length of stay, refeeding rate, type of nutritional treatment and outcome.

3. Results

As a result of the literature review, this article will cover the following topics: Characteristics of malnutrition and changes in body composition, energy and protein requirements, nutritional treatment, physical activity programmes, models of organisation of the nutritional treatment, and nutritional support related outcomes in AN patients.

3.1. Malnutrition and Body Composition in AN

According to the Global Leadership Initiative on Malnutrition (GLIM) classification, the patients with AN present chronic disease related malnutrition without inflammation with different degrees of severity. This means that the main etiological factor of malnutrition is starvation. However, if these patients suffer from an acute illness, the inflammatory process will rapidly deteriorate their nutritional status, jeopardising their clinical outcome [9].

Based on DSM-5 severity definition, patients with AN can be classified into mild BMI (BMI ≥ 17.0 kg/m^2), moderate (BMI = 16.0–16.99 kg/m^2), severe (BMI = 15.0–15.99 kg/m^2) and extreme (BMI < 15.0 kg/m^2) malnutrition [1].

The patients with AN may present with a low-fat mass and fat-free mass, however they usually maintain plasmatic visceral proteins in the normal range. It has been shown that low prealbumin is a predictor of medical complications [10].

The body composition of these patients can be evaluated with anthropometry, Bioelectrical Impedance Analysis (BIA) and Dual-Energy X-ray Absorptiometry (DEXA) as the gold standard. BIA has proved to be one of the most useful in clinical practice, although in severely malnourished patients (BMI < 15.0 kg/m^2) may not be sufficiently accurate [11].

Phase angle is one of BIA measurements that has been associated with poor outcome in some diseases (HIV, cancer). In patients with low body weight, including healthy individuals, ballet dancers and AN patients, phase angle could be a useful marker of qualitative changes [12].

The use of BIA gives clinicians and researchers the advantage of monitoring the compartmental weight gain, ideally achieving an approximate 20/80%–25/75% fat/lean body mass ratio. Moreover, each patient can act as their own "control" that could potentially allow for a more effective, individualised nutrition regimen. Nevertheless, this information must be cautiously interpreted by qualified clinicians who understand this technique and its limitations [13].

The patients with AN present micronutrient deficiencies due to low food intake that can be aggravated in patients with purging habits and during the refeeding process. In a systematic review by Hanachi et al. including 374 patients with AN (restricting (AN-R) and binge-eating/purging (AN-BP) type), it was found that zinc deficiency had the highest prevalence (64.3%), followed by vitamin D (54.2%), copper (37.1%), selenium (20.5%), vitamin B1 (15%), vitamin B12 (4.7%), and vitamin B9 (8.9%).

The AN-BP subgroup had lower selenium ($p < 0.001$) and vitamin B12 plasma concentration ($p < 0.036$), whereas lower copper plasma concentration was observed in patients with AN-R type ($p < 0.022$) [14].

3.2. Energy and Protein Requirements

The refeeding process of patients with AN can be challenging since it must allow a weight gain without developing a refeeding syndrome (RS). On top of that, physicians must deal with the difficult personalities of a psychiatric disorder which in this case shows itself as a fear of weight gain.

In order to obtain the energy requirements, there are equations that estimate the resting energy expenditure (REE) or basal energy expenditure (BEE) and methods that directly measure REE with different types of indirect calorimetry. All of these are applicable to clinical practice as well as research. Additionally, the use of indirect calorimetry can be used to monitor the nutritional treatment in hospitalised patients. Sometimes this helps to uncover patients that are not gaining weight accordingly.

In the study conducted by Cuerda et al., 22 female inpatients were studied. REE was measured by indirect calorimetry (Deltatrac II MBM-200, Aldershot, UK) and was estimated by several predictive formulas (Fleisch, Harris–Benedict, FAO, Schofield–HW, Schebendach). All formulas overestimated REE compared to indirect calorimetry, except the Schebendach formula [15].

In another study by El Ghoch et al., the REE measured by indirect calorimetry by the Douglas bag method and FitMate method was compared to the Harris–Benedict and Müller et al. equations in 15 patients with AN. Using the Douglas Bag method as the gold standard (that measures VCO2/VO2), the authors found an accurate REE estimation with the FitMate method and the Müller et al. equation. Meanwhile, the Harris–Benedict equation overestimated the REE [16].

The literature regarding protein requirements is scarce. There is no evidence that these patients have specific requirements for protein intake. The refeeding process is based on the recommendations for the general population (0.8 g/kg of body weight/day; 10%–15% of energy requirements).

3.3. Nutritional Treatment in AN

Nutritional rehabilitation is probably the most important part of the treatment of patients with AN. Its objectives focus on [6]: Restore body weight; correct the physical complications of malnutrition; improve the patients' motivation to normalise their dietary habits and collaborate in the treatment; educate the patients about healthy nutrition and proper eating patterns; and correct wrong thoughts, attitudes, and feelings about the disorder.

Many of the cognitive and behavioural alterations of malnourished AN patients (food anxiety, taste alterations, binge eating, depression, obsessions, apathy, irritability) improve with the weight gain. Moreover, it increases the effectiveness of other treatments such as psychotherapy or psychotropic drugs [17].

Depending on the setting (outpatients, day hospital, inpatients), nutritional rehabilitation varies in terms of refeeding rate and type of nutritional treatment.

The restoration of body weight is done until the patient reaches a healthy weight in which women recover menstruation and ovulation, men normalise their sexual desire and hormone levels and children and adolescents normalise their growth and sexual development. This requires long treatments, sometimes with repeated hospitalisations followed by a continuity of care in the different settings.

The refeeding process is made according to the patient in a phased manner, agreeing on weight gains during hospitalisation and weight upon discharge. There are no clear criteria for hospitalisation. Some of the usual criteria are summarised in Table 3, even though this depends on the availability of a day hospital in the centre.

Table 3. Criteria for hospitalisation in anorexia nervosa.

	Medical Indications
Adults	Bradycardia < 40 bpm or tachycardia > 110 bpm. Blood pressure < 90/60 mmHg. Symptomatic hypoglycaemia. Hypokalaemia < 3 mmol/l. Hypothermia < 36.1 °C. Dehydration. Uncontrolled vomiting or purging behaviour. Weight < 75% of ideal body weight. Rapid loss of weight (several kgs in a week). Lack of improvement or worsening despite treatment as an outpatient.
Children and adolescents	Bradycardia < 50 bpm. Orthostatic hypotension (increase of >20 bpm in heart rate or drop in blood pressure > 10–20 mmHg with orthostatism). Blood pressure < 80/50 mmHg. Hypokalaemia or hypophosphataemia Rapid weight loss even if the weight is >75% of the ideal body weight. Symptomatic hypoglycaemia. Lack of improvement or worsening despite treatment as an outpatient.
	Psychiatric Indications
All ages	Suicidal ideation. Serious concomitant psychiatric illness. Impossibility to eat independently or needs tube feeding. Unfavourable family environment. Lack of cooperation despite treatment as an outpatient.

Generally, a weight gain of 0.5–1.4 kg/week in hospitalised patients and 250–500 g/week in outpatients is established to avoid the appearance of RS [6,17,18].

Table 4 summarises the recommendations of different clinical guidelines on how to perform the refeeding in malnourished AN patients. Since very few high evidence level studies (RCT) are available, these recommendations are based mainly on clinical experience [6,19–23]. These guidelines differ in the number of calories administered at the beginning of the refeeding (from the most conservative ones that recommend 5–20 kcal/kg at hospital admission [24], to the most permissive ones that begin with 30–40 kcal/kg) [6]. The caloric intake will increase progressively to allow adequate weight gain, sometimes being necessary to reach 70–100 kcal/kg. Patients who have higher caloric requirements usually present inappropriate behaviours (throwing or hiding food, vomiting, intense exercise, etc.).

Table 4. Guidelines for the refeeding of malnourished anorexia nervosa patients.

Guideline	Population	Kcal/kg
United Kingdom: National Institute for Health and Clinical Excellence (NICE), 2017 [24]	Adults	5–20
United Kingdom: MARSIPAN: Management of Really Sick Patients with Anorexia Nervosa, 2014 [20]	Adults	5–20
United Kingdom: Junior MARSIPAN: Management of Really Sick Patients under 18 with Anorexia Nervosa, 2012 [21]	<18 years	15–20
American Psychiatric Association (APA), 2006 [6]	Adults	30–40
American Dietetic Association (ADA), 2006 [22]	Adults	30–40
Australia and New Zealand, 2004 [23]	Adults	15–20 (600–800 kcal/d)

An example of the progressive refeeding of macronutrients and micronutrients in hospitalised patients is shown in Table 5 [19].

Table 5. Example of a refeeding process in terms of macronutrient and micronutrient intake [19].

Days	Recommendations
Day 1–3	• Start with 10–15 kcal/kg (600–1000 kcal/day). • Prophylactic electrolyte supplementation (P, K, Mg). • Thiamine (200–300 mg/day). • Vitamins (200% RDI). • Minerals and trace elements (100% RDI). • Restrict the contribution of fluids to a zero balance. • Restrict sodium to <1 mmol/kg/day. • Glucose and electrolyte levels and the appearance of oedema should be adequately monitored, since the highest risk of RS occurs in these early days.
Day 4–10	• Calorie intake will increase to allow weight gain, continuing with electrolyte, vitamin and mineral supplementation and close monitoring.

In the last decades, many studies have been published regarding nutritional treatment in AN inpatients following different rates of refeeding. Some of them favour the side of "start slow, advance slow", which translates to a slow rate of refeeding especially in patients with very low BMI at admission. On the other hand, some groups follow the "start higher, advance faster", which means a more aggressive refeeding process generally in patients with moderate malnutrition with additional phosphate supplements. This usually conducts to a shorter hospital stay. In general, the results of these studies show that the refeeding is safe and effective in these patients if the supervision is adequate and follows a specific protocol [25–40].

By following any of the above recommendations the weight gain is progressive, and it avoids the appearance of RS (especially in patients weighing less than 70% of their ideal body weight). An algorithm of the nutritional treatment is shown in Figure 1.

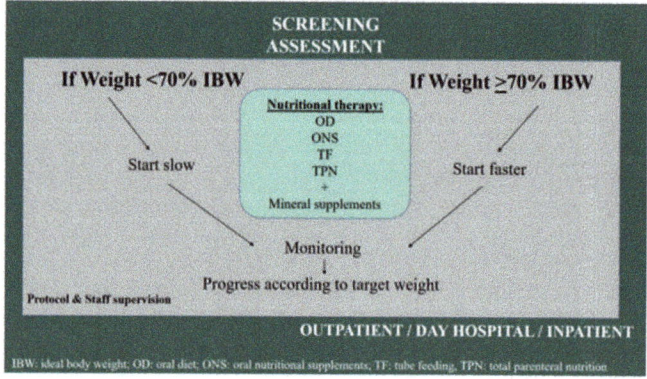

Figure 1. Algorithm of the nutritional treatment in AN.

The refeeding process can include oral diet (OD) as well as medical nutritional therapy.

OD should be the first option for the refeeding, even though there is no evidence of the best food choices and macronutrients distribution in the diet of these patients. The dietary plan should follow a healthy diet model, in which the portion size is personalised according to the patient's requirements and weight gain. Standardisation against personalised caloric prescriptions may confer advantages by facilitating accelerated early weight gain and lower the incidence of bed rest without increasing the incidence of RS [41].

No association between different nutrient contents (e.g. high-protein diet, diets with higher omega-3 polyunsaturated fatty-acid content, low-sodium versus normal-sodium diets) and refeeding outcome has been identified [18,42].

According to each protocol, oral nutritional supplements (ONS) is added if the patients' nutritional requirements are not met, or their weight is stagnating. However, some groups use ONS since the first day of hospital admission in order to shorten the hospital stay. Complete hypercaloric polymeric diets, with a caloric density of 1.5 kcal/ml or even higher, are generally used [27,29,34,38–40].

Tube feeding (TF) is indicated in those patients with severe malnutrition who refuse to eat [36]. Some patients with AN may reject this treatment, especially in the beginning, considering it as an aggression that increases their sense of lack of control over their own diet. Usually, polymeric, lactose free and fibre-enriched formulas are employed. The administration rate is progressively increased to favour tolerance. The use of infusion pumps allows a better control and it impedes the manipulation of the treatment by the patient.

Percutaneous endoscopic gastrostomy (PEG) remains a limited choice of refeeding, however, it may be necessary in patients who need a prolonged treatment. In a study conducted by Born et al. there was no increase in the rate of complications reported for patients using PEG feedings in comparison with those receiving TF [43].

Parenteral nutrition (PN) is used even less in patients with AN, although, it could be a solution in patients with severe malnutrition in whom the digestive tract is not functional (digestive haemorrhage, intestinal obstruction, intestinal perforation, ileus, etc.) [44]. PN is associated with more severe complications than TF, and there is a need to tailor the formulas with special emphasis on volume, macronutrient distribution, micronutrients, and minerals supplementation. There have been published cases with patients treated with home PN [45].

In any of the refeeding modalities, a close supervision by the ward staff is required. A detailed protocol of the steps to follow improves the daily management of the treatment of these patients and may facilitate the weight gain process.

3.4. Physical Activity Programmes

The addition of physical activity in the treatment of patients with AN is exponentially growing, even though these programmes have been characterised as controversial [46–48]. Excessive exercise is often suggested as a causal factor in AN [47], and thus, it is not often prescribed in their clinical management [48]. However, prolonged restraint from physical activity may contribute to decreased bone mass, increased risk of atherosclerosis, and decreasing compliance with the treatment programme [49]. An increasing body of literature demonstrates that individuals suffering from AN could benefit from supervised exercise sessions in combination with nutritional assistance.

Several studies that integrated exercise programmes in the treatment of AN did not interfere with weight gain [50–53] or body fat [49] progression. Different types of exercises have been suggested as beneficial. For example, individualised yoga treatment resulted in reduced food preoccupation after each session [53]. A light resistance exercise programme for a period of 8 weeks showed positive effects on physical strength, body composition, and psychological well-being of hospitalised patients with AN [54]. Furthermore, a high-intensity resistance exercise training programme effectively and safely improved participants' muscular strength as well as their ability to execute daily tasks [47]. In general, a programme incrementally going from mild to moderate exercise speed should be implemented, followed by the interrogation of emotions and thoughts after exercise [46].

Other benefits included less obligatory attitudes and distorted feelings towards exercise [51], less irregular or disorganised eating patterns [55], less drive for thinness, and reduction of the frequency of dangerous eating behaviours such as laxative abuse [56]. In addition, advantages include increased compliance with treatment [49], improved body satisfaction, positive mood states, and quality of life [52]. Physical strength [54] and cardiovascular fitness [48] also improve.

Notably, patients should only undertake physical training once weight stabilisation and nutritional status have progressed sufficiently in caloric and nutritional consumption in order to be able to support the chosen activities [46,54].

To date, there is no consensus or guideline for use of exercise in the treatment of AN [57]. The majority of studies were of small sample size and suggested training programmes varied, thus restricting generalisability of the findings. Moreover, the interventions are relatively short; there is limited follow-up, and most lack an assessment of the participants' fitness.

Nonetheless, when performed in a therapeutic setting, where training is supervised, exercise is safe and may improve treatment outcomes in some AN patients.

3.5. Models of Organisation of the Nutritional Treatment

There is a need for a multidisciplinary team in the organisation model that may differ between centres. Regardless of this, having a written protocol may help to standardise treatment and improve clinical outcome. The protocol should establish the functions of each member of the team and it will determine the options each step of the way.

Close staff supervision is needed during hospitalisation, especially during mealtimes. Some authors have identified two main types of patterns: Rule adherence and rule bending when describing how staff choose how to intervene in different situations [58].

In the day hospital, the patients receive care without being hospitalised, including medical treatment, nutritional therapy, psychiatric and psychological care in individual and/or group modality, occupational therapy and social support. This resource of treatment may be indicated in some outpatients prior or after hospitalisation [59].

Continuity of care has proven to be useful to improve long term outcomes in these patients [60].

3.6. Nutritional Support Related Outcomes

The main clinical outcomes related to the refeeding process in patients with AN are weight gain, the length of hospitalisation and rehospitalisation rate, RS, and mortality. A summary of the nutritional support related outcomes published in different studies is shown in Table 6.

Table 6. Studies in patients with anorexia nervosa reporting clinical outcomes of the nutritional treatment.

Study	Study Type	N° Patients	Mean Age (years)	Weight (kg) or BMI (kg/m²) at Admission	Weight (kg) or BMI (kg/m²) at Discharge	Length of Stay (days)	Kcal/kg or kcal/day at Admission	Type of Nutritional Treatment	Outcome
Rigaud et al., 2007 [25]	RCT a: TF b: control	a: 41 b: 40	a: 22.5 b: 24.2	a: 12.1 b: 12.8	a: 17.9 b: 15.9	60	a: 1000 (D0)–2450 (D14) b: 1000 (D0)–1850 (D14)	a: OD + TF b: OD	No RS 1-year relapse: a: 44% b: 52%
Diamanti et al., 2008 [44]	Retrospective	a: 104 b: 94	15	a: 36.3 b: 41	a: 39.6 b: 41.5	a: 30.7 b: 15.6	40 kcal/kg	a: OD + PN b: OD	No RS a: Hypophosphataemia (6 cases), Hypopotassaemia (3 cases)
Gentile et al., 2010 [26]	Retrospective	33	22.8	11.3	13.5	60	1408	OD + TF + iv. glucose	No RS
Vignaud et al., 2010 [33]	Retrospective	68	31	12	-	7.6 (in ICU)	22.3 kcal/kg	OD + TF + TPN	RS (10%) Mortality (10%)
Whitelaw et al., 2010 [34]	Retrospective	29	15.7	72.9% IBW	-	-	1900–2200 (89% of patients)	OD + ONS + TF (7 patients)	Mild hypophosphataemia (37%)
Garber et al., 2012 [35]	Prospective	35	16.2	16.3	-	17	1205	OD	Hypophosphataemia (20%)
Gentile et al., 2012 [36]	Retrospective	10	22	11.2	17.3	90	1199	OD + TF + iv. glucose	No RS
Agostino et al., 2013 [37]	Retrospective cohort study: a: Nasogastric cohort b: bolus-fed cohort	165	14.9	a: 16.6 b: 16.7	-	a: 33.8 b: 50.9	a: 1617 b: 1069	a: 31 patients b: 134 patients	No RS a: Hypopotassaemia (1 case); readmissions at 6 months (12.9%) b: Hypopotassaemia (1 case); mild-moderate hypophosphataemia (8 cases); readmissions at 6 months (23%)
Garber et al., 2013 [38]	Prospective cohort: a: high calorie b: low calorie	56	16.2	a: 16.6 b: 15.8	-	14.9	a: 1700 b: 1093	OD + ONS	No RS Hypophosphataemia (45%) Length of stay: a: 11.9 days b: 17.6 days
Golden et al., 2013 [39]	Retrospective a: low calorie b: high calorie	a: 88 b: 222	16.1	a: 15.9 b: 16.1	a: 17.2 b: 17.1	a: 16.6 b: 13	a: 1163 b: 1557	OD + ONS + TF (occasionally)	No RS Hypophosphataemia (15.8%) Hypomagnesaemia (15.2%) Hypopotassaemia (20%)
Leclerc et al., 2013 [40]	Retrospective	29	14.7	16.4	-	35.8	1500	OD + ONS	Hypophosphataemia (3.5%)
Hofer et al., 2014 [27]	Retrospective	65	27.9	13.7	15	49.5	10 kcal/kg	OD (mostly) OD + ONS (8.1%) OD + TF (8.1%) TF (5%) OD + TPN (1.2%)	Mild RS (10.5%) Severe hypopotassaemia (4.7%)

Table 6. Cont.

Study	Study Type	N° Patients	Mean Age (years)	Weight (kg) or BMI (kg/m²) at Admission	Weight (kg) or BMI (kg/m²) at Discharge	Length of Stay (days)	Kcal/kg or kcal/day at Admission	Type of Nutritional Treatment	Outcome
Brown et al., 2015 [28]	Retrospective case-control	123	28	13	13.9	13	1200	OD	Hypophosphataemia (33%)
O'Connor et al., 2016 [61]	RCT a: intervention b: control	a: 18 b: 18	13.8	a: 32.4 b: 34.6	a: 34.1 b: 35.6	10	a: 38 kcal/kg/d b: 16 kcal/kg/d	OD + TF	a: Hypophosphataemia (28%) b: Hypophosphataemia (11%)
Marugán et al., 2016 [29]	Retrospective	50	14.5	15.45	17.58	44.54	1000	OD ONS (16%) TF (8%)	No symptoms of RS
Kameoka et al., 2016 [30]	Retrospective	99	30.9	<17.5	-	82.7	Low calorie diet	OD	Hypophosphataemia (21.2%)
Smith et al., 2016 [62]	Retrospective	129	15.8	15.8	17.1	14.9	1585	OD + ONS	No RS Hypophosphataemia (47.3%) Hypokalaemia (12%)
Davies et al., 2017 [31]	Retrospective	65	24	12.8	14.4	60	20-30	OD, ONS (infrequently)	Mild hypophosphataemia (<0.8 mmol/L) (6.5%) Hypokalaemia (1 case). No RS
Peebles et al., 2017 [32]	Retrospective	215	15.3	17.1	18.2	11	1466	OD, TF (10%)	No RE: Hypophosphataemia (14%) 3.8% and 17.2% rehospitalisations after 30 days and 1 year, respectively

TF: Tube Feeding, OR: Oral Diet, ONS: Oral Nutritional Supplements, RS: Refeeding Syndrome, PN: Parenteral Nutrition, TPN: Total Parenteral Nutrition, RCT: Randomised Controlled Trial.

3.7. Weight Gain

The weight gain is the main objective in the nutritional rehabilitation of patients with AN. Achieving this is possible with any of the modalities of nutritional treatment. Some studies show that the greater the weight achieved by the patient up to hospital discharge, the lower the likelihood of relapse. This usually translates to a longer hospitalisation stay [6,63].

In a systematic review which included 10 studies with TF in AN patients, this treatment was considered safe and well tolerated, and effectively enhanced caloric intake and rate of weight gain in patients with AN [64].

In another systematic review, which included 7 observational studies with a total of 403 patients (children and adolescents), the prescribed calorie range varied between 1000–1900 kcal/day with progressive increase during hospitalisation. Additional TF increased the maximum energy intake and led to greater interim or discharge weight; however, this was also associated with a higher incidence of adverse effects [65].

Lastly, in the most recent systematic review by Hale et al., 19 out of 22 studies reported that significant short-term weight gain was achieved when TF was used for refeeding malnourished AN patients; however, results varied in the long-term weight gain, maintenance and recovery [66].

3.8. Hospital Stay and Rehospitalisation

Hospital stay as an outcome is closely related to the weight gain. In many cases, the length of hospitalisation is carefully monitored by the hospital management. One of the strategies to shorten the hospitalisation period in patients with AN includes the use of more aggressive refeeding consisting of diets with lower carbohydrate load (<40% total calories), in continuous administration, accompanied by an adequate supplementation of phosphate and potassium [37,67].

In a retrospective study including 2015 children and adolescents with AN, the authors refer a rehospitalisation rate of 3.8% and 17.2% after 30 days and 1 year after discharge, respectively [32].

In an RCT study with TF versus OD in AN, the results in terms of weight gain and rehospitalisation rate were better in patients with enteral nutrition [25].

In another RCT aimed to compare the effectiveness of hospitalisation for weight restoration to medical stabilisation in adolescent AN patients, the number of rehospitalisations and their respective length of stay (after the first hospital admission), within 12 months, were similar in the two groups when the treatment included family-based therapy [68].

3.9. Refeeding Syndrome

RS has been described in malnourished patients with AN and mainly involves mineral deficiencies (hypophosphataemia, hypokalaemia and hypomagnesaemia), as well as vitamin (thiamine) deficiencies, and volume overload. It can be presented as a symptomatic or asymptomatic clinical case, which implies that a close monitoring of laboratory parameters is necessary, especially during the first week of refeeding. The RS has been described with all feeding modalities (OD, TF, and PN) [66].

Table 7 summarises the main risk factors for developing a RS. There is no clear consensus on supplementing phosphorus in all patients starting refeeding, just in those who develop hypophosphataemia or in those severely malnourished [67].

Hypophosphataemia has been described as a hallmark in studies on RS. In a systematic review of 17 publications, an incidence of hypophosphataemia of 14% (0–38%) was reported, with the degree of malnutrition at admission being the main risk factor, without finding correlation with the refeeding rate (kcal/day) [34,69].

Table 7. Identification of patients with high risk of refeeding syndrome.

Patients with 1 or more of the following:	• BMI < 16 kg/m² • Unintentional weight loss of >15% in the previous 3–6 months. • Minimum or no intake for >10 days. • Low levels of K, P, or Mg before refeeding.
Or, patients with 2 or more of the following:	• BMI < 18.5 kg/m² • Unintentional weight loss of >10% in the previous 3–6 months • Minimum or no intake for >5 days. • History of alcohol abuse, drugs, insulin treatment, chemotherapy, antacids, or diuretics.

In a case-control study with 123 AN patients, the prevalence of hypophosphataemia was 33%, with the nadir occurring at the second day of admission. In this study, higher haemoglobin was the only risk factor associated with higher odds of developing hypophosphataemia; meanwhile a higher BMI, a higher serum potassium, and a higher serum prealbumin were protective factors against the development of hypophosphatemia [28].

3.10. Mortality

Classically, AN has been associated with a high mortality within the psychiatric disorders. In a series of 484 patients followed for 13 years, the authors refer a mortality rate of 1.2% [63].

In most of the revised articles in inpatients, the authors do not refer mortality rates during the refeeding process, even though the patients were severely malnourished [25–28,31,34,36,44].

On the other hand, in a retrospective study performed in France in 30 randomly selected ICUs including 68 patients with AN (average BMI at admission of 12 ± 3 kg/m²), the authors mention a RS rate of 10% and a mortality rate of 10%. The causes included acute respiratory distress syndrome and multiorgan-failure associated with major hydro-electrolytic problems [33].

As exemplified in the refeeding of other malnourished patients, a higher awareness of the risk associated with refeeding may decrease the risk of mortality [70,71].

4. Discussion

The treatment of AN patients is challenging, especially regarding weight gain recovery, which is the most important part of it. In severely malnourished patients, closely related to the weight gain is the risk of RS, which must be accordingly monitored. Moreover, there are factors that interfere with the recovery process, which are mainly related to the patient´s attitudes and fears.

There is a high variability in the treatment between centres, both in the feeding rate and type of nutritional treatment. One of the reasons is the lack of good scientific evidence in this topic.

There are two established pathways when feeding the patients: "start low, advance slow" versus "start higher, advance faster". Both ways have proven to be safe and effective in terms of the in appearance of RS and weight recovery, respectively [25,27,29,40,44]. However, the main difference between them is the length of hospital stay and costs. On this basis, some centres prefer the "start higher, advance faster" method in patients without severe malnutrition.

Regarding the refeeding process, all modalities of feeding (mainly OD, ONS, and TF) can be used in a safe and effective way. In a recent systematic review, no significant differences were found between TF and oral refeeding cohorts regarding gastrointestinal disturbance, RS, or electrolyte abnormalities. However, TF has proved a slight superiority achieving a higher weight at discharge and in the short term [66].

The reviewed literature does not show a high rate of RS during the treatment of these patients, probably due to a close supervision of the feeding process. However, hydro-electrolytic alterations especially hypophosphataemia is frequently reported and up to 40%. Moreover, these studies show that the degree of malnutrition at hospitalisation is the main risk factor for developing hypophosphatemia and it is not related to the refeeding rate [34,69]. Hypophosphatemia is mainly reported in the first days of refeeding. There is no agreement on the use of phosphate supplement as a prophylactic option or after an already established hypophosphatemia.

Patients with less than 70% of IBW, may benefit out of a slow refeeding process with additional mineral supplements because of their potential high risk of RS. However, in patients with higher body weight a faster refeeding rate could be an option in order to rapidly improve weight gain and shorten the hospital stay.

Even though mortality during hospitalisation is rarely reported, this fatal outcome cannot be neglected in the short term nor in the long-term [33].

As a novelty in the management of these patients, physical activity may play an important role. Supervised exercise seems to be safe and may improve treatment outcomes in some patients.

This article contains a large number of studies and systematic reviews focused on the refeeding process of AN patients; however, the main limitation of the review is the quality of the studies. Most of them were observational, case-control, and only two were RCTs. This lowers the strength of recommendation of the results.

Evidence-based standards for clinical practice with clear outcomes (weight gain rate, hospital stay and rehospitalisation, RS, mortality) are needed to improve the management of these patients and standardise the healthcare process.

5. Conclusions

This review focuses on evidence of the refeeding process of malnourished inpatients with AN with emphasis on the clinical outcome (weight gain, hospital stay and rehospitalisation, RS and mortality). Firstly, patients with AN frequently present malnutrition and usually are at high risk of RS. Secondly, literature shows that RS risk mostly depends on the baseline nutritional status and is not associated with the refeeding rate and the type of nutritional treatment. Thirdly, TF seems to have better outcomes, especially in the short-term, though more studies are needed. Lastly, evidence-based standards for clinical practice with coherent outcomes are required to improve the management of these patients and standardise the healthcare process.

Author Contributions: Conceptualization, C.C., M.F.V., and L.A.; Writing—original draft Preparation, C.C., M.F.V., and L.A.; Writing—review and editing, C.C., M.F.V., and L.A.

Funding: The APC was funded by the Research Found of the Department of Diabetes, Endocrinology, Nutritional medicine and Metabolism, Bern University Hospital, Switzerland, and in parts by Nestlé Health Science (grant to the institution).

Conflicts of Interest: The authors declare no conflicts of interest.

References

1. American Psychiatric Association. *Diagnostic and Statistical Manual of Mental Disorders*; American Psychiatric Association: Washington, DC, USA, 2013; ISBN 9780890425572.
2. Ozier, A.D.; Henry, B.W. Position of the American dietetic association: Nutrition intervention in the treatment of eating disorders. *J. Am. Diet. Assoc.* **2011**, *111*, 1236–1241. [CrossRef] [PubMed]
3. Baker, J.H.; Schaumberg, K.; Munn-Chernoff, M.A. Genetics of anorexia nervosa. *Curr. Psychiatry Rep.* **2017**, *19*, 84. [CrossRef] [PubMed]
4. Urwin, R.E.; Nunn, K.P. Epistatic interaction between the monoamine oxidase A and serotonin transporter genes in anorexia nervosa. *Eur. J. Hum. Genet.* **2005**, *13*, 370–375. [CrossRef]
5. Kaye, W.H.; Wierenga, C.E.; Bailer, U.F.; Simmons, A.N.; Bischoff-Grethe, A. Nothing tastes as good as skinny feels: The neurobiology of anorexia nervosa. *Trends Neurosci.* **2013**, *36*, 110–120. [CrossRef] [PubMed]

6. Yager, J.; Michael Devlin, C.J.; Halmi, K.A.; Herzog, D.B.; Mitchell, J.E., III; Powers, P.; Zerbe, K.J.; McIntyre, J.S.; Anzia, D.J.; Cook, I.A.; et al. *Practice Guideline for the Treatment of Patients with Eating Disorders*, 3rd ed.; Work Group on Eating Disorders, American Psychiatric Association Steering Committee on Practice Guidelines Area and Component Liaisons Staff: Washington, DC, USA, 2006.
7. Mehler, P.S.; Krantz, M.J.; Sachs, K.V. Treatments of medical complications of anorexia nervosa and bulimia nervosa. *J. Eat. Disord.* **2015**, *3*, 15. [CrossRef] [PubMed]
8. Støving, R.K. Anorexia nervosa and endocrinology: A clinical update. *Eur. J. Endocrinol.* **2019**, *180*, R9–R27. [CrossRef] [PubMed]
9. Cederholm, T.; Jensen, G.L.; Correia, M.I.T.D.; Gonzalez, M.C.; Fukushima, R.; Higashiguchi, T.; Baptista, G.; Barazzoni, R.; Blaauw, R.; Coats, A.; et al. GLIM criteria for the diagnosis of malnutrition—A consensus report from the global clinical nutrition community. *Clin. Nutr.* **2019**, *38*, 1–9. [CrossRef]
10. Gaudiani, J.L.; Sabel, A.L.; Mehler, P.S. Low prealbumin is a significant predictor of medical complications in severe anorexia nervosa. *Int. J. Eat. Disord.* **2014**, *47*, 148–156. [CrossRef]
11. Piccoli, A.; Codognotto, M.; di Pascoli, L.; Boffo, G.; Caregaro, L. Body mass index and agreement between bioimpedance and anthropometry estimates of body compartments in anorexia nervosa. *JPEN J. Parenter. Enteral Nutr.* **2005**, *29*, 148–156. [CrossRef]
12. Marra, M.; Sammarco, R.; de Filippo, E.; de Caprio, C.; Speranza, E.; Contaldo, F.; Pasanisi, F. Resting energy expenditure, body composition and phase angle in anorectic, ballet dancers and constitutionally lean males. *Nutrients* **2019**, *11*, 502. [CrossRef]
13. Saladino, C.F. The efficacy of bioelectrical impedance analysis (BIA) in monitoring body composition changes during treatment of restrictive eating disorder patients. *J. Eat. Disord.* **2014**, *2*, 34. [CrossRef] [PubMed]
14. Hanachi, M.; Dicembre, M.; Rives-Lange, C.; Ropers, J.; Bemer, P.; Zazzo, J.-F.; Poupon, J.; Dauvergne, A.; Melchior, J.-C. Micronutrients deficiencies in 374 severely malnourished anorexia nervosa inpatients. *Nutrients* **2019**, *11*, 792. [CrossRef] [PubMed]
15. Cuerda, C.; Ruiz, A.; Velasco, C.; Bretón, I.; Camblor, M.; García-Peris, P. How accurate are predictive formulas calculating energy expenditure in adolescent patients with anorexia nervosa? *Clin. Nutr.* **2007**, *26*, 100–106. [CrossRef] [PubMed]
16. El Ghoch, M.; Alberti, M.; Capelli, C.; Calugi, S.; Dalle Grave, R. Resting energy expenditure in anorexia nervosa: Measured versus estimated. *J. Nutr. Metab.* **2012**, *2012*, 1–6. [CrossRef] [PubMed]
17. Mehler, P.S.; Winkelman, A.B.; Andersen, D.M.; Gaudiani, J.L. Nutritional rehabilitation: Practical guidelines for refeeding the anorectic patient. *J. Nutr. Metab.* **2010**, *2010*, 1–7. [CrossRef] [PubMed]
18. Bargiacchi, A.; Clarke, J.; Paulsen, A.; Leger, J. Refeeding in anorexia nervosa. *Eur. J. Pediatr.* **2019**, *178*, 413–422. [CrossRef] [PubMed]
19. Stanga, Z.; Brunner, A.; Leuenberger, M.; Grimble, R.F.; Shenkin, A.; Allison, S.P.; Lobo, D.N. Nutrition in clinical practice—The refeeding syndrome: Illustrative cases and guidelines for prevention and treatment. *Eur. J. Clin. Nutr.* **2008**, *62*, 687–694. [CrossRef]
20. MARSIPAN. *Management of Really Sick Patients with Anorexia Nervosa*, 2nd ed.; Royal College Psychiatrists and Royal College of Physicians London: London, UK, 2014.
21. Marsipan, J. *Management of Really Sick Patients under 18 with Anorexia Nervosa*; Royal College Psychiatrists and Royal College of Physicians London: London, UK, 2012.
22. American Dietetic Association Position of the American Dietetic Association. Nutrition intervention in the treatment of anorexia nervosa, bulimia nervosa, and other eating disorders. *J. Am. Diet. Assoc.* **2006**, *106*, 2073–2082. [CrossRef]
23. Beumont, P.; Hay, P.; Beumont, D.; Birmingham, L.; Derham, H.; Jordan, A.; Kohn, M.; McDermott, B.; Marks, P.; Mitchell, J.; et al. Australian and New Zealand clinical practice guidelines for the treatment of anorexia nervosa. *Aust. N. Z. J. Psychiatry* **2004**, *38*, 659–670.
24. National Institute for Health and Care Excellence (NICE). *Eating Disorders: Recognition and Treatment*; National Institute for Health and Care Excellence (NICE): London, UK, 2017.
25. Rigaud, D.; Brondel, L.; Poupard, A.T.; Talonneau, I.; Brun, J.M. A randomized trial on the efficacy of a 2-month tube feeding regimen in anorexia nervosa: A 1-year follow-up study. *Clin. Nutr.* **2007**, *26*, 421–429. [CrossRef]

26. Gentile, M.G.; Pastorelli, P.; Ciceri, R.; Manna, G.M.; Collimedaglia, S. Specialized refeeding treatment for anorexia nervosa patients suffering from extreme undernutrition. *Clin. Nutr.* **2010**, *29*, 627–632. [CrossRef] [PubMed]
27. Hofer, M.; Pozzi, A.; Joray, M.; Ott, R.; Hähni, F.; Leuenberger, M.; von Känel, R.; Stanga, Z. Safe refeeding management of anorexia nervosa inpatients: An evidence-based protocol. *Nutrition* **2014**, *30*, 524–530. [CrossRef] [PubMed]
28. Brown, C.A.; Sabel, A.L.; Gaudiani, J.L.; Mehler, P.S. Predictors of hypophosphatemia during refeeding of patients with severe anorexia nervosa. *Int. J. Eat. Disord.* **2015**, *48*, 898–904. [CrossRef] [PubMed]
29. De Marugán Miguelsanz, J.M.; Torres Hinojal, M.D.C.; Geijo Uribe, M.S.; Redondo Del Río, M.P.; Mongil López, B.; de Brito García-Sousa, I.; Caballero Sanz, I.; Eiros Bouza, J.M. Abordaje nutricional de pacientes ingresados con anorexia nerviosa. *Nutr. Hosp.* **2016**, *33*, 258. [CrossRef]
30. Kameoka, N.; Iga, J.; Tamaru, M.; Tominaga, T.; Kubo, H.; Watanabe, S.-Y.; Sumitani, S.; Tomotake, M.; Ohmori, T. Risk factors for refeeding hypophosphatemia in Japanese inpatients with anorexia nervosa. *Int. J. Eat. Disord.* **2016**, *49*, 402–406. [CrossRef]
31. Davies, J.E.; Cockfield, A.; Brown, A.; Corr, J.; Smith, D.; Munro, C. The medical risks of severe anorexia nervosa during initial re-feeding and medical stabilisation. *Clin. Nutr. ESPEN* **2017**, *17*, 92–99. [CrossRef]
32. Peebles, R.; Lesser, A.; Park, C.C.; Heckert, K.; Timko, C.A.; Lantzouni, E.; Liebman, R.; Weaver, L. Outcomes of an inpatient medical nutritional rehabilitation protocol in children and adolescents with eating disorders. *J. Eat. Disord.* **2017**, *5*, 7. [CrossRef]
33. Vignaud, M.; Constantin, J.-M.; Ruivard, M.; Villemeyre-Plane, M.; Futier, E.; Bazin, J.-E.; Annane, D.; AZUREA group (AnorexieRea Study Group). Refeeding syndrome influences outcome of anorexia nervosa patients in intensive care unit: An observational study. *Crit. Care* **2010**, *14*, R172. [CrossRef]
34. Whitelaw, M.; Gilbertson, H.; Lam, P.-Y.; Sawyer, S.M. Does aggressive refeeding in hospitalized adolescents with anorexia nervosa result in increased hypophosphatemia? *J. Adolesc. Health* **2010**, *46*, 577–582. [CrossRef]
35. Garber, A.K.; Michihata, N.; Hetnal, K.; Shafer, M.-A.; Moscicki, A.-B. A prospective examination of weight gain in hospitalized adolescents with anorexia nervosa on a recommended refeeding protocol. *J. Adolesc. Health* **2012**, *50*, 24–29. [CrossRef]
36. Gentile, M.G. Enteral Nutrition for feeding severely underfed patients with anorexia nervosa. *Nutrients* **2012**, *4*, 1293–1303. [CrossRef] [PubMed]
37. Agostino, H.; Erdstein, J.; di Meglio, G. Shifting paradigms: Continuous nasogastric feeding with high caloric intakes in anorexia nervosa. *J. Adolesc. Health* **2013**, *53*, 590–594. [CrossRef] [PubMed]
38. Garber, A.K.; Mauldin, K.; Michihata, N.; Buckelew, S.M.; Shafer, M.-A.; Moscicki, A.-B. Higher calorie diets increase rate of weight gain and shorten hospital stay in hospitalized adolescents with anorexia nervosa. *J. Adolesc. Health* **2013**, *53*, 579–584. [CrossRef] [PubMed]
39. Golden, N.H.; Keane-Miller, C.; Sainani, K.L.; Kapphahn, C.J. Higher caloric intake in hospitalized adolescents with anorexia nervosa is associated with reduced length of stay and no increased rate of refeeding syndrome. *J. Adolesc. Health* **2013**, *53*, 573–578. [CrossRef] [PubMed]
40. Leclerc, A.; Turrini, T.; Sherwood, K.; Katzman, D.K. Evaluation of a nutrition rehabilitation protocol in hospitalized adolescents with restrictive eating disorders. *J. Adolesc. Health* **2013**, *53*, 585–589. [CrossRef] [PubMed]
41. Haynos, A.F.; Snipes, C.; Guarda, A.; Mayer, L.E.; Attia, E. Comparison of standardized versus individualized caloric prescriptions in the nutritional rehabilitation of inpatients with anorexia nervosa. *Int. J. Eat. Disord.* **2016**, *49*, 50–58. [CrossRef]
42. Garber, A.K.; Sawyer, S.M.; Golden, N.H.; Guarda, A.S.; Katzman, D.K.; Kohn, M.R.; le Grange, D.; Madden, S.; Whitelaw, M.; Redgrave, G.W. A systematic review of approaches to refeeding in patients with anorexia nervosa. *Int. J. Eat. Disord.* **2016**, *49*, 293–310. [CrossRef]
43. Born, C.; de la Fontaine, L.; Winter, B.; Müller, N.; Schaub, A.; Früstück, C.; Schüle, C.; Voderholzer, U.; Cuntz, U.; Falkai, P.; et al. First results of a refeeding program in a psychiatric intensive care unit for patients with extreme anorexia nervosa. *BMC Psychiatry* **2015**, *15*, 57. [CrossRef]
44. Diamanti, A.; Basso, M.S.; Castro, M.; Bianco, G.; Ciacco, E.; Calce, A.; Caramadre, A.M.; Noto, C.; Gambarara, M. Clinical efficacy and safety of parenteral nutrition in adolescent girls with anorexia nervosa. *J. Adolesc. Health* **2008**, *42*, 111–118. [CrossRef]

45. Hotta, M.; Araki, M.; Urano, A.; Ohwada, R. Home parenteral nutrition therapy in seven patients with anorexia nervosa: The role and indications. *Intern. Med.* **2014**, *53*, 2695–2699. [CrossRef]
46. Cook, B.J.; Wonderlich, S.A.; Mitchell, J.E.; Thompson, R.; Sherman, R.; McCallum, K. Exercise in eating disorders treatment: Systematic review and proposal of guidelines. *Med. Sci. Sports Exerc.* **2016**, *48*, 1408–1414. [CrossRef] [PubMed]
47. Fernandez-del-Valle, M.; Larumbe-Zabala, E.; Villaseñor-Montarroso, A.; Cardona Gonzalez, C.; Diez-Vega, I.; Lopez Mojares, L.M.; Perez Ruiz, M. Resistance training enhances muscular performance in patients with anorexia nervosa: A randomized controlled trial. *Int. J. Eat. Disord.* **2014**, *47*, 601–609. [CrossRef] [PubMed]
48. Ng, L.W.C.; Ng, D.P.; Wong, W.P. Is supervised exercise training safe in patients with anorexia nervosa? A meta-analysis. *Physiotherapy* **2013**, *99*, 1–11. [CrossRef] [PubMed]
49. Thien, V.; Thomas, A.; Markin, D.; Birmingham, C.L. Pilot study of a graded exercise program for the treatment of anorexia nervosa. *Int. J. Eat. Disord.* **2000**, *28*, 101–106. [CrossRef]
50. Danielsen, M.; Rø, Ø.; Bjørnelv, S. How to integrate physical activity and exercise approaches into inpatient treatment for eating disorders: Fifteen years of clinical experience and research. *J. Eat. Disord.* **2018**, *6*, 34. [CrossRef]
51. Calogero, R.M.; Pedrotty, K.N. The practice and process of healthy exercise: An investigation of the treatment of exercise abuse in women with eating disorders. *Eat. Disord.* **2004**, *12*, 273–291. [CrossRef] [PubMed]
52. Hausenblas, H.A.; Cook, B.J.; Chittester, N.I. Can exercise treat eating disorders? *Exerc. Sport Sci. Rev.* **2008**, *36*, 43–47. [CrossRef]
53. Carei, T.R.; Fyfe-Johnson, A.L.; Breuner, C.C.; Brown, M.A. Randomized controlled clinical trial of yoga in the treatment of eating disorders. *J. Adolesc. Health* **2010**, *46*, 346–351. [CrossRef]
54. Chantler, I.; Szabo, C.P.; Green, K. Muscular strength changes in hospitalized anorexic patients after an eight week resistance training program. *Int. J. Sports Med.* **2006**, *27*, 660–665. [CrossRef]
55. Bakland, M.; Rosenvinge, J.H.; Wynn, R.; Sundgot-Borgen, J.; Fostervold Mathisen, T.; Liabo, K.; Hanssen, T.A.; Pettersen, G. Patients' views on a new treatment for Bulimia nervosa and binge eating disorder combining physical exercise and dietary therapy (the PED-t). A qualitative study. *Eat. Disord.* **2019**, 1–18. [CrossRef]
56. Sundgot-Borgen, J.; Rosenvinge, J.H.; Bahr, R.; Schneider, L.S. The effect of exercise, cognitive therapy, and nutritional counseling in treating bulimia nervosa. *Med. Sci. Sports Exerc.* **2002**, *34*, 190–195. [CrossRef] [PubMed]
57. Bratland-Sanda, S.; Andersson, E.; Best, J.; Høegmark, S.; Roessler, K.K. The use of physical activity, sport and outdoor life as tools of psychosocial intervention: The Nordic perspective. *Sport Soc.* **2019**, *22*, 654–670. [CrossRef]
58. Hage, T.W.; Rø, Ø.; Moen, A. To bend or not to bend? Rule adherence among staff at an eating disorder unit. *Eat. Disord.* **2017**, *25*, 134–150. [CrossRef]
59. Gómez-Candela, C.; Palma Milla, S.; Miján-de-la-Torre, A.; Rodríguez Ortega, P.; Matía Martín, P.; Loria Kohen, V.; Campos Del Portillo, R.; Martín-Palmero, Á.; Virgili Casas, M.A.N.; Martínez Olmos, M.; et al. Consenso sobre la evaluación y el tratamiento nutricional de los trastornos de la conducta alimentaria: Anorexia nerviosa. *Nutr. Hosp.* **2018**, *35*, 11–48. [CrossRef] [PubMed]
60. Long, C.G.; Fitzgerald, K.-A.; Hollin, C.R. Treatment of chronic anorexia nervosa: A 4-year follow-up of adult patients treated in an acute inpatient setting. *Clin. Psychol. Psychother.* **2012**, *19*, 1–13. [CrossRef] [PubMed]
61. O'Connor, G.; Nicholls, D.; Hudson, L.; Singhal, A. Refeeding low weight hospitalized adolescents with anorexia nervosa: A multicenter randomized controlled trial. *Nutr. Clin. Pract.* **2016**, *31*, 681–689. [CrossRef] [PubMed]
62. Smith, K.; Lesser, J.; Brandenburg, B.; Lesser, A.; Cici, J.; Juenneman, R.; Beadle, A.; Eckhardt, S.; Lantz, E.; Lock, J.; et al. Outcomes of an inpatient refeeding protocol in youth with anorexia nervosa and atypical anorexia nervosa at children's hospitals and clinics of minnesota. *J. Eat. Disord.* **2016**, *4*, 35. [CrossRef]
63. Rigaud, D.; Pennacchio, H.; Bizeul, C.; Reveillard, V.; Vergès, B. Outcome in an adult patients: A 13-year follow-up in 484 patients. *Diabetes Metab.* **2011**, *37*, 305–311. [CrossRef]
64. Rizzo, S.M.; Douglas, J.W.; Lawrence, J.C. enteral nutrition via nasogastric tube for refeeding patients with anorexia nervosa: A systematic review. *Nutr. Clin. Pract.* **2019**, *34*, 359–370. [CrossRef]
65. Rocks, T.; Pelly, F.; Wilkinson, P. Nutrition therapy during initiation of refeeding in underweight children and adolescent inpatients with anorexia nervosa: A systematic review of the evidence. *J. Acad. Nutr. Diet.* **2014**, *114*, 897–907. [CrossRef]

66. Hale, M.D.; Logomarsino, J.V. The use of enteral nutrition in the treatment of eating disorders: A systematic review. *Eat. Weight Disord. Stud. Anorex. Bulim. Obes.* **2019**, *24*, 179–198. [CrossRef] [PubMed]
67. Leitner, M.; Burstein, B.; Agostino, H. Prophylactic phosphate supplementation for the inpatient treatment of restrictive eating disorders. *J. Adolesc. Health* **2016**, *58*, 616–620. [CrossRef] [PubMed]
68. Madden, S.; Miskovic-Wheatley, J.; Wallis, A.; Kohn, M.; Lock, J.; Le Grange, D.; Jo, B.; Clarke, S.; Rhodes, P.; Hay, P.; et al. A randomized controlled trial of in-patient treatment for anorexia nervosa in medically unstable adolescents. *Psychol. Med.* **2015**, *45*, 415–427. [CrossRef] [PubMed]
69. O'Connor, G.; Nicholls, D. Refeeding hypophosphatemia in adolescents with anorexia nervosa: A systematic review. *Nutr. Clin. Pract.* **2013**, *28*, 358–364. [CrossRef] [PubMed]
70. Schuetz, P.; Zurfluh, S.; Stanga, Z. Mortality due to refeeding syndrome? You only find what you look for, and you only look for what you know. *Eur. J. Clin. Nutr.* **2018**, *72*, 307–308. [CrossRef] [PubMed]
71. Matthews, K.L.; Capra, S.M.; Palmer, M.A. Throw caution to the wind: Is refeeding syndrome really a cause of death in acute care? *Eur. J. Clin. Nutr.* **2018**, *72*, 93–98. [CrossRef] [PubMed]

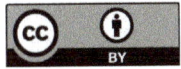

© 2019 by the authors. Licensee MDPI, Basel, Switzerland. This article is an open access article distributed under the terms and conditions of the Creative Commons Attribution (CC BY) license (http://creativecommons.org/licenses/by/4.0/).

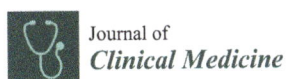

Review

Clinical Value of Muscle Mass Assessment in Clinical Conditions Associated with Malnutrition

Julie Mareschal [1,*], Najate Achamrah [2], Kristina Norman [3,4] and Laurence Genton [5,*]

1. Clinical Nutrition, Geneva University Hospitals, 1205 Geneva, Switzerland
2. Department of Clinical Nutrition, Rouen University Hospital, Normandie University, 76000 Rouen, France
3. Research Group on Geriatrics, Charité Universitätsmedizin Berlin, Corporate Member of Freie Universität Berlin, Humboldt-Universität zu Berlin, and Berlin Institute of Health, 13347 Berlin, Germany
4. Department of Nutrition and Gerontology, German Institute for Human Nutrition Potsdam-Rehbrücke, 14558 Nuthetal, Germany
5. Clinical Nutrition, Geneva University Hospital, 1205 Geneva, Switzerland
* Correspondence: julie.mareschal@hcuge.ch (J.M.); laurence.genton@hcuge.ch (L.G.)

Received: 29 May 2019; Accepted: 16 July 2019; Published: 17 July 2019

Abstract: Malnutrition results from a reduction of food intake or an alteration of nutrient assimilation and leads to decreased lean mass. Strong evidence shows that malnutrition associated with loss of muscle mass negatively impacts clinical outcomes. The preservation or improvement of muscle mass represents a challenge. This review aims to (1) describe current methods to assess muscle mass in clinical practice, (2) describe the associations between muscle mass and clinical outcomes, and (3) describe the impact of interventions aiming at increasing muscle mass on clinical outcomes. It highlights the importance of assessing muscle mass as part of the screening and the follow-up of malnutrition in clinical practice.

Keywords: mid-arm muscle circumference; bioelectrical impedance analysis; dual-energy X-ray absorptiometry; computed tomography; fat-free mass; appendicular skeletal muscle mass; lean soft tissue; skeletal muscle index; chronic disease; old

---

1. Introduction

Malnutrition results from a reduction of food intake or alteration of nutrient assimilation and leads to decreased lean mass, either combined or not with the loss of fat mass. Potential causes include diseases, starvation, or aging. This condition may be associated with other homeostasis disorders such as inflammation [1]. Malnutrition negatively impacts clinical outcomes, mortality, length of stay, and costs [2]. In hospitalized patients, the prevalence ranges from 20 to 50% [3].

To standardize the definition of malnutrition and its diagnostic criteria, the Global Leadership Initiative on Malnutrition (GLIM) has recently convened experts of major worldwide clinical nutrition societies. They suggested defining malnutrition with one phenotypic criterion (bodyweight loss, low body mass index (BMI), or reduced muscle mass) associated to one etiologic criterion (reduced food intake/assimilation or inflammation/disease burden) [4]. Thus, the experts promote the use of body composition measurement as part of a nutritional assessment to evaluate muscle mass.

This narrative review aims to (1) describe current methods to assess muscle mass in clinical practice, (2) describe the associations between muscle mass and clinical outcomes, and (3) describe the impact of interventions aiming at increasing muscle mass on clinical outcomes.

2. Methods to Assess Muscle Mass in Clinical Practice

In clinical practice, several tools and techniques are available to assess body composition. BMI is often used due to its simplicity. Indeed, the U-shaped association between BMI and all-cause mortality has been well described, as subjects with the highest and lowest BMIs have the highest mortality rates [5]. However, BMI does not allow the measurement of body composition compartments and tends to underestimate fat-free mass (FFM) depletion [6–8]. Other anthropometric measurements such as skinfold thickness and waist-hip ratio can also be used. Even though these tools are convenient, quick, and inexpensive, they do not provide direct information on muscle mass [9,10]. Therefore, other methods are required to assess muscle mass in clinical practice. In this section, we focused on portable techniques which can be used at patient bedsides, such as mid-arm muscle circumference and bioelectrical impedance analysis. We concentrated also on dual-energy X-ray absorptiometry and computed tomography, non-portable techniques used for other clinical diagnostic purposes, but allows for the simultaneous assessment of body composition. The characteristics of each method are compared in Table 1. Other methods to assess muscle mass were not introduced because they are rarely used in clinical practice.

Table 1. Principal characteristics of main clinical methods to assess muscle mass.

	MAMC	BIA	DXA	CT
Accuracy	-	+	++	+++
Interobserver variability	+++	+	-	-
Simplicity	++	++	+	-
Radiation	-	-	+	+++
Cost				
If device already available	-	-	-[1]	+[2]
If device not available	-	+	++	+++
Time to measurement	5 min	5 min	5–10 min[3]	10–15 min[3]

"-": weak/low; "+": high; [1] Body composition software usually included in the device; [2] Related to the purchase of the software; [3] To obtain body composition analysis in addition to a routine exam; MAMC: mid-arm muscle circumference; BIA: bioelectrical impedance analysis; DXA: dual-energy X-ray absorptiometry; CT: computed tomography; Adapted from Guglielmi and al. [11].

2.1. Mid-Arm Muscle Circumference

Mid-arm muscle circumference (MAMC) is obtained by using the formula: MAMC (mm) = mid-arm circumference (mm) − (3.14 × triceps skinfold(mm)) [12]. Measurements are usually performed in standing position, on the dominant arm, at the mid-point between the acromion and the olecranon. Mid-arm circumference is measured using a plastic metric tape and triceps skinfold using a skinfold caliper. For both parameters, the average of three consecutive measurements is recorded [12]. MAMC provides an estimation of upper extremity skeletal muscle mass, which strongly correlates to dual-energy X-ray absorptiometry results [13,14].

This method is quick, portable, inexpensive, and easy to perform. It requires simple equipment, minimal training, and is useful in patients with ascites and edema. The main disadvantages are interobserver variations [15]. For instance, in obese people, accuracy is low due to the difficulty of the required triceps skinfold measurement [16].

2.2. Bioelectrical Impedance Analysis

Several bioelectrical impedance analysis (BIA) methods are available (single frequency, multi-frequency, segmental, or vector BIA). We focused on single-frequency 50 kHz tetrapolar BIA, as this is the most used method in clinical practice, and on BIA devices with hand-to-foot surface electrodes, as these BIA devices provide raw electrical data. BIA allows to obtain whole FFM, which refers to all body compartments except fat mass, and appendicular skeletal muscle mass (ASMM) defined as the sum of the lean soft tissue of the four limbs.

Principles and methods of BIA have been previously detailed in the guidelines of the European Society for Clinical Nutrition and Metabolism [17]. BIA is based on the concept that adipose tissue is more resistant to the conduction of the current compared to other tissues and fluids. Briefly, the patient, lying on the back, is exposed to a low-intensity alternating current between surface electrodes. The BIA device measures resistance and reactance, or impedance and phase angle. To estimate FFM and ASMM, several population-specific equations using these electrical parameters in addition to age, sex, weight, and height have been developed and validated against dual-energy X-ray absorptiometry (DXA) [18–21]. FFM and ASMM can be divided by height squared to be converted into FFM index (FFMI) and ASMM index (ASMMI), in order to compare people of different heights.

As a portable non-invasive bedside method, BIA is convenient in clinical practice. It is safe, cheap and not technically demanding. The small interobserver variability, 0.02 kg for FFM, is an advantage compared to anthropometry methods [22,23]. This device also allows the calculation of phase angle, supposed to be an indicator of cellular integrity, associated with clinical prognosis [24]. FFM assessment using BIA does, however, bear some limitations. BIA is not accurate in patients with altered hydration (e.g., ascites, edema, fluid loss) and with extreme BMI (<16 kg/m^2 and >34 kg/m^2) [25]. BIA formulas are population-specific. Finally, multiple devices of BIA are commercially available, but integrated algorithms are not always released by the manufacturer, thus questioning the reliability of the results measured by these devices [26,27].

2.3. Dual-Energy X-ray Absorptiometry

Dual-energy X-ray absorptiometry (DXA) allows the measurement of bone, lean soft tissue, and fat mass. Compared to FFM, lean soft tissue contains essential and non-essential lipids, but not bone mass. DXA device uses X-rays of low- and high-photon energy. As they cross the body, they are attenuated according to the composition and thickness of the encountered body tissues. A detector on the opposite side of the body analyzes the transmitted photon intensity. Complex algorithms allow then to differentiate bone, fat mass, and lean soft tissue, as detailed previously [28]. This method, initially used for bone density measurement, is often considered as the reference method to assess body composition in clinical research [29].

In clinical practice, DXA allows accurate, fast, and non-invasive lean soft tissue assessment. This device is often available in developed countries. Measurement is achieved in supine position. Irradiation is acceptable (2–5 µSv), which is low compared to the daily background radiation of 5–7 µSv [28]. Besides whole-body composition, DXA also allows for the measurement of ASMM. As DXA calculations are based on a constant hydration of lean soft tissue, hydration level variations may impact the results. However, this effect seems to be negligible [30]. Finally, measurements may be influenced by the thickness of the tissue with potential underestimation of fat mass and overestimation of muscle mass in obese patients [31].

2.4. Computed Tomography

Computed tomography (CT) to assess muscle mass is becoming more common [32]. As cutoff values have been defined at the third lumbar vertebrae (L3) level, an area reflective of whole-body tissue distribution, we focused only on muscle assessment at this anatomic landmark [33,34]. L3 muscle mass area is usually normalized to the patients' height squared to determine skeletal muscle index (SMI).

CT is a medical imaging technique, performed in supine position, which measures tissue absorption of X-rays emitted through a rotating beam. Computer processing then reconstructs cross-sectional images of anatomical structures by 2D and 3D maps of pixels. According to the attenuation of the different tissues, each pixel is associated with a numerical value (Hounsfield Unit). Tissues are identified in the cross-sectional images by their specific absorption Hounsfield Unit ranges [35,36]. Muscle mass area is obtained by cross-sectional analysis using standard radiology software [37].

CT provides high-quality images and precise assessment of muscle mass [38,39]. Its advantages compared to other methods are to evaluate muscle mass quality by measuring fat infiltration in muscle. CT images are frequently available in cancer and other chronic disease patients, as part of the routine diagnosis or follow-up of these diseases [26]. Major drawbacks are high radiation exposure (10 mSv), cost, non-portability, and need for qualified technicians and specific software. Moreover, a recent systematic review highlighted the lack of consensus and high variability of CT-based methods of muscle mass assessment [32].

3. Impact of Muscle Mass on Clinical Outcomes

The impact of muscle mass on clinical outcomes is well described in different populations. In this section, we focused on chronic diseases such as chronic obstructive pulmonary disease (COPD), chronic heart failure (CHF), cancer, and on older adults. This choice was related to the fact that the prevalence of malnutrition is particularly high in these populations [40–42]. We made an update of the latest observational studies and subjectively considered articles from the last three years.

3.1. Chronic Diseases

The prevalence of malnutrition is significant in patients with chronic diseases, such as for instance, COPD, CHF or solid tumors cancer. It ranges respectively from 20–35%, 60–69% and 14–66% according to the tumor site [43–45].

3.1.1. Chronic Obstructive Pulmonary Disease

In patients with COPD, the influence of muscle mass on the severity of the disease and the prognosis has been described by Munhoz et al. [46]. In this study, disease severity was evaluated with the Global Initiative for Obstructive Lung Disease (GOLD) index based on airflow limitation, exacerbation history, symptom burden, and prognosis with the body mass index/airflow obstruction/dyspnea/exercise capacity score (BODE), known to predict disease severity and mortality. Interestingly, ASMMI assessed by DXA decreased significantly according to the worsening of GOLD and BODE indexes. In another study, Matkovic et al. have been interested in the association between body composition and physical performance [47]. In 111 moderate to very severe COPD patients, FFMI, assessed by DXA, were significantly associated with a low capacity exercise and physical activity defined, respectively, by a 6-minute walk distance ≤350 m and a daily step count ≤7128 steps/day (=median). Finally, emphysema severity in COPD patients, characterized by a loss of lung tissue, seems to be related to muscle mass and prognosis [48]. Patients in the higher quartiles of emphysema severity had lower FFMI, evaluated by BIA, and a worse BODE index. Thus, in patients with COPD, muscle mass is associated with disease severity, prognosis, and physical performance.

3.1.2. Chronic Heart Failure

As for patients with COPD, muscle mass also appears to be a good predictor of exercise capacity in patients with chronic heart failure [49]. In 117 patients with heart failure and preserved left ventricular ejection fraction, ASMM measured by DXA was significantly associated with a 6-minute walk test <400 m. Tsuchida et al. have studied the association between muscle mass obtained by DXA and severity of acute decompensated heart failure characterized by brain natriuretic peptide (BNP) > 500 pg/mL [50]. Low ASMMI was defined as two standard deviations below the mean reference values of healthy Japanese subjects [51]. After adjustment for anemia and atrial fibrillation, a low ASMMI was related to a higher BNP level, indicative of poor prognosis in CHF patients [52]. In patients with heart failure, muscle mass is associated with physical performance, severity of the disease, and prognosis.

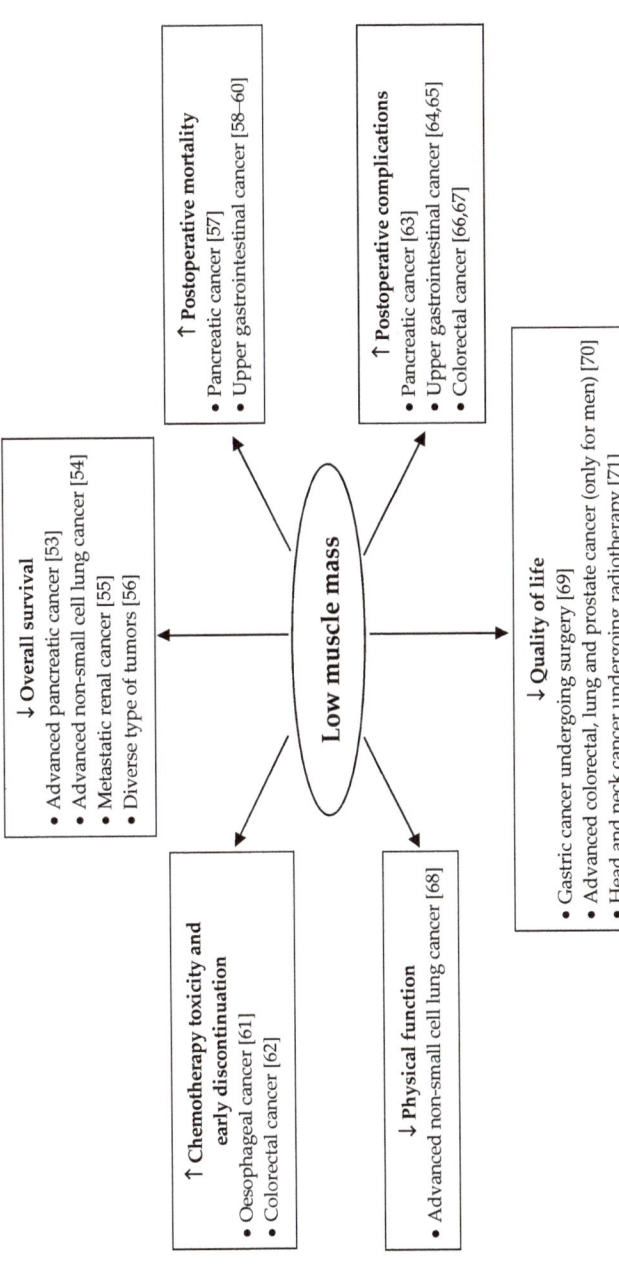

Figure 1. Association between low muscle mass and clinical outcomes in solid tumor cancer patients [53–71]. Muscle mass was quantified by computed tomography at the L3 level except for references [56] and [71] for which bioelectrical impedance analysis and mid-arm muscle circumference were respectively used.

3.1.3. Cancer

Figure 1 highlights the association between muscle mass and clinical outcomes in patients with cancer. In diverse solid tumor types, muscle mass is related with mortality, surgical complications, and quality of life. For advanced cell lung cancer, an association between muscle mass and physical function has been reported. Interestingly, early chemotherapy discontinuation and delayed chemotherapy also appear to be related to the amount of muscle mass. In summary, maintaining muscle mass is essential in cancer patients to improve overall survival, quality of life, physical exercise capacity, tolerance to cancer treatments, and to decrease postoperative mortality as well as complications.

3.2. Older Adults

Due to aging, the risk of muscle mass depletion is high in older adults. In this population, malnutrition ranges from 29% to 61% according to the diagnostic criteria [40]. Recently, muscle mass has been included in the definition of sarcopenia published by the European Working Group on Sarcopenia in Older People [72]. Over the last three years, we found over 80 studies dealing with muscle mass in older adults. Due to the large amount of publications, Figure 2 considers studies including more than 100 participants and illustrates the effect of low muscle mass according to the clinical setting. Studies including fewer participants showed a similar impact.

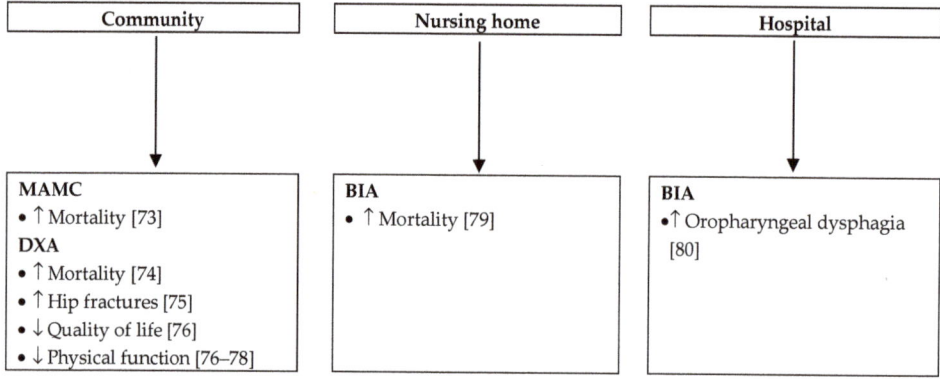

Figure 2. Impact of low muscle mass according to clinical setting [73–80]. MAMC: mid-arm muscle circumference; DXA: dual-energy X-ray absorptiometry; BIA: bioelectrical impedance analysis.

4. Improvement in Muscle Mass: Strategies and Clinical Benefits

Considering the negative effects of muscle mass loss, preserving or increasing muscle mass could lead to improvement of clinical outcomes. Therapeutic strategies to achieve this goal may include nutritional intervention, physical exercise, anabolic steroids, and growth hormone. Nutritional support is recommended for every malnourished patient, as defined by the GLIM [4]. Regular physical exercise is promoted for patients with COPD, chronic heart failure, and cancer as it improves cardiorespiratory fitness, muscle mass and strength, quality of life, and decreases COPD exacerbation and chemotherapy toxicity [81–84]. Anabolic steroids and growth hormone have been considered in malnourished patients, but no clinical practice guideline has been published yet [85,86]. These strategies are used either individually or as a multimodal treatment in clinical research with the aim to prevent muscle mass loss. In this section, we focused on non-pilot randomized controlled trials published during the last three years. We did not find new relevant studies with growth hormone supplementation.

4.1. Chronic Diseases

4.1.1. Chronic Obstructive Pulmonary Disease

Calder et al. evaluated the benefits of a 12-week specific oral nutritional supplementation (~230 kcal, 10 g whey proteins, enriched with omega 3 and vitamin D) vs. milk comparator (~200 kcal, 10 g proteins) in moderate to severe COPD with a BMI between 16–18 kg/m^2 and involuntary weight loss [87]. Although improvement in dyspnea was demonstrated in the intervention group, no modification of muscle mass was observed in either group. In another study, Van de Bool et al. demonstrated the interest of a 4-month multimodal rehabilitation, including nutritional supplementation and physical activity in moderate airflow limitation COPD patients with low muscle mass [88]. Low muscle mass was defined as a lean soft tissue index measured by DXA, under the sex and age-specific 25th percentile values published by Schutz et al. [89]. The intervention group consumed each day two or three oral nutritional supplements enriched in leucine, omega 3 and vitamin D (1 unit = 187.5 kcal, 9.4 g proteins) and underwent a supervised endurance/resistance training two to three times a week. Patients in the control group were only assigned to a supervised exercise program. In both groups, improvement in ASMM, quadriceps muscle strength, and endurance performance were observed. Inspiratory muscle strength, physical activity level, plasma vitamin D, eicosapentaenoic, and docosahexaenoic acids were improved only in the intervention group.

4.1.2. Chronic Heart Failure

Dos Santos et al. randomized CHF patients with testosterone deficiency in a 4-month exercise program, testosterone injection, or combined exercise program and testosterone injection groups [90]. The exercise program consisted of 60 min sessions, three times a week, with stretching, endurance and resistance exercises. Patients with testosterone injection received one testosterone intramuscular injection (1000 mg of testosterone undecyclate) at the beginning of the study. Lean mass was assessed by DXA before and at the end of the intervention. The exercise program, isolated or combined with testosterone injection, increased significantly lean mass ($p < 0.01$) while testosterone injection alone was associated with decreased lean mass ($p < 0.01$). Nutritional intake has not been evaluated.

4.1.3. Cancer

Randomized controlled trials studying the effects of diverse interventions on muscle mass are presented in Table 2. Only randomized controlled trials with nutritional or physical exercise interventions were found. Results are heterogeneous, probably due to significant differences in types of intervention and population. However, most studies show an increase in muscle mass and other outcomes such as muscle strength.

Under different conditions, interventions such as nutrition, physical exercise, and anabolic steroids are efficient to prevent the decrease of muscle mass and improve functional and biological parameters. In clinical practice, a body composition assessment should be used to monitor the effects of these interventions.

4.2. Older Adults

Table 3 shows randomized controlled trials studying the effects of nutritional or combined nutritional and physical interventions on muscle mass in older adults. To limit the size of the table and facilitate the reading, we reported studies including over 100 participants, but the results were similar in studies with fewer participants. As for cancer patients, population and results are heterogeneous. However, most studies demonstrated positive effects of interventions on physical function but not on muscle mass. In older adults, muscle mass quality and cardiorespiratory capacities could be more essential than muscle mass quantity to improve physical function.

Table 2. Randomized controlled trials: effects of nutritional or physical interventions on muscle mass in patients with cancer.

	Studies	Population	Intervention Group	Comparison Group	Muscle Mass	Significant Results
Nutrition	Ritch et al. 2019 [91]	Urothelial bladder carcinoma undergoing radical cystectomy INT = 31/CO = 30	Daily oral nutritional supplement with ω-3 and HMB(700 kcal, 26 g proteins) 4 weeks before and after surgery	Oral micronutrients 2×/day	CT	30 days post-operatively: - ↓ patients with SMI loss - No impact on hospital length of stay, postoperative complications, readmissions and mortality
	Burden et al. 2017 [92]	Colorectal cancer INT = 55/CO = 46	Daily oral nutritional supplement (600 kcal, 24 g proteins) ≥5 days before surgery+ dietary advice	Dietary advice	BIA	5-7 days post-operatively: - No impact on FFMI and postoperative complications - ↓ % weight loss and surgical site infection
Physical exercise	Galvao et al. 2018 [93]	Metastatic prostate cancer INT = 28/CO = 29	Supervised endurance, resistance and flexibility exercises 3 months, 3×/week, 60 min	Usual physical activity	DXA	After 3-month intervention: - No impact on lean soft tissue - ↑ self reporting physical functioning and leg strength
	Taaffe et al. 2018 [94]	Prostate cancer with previous androgen deprivation therapy and radiotherapy INT = 50/CO = 50	Supervised endurance and resistance exercises 6 months, 2×/week, 60 min followed by home-based endurance, resistance and flexibility exercises 6 months, 2×/week, 60 min	Recommendation for 150 min/week of moderate intensity physical exercise for 12 months based on educational material	DXA	After 6-month intervention: - ↑ ASMM, chair rise time, leg and arm strength - No impact on for lean soft tissue After 12-month intervention: - No impact on ASMM, leg strength and lean soft tissue - ↑ chair rise time and arm strength
	Wall et al. 2017 [32]	Prostate cancer undergoing androgen deprivation therapy INT = 60/CO = 47	Supervised endurance and resistance exercises 6 months, 2×/week, 60 min + home-based endurance exercise 6 months, 150 min/week	Usual physical activity	DXA	After 6-month intervention: - ↑ lean soft tissue, VO_{2max}, fat oxidation - No impact on resting metabolic rate, carbohydrate oxidation and body weight
	Adams et al. 2016 [95]	Breast cancer undergoing adjuvant chemotherapy INT endurance = 66 INT resistance = 64 CO = 70	During chemotherapy: INT endurance 3×/week, 105 min INT resistance 3×/week	Usual physical activity	DXA	At the end of chemotherapy: INT resistance VS CO: - ↑ lean soft tissue index, leg and arm strength INT endurance VS CO: - No impact on lean soft tissue, leg and arm strength INT resistance VS INT endurance:- No impact on lean soft tissue - ↑ leg and arm strength

INT: intervention group, CO: control group, ω-3: omega-3 fatty acids, HMB: β-hydroxy β-methyl butyrate, CT: computed tomography, BIA: bioelectrical impedance analysis, DXA: dual-energy X-ray absorptiometry, SMI: skeletal muscle index, FFMI: fat-free mass index, ASMM: appendicular skeletal muscle mass.

Table 3. Randomized controlled trials (>100 participants): effects of nutritional or combined nutritional and physical interventions on muscle mass in older adults.

	Studies	Population	Intervention Group	Comparison Group	Muscle Mass	Significant Results
Nutrition	Cramer et al. 2016 [96]	Malnutrition and sarcopenia in the community INT = 165/CO = 165	Daily oral nutritional supplement with HMB (660 kcal, 40 g proteins) + Usual diet during 24 weeks	Daily oral nutritional supplement (660 kcal, 28 g proteins) + Usual diet	DXA	After 24-week intervention, in both groups: - No impact on lean soft tissue - ↑ FM, handgrip strength, gait speed, muscle quality and isokenetic peak torque leg strength - No outcome difference between groups
Nutrition	Malafarina et al. 2017 [97]	Traumatic hip fracture in rehabilitation hospital INT = 55/CO = 52	Daily oral nutritional supplement with HMB (660 kcal, 40 g proteins) + Standard diet 1500 kcal, 87.4 g protein during rehabilitation stay	Standard diet 1500 kcal, 87.4 g protein	BIA	At the end of the rehabilitation: - ↓ FFM, ASMM and BMI decrease - No impact on handgrip strength, gait speed
Nutrition and physical exercise	Englund et al. 2017 [98] Fielding et al. 2017 [99]	Mobility-limitation and vitamin D insufficiency in the community INT = 74/CO = 75	Daily oral nutritional supplement (150 kcal, 20 g whey protein, 800UI vit D) + Supervised endurance, resistance, balance and flexibility exercises 3x/week, 60 min during 6 months	Daily placebo (30 kcal) + Supervised endurance, resistance, balance and flexibility exercises 3x/week, 60 min during 6 months	DXA	After 6-month intervention, in both groups: - No impact on ASMM - ↑ muscle strength, thigh muscle composition, gait speed, short physical performance battery score - ↓ FM - ↑ lean soft tissue only for control group - ↑ 25(OH)D only for intervention group - No outcome difference between groups

INT: Intervention group, CO: Control group, HMB: β-hydroxy β-methyl butyrate, DXA: dual-energy X-ray absorptiometry, BIA: bioelectrical impedance analysis, FM: fat mass, FFM: fat-free mass, ASMM: appendicular skeletal muscle mass, BMI: body mass index.

5. Use of Body Composition in Clinical Practice

Current trends towards the aging population and increased prevalence of chronic diseases will continue to rise in the next decades [100]. Malnutrition will thus likely become more problematic on a large scale and standardized care of this condition is needed. Although convenient and quick, BMI has shown limitations in the screening and the follow-up of malnutrition with a tendency to underestimate muscle mass [6–8]. The disparity between BMI and FFM raise the need for a precise quantitative evaluation of muscle mass or muscle function to both direct and validate the effects of clinical interventions in malnourished patients. Indeed, it has been established that a loss of muscle mass is associated with a decrease in physical function or muscle strength [101]. Thus, body composition evaluation should be used for the screening and diagnosis of malnutrition in clinical practice, but also for its follow-up, such as in investigation of weight loss composition following surgery or cancer therapy [4,72,84,102]. Repeated measurements of body composition will allow for the tailoring multimodal therapy. Examples of patient samples are presented in Figure 3. They highlight the clinical importance of body composition assessment to detect changes in muscle mass according to every specific patient event. Furthermore, these examples illustrate the advantage of body composition over BMI. For example, Figure 3a shows a stabilization of FFM but a decrease of total body weight and thus of BMI between July and September 2018. In Figure 3c, BMI tends to decrease as MAMC increases.

To date, MAMC, DXA, BIA, and CT at the L3 level seem to be more relevant to assess body composition in clinical practice. Figure 4 summarizes the best methods to evaluate muscle mass according to techniques availability, patient's hydration, and BMI. CT is highly precise, but, due to radiation exposure and the existence of less irradiating body composition methods, this technique should only be used in patients who undergo CT scan for other purposes such as diagnosis or follow-up [103]. Of note, deriving body composition from pre-existing clinical images is an opportunity to improve diagnosis and treatment without additional cost or patient burden. Clinical research in this area is warranted. The same applies to DXA, which can be performed without additional radiation, costs, and logistical constraints in patients who already benefit from repetitive measurement of bone density in routine care [11]. These two methods are, however, rarely used for body composition assessment in clinical routine, probably because clinical practitioners and radiologists lack information on these techniques. In other situations, BIA appears to be the most suitable method. Indeed, BIA is a portable non-invasive bedside method, quick, cheap, and reproducible [25]. Finally, MAMC will be useful especially in patients with variations in hydration level (e.g., ascites and edemas) or extreme BMI which are BIA limitations [104]. Furthermore, body composition should be integrated into routine clinical practice for a personalized nutritional support. FFM, including muscle mass, is the primary determinant of resting energy expenditure (REE) [105]. In clinical routine, indirect calorimetry is used to assess REE that reflects vital activities (cardiac, respiratory, secretory, cellular, basal muscle tone). The effect of FFM on REE depends on its quantity, assessed by body composition, and its metabolic activity [106]. Clinical conditions associated with muscle wasting, hypercatabolism and/or immobilization, lead to REE variations. Thus, in clinical practice, combining the measurement of body composition with indirect calorimetry may be useful to optimize the nutritional prescription and for the interpretation of feeding energy needs over time. Finally, clinicians should be trained to routinely use body composition in their practice, and interpreting the results should be included in pre- and post-graduate educational programs, as proposed by the European Society for Clinical Nutrition and Metabolism Life Long Learning (LLL) program. The awareness and the training of clinicians to body composition assessment may be a great opportunity to improve interdisciplinary care in the screening and management of malnutrition.

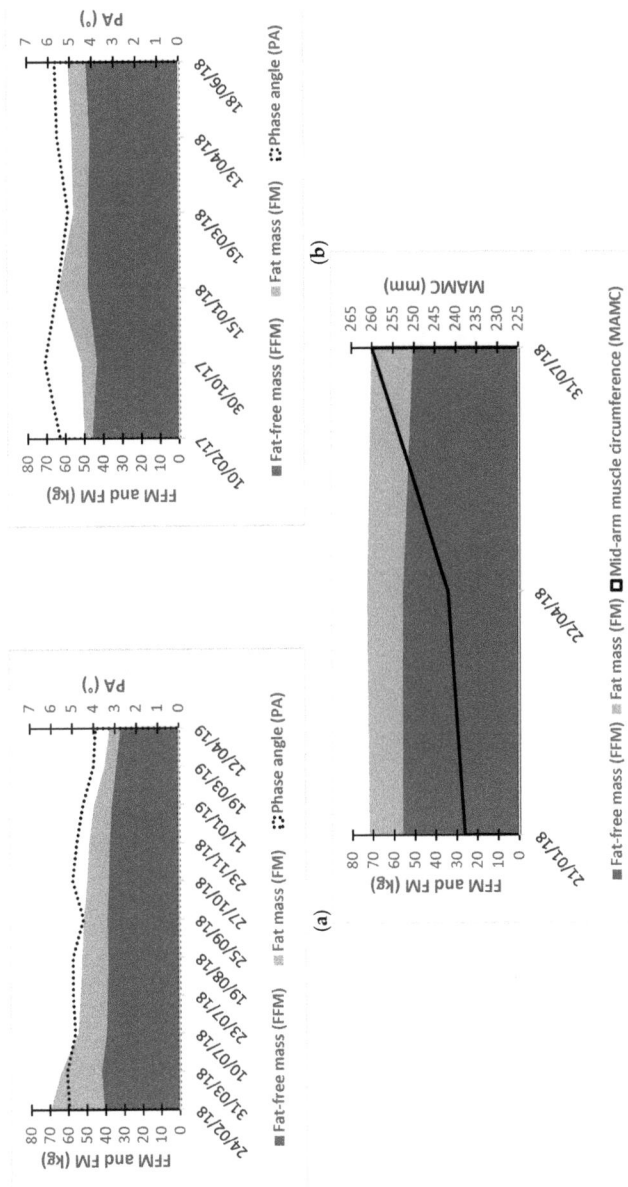

Figure 3. Patients samples (personal data). Evaluation of body composition by 50 kHz bioelectrical impedance analysis: (**a**) Obese patient with gastric cancer. February 2018: total gastrectomy. March to July 2018: severe diarrhea. October 2018: severe nausea. January 2019: tumor recurrence and beginning of a new cycle of chemotherapy until death in April 2019. A decrease in fat-free mass, fat mass and phase angle is observed for each new event and until patient's death. This example illustrates the association between muscle mass drop and mortality. (**b**) Malnourished COPD patient GOLD stage IV. October 2017: Start of multimodal therapy including enteral support, resistance and endurance physical training and anabolic steroids. An increase of fat-free mass, fat mass and phase angle is observed during the time of multimodal therapy. This example illustrates the importance of body composition assessment to monitor the effects of intervention(s). Evaluation of body composition by 50 kHz bioelectrical impedance analysis and mid-arm muscle circumference: (**c**) Cirrhotic patient with ascites. July 2018: Documented ascites. A decrease of fat-free mass but an increase of mid-arm muscle circumference are observed. This case illustrates BIA limitation in the presence of hydration level variations.

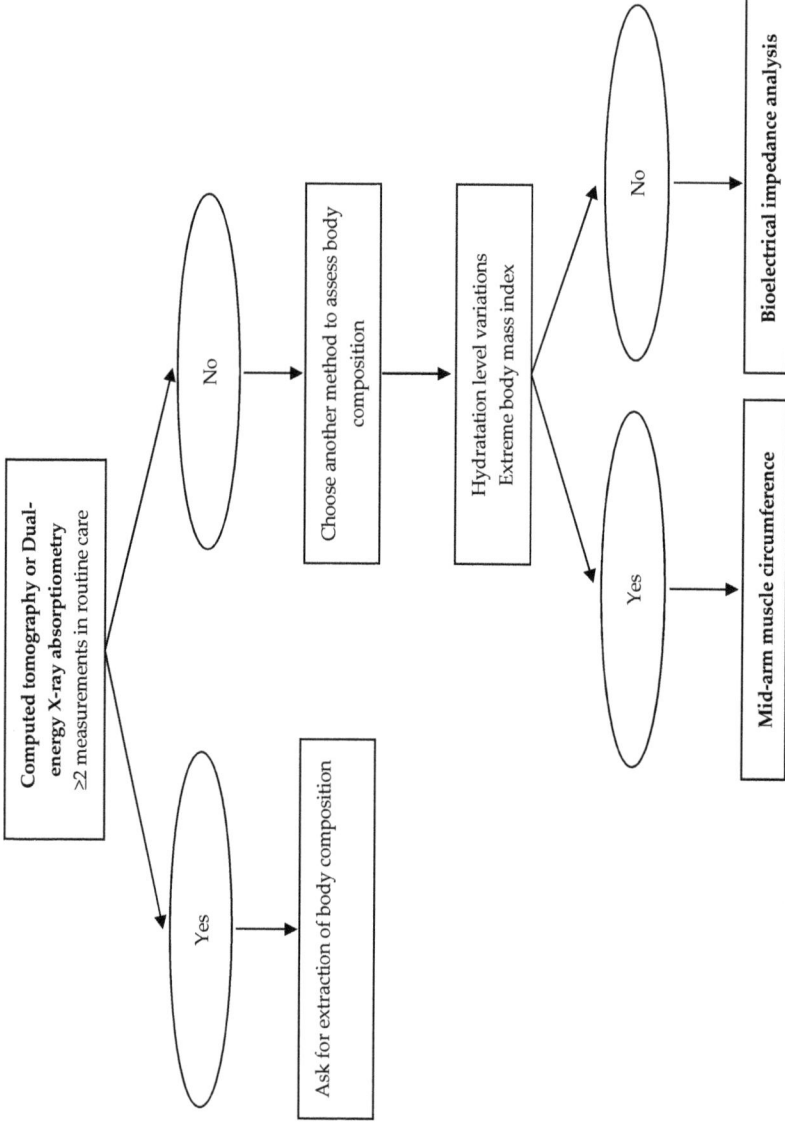

Figure 4. Muscle mass assessment in clinical practice: which method?

6. Conclusions

Available data suggest that precise assessment of body composition might be clinically relevant in the management of malnourished patients. Various methods have been validated to measure muscle mass. The method selection should be driven by the clinical situation, the patient's characteristics, and logistic and economic parameters. Standard measures of body composition such as BMI are valuable for their simplicity in daily practice. They do, however, not reflect body composition compartments. There is growing evidence in the literature that repartition of muscle mass is a more valuable tool in this assessment. Knowing this repartition allows a tailored approach to the nutritional treatment of malnourished patients and, according to the literature, led to improved clinical outcomes in various chronic diseases as well as in the older adult. Therefore, there is a need for more systematized data to orientate upcoming clinical guidelines of body composition assessment in malnourished patients.

Author Contributions: Conceptualization, J.M., N.A., K.N. and L.G.; methodology J.M. and L.G.; writing—original draft preparation, J.M.; writing—review and editing, N.A., K.N. and L.G.; supervision, L.G.

Conflicts of Interest: The authors declare no conflict of interest.

Abbreviations

GLIM	Global Leadership Initiative on Malnutrition
BMI	body mass index
MAMC	mid-arm muscle circumference
BIA	bioelectrical impedance analysis
DXA	dual-energy X-ray absorptiometry
CT	computed tomography
FFM	fat-free mass
ASMM	appendicular skeletal muscle mass
FFMI	fat-free mass index
ASMMI	appendicular skeletal muscle mass index
SMI	skeletal muscle index
COPD	chronic obstructive pulmonary disease
CHF	chronic heart failure
BNP	brain natriuretic peptide
GOLD	Global Initiative for Obstructive Lung Disease
BODE	Body mass index/Airflow obstruction/Dyspnea/Exercise capacity
REE	resting energy expenditure

References

1. Cederholm, T.; Barazzoni, R.; Austin, P.; Ballmer, P.; Biolo, G.; Bischoff, S.C.; Compher, C.; Correia, I.; Higashiguchi, T.; Holst, M.; et al. ESPEN guidelines on definitions and terminology of clinical nutrition. *Clin. Nutr.* **2017**, *36*, 49–64. [CrossRef] [PubMed]
2. Ljungqvist, O.; Van Gossum, A.; Sanz, M.L.; De Man, F. The European fight against malnutrition. *Clin. Nutr.* **2010**, *29*, 149–150. [CrossRef] [PubMed]
3. Norman, K.; Pichard, C.; Lochs, H.; Pirlich, M. Prognostic impact of disease-related malnutrition. *Clin. Nutr.* **2008**, *27*, 5–15. [CrossRef] [PubMed]
4. Cederholm, T.; Jensen, G.; Correia, M.; Gonzalez, M.; Fukushima, R.; Higashiguchi, T.; Baptista, G.; Barazzoni, R.; Blaauw, R.; Coats, A.; et al. GLIM criteria for the diagnosis of malnutrition—A consensus report from the global clinical nutrition community. *J. Cachexia Sarcopenia Muscle* **2019**, *10*, 207–217. [CrossRef] [PubMed]
5. Bigaard, J.; Frederiksen, K.; Tjønneland, A.; Thomsen, B.L.; Overvad, K.; Heitmann, B.L.; Sørensen, T.I. Body Fat and Fat-Free Mass and All-Cause Mortality. *Obes. Res.* **2004**, *12*, 1042–1049. [CrossRef] [PubMed]
6. Gonzalez, M.C.; Pastore, C.A.; Orlandi, S.P.; Heymsfield, S.B. Obesity paradox in cancer: New insights provided by body composition. *Am. J. Clin. Nutr.* **2014**, *99*, 999–1005. [CrossRef] [PubMed]

7. Kyle, U.G.; Janssens, J.-P.; Rochat, T.; Raguso, C.A.; Pichard, C. Body composition in patients with chronic hypercapnic respiratory failure. *Respir. Med.* **2006**, *100*, 244–252. [CrossRef] [PubMed]
8. Leal, V.O.; Moraes, C.; Stockler-Pinto, M.B.; Lobo, J.C.; Farage, N.E.; Velarde, L.G.; Fouque, D.; Mafra, D. Is a body mass index of 23 kg/m2 a reliable marker of protein–energy wasting in hemodialysis patients? *Nutrition* **2012**, *28*, 973–977. [CrossRef] [PubMed]
9. Scafoglieri, A.; Provyn, S.; Bautmans, I.; Van Roy, P.; Clarys, J.P. Direct relationship of body mass index and waist circumference with body tissue distribution in elderly persons. *J. Nutr. Health Aging* **2011**, *15*, 924–931. [CrossRef]
10. Seidell, J.C.; Oosterlee, A.; Thijssen, M.A.; Burema, J.; Deurenberg, P.; Hautvast, J.G.; Ruijs, J.H. Assessment of intra-abdominal and subcutaneous abdominal fat: Relation between anthropometry and computed tomography. *Am. J. Clin. Nutr.* **1987**, *45*, 7–13. [CrossRef]
11. Guglielmi, G.; Ponti, F.; Agostini, M.; Amadori, M.; Battista, G.; Bazzocchi, A. The role of DXA in sarcopenia. *Aging Clin. Exp. Res.* **2016**, *28*, 1047–1060. [CrossRef] [PubMed]
12. Antonelli Incalzi, R.; Landi, F.; Cipriani, L.; Bruno, E.; Pagano, F.; Gemma, A.; Capparella, O.; Carbonin, P. Nutritional assessment: A primary component of multidimensional geriatric assessment in the acute care setting. *J. Am. Geriatr. Soc.* **1996**, *44*, 166–174. [CrossRef] [PubMed]
13. Carnevale, V.; Castriotta, V.; Piscitelli, P.A.; Nieddu, L.; Mattera, M.; Guglielmi, G.; Scillitani, A. Assessment of Skeletal Muscle Mass in Older People: Comparison Between 2 Anthropometry-Based Methods and Dual-Energy X-ray Absorptiometry. *J. Am. Med. Dir. Assoc.* **2018**, *19*, 793–796. [CrossRef] [PubMed]
14. Noori, N.; Kopple, J.D.; Kovesdy, C.P.; Feroze, U.; Sim, J.J.; Murali, S.B.; Luna, A.; Gomez, M.; Luna, C.; Bross, R.; et al. Mid-Arm Muscle Circumference and Quality of Life and Survival in Maintenance Hemodialysis Patients. *Clin. J. Am. Soc. Nephrol.* **2010**, *5*, 2258–2268. [CrossRef] [PubMed]
15. Wijnhoven, H.A.; de Boer, M.R.; van Maanen, M.J.; van Dongen, D.M.; Kraaij, S.F.; Smit, T.; Visser, M. Reproducibility of measurements of mid-upper arm circumference in older persons. *J. Hum. Nutr. Diet.* **2013**, *26*, 24–31. [CrossRef] [PubMed]
16. Duren, D.L.; Sherwood, R.J.; Czerwinski, S.A.; Lee, M.; Choh, A.C.; Siervogel, R.M.; Chumlea, W.C. Body Composition Methods: Comparisons and Interpretation. *J. Diabetes Sci. Technol.* **2008**, *2*, 1139–1146. [CrossRef] [PubMed]
17. Kyle, U.G.; Bosaeus, I.; De Lorenzo, A.D.; Deurenberg, P.; Elia, M.; Gómez, J.M.; Heitmann, B.L.; Kent-Smith, L.; Melchior, J.-C.; Pirlich, M.; et al. Bioelectrical impedance analysis?part I: Review of principles and methods. *Clin. Nutr.* **2004**, *23*, 1226–1243. [CrossRef] [PubMed]
18. Kyle, U.G.; Genton, L.; Karsegard, L.; Slosman, D.O.; Pichard, C. Single prediction equation for bioelectrical impedance analysis in adults aged 20–94 years. *Nutr.* **2001**, *17*, 248–253. [CrossRef]
19. Kyle, U.; Genton, L.; Hans, D.; Pichard, C. Validation of a bioelectrical impedance analysis equation to predict appendicular skeletal muscle mass (ASMM). *Clin. Nutr.* **2003**, *22*, 537–543. [CrossRef]
20. Bosaeus, I.; Wilcox, G.; Rothenberg, E.; Strauss, B.J. Skeletal muscle mass in hospitalized elderly patients: Comparison of measurements by single-frequency BIA and DXA. *Clin. Nutr.* **2014**, *33*, 426–431. [CrossRef] [PubMed]
21. Peniche, D.B.R.; Giorguli, G.R.; Alemán-Mateo, H. Accuracy of a predictive bioelectrical impedance analysis equation for estimating appendicular skeletal muscle mass in a non-Caucasian sample of older people. *Arch. Gerontol. Geriatr.* **2015**, *61*, 39–43. [CrossRef] [PubMed]
22. Diaz, E.O.; Villar, J.; Immink, M.; Gonzales, T. Bioimpedance or anthropometry? *Eur. J. Clin. Nutr.* **1989**, *43*, 129–137. [PubMed]
23. Kyle, U.G.; Genton, L.; Slosman, D.O.; Pichard, C. Fat-free and fat mass percentiles in 5225 healthy subjects aged 15 to 98 years. *Nutrition* **2001**, *17*, 534–541. [CrossRef]
24. Norman, K.; Stobäus, N.; Pirlich, M.; Bosy-Westphal, A. Bioelectrical phase angle and impedance vector analysis—Clinical relevance and applicability of impedance parameters. *Clin. Nutr.* **2012**, *31*, 854–861. [CrossRef] [PubMed]
25. Kyle, U.G.; Bosaeus, I.; De Lorenzo, A.D.; Deurenberg, P.; Elia, M.; Gómez, J.M.; Heitmann, B.L.; Kent-Smith, L.; Melchior, J.-C.; Pirlich, M.; et al. Bioelectrical impedance analysis—part II: Utilization in clinical practice. *Clin. Nutr.* **2004**, *23*, 1430–1453. [CrossRef] [PubMed]
26. Andreoli, A.; Garaci, F.; Cafarelli, F.P.; Guglielmi, G. Body composition in clinical practice. *Eur. J. Radiol.* **2016**, *85*, 1461–1468. [CrossRef] [PubMed]

27. Deutz, N.E.; Ashurst, I.; Ballesteros, M.D.; Bear, D.E.; Cruz-Jentoft, A.J.; Genton, L.; Landi, F.; Laviano, A.; Norman, K.; Prado, C.M. The Underappreciated Role of Low Muscle Mass in the Management of Malnutrition. *J. Am. Med. Dir. Assoc.* **2019**, *20*, 22–27. [CrossRef]
28. Genton, L.; Hans, D.; Kyle, U.G.; Pichard, C. Dual-Energy X-ray absorptiometry and body composition: Differences between devices and comparison with reference methods. *Nutrition* **2002**, *18*, 66–70. [CrossRef]
29. Andreoli, A.; Scalzo, G.; Masala, S.A.; Tarantino, U.; Guglielmi, G. Body composition assessment by dual-energy X-ray absorptiometry (DXA). *La Radiol. Med.* **2009**, *114*, 286–300. [CrossRef]
30. Kelly, T.; Berger, N.; Richardson, T. DXA body composition: Theory and practice. *Appl. Radiat. Isot.* **1998**, *49*, 511–513. [CrossRef]
31. Bredella, M.A.; Ghomi, R.H.; Thomas, B.J.; Torriani, M.; Brick, D.J.; Gerweck, A.V.; Misra, M.; Klibanski, A.; Miller, K.K. Comparison of DXA and CT in the Assessment of Body Composition in Premenopausal Women with Obesity and Anorexia Nervosa. *Obesity* **2010**, *18*, 2227–2233. [CrossRef] [PubMed]
32. Amini, B.; Boyle, S.P.; Boutin, R.D.; Lenchik, L. Approaches to Assessment of Muscle Mass and Myosteatosis on Computed Tomography (CT): A Systematic Review. *J. Gerontol. Ser. A* **2019**. [CrossRef] [PubMed]
33. Fearon, K.; Strasser, F.; Anker, S.D.; Bosaeus, I.; Bruera, E.; Fainsinger, R.L.; Jatoi, A.; Loprinzi, C.; Macdonald, N.; Mantovani, G.; et al. Definition and classification of cancer cachexia: An international consensus. *Lancet Oncol.* **2011**, *12*, 489–495. [CrossRef]
34. Shen, W.; Punyanitya, M.; Wang, Z.; Gallagher, D.; St-Onge, M.P.; Albu, J.; Heymsfield, S.B.; Heshka, S. Total body skeletal muscle and adipose tissue volumes: Estimation from a single abdominal cross-sectional image. *J. Appl. Physiol.* **2004**, *97*, 2333–2338. [CrossRef] [PubMed]
35. Mattsson, S.; Thomas, B.J. Development of methods for body composition studies. *Phys. Med. Boil.* **2006**, *51*, R203–R228. [CrossRef] [PubMed]
36. Heymsfield, S.B.; Wang, Z.; Baumgartner, R.N.; Ross, R. Human Body Composition: Advances in Models and Methods. *Annu. Rev. Nutr.* **1997**, *17*, 527–558. [CrossRef] [PubMed]
37. Prado, C.M.; Heymsfield, S.B. Lean tissue imaging: A new era for nutritional assessment and intervention. *JPEN J. Parenter Enter. Nutr.* **2014**, *38*, 940–953. [CrossRef] [PubMed]
38. Prado, C.M.; Birdsell, L.A.; Baracos, V.E. The emerging role of computerized tomography in assessing cancer cachexia. *Curr. Opin. Support. Palliat. Care* **2009**, *3*, 269–275. [CrossRef]
39. Visser, M.; Fuerst, T.; Lang, T.; Salamone, L.; Harris, T.B. Validity of fan-beam dual-energy X-ray absorptiometry for measuring fat-free mass and leg muscle mass. Health, aging, and body composition study–dual-energy X-ray absorptiometry and body composition working group. *J. Appl. Physiol.* **1999**, *87*, 1513–1520. [CrossRef]
40. Hickson, M. Malnutrition and ageing. *Postgrad. Med. J.* **2006**, *82*, 2–8. [CrossRef]
41. Von Haehling, S.; Anker, M.S.; Anker, S.D. Prevalence and clinical impact of cachexia in chronic illness in Europe, USA, and Japan: Facts and numbers update 2016. *J. Cachexia Sarcopenia Muscle* **2016**, *7*, 507–509. [CrossRef] [PubMed]
42. Murray, C.J.; Lopez, A.D. Measuring the Global Burden of Disease. *N. Engl. J. Med.* **2013**, *369*, 448–457. [CrossRef] [PubMed]
43. Narumi, T.; Arimoto, T.; Funayama, A.; Kadowaki, S.; Otaki, Y.; Nishiyama, S.; Takahashi, H.; Shishido, T.; Miyashita, T.; Miyamoto, T.; et al. The prognostic importance of objective nutritional indexes in patients with chronic heart failure. *J. Cardiol.* **2013**, *62*, 307–313. [CrossRef] [PubMed]
44. Montes de Oca, M.; Talamo, C.; Perez-Padilla, R.; Jardim, J.R.; Muino, A.; Lopez, M.V.; Valdivia, G.; Pertuzé, J.; Moreno, D.; Halbert, R.J.; et al. Chronic obstructive pulmonary disease and body mass index in five Latin America cities: The PLATINO study. *Respir. Med.* **2008**, *102*, 642–650. [CrossRef] [PubMed]
45. Michallet, M.; De Montreuil, C.B.; Hébuterne, X.; Lemarié, E.; Schneider, S.M.; Goldwasser, F. Prevalence of Malnutrition and Current Use of Nutrition Support in Patients with Cancer. *J. Parenter. Enter. Nutr.* **2014**, *38*, 196–204. [CrossRef]
46. Costa, T.M.R.L.; Costa, F.M.; Jonasson, T.H.; Moreira, C.A.; Boguszewski, C.L.; Borba, V.Z.C. Body composition and sarcopenia in patients with chronic obstructive pulmonary disease. *Endocrine* **2018**, *60*, 95–102. [CrossRef]
47. Matkovic, Z.; Cvetko, D.; Rahelic, D.; Esquinas, C.; Zarak, M.; Miravitlles, M.; Tudoric, N. Nutritional Status of Patients with Chronic Obstructive Pulmonary Disease in Relation to their Physical Performance. *COPD J. Chronic Obstr. Pulm. Dis.* **2017**, *14*, 626–634. [CrossRef]

48. Celli, B.R.; Locantore, N.; Tal-Singer, R.; Riley, J.; Miller, B.; Vestbo, J.; Yates, J.C.; Silverman, E.K.; Owen, C.A.; Divo, M.; et al. Emphysema and extrapulmonary tissue loss in COPD: A multi-organ loss of tissue phenotype. *Eur. Respir. J.* **2018**, *51*. [CrossRef]
49. Bekfani, T.; Pellicori, P.; Morris, D.A.; Ebner, N.; Valentova, M.; Steinbeck, L.; Wachter, R.; Elsner, S.; Sliziuk, V.; Schefold, J.C.; et al. Sarcopenia in patients with heart failure with preserved ejection fraction: Impact on muscle strength, exercise capacity and quality of life. *Int. J. Cardiol.* **2016**, *222*, 41–46. [CrossRef]
50. Tsuchida, K.; Fujihara, Y.; Hiroki, J.; Hakamata, T.; Sakai, R.; Nishida, K.; Sudo, K.; Tanaka, K.; Hosaka, Y.; Takahashi, K.; et al. Significance of Sarcopenia Evaluation in Acute Decompensated Heart Failure. *Int. Heart J.* **2018**, *59*, 143–148. [CrossRef]
51. Sanada, K.; Miyachi, M.; Tanimoto, M.; Yamamoto, K.; Murakami, H.; Okumura, S.; Gando, Y.; Suzuki, K.; Tabata, I.; Higuchi, M. A cross-sectional study of sarcopenia in Japanese men and women: Reference values and association with cardiovascular risk factors. *Eur. J. Appl. Physiol.* **2010**, *110*, 57–65. [CrossRef] [PubMed]
52. Doust, J.A.; Pietrzak, E.; Dobson, A.; Glasziou, P. How well does B-type natriuretic peptide predict death and cardiac events in patients with heart failure: Systematic review. *BMJ* **2005**, *330*, 625. [CrossRef] [PubMed]
53. Bian, X.; Dai, H.; Feng, J.; Ji, H.; Fang, Y.; Jiang, N.; Li, W.; Liu, Y. Prognostic values of abdominal body compositions on survival in advanced pancreatic cancer. *Medicine* **2018**, *97*, e10988. [CrossRef] [PubMed]
54. Sjøblom, B.; Grønberg, B.H.; Wentzel-Larsen, T.; Baracos, V.E.; Hjermstad, M.J.; Aass, N.; Bremnes, R.M.; Fløtten, Ø.; Bye, A.; Jordhøy, M. Skeletal muscle radiodensity is prognostic for survival in patients with advanced non-small cell lung cancer. *Clin. Nutr.* **2016**, *35*, 1386–1393. [CrossRef] [PubMed]
55. Gu, W.; Wu, J.; Liu, X.; Zhang, H.; Shi, G.; Zhu, Y.; Ye, D. Early skeletal muscle loss during target therapy is a prognostic biomarker in metastatic renal cell carcinoma patients. *Sci. Rep.* **2017**, *7*, 7587. [CrossRef] [PubMed]
56. Otten, L.; Stobäus, N.; Franz, K.; Genton, L.; Müller-Werdan, U.; Wirth, R.; Norman, K. Impact of sarcopenia on 1-year mortality in older patients with cancer. *Age Ageing* **2019**, *48*, 413–418. [CrossRef] [PubMed]
57. El Amrani, M.; Vermersch, M.; Fulbert, M.; Prodeau, M.; Lecolle, K.; Hebbar, M.; Ernst, O.; Pruvot, F.-R.; Truant, S. Impact of sarcopenia on outcomes of patients undergoing pancreatectomy: A retrospective analysis of 107 patients. *Medicine* **2018**, *97*, e12076. [CrossRef]
58. Choi, M.H.; Kim, K.A.; Hwang, S.S.; Byun, J.Y.; Schaller, B. CT-quantified muscle and fat change in patients after surgery or endoscopic resection for early gastric cancer and its impact on long-term outcomes. *Medicine* **2018**, *97*, e13878. [CrossRef]
59. Kudou, K.; Saeki, H.; Nakashima, Y.; Edahiro, K.; Korehisa, S.; Taniguchi, D.; Tsutsumi, R.; Nishimura, S.; Nakaji, Y.; Akiyama, S.; et al. Prognostic Significance of Sarcopenia in Patients with Esophagogastric Junction Cancer or Upper Gastric Cancer. *Ann. Surg. Oncol.* **2017**, *24*, 1804–1810. [CrossRef]
60. Park, H.S.; Kim, H.S.; Beom, S.H.; Rha, S.Y.; Chung, H.C.; Kim, J.H.; Chun, Y.J.; Lee, S.W.; Choe, E.-A.; Heo, S.J.; et al. Marked Loss of Muscle, Visceral Fat, or Subcutaneous Fat After Gastrectomy Predicts Poor Survival in Advanced Gastric Cancer: Single-Center Study from the CLASSIC Trial. *Ann. Surg. Oncol.* **2018**, *25*, 3222–3230. [CrossRef]
61. Anandavadivelan, P.; Brismar, T.B.; Nilsson, M.; Johar, A.M.; Martin, L. Sarcopenic obesity: A probable risk factor for dose limiting toxicity during neo-adjuvant chemotherapy in oesophageal cancer patients. *Clin. Nutr.* **2016**, *35*, 724–730. [CrossRef] [PubMed]
62. Feliciano, E.M.C.; Lee, V.S.; Prado, C.M.; Meyerhardt, J.A.; Alexeeff, S.; Kroenke, C.H.; Xiao, J.; Castillo, A.L.; Caan, B.J. Muscle mass at diagnosis of non-metastatic colon cancer and early discontinuation of chemotherapy, delays and dose reductions on adjuvant FOLFOX: The C-SCANS Study. *Cancer* **2017**, *123*, 4868–4877. [CrossRef] [PubMed]
63. Pecorelli, N.; Capretti, G.; Sandini, M.; Damascelli, A.; Cristel, G.; De Cobelli, F.; Gianotti, L.; Zerbi, A.; Braga, M. Impact of sarcopenic obesity on failure to rescue from major complications following pancreaticoduodenectomy for cancer: Results from a multicenter study. *Ann. Surg. Oncol.* **2018**, *25*, 308–317. [CrossRef] [PubMed]
64. Zhou, C.-J.; Zhang, F.-M.; Zhang, F.-Y.; Yu, Z.; Chen, X.-L.; Shen, X.; Zhuang, C.-L.; Chen, X.-X. Sarcopenia: A new predictor of postoperative complications for elderly gastric cancer patients who underwent radical gastrectomy. *J. Surg. Res.* **2017**, *211*, 137–146. [CrossRef] [PubMed]
65. Elliott, J.A.; Doyle, S.L.; Murphy, C.F.; King, S.; Guinan, E.M.; Beddy, P.; Ravi, N.; Reynolds, J.V. Sarcopenia: Prevalence, and impact on operative and oncologic outcomes in the multimodal management of locally advanced esophageal cancer. *Ann. Surg.* **2017**, *266*, 822–830. [CrossRef] [PubMed]

66. Van Vugt, J.L.A.; Coebergh van den Braak, R.R.J.; Lalmahomed, Z.S.; Vrijland, W.W.; Dekker, J.W.T.; Zimmerman, D.D.E.; Vles, W.J.; Coene, P.-P.L.O.; IJzermans, J.N.M. Impact of low skeletal muscle mass and density on short and long-term outcome after resection of stage I–III colorectal cancer. *Eur. J. Surg. Oncol.* **2018**, *44*, 1354–1360. [CrossRef]
67. Reisinger, K.W.; Derikx, J.P.; Van Vugt, J.L.; Von Meyenfeldt, M.F.; Hulsewé, K.W.; Damink, S.W.O.; Stoot, J.H.; Poeze, M.; Information, P.E.K.F.C. Sarcopenia is associated with an increased inflammatory response to surgery in colorectal cancer. *Clin. Nutr.* **2016**, *35*, 924–927. [CrossRef] [PubMed]
68. Naito, T.; Okayama, T.; Aoyama, T.; Ohashi, T.; Masuda, Y.; Kimura, M.; Shiozaki, H.; Murakami, H.; Kenmotsu, H.; Taira, T.; et al. Skeletal muscle depletion during chemotherapy has a large impact on physical function in elderly Japanese patients with advanced non–small-cell lung cancer. *BMC Cancer* **2017**, *17*, 571. [CrossRef]
69. Huang, D.-D.; Ji, Y.-B.; Zhou, D.-L.; Li, B.; Wang, S.-L.; Chen, X.-L.; Yu, Z.; Zhuang, C.-L. Effect of surgery-induced acute muscle wasting on postoperative outcomes and quality of life. *J. Surg. Res.* **2017**, *218*, 58–66. [CrossRef]
70. Neefjes, E.C.; Hurk, R.M.V.D.; Blauwhoff-Buskermolen, S.; Van Der Vorst, M.J.; Becker-Commissaris, A.; De Van Der Schueren, M.A.; Buffart, L.M.; Verheul, H.M.; Vorst, M.J.; Schueren, M.A. Muscle mass as a target to reduce fatigue in patients with advanced cancer. *J. Cachexia Sarcopenia Muscle* **2017**, *8*, 623–629. [CrossRef]
71. Citak, E.; Tulek, Z.; Uzel, O. Nutritional status in patients with head and neck cancer undergoing radiotherapy: A longitudinal study. *Support. Care Cancer* **2019**, *27*, 239–247. [CrossRef] [PubMed]
72. Cruz-Jentoft, A.J.; Bahat, G.; Bauer, J.; Boirie, Y.; Bruyere, O.; Cederholm, T.; Cooper, C.; Landi, F.; Rolland, Y.; Aihie Sayer, A.; et al. Sarcopenia: Revised European consensus on definition and diagnosis. *Age Ageing* **2019**, *48*, 16–31. [CrossRef] [PubMed]
73. Landi, F.; Calvani, R.; Tosato, M.; Martone, A.M.; Bernabei, R.; Onder, G.; Marzetti, E. Impact of physical function impairment and multimorbidity on mortality among community-living older persons with sarcopaenia: Results from the ilSIRENTE prospective cohort study. *BMJ Open* **2016**, *6*, e008281. [CrossRef] [PubMed]
74. Kim, Y.H.; Kim, K.I.; Paik, N.J.; Kim, K.W.; Jang, H.C.; Lim, J.Y. Muscle strength: A better index of low physical performance than muscle mass in older adults. *Geriatr. Gerontol. Int.* **2016**, *16*, 577–585. [CrossRef] [PubMed]
75. Zaslavsky, O.; Li, W.; Going, S.; Datta, M.; Snetselaar, L.; Zelber-Sagi, S. Association between body composition and hip fractures in older women with physical frailty. *Geriatr. Gerontol. Int.* **2017**, *17*, 898–904. [CrossRef] [PubMed]
76. Verlaan, S.; Aspray, T.J.; Bauer, J.M.; Cederholm, T.; Hemsworth, J.; Hill, T.R.; McPhee, J.S.; Piasecki, M.; Seal, C.; Sieber, C.C.; et al. Nutritional status, body composition, and quality of life in community-dwelling sarcopenic and non-sarcopenic older adults: A case-control study. *Clin. Nutr.* **2017**, *36*, 267–274. [CrossRef] [PubMed]
77. Chiles Shaffer, N.; Ferrucci, L.; Shardell, M.; Simonsick, E.M.; Studenski, S. Agreement and predictive validity using less-conservative foundation for the national institutes of health sarcopenia project weakness cutpoints. *J. Am. Geriatr. Soc.* **2017**, *65*, 574–579. [CrossRef] [PubMed]
78. Resnick, B.; Hebel, J.R.; Gruber-Baldini, A.L.; Hicks, G.E.; Hochberg, M.C.; Orwig, D.; Eastlack, M.; Magaziner, J. The impact of body composition, pain and resilience on physical activity, physical function and physical performance at 2 months post hip fracture. *Arch. Gerontol. Geriatr.* **2018**, *76*, 34–40. [CrossRef]
79. Yalcin, A.; Aras, S.; Atmis, V.; Cengiz, O.K.; Cinar, E.; Atli, T.; Varli, M. Sarcopenia and mortality in older people living in a nursing home in Turkey. *Geriatr. Gerontol. Int.* **2017**, *17*, 1118–1124. [CrossRef]
80. Carrión, S.; Roca, M.; Costa, A.; Arreola, V.; Ortega, O.; Palomera, E.; Serra-Prat, M.; Cabré, M.; Clavé, P. Nutritional status of older patients with oropharyngeal dysphagia in a chronic versus an acute clinical situation. *Clin. Nutr.* **2017**, *36*, 1110–1116. [CrossRef]
81. Coats, A.J.S. Clinical utility of exercise training in chronic systolic heart failure. *Nat. Rev. Cardiol.* **2011**, *8*, 380–392. [CrossRef] [PubMed]
82. Maltais, F.; Decramer, M.; Casaburi, R.; Barreiro, E.; Burelle, Y.; Debigare, R.; Dekhuijzen, P.N.R.; Franssen, F.; Gayan-Ramirez, G.; Gea, J.; et al. An Official American Thoracic Society/European Respiratory Society Statement: Update on Limb Muscle Dysfunction in Chronic Obstructive Pulmonary Disease. *Am. J. Respir. Crit. Care Med.* **2014**, *189*, e15–e62. [CrossRef] [PubMed]

83. Fong, D.Y.T.; Ho, J.W.C.; Hui, B.P.H.; Lee, A.M.; Macfarlane, D.J.; Leung, S.S.K.; Cerin, E.; Chan, W.Y.Y.; Leung, I.P.F.; Lam, S.H.S.; et al. Physical activity for cancer survivors: Meta-analysis of randomised controlled trials. *BMJ* **2012**, *344*, e70. [CrossRef] [PubMed]
84. Arends, J.; Bachmann, P.; Baracos, V.; Barthelemy, N.; Bertz, H.; Bozzetti, F.; Fearon, K.; Hütterer, E.; Isenring, E.; Kaasa, S.; et al. ESPEN guidelines on nutrition in cancer patients. *Clin. Nutr.* **2017**, *36*, 11–48. [CrossRef] [PubMed]
85. Gullett, N.P.; Hebbar, G.; Ziegler, T.R. Update on clinical trials of growth factors and anabolic steroids in cachexia and wasting1234. *Am. J. Clin. Nutr.* **2010**, *91*, 1143S–1147S. [CrossRef] [PubMed]
86. Liu, H.; Bravata, D.M.; Olkin, I.; Nayak, S.; Roberts, B.; Garber, A.M.; Hoffman, A.R. Systematic Review: The Safety and Efficacy of Growth Hormone in the Healthy Elderly. *Ann. Internal Med.* **2007**, *146*, 104. [CrossRef]
87. Calder, P.C.; Laviano, A.; Lonnqvist, F.; Muscaritoli, M.; Ohlander, M.; Schols, A. Targeted medical nutrition for cachexia in chronic obstructive pulmonary disease: A randomized, controlled trial. *J. Cachexia Sarcopenia Muscle* **2018**, *9*, 28–40. [CrossRef]
88. Van De Bool, C.; Rutten, E.P.; Van Helvoort, A.; Franssen, F.M.; Wouters, E.F.; Schols, A.M.; Bool, C.; Helvoort, A. A randomized clinical trial investigating the efficacy of targeted nutrition as adjunct to exercise training in COPD. *J. Cachexia Sarcopenia Muscle* **2017**, *8*, 748–758. [CrossRef]
89. Schutz, Y.; Kyle, U.U.G.; Pichard, C. Fat-free mass index and fat mass index percentiles in Caucasians aged 18–98 y. *Int. J. Obes.* **2002**, *26*, 953–960. [CrossRef]
90. Dos Santos, M.R.; Sayegh, A.L.; Bacurau, A.V.; Arap, M.A.; Brum, P.C.; Pereira, R.M.; Takayama, L.; Barretto, A.C.P.; Negrão, C.E.; de Nazaré NunesAlves, M.L. Effect of exercise training and testosterone replacement on skeletal muscle wasting in patients with heart failure with testosterone deficiency. *Mayo Clin. Proc.* **2016**, *91*, 575–586. [CrossRef]
91. Ritch, C.R.; Cookson, M.S.; Clark, P.E.; Chang, S.S.; Fakhoury, K.; Ralls, V.; Thu, M.H.; Penson, D.F.; Smith, J.A.; Silver, H.J. Perioperative Oral Nutrition Supplementation Reduces Prevalence of Sarcopenia following Radical Cystectomy: Results of a Prospective Randomized Controlled Trial. *J. Urol.* **2019**, *201*, 470–477. [CrossRef] [PubMed]
92. Burden, S.T.; Gibson, D.J.D.J.; Lal, S.; Hill, J.; Pilling, M.; Soop, M.; Ramesh, A.; Todd, C.; Burden, S.T.S.T. Pre-operative oral nutritional supplementation with dietary advice versus dietary advice alone in weight-losing patients with colorectal cancer: Single-blind randomized controlled trial. *J. Cachexia Sarcopenia Muscle* **2017**, *8*, 437–446. [CrossRef] [PubMed]
93. Galvao, D.A.; Taaffe, D.R.; Spry, N.; Cormie, P.; Joseph, D.; Chambers, S.K.; Chee, P.; Peddle-Mcintyre, C.J.; Hart, N.H.; Baumann, F.T.; et al. Exercise preserves physical function in prostate cancer patients with bone metastases. *Med. Sci. Sports Exerc.* **2018**, *50*, 393–399. [CrossRef] [PubMed]
94. Taaffe, D.R.; Buffart, L.M.; Newton, R.U.; Spry, N.; Denham, J.; Joseph, D.; Lamb, D.; Chambers, S.K.; Galvão, D.A. Time on androgen deprivation therapy and adaptations to exercise: Secondary analysis from a 12-month randomized controlled trial in men with prostate cancer. *BJU Int.* **2018**, *121*, 194–202. [CrossRef] [PubMed]
95. Adams, S.C.; Segal, R.J.; McKenzie, D.C.; Vallerand, J.R.; Morielli, A.R.; Mackey, J.R.; Gelmon, K.; Friedenreich, C.M.; Reid, R.D.; Courneya, K.S. Impact of resistance and aerobic exercise on sarcopenia and dynapenia in breast cancer patients receiving adjuvant chemotherapy: A multicenter randomized controlled trial. *Breast Cancer Res. Treat.* **2016**, *158*, 497–507. [CrossRef] [PubMed]
96. Cramer, J.T.; Cruz-Jentoft, A.J.; Landi, F.; Hickson, M.; Zamboni, M.; Pereira, S.L.; Hustead, D.S.; Mustad, V.A. Impacts of High-Protein Oral Nutritional Supplements Among Malnourished Men and Women with Sarcopenia: A Multicenter, Randomized, Double-Blinded, Controlled Trial. *J. Am. Med. Dir. Assoc.* **2016**, *17*, 1044–1055. [CrossRef] [PubMed]
97. Malafarina, V.; Uriz-Otano, F.; Malafarina, C.; Martinez, J.A.; Zulet, M.A. Effectiveness of nutritional supplementation on sarcopenia and recovery in hip fracture patients. A multi-centre randomized trial. *Maturitas* **2017**, *101*, 42–50. [CrossRef]
98. Englund, D.A.; Kirn, D.R.; Koochek, A.; Zhu, H.; Travison, T.G.; Reid, K.F.; Von Berens, Å.; Melin, M.; Cederholm, T.; Gustafsson, T.; et al. Nutritional Supplementation with Physical Activity Improves Muscle Composition in Mobility-Limited Older Adults, The VIVE2 Study: A Randomized, Double-Blind, Placebo-Controlled Trial. *J. Gerontol. Ser. A* **2017**, *73*, 95–101. [CrossRef]

99. Fielding, R.A.; Travison, T.G.; Kirn, D.R.; Koochek, A.; Reid, K.F.; Von Berens, Å.; Zhu, H.; Folta, S.C.; Sacheck, J.M.; Nelson, M.E.; et al. Effect of structured physical activity and nutritional supplementation on physical function in mobility-limited older adults: Results from the VIVE2 randomized trial. *J. Nutr. Health Aging* **2017**, *21*, 936–942. [CrossRef]
100. Van Oostrom, S.H.; Gijsen, R.; Stirbu, I.; Korevaar, J.C.; Schellevis, F.G.; Picavet, H.S.J.; Hoeymans, N. Time trends in prevalence of chronic diseases and multimorbidity not only due to aging: Data from general practices and health surveys. *PLoS ONE* **2016**, *11*, e0160264. [CrossRef]
101. Health AgingBody Composition Study; Delmonico, M.J.; Harris, T.B.; Visser, M.; Park, S.W.; Conroy, M.B.; Velasquez-Mieyer, P.; Boudreau, R.; Manini, T.M.; Nevitt, M.; et al. Longitudinal study of muscle strength, quality, and adipose tissue infiltration. *Am. J. Clin. Nutr.* **2009**, *90*, 1579–1585. [CrossRef] [PubMed]
102. Kiyama, T.; Mizutani, T.; Okuda, T.; Fujita, I.; Tokunaga, A.; Tajiri, T.; Barbul, A. Postoperative Changes in Body Composition after Gastrectomy. *J. Gastrointest. Surg.* **2005**, *9*, 313–319. [CrossRef] [PubMed]
103. Mourtzakis, M.; Prado, C.M.; Lieffers, J.R.; Reiman, T.; McCargar, L.J.; Baracos, V.E. A practical and precise approach to quantification of body composition in cancer patients using computed tomography images acquired during routine care. *Appl. Physiol. Nutr. Metab.* **2008**, *33*, 997–1006. [CrossRef] [PubMed]
104. Raman, M.; Mourtzakis, M.; Merli, M.; Tandon, P. A practical approach to nutritional screening and assessment in cirrhosis. *Hepatology* **2017**, *65*, 1044–1057. [CrossRef]
105. Hopkins, M.; Finlayson, G.; Duarte, C.; Whybrow, S.; Ritz, P.; Horgan, G.W.; Blundell, J.E.; Stubbs, R.J. Modelling the associations between fat-free mass, resting metabolic rate and energy intake in the context of total energy balance. *Int. J. Obes.* **2016**, *40*, 312–318. [CrossRef]
106. Cunningham, J.J. Body composition as a determinant of energy expenditure: A synthetic review and a proposed general prediction equation. *Am. J. Clin. Nutr.* **1991**, *54*, 963–969. [CrossRef]

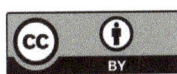

© 2019 by the authors. Licensee MDPI, Basel, Switzerland. This article is an open access article distributed under the terms and conditions of the Creative Commons Attribution (CC BY) license (http://creativecommons.org/licenses/by/4.0/).

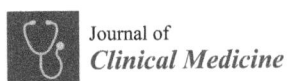

Review

Management of Malnutrition in Older Patients—Current Approaches, Evidence and Open Questions

Dorothee Volkert [1,*], Anne Marie Beck [2,3], Tommy Cederholm [4,5], Emanuele Cereda [6], Alfonso Cruz-Jentoft [7], Sabine Goisser [8], Lisette de Groot [9], Franz Großhauser [1], Eva Kiesswetter [1], Kristina Norman [10,11,12], Maryam Pourhassan [13], Ilse Reinders [14], Helen C. Roberts [15], Yves Rolland [16], Stéphane M. Schneider [17], Cornel C. Sieber [1,18], Ulrich Thiem [19], Marjolein Visser [14], Hanneke A.H. Wijnhoven [14] and Rainer Wirth [13]

1. Institute for Biomedicine of Aging, Friedrich-Alexander-Universität Erlangen-Nürnberg, 90408 Nuremberg, Germany
2. Department Nutrition and Health, University College Copenhagen, 2200 Copenhagen, Denmark
3. Herlev and Gentofte University Hospital, 2703 Herlev, Denmark
4. Clinical Nutrition and Metabolism, Department of Public Health and Caring Sciences, Uppsala University, 701 05 Uppsala, Sweden
5. Theme Ageing, Karolinska University Hospital, 171 76 Stockholm, Sweden
6. Clinical Nutrition and Dietetics Unit, Fondazione IRCCS Policlinico San Matteo, 27100 Pavia, Italy
7. Servicio de Geriatría, Hospital Universitario Ramón y Cajal (IRYCIS), 28034 Madrid, Spain
8. Heidelberg University Centre for Geriatric Medicine and Network Aging Research (NAR), University of Heidelberg, 69126 Heidelberg, Germany
9. Division of Human Nutrition, Wageningen University, 6708 WE Wageningen, The Netherlands
10. German Institute for Human Nutrition Potsdam-Rehbrücke, Department of Nutrition and Gerontology, 14558 Nuthetal, Germany
11. Research Group on Geriatrics, Charité Universitätsmedizin Berlin, corporate member of Freie Universität Berlin, Humboldt-Universität zu Berlin, and Berlin Institute of Health, 10117 Berlin, Germany
12. Institute of Nutritional Science, University of Potsdam, 14558 Nuthetal, Germany
13. Department for Geriatric Medicine, Marien Hospital Herne—University Hospital, Ruhr-Universität Bochum, 44625 Herne, Germany
14. Department of Health Sciences, Faculty of Science, and Amsterdam Public Health Research Institute, Vrije Universiteit Amsterdam, 1081 HV Amsterdam, The Netherlands
15. Southampton NIHR Biomedical Research Centre, University of Southampton, Southampton General Hospital, Southampton SO16 6YD, UK
16. Gérontopôle, Centre Hospitalo-Universitaire de Toulouse, 31059 Toulouse, France
17. Nutritional Support Unit, Centre Hospitalier Universitaire de Nice, Université Côte d'Azur, 06200 Nice, France
18. Department of Medicine, Kantonsspital Winterthur, 8401 Winterthur, Switzerland
19. Centre of Geriatrics and Gerontology, Albertinen-Haus, Hamburg, and Chair of Geriatrics and Gerontology, University Medical Centre Eppendorf, 20246 Hamburg, Germany
* Correspondence: dorothee.volkert@fau.de; Tel.: +49-911-5302-96168

Received: 4 June 2019; Accepted: 1 July 2019; Published: 4 July 2019

Abstract: Malnutrition is widespread in older people and represents a major geriatric syndrome with multifactorial etiology and severe consequences for health outcomes and quality of life. The aim of the present paper is to describe current approaches and evidence regarding malnutrition treatment and to highlight relevant knowledge gaps that need to be addressed. Recently published guidelines of the European Society for Clinical Nutrition and Metabolism (ESPEN) provide a summary of the available evidence and highlight the wide range of different measures that can be taken—from the identification and elimination of potential causes to enteral and parenteral nutrition—depending on the patient's abilities and needs. However, more than half of the recommendations therein are based on expert consensus because of a lack of evidence, and only three are concern patient-centred outcomes. Future research should further clarify the etiology of malnutrition and identify the most relevant causes in order to prevent malnutrition. Based on limited and partly conflicting evidence and the limitations of existing studies, it remains unclear which interventions are most effective in which patient groups, and if specific situations, diseases or etiologies of malnutrition require specific approaches. Patient-relevant outcomes such as functionality and quality of life need more attention, and research methodology should be harmonised to allow for the comparability of studies.

Keywords: Geriatric patients; older persons; malnutrition; therapy; interventions

1. Malnutrition in Geriatric Patients

Although geriatric patients are usually at an advanced age, a geriatric patient is not defined by a specific age, but rather by a high degree of frailty and the presence of chronic disease. Functional reserves are reduced and vulnerability to stress increased as a consequence of a cumulative decline in many physiological systems during ageing. Limitations are, however, not restricted to physical functions, but may also affect mental and/or social integrity, leading to the need of comprehensive treatment to maintain or restore independence in everyday life as far as possible.

Among other typical geriatric syndromes, such as dementia, delirium, falls or incontinence, which are characterised by high prevalence, multifactorial origin and poor outcomes [1], malnutrition (i.e., protein-energy-malnutrition or undernutrition) merits attention.

1.1. Prevalence

Malnutrition is reported in up to 50% of older adults, although prevalence estimates vary substantially depending on the population considered, the healthcare setting, and the tool used for its assessment [2–4]. A recent systematic review and meta-analysis of studies using the Mini Nutritional Assessment®— the most widespread malnutrition screening tool for older people—has summarised the following estimates according to the setting of care: community, 3%; outpatients, 6%; home-care services, 9%; nursing homes, 17.5%; hospital, 22%; long-term care, 29%; rehabilitation/sub-acute care, 29%. In addition, a high proportion of older adults are at risk of malnutrition, with estimates ranging between 27% (community/outpatients) and 50% (all other healthcare settings) [2]. These figures are in accordance with other studies and reviews, describing an increasing prevalence of malnutrition with decreasing health and functional status and increasing dependency and disability [5,6]. Prevalence rates may however vary widely between study samples even when using the same definition in the same health-care setting [2,7].

Since low muscle mass is now included as one important phenotypic criterion in the new global definition of malnutrition [8,9], and older adults are characterised by a decline of muscle mass not only due to ageing and poor physical activity but also to a poor adaptation to nutritional deficits [10], it is reasonable to argue that prevalence estimates may be even higher than previously reported.

1.2. Etiology

Due to a variety of factors, older people and specifically in-patients are at increased risk of malnutrition. A decrease in food intake is common [11] and often associated with a disease, acute or chronic, which is increasing energy needs. The combination of a decrease in dietary intake and increased needs during an illness places the older person in a group of particular risk.

The decrease in food intake is often associated with a loss of the sensory abilities of taste and smell, that results in anorexia and is termed "anorexia of ageing" [12,13], but may also be caused by a poor oral health, difficulties in chewing and swallowing, side effects of pharmacological treatment, cognitive limitations, social isolation, loneliness or depression. Many acute conditions (e.g., infections, surgery) often occur on a background of chronic co-morbidities (e.g., heart failure, respiratory disease, cancer, renal failure) and increase energy needs and precipitate malnutrition in already vulnerable older people.

Besides these individual aspects, external factors such as the quality of meals, meal ambience, and the quality of (medical and nutritional) care may affect dietary intake and contribute to malnutrition, in particular in hospitals and care homes.

Many other factors may be involved [14–16], which may be of different relevance in different health-care settings, and may also differ from person to person. Thus, without doubt, the development of malnutrition in older persons is multifactorial and complex, and presently, only partly understood.

1.3. Consequences

It is well established that malnutrition is associated with increased morbidity and mortality both in acute and chronic disease and has serious implications for recovery from disease, trauma and surgery [17]. Loss of body protein resulting from insufficient protein intake or increased requirements in disease is one hallmark of malnutrition, followed by an impaired immune status and loss of muscle mass, which contribute in large part to the increased morbidity observed in malnutrition. In old and sick individuals in particular, decreased muscle mass and strength, referred to as sarcopenia, in turn lead to impaired physical status, loss of independence and increased risk of falls and subsequent fractures which have a debilitating impact on quality of life [18]. Recovery from disease is delayed in malnutrition with longer convalescence periods. Not surprisingly, malnourished patients therefore have significantly longer hospital stays with more infectious and non-infectious complications, an increased rate of unplanned readmissions to hospital and higher health resource utilisation in the outpatient setting. These consequences not only increase the burden for the individuals concerned, but ultimately also increase the economic burden for the health care system [19]. A prospective study in adults aged over 70 recently showed that adjusted healthcare costs were 714 € per year greater in patients with malnutrition or malnutrition risk compared to well-nourished patients, mainly due to hospital admission costs [20].

In summary, malnutrition is widespread in older people and represents a major geriatric syndrome with multifactorial etiology and severe consequences. In the following section, we aim to describe current approaches and evidence regarding malnutrition treatment, and to highlight relevant knowledge gaps that need to be addressed.

2. Management of Malnutrition

2.1. General Aims and Options

Nutritional interventions in the older adult may have several complementary aims [21]:

- Maintenance or improvement of nutritional status, which may replenish the protein and energy storage that is necessary to accommodate the needs induced by a metabolic stress;
- Maintenance or improvement of function and capacity for rehabilitation; this is mostly related to the muscle compartment including muscle mass. Activities of daily living but also community living may therefore be secondary aims;
- Maintenance or improvement of health-related quality of life, probably more important, compared to the reduction in mortality, than in younger adults; restoring food intake may play a direct role as being an important mediator of pleasure and well-being;
- Reduction of morbidity, including an improved outcome of underlying chronic diseases;
- Reduction of mortality as a consequence of morbidity reduction but also by increasing treatment tolerability of the underlying chronic disease (e.g., cancer);
- Reduction of malnutrition-associated costs (reduction of the hospital length of stay, the need for subacute care stays, reduction of nursing home admissions, the number of medical examinations and prescriptions).

Thus, the aims and approaches of malnutrition treatment in older patients do not generally differ from those in younger patients, but maintenance of function and quality of life gain in importance compared to reduction of mortality.

Nutritional interventions for older people cover a broad range of different measures, which all may contribute to support adequate intake and go far beyond just providing adequate amounts of energy and nutrients. As with any geriatric syndrome, the identification and management of multiple causes constitutes the basis of appropriate nutritional care. Furthermore, adequate intake may be supported by various strategies—first of all but not only by help with eating if required. Regarding direct nutritional measures, oral strategies are always the first choice. These include various modifications of usual foods as well as offering oral nutritional supplements. Moreover, enteral and parenteral nutrition are important options also for older patients, although less often indicated.

2.2. Current Recommendations and Evidence: ESPEN Guidelines 2019

Current knowledge about the effectiveness of nutritional interventions is summarised in the updated 'ESPEN guidelines on clinical nutrition and hydration in geriatrics', which were developed in a multidisciplinary group of 13 experienced experts from 9 European countries [21]. In contrast to the previous guidelines from 2006 [22] and 2009 [23], they focus on systematic reviews, where available, and for the first time also cover the topic of dehydration, a very relevant, frequent and serious aspect of malnutrition in older persons.

Central recommendations of the ESPEN guideline for the management of malnutrition and corresponding evidence are summarised in Table 1 and described in the following Sections 2.2.1–2.2.7.

Table 1. Intervention strategies for the management of malnutrition (based on [21]).

Basic recommendations
• Routine screening for malnutrition with validated tool (GPP) followed by assessment, individualised intervention, monitoring and adjustment of interventions (GPP)
• Individualised and comprehensive nutritional care (A)
• Nutritional interventions as part of a multimodal and multidisciplinary team intervention (B)
• Identification and elimination of potential causes of malnutrition (GPP)
• Avoidance of dietary restrictions (GPP)
Supportive interventions
• Pleasant eating environment in institutions (A)
• Mealtime assistance in case of eating dependency (A in institutions, GPP in home-care)
• Sharing mealtimes with others (GPP)
• Energy-dense meals on wheels with additional meals (B)
• Nutritional information and education (B)
• Easy access to food *
Nutritional counselling
• for older persons/care givers—individualised (B)
• by a qualified person in several sessions (GPP)
Food modification
• food fortification (B)
• additional snacks/meals*, finger food (GPP)
• texture-modified, enriched foods (GPP)
• organoleptic enhancement (flavor/taste/visual appearance) *
• increasing variety of diet *
• considering individual preferences *
Oral nutritional supplements (ONS) (3 A, 3 GPP)
Enteral/parenteral nutrition (12 GPP)
Grades of recommendation: A = based on strong evidence (at least one high-quality RCT), B = based on medium evidence (high quality case-control or cohort studies); GPP = good practice point/expert consensus: Recommended best practice based on the clinical experience of the guideline development group.* topic not addressed in the ESPEN Guideline 2019 [21]).

2.2.1. Basic Recommendations

It is common sense that, as a first step in the management of malnutrition, those affected and also those at risk need to be identified. Thus, routine-screening for (risk of) malnutrition is recommended in all older people in institutions and in the community (at admission/initial contact and at regular intervals) independent of their diagnosis and the presence of overweight or obesity [21]. The use of a validated tool is considered to be good clinical practice, confirmed by recent study results indicating an association of the use of validated tools with lower prevalence of malnutrition and better nutritional care in hospitals [24]. The most common screening tool developed and validated for older persons is the short-form of the Mini Nutritional Assessment (MNA), which can be applied in all geriatric settings [2,21,25]. There are, however, many other tools available. Among 48 tools used to screen for risk of malnutrition in older adults, and recently rated with respect to validation, parameters and practicability, the highest scoring tools were: i) DETERMINE your health checklist for the community setting; ii) the Nutritional Form for the Elderly (NUFFE) for the rehabilitation setting; iii) the Short Nutritional Assessment Questionnaire-Residential Care (SNAQ^{RC}) for residential care and iv) both the Malnutrition Screening Tool (MST) and the Mini Nutritional Assessment Short Form Version 1 (MNA-SF-V1) for the hospital setting [26].

In people with a positive screening result, a comprehensive nutritional assessment should follow as the basis for targeted interventions [21]. The assessment should focus on the identification of potential underlying causes of malnutrition as well as of individual preferences, resources and expectations, evaluation of the severity of the nutritional deficit, and a critical review of existing dietary prescriptions. To check whether intervention goals have been reached, a close monitoring is necessary in clinical practice [21].

Regarding interventions, due to the huge heterogeneity of older people and the multitude of potential causes of malnutrition [14,15], individualised and comprehensive approaches are recommended to optimally tackle malnutrition [21]. Beneficial effects on several outcomes are documented in quite a few randomised controlled trials, interestingly all reporting benefits with respect to quality of life [21].

It is recognised that identifying and eliminating potential causes as far as possible is fundamental, although scientific evidence for this recommendation is unfortunately lacking. In older patients, adequate medical treatment is certainly of central importance, preferably avoiding medication with potentially harmful side effects on appetite, taste and smell perception, salivation or cognition.

Comprehensive approaches and treatment focused on potential causes from all areas of life require the involvement of different professional disciplines namely dietitians, nurses, nurse-aids, kitchen staff, medical doctors including dentists, and all types of therapists (e.g., speech-/swallowing, occupational, physio- and psycho-). This team effort is regarded an important factor for successful nutrition interventions. Positive effects on body weight, functional and clinical outcome have been shown in several trials, although results are partly inconsistent [21].

2.2.2. Supportive Interventions

Several recommendations in the ESPEN guideline address supportive interventions, which were highlighted more than 15 years ago in the resolution of the Council of Europe on food and nutritional care in hospitals [27]. Beneficial effects of assistance with eating, as far as required, and of a pleasant eating environment in institutions on dietary intake of older persons with malnutrition or at risk of malnutrition are well documented in several systematic reviews. A home-like dining environment has been shown also to contribute to quality of life. Based on expert consensus, it is also recommended to encourage older persons to share their mealtimes with others, since eating in company is known to stimulate dietary intake and may also be an important aspect with respect to quality of life [21].

In addition, the ability to access the meal (in case of mobility limitations) and the food (e.g., in packages that are difficult to open) may be relevant [28]. Of course, food should be easily accessible—also between meals—and support with shopping and preparing meals, reaching the dining room and opening packages should be provided as needed. In individual cases, it may be sensible to provide specially adapted cutlery or cups with special shapes.

The need for education regarding nutrition among all staff groups and the need for knowledge among patients about the importance of a good nutritional status are well recognised [27]. Several systematic reviews document that older persons with malnutrition or who are at risk of malnutrition, as well as their care givers, should be offered nutritional information and education as part of a comprehensive intervention concept in order to improve awareness of and basic knowledge about nutritional problems, and thus promote adequate dietary intake, albeit based on partly conflicting and fragmentary evidence [21].

2.2.3. Nutritional Counselling

Nutritional counselling goes beyond information and education with the aim to develop a sound understanding of nutritional topics and to support sustainable health-promoting eating habits, and is regarded as the first line of nutrition therapy. Current guidelines recommend that older people with or at risk of malnutrition and/or their caregivers should be offered individualised nutritional counselling by a qualified dietician in several sessions to develop their understanding of the importance of nutrition and support healthy eating habits [21]. Individual sessions may be combined with group sessions, telephone contacts and written advice.

Counselling by a dietician or nutritionist is recommended, but in practice this may be impractical for all and reserved for those patients at highest risk. Many older people at risk of malnutrition live at home and will have initial contact with their primary healthcare team who could review their nutritional status and deliver appropriate advice, supported by local care pathways that include dietetic referral where appropriate [29]. However, it is unclear how to train these healthcare teams to best deliver the nutritional counselling. Group educational sessions for older people can be cost-effective but difficult to access for those with limited mobility. Older people may have difficulty accessing advice delivered in electronic formats but telephone consultations can effectively offer nutritional support for older people [30] and for family carers of those with dementia at risk of malnutrition [31].

2.2.4. Food Modification

Food modifications include adjustments of macro- and/or micronutrient content, or the avoidance of specific allergens as well as modifications of food texture or of flavor, taste and/or visual appearance (organoleptic enhancement). Nutrients or additional ingredients can be added to regular foods in order to increase energy and/or nutrient density (fortified or enriched food) or to yield specific beneficial health effects (functional food) [32].

It has been shown in several studies and summarised in two systematic reviews that food fortification—i.e., by means of natural foods (e.g., oil, cream, butter, eggs) and/or specific nutrient preparations (e.g., maltodextrin, protein powder)—can enable increased intake while eating similar amounts of food [21]. Snacks between meals and/or finger foods can also help to increase intake, in particular for people who have difficulties using cutlery or remaining at the table for the meal; this is, however, not well studied [21].

Texture-modified foods are available in various qualities (e.g., liquidised/thin puree, thick puree/ soft and smooth, finely minced) [32] and intend to compensate for chewing and swallowing problems, which are widespread in older people and related to poor food intake [33]. Since evidence regarding the effects of texture-modified food is scarce [21], it was concluded that it is 'good clinical practice' to offer texture-modified, enriched foods to older persons with malnutrition or at risk of malnutrition and signs of oropharyngeal dysphagia and/or chewing problems as a compensatory strategy to support adequate dietary intake [21,34]. Based on positive effects of enrichment of regular texture diets it was assumed that enrichment could have similar effects in texture-modified diets for patients with chewing and/or swallowing problems [21]. Since insufficient dietary and fluid intake is described in older people receiving texture-modified diets, it seems reasonable to monitor nutritional intake closely [21].

Due to little expense and no risk of harm, these recommendations were made despite presently very limited scientific evidence [21].

In addition, it seems logical that increasing the variety of foods offered and considering individual food preferences could help to ensure adequate intake of older persons—this is however not studied up to now and not addressed in current guidelines.

2.2.5. Oral Nutritional Supplements (ONS)

Several recommendations of the ESPEN guideline on clinical nutrition and hydration in geriatrics address whether older people with malnutrition or at risk of malnutrition should be offered ONS. Such supplements provide both macro- and micronutrients which are delivered as ready to drink liquids, or as semi-solids or powders that can be prepared as drinks or added to drinks or foods. According to a vast body of high-level evidence and strong consensus among experts, these supplements should provide at least 400 kcal and a minimum of 30 g of protein per day. They should be given to all older people with (risk of) malnutrition when nutritional goals cannot be met through dietary counselling for enhancing (fortified) food consumption, to improve dietary intake, body weight and to lower the risk of complications and readmission and to lower the risk of functional decline after discharge. Once offered, ONS should be given for at least one month with concurrent monthly assessment of presumed benefits and compliance evaluation, thereby tailoring ONS-type, flavour, texture and timing of supply to the older person's characteristics [21].

2.2.6. Enteral and Parenteral Nutrition

Enteral nutrition (EN)—mostly via nasogastric tubes or percutaneous endoscopic gastrostomy (PEG)—and parenteral nutrition (PN) via central or peripheral veins are important options also for old and very old patients. These invasive measures should however be reserved for those who are unable to meet their nutritional requirements by the oral or enteral route, respectively, but have a reasonable prospect of general recovery or at least stabilisation of health and well-being. Twelve recommendations in the ESPEN guideline refer to this topic, all based on available descriptive studies and expert consensus, since randomised trials would be unethical in this field. Application of these techniques always requires careful weighing of expected individual benefits and risks [21].

2.2.7. Relevance of the Refeeding Syndrome (RFS)

Based on recent research activities, management of malnutrition in older persons cannot be described without pointing out the RFS, a serious metabolic complication after reinitiating nutrition in malnourished patients [35,36]. If patients with RFS are not adequately treated, adverse effects may range from muscle weakness and peripheral oedema to multi-organ dysfunction and death [36].

The risk of developing RFS is suggested to be high especially among malnourished older patients, and is not restricted to enteral or parenteral nutrition. However, due to nonspecific initial symptoms [36] but also due to a lack of knowledge among many physicians [37], the RFS is frequently not diagnosed and consequently not treated in these patients [38]. A recent cross-sectional multicentre-study showed that nearly three-quarters of 342 geriatric hospitalised patients who were at risk of malnutrition demonstrated significant risk of RFS [39]. Like malnutrition, RFS remains a widely unrecognised and undertreated condition in clinical practice.

The key to improved patient care in this context is to raise awareness of RFS among physicians involved in nutritional care in order to identify at-risk patients and to recognise the occurrence of the RFS. In the ESPEN guideline, it is recommended to pay special attention during the first three days of EN and PN therapy in malnourished individuals to serum levels of phosphate, magnesium potassium and thiamine, which decline in RFS and should be supplemented where appropriate [21]. Accordingly, a recent review [38] also recommends close monitoring of vital parameters, fluid, serum electrolytes and thiamine in older patients at risk of RFS, whereas nutrition repletion should be started slowly and increased cautiously to reach nutritional goals after four to seven days. Using this strategy in a randomised clinical trial, mortality risk was reduced among critically ill patients [40].

2.3. New Evidence after the ESPEN Guidelines

After the literature review for the ESPEN guideline was completed, a number of new systematic reviews and clinical trials addressing different nutritional interventions in different setting have been published.

A systematic review and meta-analysis considered studies that only included older persons with malnutrition and found no beneficial effects of ONS in changing body weight, body mass index, MNA score, muscle strength, activities of daily living, Timed Up&Go test, quality of life and mortality. Results of other interventions (dietary counselling and ONS, ONS combined with exercise, new ONS nutrition delivery systems) were inconsistent [41]. Another systematic review that explored the role of exercise added to oral nutritional support reported improvements in muscle strength but not in any other outcome, however mostly based on low or very low quality evidence [42]. An interesting analysis showed that nutritional support performed by a multidisciplinary team—as recommended in the ESPEN guideline—might fare better than simple interventions in reducing mortality risk and improving quality of life [43]. A systematic review looking at studies performed in nursing homes found an effect on handgrip strength only and not in other functional parameters [44]. A further recent review focused on various treatments for anorexia of ageing, also including pharmacologic approaches and flavour enhancement, suggests that some interventions may have an impact on energy intake and body weight, but calls for methodological improvements in the field [45]. Based on a systematic review and meta-analysis, the use of telehealth interventions seems to be a new, promising strategy also for malnutrition in older people. Improved protein intake and quality of life are reported, but further research is demanded [30].

Thus, the number of systematic reviews is rapidly increasing with only few remarkable original studies. Among these, a pooled analysis of individual data from nine RCTs in older adults at risk of malnutrition merits attention. Positive intervention effects on energy intake and body weight were found, whereby the combination of nutritional counselling and ONS showed the strongest effects [46]. Pooled data from studies targeting muscle strength and mortality, however, revealed no intervention effect [47]. In contrast, the recently published large multicentre EFFORT trial demonstrated beneficial effects on important clinical outcomes by routine malnutrition screening connected with individualised nutrition support in medical inpatients managed by a dietician during hospital stay [48].

3. Knowledge Gaps

3.1. Lacking Evidence in Many Fields

Despite increasing numbers of systematic reviews on the topic, more than half of the recommendations in the ESPEN guideline are "good practice points", meaning that they are based on the clinical experience of the guideline development group because of a lack of studies [49]. The level of evidence of only 15 of the 82 recommendations justifies a grade A recommendation, and only three recommendations are directed towards patient-centered outcomes [21].

Regarding outcome parameters, most studies testing the effects of supportive interventions or food modification focus on dietary intake but do not include functional or clinical outcomes.

Most randomised clinical trials performed have examined the effects of ONS in (malnourished) older adults. Given the large number of studies and the generally quite good compliance (78%) [50], this study and intervention type currently provides the strongest evidence in the field. Besides positive effects on intake, positive effects on nutritional status are also reported, and a couple of studies also look at functional and clinical outcomes. Unfortunately, findings in this latter respect are inconsistent and often negative [21], and benefits were generally questioned just recently [41].

A general lack of scientific evidence on the effects of nutritional interventions on functional or clinical outcomes in malnourished older adults is also concluded in multiple systematic reviews [21,41,51–55].

3.2. Limitations of Existing Studies

The conflicting evidence regarding effects of nutritional interventions on functional and clinical outcomes of malnourished older adults may be explained by various limitations of previous studies. The limitations frequently addressed in the literature are summarised in Figure 1, categorised according to sample selection, design of the study, adherence to the intervention, outcome assessment, and data analyses and reporting. Some of these limitations result in a high risk of bias [56,57], thereby reducing the internal validity of previous studies.

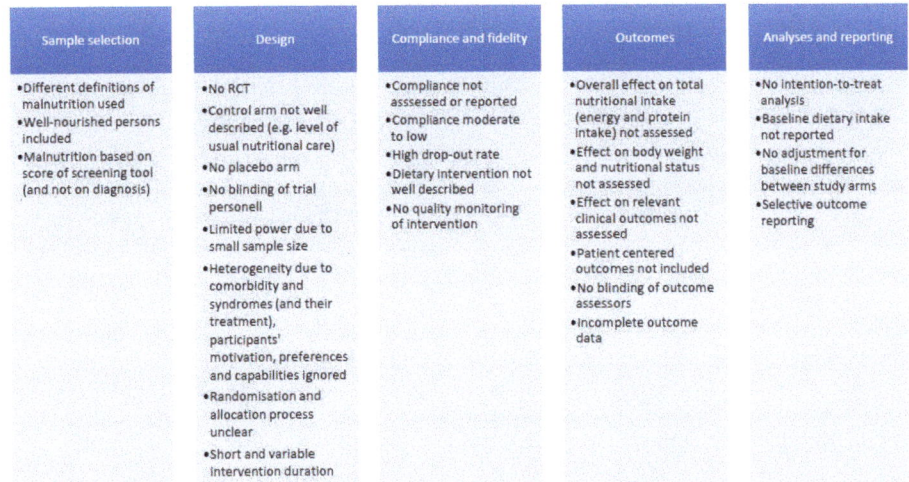

Figure 1. Limitations of previous studies investigating the effect of nutritional interventions in malnourished older people.

With regard to sample selection, some previous studies have not only included malnourished persons but older adults without malnutrition as well, which likely dilutes the potential effect of treatment on outcomes [55]. Different definitions of malnutrition were used to select participants, reducing comparability between studies. Among frequently occurring limitations of study design are a small sample size and/or lack of a proper power calculation based on a primary outcome variable, thus limiting the power to detect an effect. Baseline nutritional intake is usually not reported. In studies using 'usual care' in the control arm, the level of nutritional care is mostly not or only poorly described, and thus the contrast between control and intervention arm remains unclear. Hence, possible differences are not attributable to the specific intervention but rather to the difference in the overall quality of nutritional care. Further, participants and study personnel are often not blinded leading to performance bias. Even in situations where a placebo intervention appears possible (for example using a low caloric, similar looking supplement when ONS is being tested) placebo is rarely used. In most studies, a single intervention is used for all selected participants, without incorporating knowledge of participants' health and functional status, other treatments, and participants' motivation and preferences, which may reduce its effect. Details regarding compliance and intervention fidelity are sometimes not reported, while low compliance and poor fidelity will likely reduce potential effects. With regard to study outcomes, some studies lack the inclusion of clinically relevant or patient-centred parameters such as quality of life. Detection bias is often present due to non-blinding of the outcome assessors [56,57]. Moreover, studies often describe the provided amounts of energy and protein but do not report the net effect on the overall daily intake (which may have increased less due to energy compensation at other meal times) [46]. Finally, when analysing the results, several previous studies did not perform intention-to-treat analyses, but used complete case analysis only, possibly inducing further bias.

Overall, due to one or more of these limitations in most of the studies, the available evidence is mostly of only low or moderate quality. Moreover, due to large heterogeneity of inclusion criteria and study populations, intervention types and outcome assessments, the pooling of individual patient data and performing meta-analyses is currently seriously hampered [47,57]. Applying a fixed definition for malnutrition in future studies could importantly increase comparability between studies. The field could also benefit from establishing a minimum dataset (MDS) for clinically relevant outcome variables, per setting when deemed necessary, and defining the preferred method for assessing these outcome variables. This MDS would stimulate the incorporation of standardised outcome variables in future trials, and would enable the pooling of data and the performance of meta-analyses in order to obtain the highest level of evidence regarding the effect of nutritional interventions on relevant clinical outcomes.

3.3. Open Questions and Research Needs

In view of the recent global malnutrition definitions, which also consider muscle mass and inflammation as part of malnutrition [8], an update of prevalence data using this definition is needed.

Validity of available screening tools remains unclear due to multiple methodological problems [58]. Setting-specific tools have been suggested based on a newly developed scoring system which was applied to 48 existing tools, but more work is still needed to derive sound recommendations regarding the optimal tool [26].

Based on limited and partly conflicting evidence and limitations of existing studies outlined above, it remains unclear which interventions are most effective in which patient groups, and if specific situations (e.g., acute malnutrition), specific diseases (e.g., dementia) or specific etiologies of malnutrition require specific approaches. Interestingly and for example, an animal study with an infection-triggered model of acute malnutrition has recently demonstrated differential effects of parenteral glucose supplementation in addition to free oral intake on survival: Whereas in mice with an experimental viral infection a significant survival benefit was observed, mortality was significantly higher in mice with an experimental bacterial infection [59]. Thus, it may be hypothesised that especially in acute malnutrition nutrition support is not always beneficial or might need a specific approach.

With regard to a causative treatment, the complex etiology of malnutrition needs further research. The etiologic relevance of the many different potential causes and therefore the priority of distinct diagnostic measures remains unclear, and a treatment, based on individually identified causative factors is probably only rarely performed. More knowledge about the most relevant causes and their common pathophysiology would increase the potential for causation-oriented treatment and could in addition contribute to enhance malnutrition awareness and preventive approaches in patients with the respective problems.

Regarding general intervention characteristics, individualised, multimodal and multi-disciplinary strategies seem to be promising and should be pursued further.

In terms of specific interventions, food fortification, additional snacks and finger food are promising options but need high-quality reassessment through further studies that provide reliable evidence. Possible beneficial effects of all different types of food modifications including also organoleptic enhancement or texture modifications need to be tested in explorative trials as well as in subsequent sufficiently powered high-quality trials.

Further research is also needed to determine which methods of delivering dietary counselling are appropriate and cost-effective for different participants and care settings. It is also unclear whether and if when the counselling should be repeated and followed up. Furthermore, the role of social care staff, such as domiciliary carers, in delivering nutritional advice and support should also be explored.

Moreover, RFS must be highlighted as an area that needs further high-quality research to develop the best preventive strategies as effective treatments for malnutrition.

Relevant outcomes for malnutrition intervention studies were recently agreed in a Delphi study among geriatric and nutrition experts [57], however more research is also needed in this regard. Clearly, patient-centred outcomes such as independence in activities of daily living and quality of life need much more attention than in the past and should be assessed using reliable and meaningful tools. Also, health and social care resource use and cost-effectiveness are important outcomes which need to be further addressed. Here, a comprehensive, cross-sectoral perspective is needed as treatment costs in one setting may only be offset by a larger cost saving in another setting.

As studies were mainly conducted in the hospital setting, further research in other health-care settings is needed.

Furthermore, the topic of dehydration urgently needs further research efforts. As one of the most frequent diagnoses of older patients, the issue of dehydration has been addressed in the current ESPEN guidelines [21], which however also uncovered many open questions and lacking evidence. For example, there is no uniform definition of dehydration, the diagnostic criteria remain vague and there is no accepted screening tool. Effective strategies to better prevent dehydration must be developed.

Last but not least, effective ways to implement current knowledge in clinical practice need to be explored.

These and other topics considered important by the authors are listed in Table 2.

Table 2. Open questions regarding management of malnutrition in older people.

Prevalence, screening and diagnosis

- How are prevalence data affected by the new global definition of malnutrition (GLIM criteria)?
- Are the new GLIM criteria appropriate for older persons?
- Are different screening tools needed in different care settings?
- Which screening tools should be used in which setting?
- Are there biomarkers that could enhance screening and diagnosis of malnutrition?

Determinants and multifactorial etiology of malnutrition

- What are the most relevant causes of malnutrition in older patients?
- What are the etiologic mechanisms?
- What is the role of medication in malnutrition and reduced appetite?
- What are the essential aspects of assessment of the causes of malnutrition in an individual?

Effectiveness and safety of interventions

- Which interventions are most effective in which patient groups?
- Should specific interventions have priority?
- What are the best outcomes to assess the effect of interventions?
- Which interventions are most cost-effective?
- What is the optimal duration of interventions in each health-care setting?
- Do specific situations (e.g., acute malnutrition), specific diseases (e.g., dementia) or specific etiologies of malnutrition require specific intervention approaches?
- Are there situations, e.g., acute disease, where increasing energy intake could be harmful?
- Which strategies are most effective to prevent RFS but effectively treat malnutrition at the same time?
- Which types of food modifications are beneficial?
- Which methods of delivering nutritional counselling are appropriate and cost-effective for different participants and care settings?
- (When) should nutritional counselling be repeated and followed up?
- What is the role of social care staff in delivering nutritional advice and support?
- At what degree of malnutrition do patients benefit from interventions?
- At what degree of malnutrition do patients benefit from (par)enteral nutrition?
- Which interventions are effective with respect to patient-centred outcomes?
- Do malnourished obese patients need a specific approach?

Table 2. *Cont.*

Natural recovery
- Are there patients who do not need treatment because of early natural recovery?
- Can early natural recovery be predicted?

Role of protein and other specific nutrients
- How much protein is required in specific situations (e.g., diseases, nutritional states, functional states)?
- How should protein intake be distributed over the day?
- Is there an optimal time of protein intake in relation to physical training?
- What is the relevance of different protein sources for meaningful outcomes?
- Which micronutrients are frequently deficient in malnourished older persons?
- Is supplementation of any micronutrient beneficial in malnourished older persons?

Dehydration
- What are reliable diagnostic criteria for dehydration?
- How could an effective screening for dehydration be performed?
- How is the overlap of dehydration with malnutrition?
- What are effective preventive approaches against dehydration?

Knowledge transfer into clinical practice
- How can knowledge about malnutrition and respective guidelines be effectively implemented in clinical practice?
- What are the effects of nutritional training for health care professionals?

GLIM = Global Leadership Initiative on Malnutrition.

4. Conclusions

In conclusion, we are faced to a wide range of unresolved issues regarding the management of malnutrition in older persons which need to be addressed. Many of these questions cannot easily be answered, and it is an important next step to develop innovative strategies and well-conceived concepts for this purpose. Altogether, high-quality research is urgently required to develop effective strategies for the prevention and treatment of malnutrition in the increasing number of old and very old patients at risk.

Author Contributions: All authors contributed to writing the manuscript and to discussing and collecting the gaps regarding management of malnutrition in older people listed in Table 2. DV developed the structure of the manuscript and collated and harmonized the manuscript sections received from the co-authors. RW critically reviewed the final manuscript. All authors read and commented on the complete manuscript and approved the final version.

Acknowledgments: We are grateful to the BANSS foundation who enabled a two-day live-meeting of all authors in Biedenkopf an der Lahn, Germany, to discuss the topic without any obligation.

Conflicts of Interest: The authors declare no conflict of interest.

References

1. Inouye, S.K.; Studenski, S.; Tinetti, M.E.; Kuchel, G.A. Geriatric Syndromes: Clinical, Research and Policy Implications of a Core Geriatric Concept. *J. Am. Geriatr. Soc.* **2007**, *55*, 780–791. [CrossRef] [PubMed]
2. Cereda, E.; Pedrolli, C.; Klersy, C.; Bonardi, C.; Quarleri, L.; Cappello, S.; Turri, A.; Rondanelli, M.; Caccialanza, R. Nutritional status in older persons according to healthcare setting: A systematic review and meta-analysis of prevalence data using MNA ®. *Clin. Nutr.* **2016**, *35*, 1282–1290. [CrossRef] [PubMed]
3. Lacau St. Guily, J.L.S.; Bouvard, É.; Raynard, B.; Goldwasser, F.; Maget, B.; Prevost, A.; Seguy, D.; Romano, O.; Narciso, B.; Couet, C.; et al. NutriCancer: A French observational multicentre cross-sectional study of malnutrition in elderly patients with cancer. *J. Geriatr. Oncol.* **2018**, *9*, 74–80. [CrossRef] [PubMed]
4. Cereda, E.; Veronese, N.; Caccialanza, R. The final word on nutritional screening and assessment in older persons. *Curr. Opin. Clin. Nutr. Metab. Care* **2018**, *21*, 24–29. [CrossRef] [PubMed]

5. Kaiser, M.J.; Bauer, J.M.; Rämsch, C.; Uter, W.; Guigoz, Y.; Cederholm, T.; Thomas, D.R.; Anthony, P.S.; Charlton, K.E.; Maggio, M.; et al. Frequency of Malnutrition in Older Adults: A Multinational Perspective Using the Mini Nutritional Assessment. *J. Am. Geriatr. Soc.* **2010**, *58*, 1734–1738. [CrossRef] [PubMed]
6. Clarke, D.M.; Strauss, B.J.G.; Wahlqvist, M.L. Undereating and undernutrition in old age: Integrating bio-psychosocial aspects. *Age Ageing* **1998**, *27*, 527–534. [CrossRef] [PubMed]
7. Wolters, M.; Volkert, D.; Streicher, M.; Kiesswetter, E.; Torbahn, G.; O'Connor, E.M.; O'Keeffe, M.; Kelly, M.; O'Herlihy, E.; O'Toole, P.W.; et al. Prevalence of malnutrition using harmonized definitions in older adults from different settings—A MaNuEL study. *Clin. Nutr.* **2018**. [CrossRef] [PubMed]
8. Cederholm, T.; Jensen, G.L.; Correia, M.I.T.D.; Gonzalez, M.C.; Fukushima, R.; Higashiguchi, T.; Baptista, G.; Barazzoni, R.; Blaauw, R.; Coats, A.; et al. GLIM criteria for the diagnosis of malnutrition–A consensus report from the global clinical nutrition community. *Clin. Nutr.* **2019**, *38*, 1–9. [CrossRef] [PubMed]
9. Cederholm, T.; Bosaeus, I.; Barazzoni, R.; Bauer, J.; Van Gossum, A.; Klek, S.; Muscaritoli, M.; Nyulasi, I.; Ockenga, J.; Schneider, S.; et al. Diagnostic criteria for malnutrition–An ESPEN Consensus Statement. *Clin. Nutr.* **2015**, *34*, 335–340. [CrossRef]
10. Schneider, S.M.; Al-Jaouni, R.; Pivot, X.; Braulio, V.B.; Rampal, P.; Hebuterne, X. Lack of adaptation to severe malnutrition in elderly patients. *Clin. Nutr.* **2002**, *21*, 499–504. [CrossRef]
11. Agarwal, E.; Miller, M.; Yaxley, A.; Isenring, E. Malnutrition in the elderly: A narrative review. *Maturitas* **2013**, *76*, 296–302. [CrossRef] [PubMed]
12. Malafarina, V.; Uriz-Otano, F.; Gil-Guerrero, L.; Iniesta, R. The anorexia of ageing: Physiopathology, prevalence, associated comorbidity and mortality. A systematic review. *Maturitas* **2013**, *74*, 293–302. [CrossRef] [PubMed]
13. Landi, F.; Picca, A.; Calvani, R.; Marzetti, E. Anorexia of Aging: Assessment and Management. *Clin. Geriatr. Med.* **2017**, *33*, 315–323. [CrossRef] [PubMed]
14. O'Keeffe, M.; Kelly, M.; O'Herlihy, E.; O'Toole, P.W.; Kearney, P.M.; Timmons, S.; O'Shea, E.; Stanton, C.; Hickson, M.; Rolland, Y.; et al. Potentially Modifiable Determinants of Malnutrition in Older Adults: A systematic review. Available online: https://www.sciencedirect.com/science/article/pii/S0261561418325755 (accessed on 28 June 219).
15. Van Der Pols-Vijlbrief, R.; Wijnhoven, H.A.; Schaap, L.A.; Terwee, C.B.; Visser, M. Determinants of protein–energy malnutrition in community-dwelling older adults: A systematic review of observational studies. *Ageing Res. Rev.* **2014**, *18*, 112–131. [CrossRef] [PubMed]
16. Volkert, D.; Kiesswetter, E.; Cederholm, T.; Donini, L.M.; Eglseer, D.; Norman, K.; Schneider, S.M.; Ströbele-Benschop, N.; Torbahn, G.; Rainer Wirth, R.; et al. Development of a model on Determinants of Malnutrition in Aged Persons (DoMAP) – a MaNuEL project. *Gerontol. Geriatr. Med.* **2019**, *5*, 1–8. [CrossRef]
17. Norman, K.; Pichard, C.; Lochs, H.; Pirlich, M. Prognostic impact of disease-related malnutrition. *Clin. Nutr.* **2008**, *27*, 5–15. [CrossRef] [PubMed]
18. Deutz, N.E.; Ashurst, I.; Ballesteros, M.D.; Bear, D.E.; Cruz-Jentoft, A.J.; Genton, L.; Landi, F.; Laviano, A.; Norman, K.; Prado, C.M. The Underappreciated Role of Low Muscle Mass in the Management of Malnutrition. *J. Am. Med Dir. Assoc.* **2019**, *20*, 22–27. [CrossRef] [PubMed]
19. Abizanda, P.; Sinclair, A.; Barcons, N.; Lizan, L.; Rodriguez-Manas, L. Costs of Malnutrition in Institutionalized and Community-Dwelling Older Adults: A Systematic Review. *J. Am. Med. Dir. Assoc.* **2016**, *17*, 17–23. [CrossRef]
20. Martínez-Reig, M.; Aranda-Reneo, I.; Peña-Longobardo, L.M.; Oliva-Moreno, J.; Barcons-Vilardell, N.; Hoogendijk, E.O.; Abizanda, P. Use of health resources and healthcare costs associated with nutritional risk: The FRADEA study. *Clin. Nutr.* **2018**, *37*, 1299–1305. [CrossRef]
21. Volkert, D.; Beck, A.M.; Cederholm, T.; Cruz-Jentoft, A.; Goisser, S.; Hooper, L.; Kiesswetter, E.; Maggio, M.; Raynaud-Simon, A.; Sieber, C.C.; et al. ESPEN guideline on clinical nutrition and hydration in geriatrics. *Clin. Nutr.* **2019**, *38*, 10–47. [CrossRef]
22. Volkert, D.; Berner, Y.N.; Berry, E.; Cederholm, T.; Coti Bertrand, P.; Milne, A.; Palmblad, J.; Schneider, S.; Sobotka, L.; Stanga, Z.; et al. ESPEN Guidelines on Enteral Nutrition: Geriatrics. *Clin. Nutr.* **2006**, *25*, 330–360. [CrossRef] [PubMed]
23. Sobotka, L.; Schneider, S.; Berner, Y.; Cederholm, T.; Krznaric, Z.; Shenkin, A.; Stanga, Z.; Toigo, G.; Vandewoude, M.; Volkert, D.; et al. ESPEN Guidelines on Parenteral Nutrition: Geriatrics. *Clin. Nutr.* **2009**, *28*, 461–466. [CrossRef] [PubMed]

24. Eglseer, D.; Halfens, R.J.; Lohrmann, C. Is the presence of a validated malnutrition screening tool associated with better nutritional care in hospitalized patients? *Nutrition.* **2017**, *37*, 104–111. [CrossRef] [PubMed]
25. Kaiser, M.J.; Bauer, J.M.; Uter, W.; Donini, L.M.; Stange, I.; Volkert, D.; Diekmann, R.; Drey, M.; Bollwein, J.; Tempera, S.; et al. Prospective Validation of the Modified Mini Nutritional Assessment Short-Forms in the Community, Nursing Home, and Rehabilitation Setting. *J. Am. Geriatr. Soc.* **2011**, *59*, 2124–2128. [CrossRef] [PubMed]
26. Power, L.; de van der Schueren, M.A.E.; Leij-Halfwerk, S.; Bauer, J.; Clarke, M.; Visser, M.; Volkert, D.; Bardon, L.; Gibney, E.; Corish, C.A. Development and application of a scoring system to rate malnutrition screening tools used in older adults in community and healthcare settings—A MaNuEL study. *Clin. Nutr.* **2018**. [CrossRef] [PubMed]
27. Council of Europe, Committee of ministers. Resolution ResAP(2003)3 on Food and Nutritional Care in Hospitals. Available online: https://www.nutritionday.org/cms/upload/pdf/11.resolution/Resolution_of_the_Council_of_Europe.pdf (accessed on 1 July 2019).
28. Keller, H.; Carrier, N.; Duizer, L.; Lengyel, C.; Slaughter, S.; Steele, C. Making the Most of Mealtimes (M3): Grounding mealtime interventions with a conceptual model. *J. Am. Med Dir. Assoc.* **2014**, *15*, 158–161. [CrossRef] [PubMed]
29. Roberts, H.C.; Lim, S.E.R.; Cox, N.J.; Ibrahim, K. The challenge of managing undernutrition in older people with Frailty. *Nutrition* **2019**, *11*, 808. [CrossRef] [PubMed]
30. Marx, W.; Kelly, J.T.; Crichton, M.; Craven, D.; Collins, J.; Mackay, H.; Isenring, E.; Marshall, S. Is telehealth effective in managing malnutrition in community—dwelling older adults? A systematic review and meta–analysis. *Maturitas* **2018**, *111*, 31–46. [CrossRef]
31. Marshall, S.; Agarwal, E.; Young, A.; Isenring, E. Role of domiciliary and family carers in individualised nutrition support for older adults living in the community. *Maturitas* **2017**, *98*, 20–29. [CrossRef]
32. Cederholm, T.; Barazzoni, R.; Austin, P.; Ballmer, P.; Biolo, G.; Bischoff, S.C.; Compher, C.; Correia, I.; Higashiguchi, T.; Holst, M.; et al. ESPEN guidelines on definitions and terminology of clinical nutrition. *Clin. Nutr.* **2017**, *36*, 49–64. [CrossRef]
33. Wirth, R.; Dziewas, R.; Beck, A.M.; Clave, P.; Hamdy, S.; Heppner, H.J.; Langmore, S.; Leischker, A.H.; Martino, R.; Pluschinski, P.; et al. Oropharyngeal dysphagia in older persons— from pathophysiology to adequate intervention: A review and summary of an international expert meeting. *Clin. Interv. Aging.* **2016**, *11*, 189–208. [CrossRef] [PubMed]
34. Beck, A.M.; Kjaersgaard, A.; Hansen, T.; Poulsen, I. Systematic review and evidence based recommendations on texture modified foods and thickened liquids for adults (above 17 years) with oropharyngeal dysphagia–An updated clinical guideline. *Clin. Nutr.* **2018**, *37*, 1980–1991. [CrossRef] [PubMed]
35. Friedli, N.; Stanga, Z.; Sobotka, L.; Culkin, A.; Kondrup, J.; Laviano, A.; Mueller, B.; Schuetz, P. Revisiting the refeeding syndrome: Results of a systematic review. *Nutrition* **2017**, *35*, 151–160. [CrossRef] [PubMed]
36. Friedli, N.; Stanga, Z.; Culkin, A.; Crook, M.; Laviano, A.; Sobotka, L.; Kressig, R.W.; Kondrup, J.; Mueller, B.; Schuetz, P. Management and prevention of refeeding syndrome in medical inpatients: An evidence-based and consensus—supported algorithm. *Nutrition* **2018**, *47*, 13–20. [CrossRef] [PubMed]
37. Janssen, G.; Pourhassan, M.; Lenzen-Großimlinghaus, R.; Jäger, M.; Schäfer, R.; Spamer, C.; Cuvelier, I.; Volkert, D.; Wirth, R.; on Behalf of the Working Group on Nutrition and Metabolism of the German Geriatric Society (DGG). The Refeeding Syndrome Revisited: You can only Diagnose What You Know. Available online: https://www.nature.com/articles/s41430-019-0441-x (accessed on 29 June 2019).
38. Aubry, E.; Friedli, N.; Schuetz, P.; Stanga, Z. Refeeding syndrome in the frail elderly population: Prevention, diagnosis and management. *Clin. Exp. Gastroenterol.* **2018**, *11*, 255–264. [CrossRef] [PubMed]
39. Pourhassan, M.; Cuvelier, I.; Gehrke, I.; Marburger, C.; Modreker, M.K.; Volkert, D.; Willschrei, H.P.; Wirth, R. Risk factors of refeeding syndrome in malnourished older hospitalized patients. *Clin. Nutr.* **2018**, *37*, 1354–1359. [CrossRef] [PubMed]

40. Doig, G.S.; Simpson, F.; Heighes, P.T.; Bellomo, R.; Chesher, D.; Caterson, I.D.; Reade, M.C.; Harrigan, P.W.J. Restricted versus continued standard caloric intake during the management of refeeding syndrome in critically ill adults: A randomised, parallel-group, multicentre, single-blind controlled trial. *Lancet Respir. Med.* **2015**, *3*, 943–952. [CrossRef]

41. Correa-Perez, A.; Abraha, I.; Cherubini, A.; Collinson, A.; Dardevet, D.; de Groot, L.; de van der Schueren, M.A.E.; Hebestreit, A.; Hickson, M.; Jaramillo-Hidalgo, J.; et al. Efficacy of non-pharmacological interventions to treat malnutrition in older persons: A systematic review and meta-analysis. The SENATOR project ONTOP series and MaNuEL knowledge hub project. *Ageing Res. Rev.* **2019**, *49*, 27–48. [CrossRef] [PubMed]

42. Wright, J.; Baldwin, C. Oral nutritional support with or without exercise in the management of malnutrition in nutritionally vulnerable older people: A systematic review and meta-analysis. *Clin. Nutr.* **2018**, *37*, 1879–1891. [CrossRef] [PubMed]

43. Rasmussen, N.M.; Belqaid, K.; Lugnet, K.; Nielsen, A.L.; Rasmussen, H.H.; Beck, A.M. Effectiveness of multidisciplinary nutritional support in older hospitalised patients: A systematic review and meta-analyses. *Clin. Nutr. ESPEN* **2018**, *27*, 44–52. [CrossRef] [PubMed]

44. Tsuboi, M.; Momosaki, R.; Vakili, M.; Abo, M. Nutritional supplementation for activities of daily living and functional ability of older people in residential facilities: A systematic review. *Geriatr. Gerontol. Int.* **2018**, *18*, 197–210. [CrossRef] [PubMed]

45. Perna, S.; Rondanelli, M.; Spadaccini, D.; Lenzi, A.; Donini, L.M.; Poggiogalle, E. Are the therapeutic strategies in anorexia of ageing effective on nutritional status? A systematic review with meta-analysis. *J. Hum. Nutr. Diet.* **2019**, *32*, 128–138. [CrossRef] [PubMed]

46. Reinders, I.; Volkert, D.; de Groot, L.C.P.G.M.; Beck, A.M.; Feldblum, I.; Jobse, I.; Neelemaat, F.; de van der Schueren, M.A.E.; Shahar, D.R.; Smeets, E.T.H.C.; et al. Effectiveness of nutritional interventions in older adults at risk of malnutrition across different health care settings: Pooled analyses of individual participant data from nine randomized controlled trials. *Clin. Nutr.* **2018**. [CrossRef] [PubMed]

47. van Zwienen-Pot, J.I.; Reinders, I.; de Groot, L.C.P.G.M.; Beck, A.M.; Feldblum, I.; Jobse, I.; Neelemaat, F.; de van der Schueren, M.A.E.; Shahar, D.R.; Smeets, E.T.H.C.; et al. The effect of nutritional intervention in older adults at risk of malnutrition on handgrip strength and mortality: Results from 9 pooled RCTs. *Clin. Nutr.* **2018**, *37*, S177.

48. Schuetz, P.; Fehr, R.; Baechli, V.; Geiser, M.; Deiss, M.; Gomes, F.; Kutz, A.; Tribolet, P.; Bregenzer, T.; Braun, N.; et al. Individualised nutritional support in medical inpatients at nutritional risk: A randomised clinical trial. *Lancet* **2019**, *393*, 2312–2321. [CrossRef]

49. Bischoff, S.C.; Singer, P.; Koller, M.; Barazzoni, R.; Cederholm, T.; Van Gossum, A. Standard operating procedures for ESPEN guidelines and consensus papers. *Clin. Nutr.* **2015**, *34*, 1043–1051. [CrossRef] [PubMed]

50. Hubbard, G.P.; Elia, M.; Holdoway, A.; Stratton, R.J. A systematic review of compliance to oral nutritional supplements. *Clin. Nutr.* **2012**, *31*, 293–312. [CrossRef] [PubMed]

51. Baldwin, C.; Weekes, C.E. Dietary advice with or without oral nutritional supplements for disease-related malnutrition in adults. *Cochrane Database Syst. Rev.* **2011**. [CrossRef] [PubMed]

52. Abbott, R.A.; Whear, R.; Thompson-Coon, J.; Ukoumunne, O.C.; Rogers, M.; Bethel, A.; Hemsley, A.; Stein, K. Effectiveness of mealtime interventions on nutritional outcomes for the elderly living in residential care: A systematic review and meta-analysis. *Ageing Res. Rev.* **2013**, *12*, 967–981. [CrossRef]

53. Collins, J.; Porter, J. The effect of interventions to prevent and treat malnutrition in patients admitted for rehabilitation: A systematic review with meta-analysis. *J. Hum. Nutr. Diet.* **2015**, *28*, 1–15. [CrossRef]

54. Poscia, A.; Milovanovic, S.; La Milia, D.I.; Duplaga, M.; Grysztar, M.; Landi, F.; Moscato, U.; Magnavita, N.; Collamati, A.; Ricciardi, W. Effectiveness of nutritional interventions addressed to elderly persons: Umbrella systematic review with meta-analysis. *Eur. J. Public Health* **2018**, *28*, 275–283. [CrossRef] [PubMed]

55. Milne, A.C.; Potter, J.; Vivanti, A.; Avenell, A. Protein and energy supplementation in elderly people at risk from malnutrition. *Cochrane Database Syst. Rev.* **2009**. [CrossRef] [PubMed]

56. Baldwin, C.; Weekes, C.E. Dietary counselling with or without oral nutritional supplements in the management of malnourished patients: A systematic review and meta-analysis of randomised controlled trials. *J. Hum. Nutr. Diet.* **2012**, *25*, 411–426. [CrossRef] [PubMed]

57. Correa-Pérez, A.; Lozano-Montoya, I.; Volkert, D.; Visser, M.; Cruz-Jentoft, A.J. Relevant outcomes for nutrition interventions to treat and prevent malnutrition in older people: A collaborative senator-ontop and manuel delphi study. *Eur. Geriatr. Med.* **2018**, *9*, 243–248. [CrossRef]
58. Power, L.; Mullally, D.; Gibney, E.R.; Clarke, M.; Visser, M.; Volkert, D.; Bardon, L.; De Van Der Schueren, M.A.; Corish, C.A. A review of the validity of malnutrition screening tools used in older adults in community and healthcare settings–A MaNuEL study. *Clin. Nutr. ESPEN* **2018**, *24*, 1–13. [CrossRef] [PubMed]
59. Wang, A.; Huen, S.C.; Luan, H.H.; Yu, S.; Zhang, C.; Gallezot, J.-D.; Booth, C.J.; Medzhitov, R. Opposing Effects of Fasting Metabolism on Tissue Tolerance in Bacterial and Viral Inflammation. *Cell* **2016**, *166*, 1512–1525.e12. [CrossRef] [PubMed]

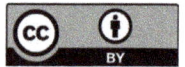

© 2019 by the authors. Licensee MDPI, Basel, Switzerland. This article is an open access article distributed under the terms and conditions of the Creative Commons Attribution (CC BY) license (http://creativecommons.org/licenses/by/4.0/).

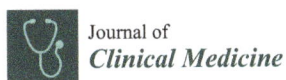

Review

Management of Glucose Control in Noncritically Ill, Hospitalized Patients Receiving Parenteral and/or Enteral Nutrition: A Systematic Review

Céline Isabelle Laesser [1], Paul Cumming [2,3], Emilie Reber [1], Zeno Stanga [1], Taulant Muka [4] and Lia Bally [1,*]

1. Department of Diabetes, Endocrinology, Clinical Nutrition, and Metabolism, Inselspital, Bern University Hospital, University of Bern, 3010 Bern, Switzerland
2. Department of Nuclear Medicine, Inselspital, Bern University Hospital, University of Bern, 3010 Bern, Switzerland
3. School of Psychology and Counselling and IHBI, Queensland University of Technology, Brisbane, QLD 4059, Australia
4. Institute of Social and Preventive Medicine, University of Bern, 3012 Bern, Switzerland
* Correspondence: lia.bally@insel.ch; Tel.: +41-316-323-677

Received: 30 May 2019; Accepted: 26 June 2019; Published: 28 June 2019

Abstract: Hyperglycemia is a common occurrence in hospitalized patients receiving parenteral and/or enteral nutrition. Although there are several approaches to manage hyperglycemia, there is no consensus on the best practice. We systematically searched PubMed, Embase, Cochrane Central, and ClinicalTrials.gov to identify records (published or registered between April 1999 and April 2019) investigating strategies to manage glucose control in adults receiving parenteral and/or enteral nutrition whilst hospitalized in noncritical care units. A total of 15 completed studies comprising 1170 patients were identified, of which 11 were clinical trials and four observational studies. Diabetes management strategies entailed adaptations of nutritional regimens in four studies, while the remainder assessed different insulin regimens and administration routes. Diabetes-specific nutritional regimens that reduced glycemic excursions, as well as algorithm-driven insulin delivery approaches that allowed for flexible glucose-responsive insulin dosing, were both effective in improving glycemic control. However, the assessed studies were, in general, of limited quality, and we see a clear need for future rigorous studies to establish standards of care for patients with hyperglycemia receiving nutrition support.

Keywords: glucose control; hyperglycemia; parenteral nutrition; enteral nutrition; nutritional support; insulin

1. Introduction

Hyperglycemia is frequently encountered during parenteral (PN) and/or enteral (EN) nutrition in hospitalized patients with and without pre-existing diabetes [1,2]. Indeed, it is estimated that more than 50% of patients on PN and 30% of patients on EN experience hyperglycemia whilst in the hospital [3,4]. Hyperglycemia arises in these patients due to one or more of the following factors: (1) diminished insulin sensitivity due to inflammation, stress hormones, and sedentarism [5]; (2) increased carbohydrate provision [6]; and (3) side-effects of medication such as glucocorticoids that interfere with glucose metabolism [7]. In patients totally reliant on PN, these factors are compounded by the loss of the physiological incretin effect on insulin release, as occurs when entirely bypassing the gastrointestinal tract with intravenous nutrient supply [8]. Furthermore, the diminished glucose-stimulated insulin secretion in diabetic patients with some residual beta-cell function increases their requirement for exogenous insulin.

Evidence from several observational studies suggests that emergent hyperglycemia during nutrition support is associated with increased morbidity and mortality [1,9]. There is an apparently linear relationship between the incidence of adverse outcomes and mean glucose levels once glycaemia surpasses a threshold of 6.3 mM [10]. In individuals on PN, the risk of any complication increases by a factor of 1.58 for each 1 mM increase in glycaemia above this threshold [11]. Conversely, treatment of hyperglycemia is shown to improve clinical outcomes [12–15]. However, striving for tight glucose control inherently increases the risk of hypoglycemia, which is similarly associated with adverse clinical outcomes [16,17].

PN and EN nutrition support are provided in a number of ways, ranging from continuous to cyclic regimens, often in combination with unpredictable and variable oral intake or additional intravenous glucose administration. Maintaining glycemic control is even more demanding in patients with unanticipated interruptions of their feeding (e.g., due to emergency surgery), or if nutrition support is suspended due to accidental removal or obstruction of tubing. Guidelines such as those from the American Diabetes Society [18] and the Endocrine Society [19] recommend that random blood glucose levels be maintained below 10.0 mM, provided that this target can be safely achieved. According to these guidelines, the mainstay of hyperglycemia management in the hospital is the administration of insulin, given its high efficacy, flexibility, and lack of interference with most other pharmacotherapies or organ dysfunctions.

Although there are some recommendations for insulin dosing tailored to the needs of patients receiving PN and/or EN, there is a lack of evidence-based support for specific insulin regimens. Insulin can be delivered via intravenous or subcutaneous routes, or in patients receiving PN, insulin may simply be mixed in the nutrition solution [20]. Intravenous insulin infusion at a rate continuously adjusted according to regular capillary blood glucose measurements helps to maintain glucose levels within the recommended limits. However, implementation of intravenous protocols imposes considerable demand on nursing staff, calling for two hours of direct nursing daily per patient [21], which substantially increases the workload of ward staff. Noncritical care nurses have to manage several patients, and staff levels are reduced at nighttime, which does not encourage constant vigilance of blood glucose and manual adjustment of insulin infusion rates. Thus, for practical and safety considerations in noncritical care settings, subcutaneous administration is the favored route for insulin delivery. However, the formulation of PN and EN support can also influence glucose levels in patients on nutrition support. Whereas glucose is the only carbohydrate source in standard PN solutions, the glycemic impact can be modulated by changing the caloric contributions of carbohydrates versus monounsaturated fatty acids (MUFAs), or by using alternate carbohydrates such as fructose. Furthermore, the addition of fibers to EN formulae can delay carbohydrate absorption, thereby attenuating the glycemic impact [22,23]. An overview of the different management strategies is provided in Figure 1.

Diabetes technology has progressed greatly over the past decade, bringing considerable improvements to the care of outpatients with type 1 and type 2 diabetes. Notably, recent development of continuous glucose monitoring (CGM) systems that measure interstitial fluid glucose concentration every few minutes allow to depict glucose profiles in higher resolution, thereby facilitating adjustment of insulin dosages [24]. CGM systems also project trends for glucose levels and feature customizable hypo- and hyperglycemia alerts. There is a growing interest in the use of this technology in hospital settings given the abundance of additional information that can guide therapy adjustments.

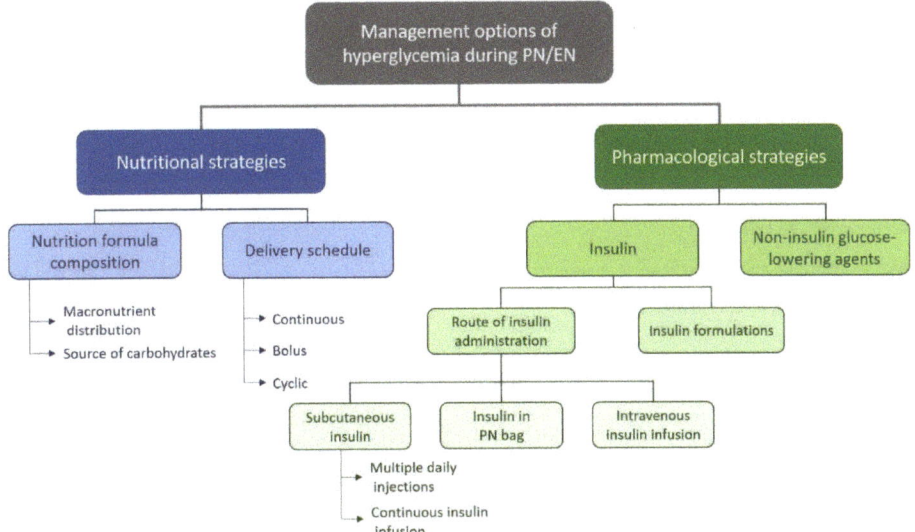

Figure 1. Management options of hyperglycemia during PN/EN. PN = parenteral nutrition, EN = enteral nutrition.

An important variable in the control of glycaemia is the modulation of insulin to meet with the continuously changing metabolic needs. Due to its inherent flexibility of insulin dose adjustment, the predominant mode of delivery in patients with type 1 diabetes is via a subcutaneous insulin pump, also known as continuous subcutaneous insulin infusion [25]. Here, a portable pump infuses rapid-acting insulin at a rate that can be altered on demand or preset to change at fixed times. This flexible adaptation of the insulin delivery profile makes the approach particularly attractive for patients under cyclic nutrition regimens who may receive large amounts of carbohydrates within predefined time windows. The combination of real-time glucose measurements from a CGM device with a control algorithm that directs insulin delivery via an insulin pump constitutes a closed-loop system, also known as the artificial pancreas [26,27]. Closed-loop systems automatically adjust insulin delivery every 10–12 min according to real-time glucose measurements. The autonomy and glucose feedback-regulation obtained through closed-loop systems hold promise in the particular context of hyperglycemia, arising along with nutritional support, while sparing an excess burden on nursing staff.

Our aim in the present review is to provide an overview of the current status and future outlook of glucose management strategies for noncritical care patients receiving PN and/or EN nutrition support.

2. Materials and Methods

2.1. Literature Search

This review was conducted and reported in accordance with the PRISMA and MOOSE guidelines [28,29]. Completed checklists can be found in Supplementary Tables S5 and S6. PubMed and Embase databases were used to identify relevant records over the past 20 years. The Cochrane Central Register of Controlled Trials and ClinicalTrials.gov were searched for published and ongoing studies. The search strategies for the databases are summarized in Supplementary Tables S1–S4. Two reviewers independently evaluated the titles and abstracts according to the selection criteria. For each potentially eligible study, two reviewers assessed the full-text. In cases of disagreement, a decision was made by consensus or, if necessary, a third reviewer was consulted.

2.2. Study Selection Criteria

Studies were included if they met the following criteria: (i) were published or registered in English language between 10 April 1999 and 10 April 2019 (date last searched); (ii) were clinical studies evaluating new treatment approaches against a comparator; (iii) included adult (age ≥ 18 years) noncritical care inpatients receiving PN and/or EN nutrition; (iv) investigated strategies to manage blood glucose control; and (v) had outcomes reflecting glucose control. Exclusion criteria were pregnancy, breast feeding, case reports, abstracts, guidelines, or literature reviews. The selection process is shown in Figure 2.

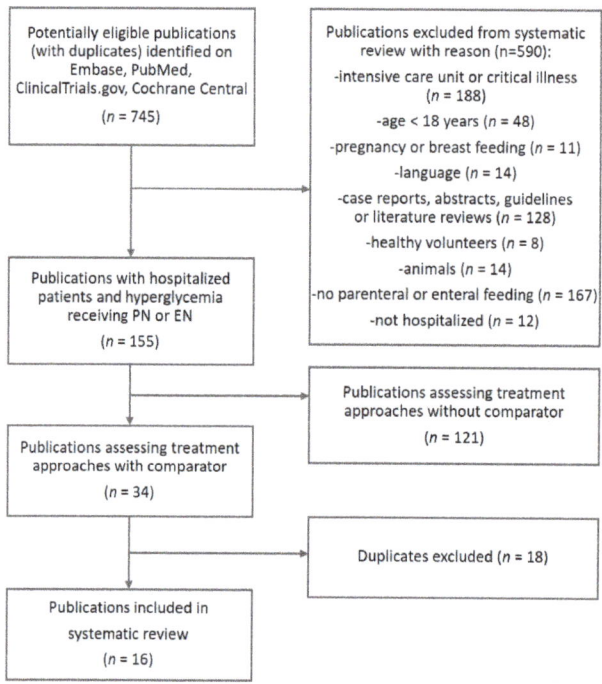

Figure 2. Flowchart illustrating the study selection process.

2.3. Data Extraction

Two reviewers extracted data independently using a predesigned form, including study design, sample size, glucose management strategy, primary outcome, and main results. If no primary outcome was specified, we obtained the endpoints deemed most relevant.

2.4. Quality Assessment

The quality of clinical trials was evaluated by two reviewers based on the "Cochrane Risk of Bias tool" [30]. According to this tool, studies are judged to be of low or high risk for bias based on criteria to evaluate random sequence generation, allocation concealment, blinding of participants/personnel and outcome assessment, incomplete outcome data, and selective reporting. Since retrospective publications have an inherently high risk of bias in most domains, and there is not a standardized assessment tool available, we refrained them from quality evaluation.

3. Results

3.1. Study Identification and Selection

We identified in total 745 potentially eligible records. Following screening based on titles and abstracts, 34 citations were selected for detailed full-text evaluation. Of those, 16 articles met the selection criteria and were included in the review (Figure 2). One ongoing study was eligible for inclusion.

3.2. Characteristics of the Included Studies

The included published publications comprised 1170 participants from 15 clinical studies, of which 11 were clinical trials (9 randomized and 2 nonrandomized) and 4 were retrospective observational studies. One study was an ongoing registered study. Seven studies were conducted in Europe, three in North America, and five in Asia. Only three studies included more than one center. The study population represented medical (20%), surgical (27%), or mixed medical and surgical (53%) noncritical care inpatients. Three studies explicitly stated the inclusion of patients with type 1 diabetes, three studies explicitly excluded patients with type 1 diabetes, five studies exclusively recruited patients with type 2 diabetes, whereas the remainder did not further characterize the diabetic state of study participants or the reason for hyperglycemia ($n = 4$). Nutrition support comprised PN in six studies, EN in seven studies, and PN and/or EN in two studies. Regarding glucose management strategies, 4 studies investigated nutritional approaches, and 11 studies explored insulin interventions. No studies were found that explored noninsulin pharmacological strategies. The study duration ranged from 36 h to 46 days. Study characteristics and findings are summarized in Tables 1 and 2.

Four of the clinical trials were considered of medium quality, indicating a low risk of bias in all domains except for performance and detection bias, which was deemed reasonable with a near impossibility of blinding [31–34]. The other studies were deemed to be of limited quality, with high risk of bias in the domains of lack of primary outcome definition and selective or incomplete reporting (Supplementary Figure S1). Since retrospective publications have an inherently high risk of bias in most domains, we refrained from a quality evaluation of the four such studies.

3.3. Studies Examining Nutritional Strategies

Four studies examined nutritional strategies to manage glycaemia in patients receiving nutrition support. The use of EN formulae with lower glycemic impacts were contrasted against conventional products in two clinical trials [35,36]. In a nonrandomized crossover study involving inpatients with type 2 diabetes, Tiyapanjanit et al. tested a formula compounded in-house to contain 50% of calories as carbohydrates, thereof 67% as fructose, in comparison with an iso-energetic control formula (53% of calories as carbohydrates and 15% as fructose). Over the study period of 36 h, lower mean glucose was achieved with the high-fructose formula compared to control (6.8 ± 1.5 vs. 8.0 ± 2.1 mM, $p = 0.022$). No insulin or antidiabetic medication was administered in these patients [35]. Similarly, a four-center randomized controlled parallel trial conducted in 104 inpatients with type 2 diabetes found a lower nutrition-induced relative change from baseline glycaemia with the use of lower glycemic impact enteral vs. standard enteral nutrition formula (10% vs. 21%, $p = 0.006$). The investigated EN formula contained a reduced amount of carbohydrates (9.4 vs. 12.5 g/100 mL, $p = $ n/a) and higher amounts of MUFAs (3.8 vs. 1.0 g/100 mL, $p = $ n/a) [36]. Similarly, an ongoing randomized clinical trial (GlyENStroke, NCT03422900) evaluates the efficacy of a diabetes-specific enteral nutrition formula to reduce hyperglycemia (glucose levels > 8.3 mM) in nondiabetic patients with hyperglycemia on nutrition support after stroke [37].

Table 1. Overview of clinical trials.

Author, Year	Study Design [1]	Sample Size	Population	Nutrition Therapy	Interventions	Primary Outcome (Study Period)	Main Results	Risk of Bias [3]
Boughton et al., 2019 [31]	RCT, parallel, two-center	43	Non-T1D surgical and medical	PN and/or EN	Insulin adaptation Fully automated s.c. closed-loop insulin delivery (closed loop, n = 21) Conventional s.c. insulin therapy according to local practice (control, n = 22)	% time in target (5.6–10.0 mM) based on CGM values (Up to 15 d or discharge)	% time in target higher in closed-loop vs. control (68% vs. 36%, $p < 0.0001$); hypoglycemia (<3.9 mM) infrequent and similar between closed-loop and control (0.5% for both), $p = $ ns	Low
Olveira et al., 2019 [32]	RCT, parallel, multi-center (26 sites)	161	T2D surgical and medical	TPN	100% regular insulin in PN bag (100% in bag, n = 80) 50% s.c. glargine + 50% regular insulin in PN bag (50% in bag, n = 81)	Mean glucose based on capillary POC BG values (Up to 15 d or until PN stop)	Mean glucose during TPN 9.2 vs. 9.6 mM 100% in bag vs. 50% in bag (ns); mean glucose 48 h post-TPN higher in 100% in bag vs. 50% in bag (8.9 vs. 7.9 mM, $p = 0.024$); number of patients with hypoglycemia (≤3.9 mM) lower in 100% in bag vs. 50% in bag (9 vs. 22, $p = 0.016$)	Medium
Li et al., 2018 [38]	RCT, parallel, single-center	102	T2D surgical	PN (cyclic)	Continuous s.c. insulin infusion (CSII, n = 50) S.c. basal-bolus glargine/aspart (basbol, n = 52)	mean amplitude of glycemic excursion (MAGE) based on CGM (4 d)	MAGE lower in CSII vs. basbol (3.7 vs. 6.2 mM, $p < 0.05$), no hypoglycemia events (<3.9 mM) occurred	High
Hakeam et al., 2017 [33]	RCT, parallel, single-center	67	Non-T1D surgical (non-cardiac)	PN	S.c. glargine (scGlarg, n = 35) Regular insulin added to PN bag (RIbag, n = 32)	Mean glucose based on capillary POC BG values from day 5 on PN and % of patients who achieved target glycaemia (7.8–10.0 mM) (9 d)	Comparable mean BG in scGlar vs. RIbag, % of values in target 52% in scGlar vs. 48% in RIbag ($p = 0.06$); no significant difference in hypoglycemia (<3.9 mM) events	Medium
Yuan et al., 2015 [12]	RCT, parallel, single-center	212	T2D surgical (gastrectomy for gastric cancer)	EN (continuous)	VRII (short-acting insulin NOS) (VRII, n = 106) S.c. conventional insulin therapy (s.c.Ins., n = 106)	PO not specified; mean glucose based on capillary POC BG values, infective and noninfective complications (8–10 d)	Mean BG lower in VRII vs. s.c.Ins. (5.4 vs. 9.5 mM, $p < 0.001$); higher rate of severe hypoglycemia (≤2.2 mM) in VRII vs. s.c.Ins. (8% vs. 1%, $p = 0.035$)	High
Kruyt et al., 2010 [39]	Single-arm intervention with historical control	23	Hyperglycemic patients (excluded patients with previous insulin use)(medical (stroke unit)	EN	Continuous feeding with computerized VRII group (continuous, n = 10) Bolus feeding with regular i.v. insulin adaptation intermediate group (inter, n = 13)	% of capillary POC BG values in target range (4.4–6.1 mM)(5 d)	Higher % values in target and mean glucose in continuous vs. inter group (55% vs. 19%, $p < 0.005$ and 5.8 vs. 7.6 mM, $p < 0.005$)	Medium

Table 1. Cont.

Author, Year	Study Design [1]	Sample Size	Population	Nutrition Therapy	Interventions	Primary Outcome (Study Period)	Main Results	Risk of Bias [3]
Korytkowski et al., 2009 [40]	RCT, parallel, single-center	50	Diabetes NOS surgical and medical	EN	S.c. SSI (regular insulin) every 4–6 h (SSRI, $n = 25$); (NPH initialized if persistent BG > 10.0 mM) S.c. SSRI plus s.c. glargine (basalPLUS, $n = 25$)	PO not specified; mean glucose based on capillary POC BG values [8 d]	mean BG similar in SSRI and basalPLUS (8.9 vs. 9.2 mM, p = ns); NPH initialized in 55% of those on SSRI	High
Tsyapanjanit et al., 2014 [35]	Non-randomized cross-over (no washout)	10	T2D (BG < 10 mM wo antidiabetic medication) medical	EN (continuous)	Nutrition adaptation: In-house prepared EN formula with 50% CHO thereof 67% fructose, (inhouse, $n = 10$) Standard diabetic EN formula with 53% CHO thereof 15% fructose and 57% maltodextrin (standard, $n = 10$)	PO not specified; mean glucose based on capillary POC BG values; glycemic variability based on CGM (3 d, each formula for 36 h)	Mean glucose lower in inhouse vs. standard group (6.8 vs. 8.0 mM, $p = 0.022$); glucose variability comparable	High
Lidder et al., 2009 [34]	RCT, parallel, single-center	30	Prediabetes (fasting BG < 7 mM) surgical (esophagectomy for esophageal cancer)	PN with or wo EN	100% of energy covered by PN (PN, $n = 14$) 70% covered by PN + 30% covered by EN (PN + EN, $n = 16$)	Mean glucose values based on CGM values [surgery until postoperative day 5]	Mean glucose comparable over entire study period, lower from day 3 post-surgery to day 5 post-surgery in PN + EN vs. PN ($p = 0.002$)	Medium
Leon-Sanz et al., 2005 [36]	RCT, parallel, multi-center (4 sites)	104	T2D surgical and medical	EN (continuous)	Low-CHO high-MUFA nutrition formula (lowCHO, $n = 51$) Energy-matched high-CHO nutrition formula (highCHO, $n = 53$)	Mean glucose based on capillary POC BG values and mean daily insulin dose [2 weeks]	BG increase from baseline lower in lowCHO than highCHO after 7 d on EN (10% vs. 21%, $p = 0.006$); mean BG identical (12.7 vs. 12.7 mM²)	Medium
Valero et al., 2001 [41]	RCT, parallel, double-blind, single-center	138	T1D (21%) and T2D (79%) surgical and medical	TPN (continuous)	Standard TPN containing glucose (PN_G, $n = 71$) Energy-matched TPN containing glucose:fructose:xylitol 2:1:1 (PN_GFX, $n = 67$)	PO not specified; number of patients with target glycemia (capillary POC BG values 8.3–11.1 mM) at end of TPN (TPN duration 5–46 d)	BG < 11.1 mM at end of TPN reached in 75% vs. 85% in PN_G and PN_GFX respectively [2]	High

RCT = randomized controlled trial, T1D = type 1 diabetes, EN = enteral nutrition, PN = parenteral nutrition, s.c. = subcutaneous, CGM = continuous glucose monitoring, T2D = type 2 diabetes, TPN = total parenteral nutrition, POC = point of care, BG = blood glucose, (ns) = not significant, CSII = continuous subcutaneous insulin infusion, VRII = variable rate intravenous insulin, excl = exclusion, NOS = not otherwise specified, PO = primary outcome, SSI = sliding scale insulin, SSRI = sliding-scale regular insulin, NPH = neutral protamine Hagedorn insulin, wo = without, i.v. = intravenous, CHO = carbohydrates, h = hours, d = day(s) and MUFA = monounsaturated fatty acids. [1] Open-label if not stated otherwise. [2] No p-value available. [3] Overall quality assessment; specific domains can be found in Supplementary Figure S1.

Table 2. Overview of observational, retrospective studies.

Author, Year	Study Design	Sample Size	Population	Nutrition Therapy	Interventions	Primary Outcome (Study Period)	Main Results
					Insulin adaptation		
Truong et al., 2019 [42]	Retrospective observational, single-center	102	Hyperglycemic patients (≥2 BG values > 10.0 mM, including T1D and T2D) surgical and medical	PN (continuous or cyclic)	Regular insulin added to PN bag (100% bag, n = 78) S.c. insulin glargine (scGlarg, n = 35)	% of patients with ≥5/6 capillary POC BG values per day <10.0 mM for ≥2 consecutive days (during PN or until target reached)	Higher % of patients with target achieved in 100%bag vs. scGlarg (72% vs. 49%, p = 0.017); ≥2 hypoglycemic events (<3.9 mM) in 9% of 100%bag and 17% of scGlarg group (p = ns); lower need for corrective insulin less in 100%bag vs. scGlarg (28 vs. 57% of patients, p = 0.003)
Hijaze et al., 2017 [43]	Retrospective observational, single-center	53	Non-T1D medical	EN (continuous)	S.c. NPH insulin 3×/day (NPH, n = 26) (Rescue bolus with 6 units rapid insulin analoga if BG > 16.7 mM) S.c. basal-bolus insulin analoga therapy (basbol, n = 27)	PO not specified; mean glucose based on capillary POC BG values and % of values in the target range (7.8–10 mM) (until discharge or stop EN)	mean BG comparable in NPH vs. basbol (10.6 vs. 11.1 mM, p = ns), 24% and 22% of values in range (p = ns)
Neff et al., 2014 [44]	Retrospective observational, single-center	53	Hyperglycemic patients (BG > 10 mM including T1D and T2D) surgical and medical	PN	Protocol-driven VRII (VRII, n = 32) S.c. basal-bolus insulin (basbol, n = 21)	PO not specified; mean glucose based on POC BG values and % of values in target range (4.0–10.0 mM) [until stop PN]	Mean glucose lower and % of values in target range higher in VRII vs. basbol (9.6 vs. 11.2 mM, p = 0.009 and 62% vs. 43%, p = 0.008)
Hsia et al., 2011 [45]	Retrospective observational, single-center	22	Diabetes NOS surgical and medical	EN (continuous)	S.c. basal-bolus with glargine/lispro (basbol, n = 8) S.c. 70/30 premixed insulin 2×/day (mixed2, n = 8) S.c. 70/30 pre-mixed insulin 3×/day (mixed3, n = 6)	PO not specified; mean glucose based on POC BG values, % of values in target range (7.8–10.0 mM) (72 h)	mean glucose comparable, % of values in target range higher in mixed3 vs. mixed2 and basbol (69% vs. 22% vs. 24%, p < 0.01); patients with hypoglycemic events (<3.9 mM) in basbol vs. mixed2 and mixed3 (5 vs. 2 vs. 1)

BG = blood glucose, vs. = versus, T1D = type 1 diabetes, T2D = type 2 diabetes, PN = parenteral nutrition, s.c. = subcutaneous, POC = point of care, EN = enteral nutrition, NPH = Neutral Protamine Hagedorn, ns = not significant, VRII = variable rate intravenous insulin, PO = primary outcome, and NOS = not otherwise specified.

There was only one study examining a modified nutritional formula in abdominal surgery patients that were entirely parenterally fed. In this randomized parallel double-blind single-center study, Valero et al. contrasted a PN formula with glucose as a sole carbohydrate source with an iso-energetic PN formulation containing a 2:1:1 glucose:fructose:xylitol carbohydrate mixture. The study population consisted of patients with type 1 diabetes (21%) or type 2 diabetes (79%). Both formulae provided a similar total amount of carbohydrates (2.9 ± 0.5 vs. 2.9 ± 0.7 g/kg/day), but the test formula under investigation contained less glucose (2.9 ± 0.5 vs. 1.5 ± 0.4 g/kg/day). Protein and fat quantity were similar. The time until attaining target glycaemia (8.3–11.1 mM) did not significantly differ (2.5 ± 1.7 vs. 2.4 ± 2.1 day, p = ns), nor did the percentage of patients attaining values below 11.1 mM (75% vs. 85%, p = ns) and total daily insulin dose (45 ± 19 vs. 45 ± 26 U/day, p = ns). However, when stratified according to the occurrence of sepsis, the nonseptic patients showed lower insulin requirements with the glucose–fructose–xylitol regime (37 ± 17 vs. 44 ± 17 U/day, p = 0.026) [41].

Managing glycaemia during PN is more demanding than during EN. In this context, the combination of PN with EN, in addition to its well-established trophic benefits on gastrointestinal function, may also confer glycemic advantages. This was shown by a randomized controlled parallel study performed by Lidder et al. in patients undergoing esophagectomy who received nutrition support for up to five days post-surgery. The study contrasted the coverage of 30% of energy needs by EN and 70% by PN feeds with 100% coverage by PN. Although no effect was seen in mean glucose over the five-day study period, the combined use of EN and PN lead to lower glycaemia three days after surgery (p = 0.002) [34].

3.4. Studies Examining Insulin Strategies

Eleven studies examined insulin-based strategies to manage glucose in patients receiving nutrition support (five with PN, five with EN, and one with combined PN/EN). A randomized controlled single-center parallel study involving 212 type 2 diabetic patients who had undergone gastrectomy for gastric cancer compared protocol-driven intravenous insulin therapy with conventional subcutaneous sliding scale insulin delivery over 8–10 days of continuous EN. Mean glucose levels were lower (5.4 ± 1.2 vs. 9.5 ± 1.8 mM, p < 0.001), and mean daily insulin doses were higher (55 ± 15 vs. 32 ± 16 U/day, p < 0.001) in patients receiving intravenous insulin compared with subcutaneous insulin. However, in the group receiving intravenous insulin, eight participants experienced episodes of severe hypoglycemia (defined as blood glucose < 2.2 mM), versus only one participant in the subcutaneous group (p = 0.010). Additionally, this study reported outcomes extending beyond glycemic control, finding a reduced incidence of surgical site infection in the intravenous insulin group [12].

A second randomized controlled trial (RCT) evaluating different insulin treatments during EN included 50 patients with non-type 1 diabetes who were randomly assigned to receive sliding scale subcutaneous regular insulin either with or without once daily subcutaneous glargine. In the group without glargine administration, subcutaneous neutral protamine Hagedorn (NPH, isophane) was given as a rescue medication when glucose levels exceeded 10.0 mM. Mean glucose as the primary outcome was comparable between groups, as were the number of hypoglycemic events and total daily insulin dose. However, NPH was required in 48% of the control participants, as their glucose levels were not sufficiently controlled with the regular sliding scale subcutaneous insulin alone [40].

A single-arm trial evaluated the efficacy of a computerized variable rate insulin infusion rate protocol in previously insulin-naïve stroke patients on continuous EN over five days. Compared to a historical control population who received enteral bolus feeds accompanied by intravenous insulin coverage, the intervention resulted in a higher percentage of values in the target range of 4.4–6.1 mM (55% vs. 19%, p < 0.005) [39].

Additionally, two retrospective observational studies evaluated insulin-based strategies to treat hyperglycemia in hospitalized patients receiving EN. Hijaze et al. found comparable mean glucose values, and similar times with glucose values within the target range (7.8–10 mM), in patients receiving subcutaneous NPH insulin thrice daily vs. basal–bolus insulin therapy with insulin analogues [43].

In the second such study, Hsia et al. retrospectively evaluated glucose control using three different insulin regimens in patients with diabetes of type not otherwise specified during at least three days of continuous EN. Treatment consisted of (1) 70/30 biphasic insulin (NPH/regular) every 8 h ($n = 6$), (2) 70/30 biphasic insulin every 12 h ($n = 8$), and (3) a basal–bolus regimen (glargine and lispro, $n = 8$). The 8 h 70/30 biphasic insulin group had the highest proportion of glucose values falling within the target range (7.8–10.0 mM) (69% vs. 22% vs. 24%, $p < 0.01$). Hypoglycemic events (<3.9 mM) occurred five times in glargine/lispro group, twice in the twice-daily biphasic group, and once in the thrice-daily biphasic group [45]. In patients receiving PN, two randomized controlled parallel trials evaluated strategies that involved the addition of regular insulin to the PN feeding bag. Olveira et al. recently compared the use of 100% coverage of insulin needs by regular insulin added to the PN bag with 50% coverage by regular insulin added to the PN bag and 50% administered subcutaneously as insulin glargine in a total of 161 mixed surgical and medical patients with type 2 diabetes recruited at 26 different sites. The glucose values of participants were evaluated while receiving total PN (maximum of 15 days) and two days after cessation of total PN. Mean glucose levels during total PN did not significantly differ between groups (9.2 ± 2.0 vs. 9.6 ± 2.4 mM, p = ns); however, mean glucose two days after cessation of total PN was higher in the group that had received 100% of their exogenous insulin requirements added to the PN feeding bag (8.9 ± 2.5 vs. 7.9 ± 2.4 mM, $p = 0.024$). The authors did not provide any details on the requirement for insulin therapy after cessation of nutrition support [32]. Another randomized controlled clinical trial of PN patients contrasted two different basal insulin regimens. Hakeam et al. compared subcutaneous basal–bolus therapy (insulin glargine + short-acting insulin analogue) with the addition of regular insulin to the PN bag in a total of 67 non-type 1 diabetic patients. Both groups received additional corrective regular subcutaneous insulin according to a sliding scale. Basal insulin delivery dose was titrated based on glucose values by a daily 40%–60% dose increase if glucose values were still above target. The percentage of glucose values within the glycemic target range (7.8–10.0 mM) tended to be higher in the group who received s.c. insulin glargine compared to those who received regular insulin added to the PN bag (52% vs. 48%, $p = 0.06$). Mean glucose levels and number of hypoglycemic events did not differ between treatment groups [33].

In contrast to these prospective findings in PN patients, a retrospective evaluation performed by Truong et al. in 102 patients on PN showed superior glucose control defined as percentage of patients with ≥5 of 6 glucose values <10 mM over 2 days in those who had received 100% of required insulin added to the PN bag ($n = 78$), compared with those treated with subcutaneous insulin glargine ($n = 35$) (72% vs. 49%, $p = 0.017$). Additionally, fewer patients receiving insulin via the PN bag experienced two or more hypoglycemic events compared to those with subcutaneous administration (9% vs. 17.1%, p = ns) [42].

As reviewed above in patients receiving EN, a protocol-driven intravenous insulin delivery approach has proven to confer glycemic benefits in PN patients, according to a retrospective analysis performed by Neff et al. A total of 53 surgical and medical patients requiring insulin therapy whilst in the hospital were treated either with protocol-driven variable rate intravenous insulin ($n = 32$), or received basal–bolus subcutaneous insulin therapy ($n = 21$). The insulin infusion group compared to the group receiving subcutaneous basal–bolus insulin therapy showed lower mean glucose levels (9.6 ± 2.1 vs. 11.2 ± 2.6 mM, $p = 0.009$) and a higher percentage of glucose values within the glycemic target of 4.0–10.0 mM (62% vs. 43%, $p = 0.008$), without increased risk of hypoglycemia [44].

Two recently performed randomized controlled parallel design trials evaluated insulin pump therapy, also known as continuous subcutaneous insulin infusion (CSII), in patients receiving nutrition support. The study performed by Li et al. compared the use of CSII ($n = 50$) to basal–bolus therapy using insulin glargine in combination with insulin aspart ($n = 52$) in patients receiving PN. Study treatment was initialized before surgery, and PN began on day 1 after surgery, with comparison of glucose control with CGM from postoperative day 1 to day 5. Glycemic variability was assessed by mean amplitude of glucose excursion (MAGE) as the primary outcome. CSII reduced glycemic variability compared to basal–bolus injection therapy (3.7 ± 2.8 vs. 6.2 ± 3.0 mM, $p < 0.05$). No hypoglycemic events occurred in either treatment group [38].

The second study evaluated CSII as part of a fully automated subcutaneous closed-loop glucose control ($n = 21$) against conventional subcutaneous insulin therapy according to local practice ($n = 22$) in two different hospitals. Randomization was stratified according to BMI, prestudy total daily insulin dose, and type of nutrition support to ensure to demographic balance between groups. The closed-loop system consisted of a subcutaneous insulin pump, a CGM device, and a control algorithm, which adjusted insulin delivery every 12 min based on real-time CGM values. An example of such fully automated closed-loop insulin delivery is illustrated in Figure 3. Participants were recruited from medical and surgical wards and received PN ($n = 13$), EN ($n = 27$), or combined PN/EN ($n = 3$). The primary outcome was the proportion of time when sensor glucose was within the target range (5.6–10.0 mM). Participants were followed for up to 15 days or until hospital discharge. The closed-loop system nearly doubled the proportion of time spent in the glycemic target range compared to control (68% ± 16% vs. 36% ± 27%, $p < 0.0001$). Time spent above target, mean glucose level, and glucose variability were all significantly lower in the closed-loop group. Hypoglycemia was infrequent in both arms, and its incidence did not differ significantly. The substantially better glycemic control in the closed-loop compared to the control group was achieved with a similar total daily insulin dose (53.9 vs. 40.3 U, $p = $ ns) [31].

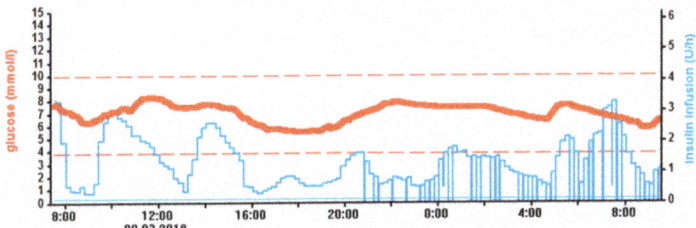

Figure 3. Profile of fully automated subcutaneous closed-loop insulin delivery over 24 h in a noncritical care patient [31]. A control algorithm modulates subcutaneous insulin delivery via an insulin pump (denoted in blue) according to interstitial sensor glucose values (denoted in red). (Kindly provided by Professor Roman Hovorka, University of Cambridge, UK).

4. Discussion

Hyperglycemia is a common occurrence in hospitalized patients receiving PN and/or EN, and its management in noncritical care settings is challenging. The present review summarized the available evidence for strategies to improve glucose control in this vulnerable population. Improved glucose control can be achieved either by lowering the glycemic impact of nutrition supply and/or matching the nutrition-induced glycemic excursions with a tailored pharmacokinetic profile of a given insulin preparation. Both approaches have been evaluated in a limited number of randomized and nonrandomized clinical trials and observational studies over the past 20 years.

Altering the macronutrient distribution (an increase of calories as MUFAs at the expense of carbohydrates) and the use of nonglucose carbohydrate sources along with high fiber content to delay absorption in EN formulae have proven effective in various studies as well as in meta-analyses [22,23]. The use of diabetes-specific enteral formulae is therefore supported by the expert group of the European Society of Clinical Nutrition and Metabolism (ESPEN) for patients with a history of diabetes [46]. With respect to PN formulae, glucose substitutes such as fructose or xylitol to lower the glycemic impact are no longer used in clinical practice. This may relate to previously reported metabolic side effects of parenteral xylitol and fructose such as formation of oxalate crystals in the kidney and lactate accumulation [47–49]. To make matters worse, life-threatening metabolic complications can occur in patients with undeclared hereditary fructose intolerance [50]. There is currently no data on the efficacy and safety of PN formulations with reduced carbohydrate content (and consequently higher protein or lipid fractions) in noncritically ill patients with hyperglycemia. In critically ill patients, however, lipid-based, compared to iso-energetic glucose-based, PN formulae showed more favorable metabolic effects [51]. Additionally, lowering the overall carbohydrate and energy provision has proven effective in reducing hyperglycemia in critically ill patients [52,53].

As an alternative to conventional routes of insulin administration, algorithm-driven intravenous insulin titration protocols during both PN and EN achieved superior glucose control compared to subcutaneous approaches with either sliding scale or basal–bolus insulin therapy. However, this approach poses logistical challenges for ward staff, given the need for frequent glucose draws and insulin dose adjustments, which are either impractical or simply unfeasible in noncritical care settings with low nurse-to-patient ratios. Regarding subcutaneous insulin regimens, administering basal plus supplemental short-acting insulin analogues showed superior efficacy compared to a sliding scale approach with short-acting insulin. The administration of intermediate or long-acting insulins can thus be recommended for PN/EN patients receiving subcutaneous insulin therapy. No data exist with regard to the use of recently introduced ultra-long acting insulins (e.g., degludec). Of note, the required time to reach steady state insulin levels with ultra-long acting formulations imposes certain constraints on the titration method, and predisposes to dysglycemia. There is a practical consideration that administering long-acting insulin in previously insulin-naïve patients brings a risk of hypoglycemia if feeding tubes are accidentally pulled or obstructed.

The admixture of insulin into the PN feeding bag is a safe and effective alternative to using short- or rapid-acting subcutaneous insulin. Moreover, further advantages lie in the lesser need for nursing time, the concomitant discontinuation of insulin delivery upon PN interruption, and the consequently lower risk of hypoglycemic events. The latter is particularly relevant for patients in whom the transient need for exogenous insulin is primarily a result of their nutrition support. However, the need for strict aseptic conditions may render the procedure impractical or not permissible. Furthermore, reservations exist regarding the diminished or highly variable efficacy of PN insulin due to interference from PN ingredients or bag surface material [54,55].

Irrespective to the chosen approach for insulin administration, a limiting factor in obtaining tight glucose control is the risk of inadvertent hypoglycemia [17]. As is the case for hyperglycemia, iatrogenic hypoglycemia is associated with increased cost and adverse medical outcomes [16]. In this context, there is an increasing interest in the use of noninsulin glucose-lowering agents (without hypoglycemia risk) for the treatment of inpatient hyperglycemia. The recent SITA-HOSPITAL randomized controlled study investigated 279 noncritical care patients with type 2 diabetes and showed that oral sitagliptin plus basal insulin led to similar glycemic control than the more labor-intensive basal–bolus insulin regimen [56]. However, challenging patients such as those with high insulin requirements, renal failure, or use of glucocorticoids were excluded from the study. Currently, there are no data on the inpatient use of noninsulin glucose-lowering treatments for hyperglycemia in noncritical care patients on PN and/or EN. Reservations apply to the common side effects of noninsulin treatments (e.g., incretin-based therapies) on the gastrointestinal tract, which is often the primary pathophysiology calling for nutrition support. Further research is needed to explore the potential risks and benefits of noninsulin pharmacotherapy for managing glucose levels in noncritical care settings with EN/PN.

The high prevalence of hyperglycemia amongst noncritical care patients on PN and/or EN support, in conjunction with the increasing workload burden placed on hospital staff, brings an urgent need for innovative approaches to improve the efficacy, efficiency, and safety of healthcare delivery in this context. The advent of novel technologies such as automated closed-loop systems that titrate insulin delivery based on real-time sensor glucose measurements could potentially address this need, whilst reducing staff workload burden. Uncertainties remain with respect to interference with certain medications and inaccurate glucose readouts related to compromised microcirculation. In addition, we concede that there are short-term costs to purchase, install, and train staff in the use of any novel technology. Ongoing studies will further document the potential role of this technology and the obstacles to its integration into clinical practice without disrupting the usual workflow.

The present systematic review turned up rather few randomized controlled trials and a limited number of retrospective observational studies addressing hyperglycemia in noncritical care patients on PN and/or EN. The studies were highly heterogeneous in terms of study population, nutrition regimen, study endpoints, and glucose measurement techniques. Patients with pre-existing diabetes already on insulin treatment before their admission to the hospital and those receiving steroids or showing impaired renal function clearly have different optimal insulin delivery profiles compared to patients without pre-existing diabetes and/or with stress-induced hyperglycemia. The particular nutrition regime (i.e., the EN/PN feeding schedule and any additional oral intake) leads to variable carbohydrate exposures with relevant impact on insulin requirements. The few studies that utilized CGM more comprehensively assessed both hyper- and hypoglycemic excursions, whilst studies adopting intermittent (i.e., six-hourly) point-of-care measurements may have missed important events such as postprandial transients. Most studies were conducted in patients on continuous PN and/or EN, which may be less demanding for insulin management compared to the less common bolus or cyclic feeding practices. The scarce evidence and the many factors (e.g., patient comorbidity, staffing level, hospital guidelines, and policies) that determine the ability and capacity to treat hyperglycemia effectively and safely challenge the provision of generalizable treatment recommendations. In Figure 4, we propose a workflow recommendation considering both nutritional and insulin adaptation to manage hyperglycemia in the noncritical care population receiving nutrition support.

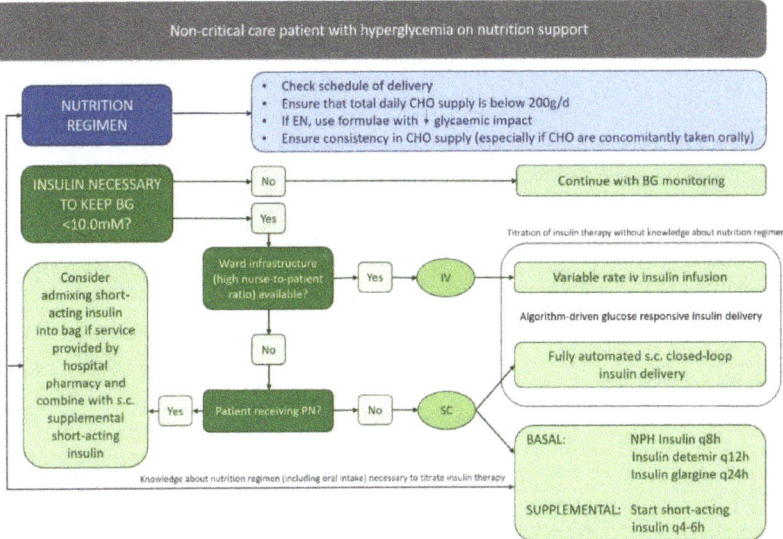

Figure 4. Approach to the management of hyperglycemia in patients receiving enteral or parenteral nutrition. CHO = carbohydrates, EN = enteral nutrition, BG = blood glucose, IV = intravenous, PN = parenteral nutrition, SC = subcutaneous, and q8h = dosing every 8 h.

The majority of the included studies scored poorly in methodology, with a high or unclear risk of biases according to Cochrane criteria. Undoubtably, it is sometimes difficult or unethical to undertake double-blind RCTs with standardized protocols. Also, some studies did not correct for multiple testing, which may have overestimated outcomes. The included retrospective observational studies were not evaluated for quality given the known risk of outcome overestimation and confounding biases inherent in that design. However, we chose to report these studies in this review to cover the widest possible range of different management possibilities.

Small sample sizes and short study durations of some studies may have led to an underestimation of effect sizes, thus hindering the sensitivity to ascertain the efficacy of potential methods to improve glycemic control or indeed to confirm the impact of superior glucose control on patient outcomes. There is clearly a need for further research in the form of well-designed and adequately powered multicenter trials of sufficient duration aiming to examine effects of glucose management strategies on glucose control, clinical outcome, and also optimization of nutritional status in patients receiving PN and/or EN.

5. Conclusions

The management of hyperglycemia in patients receiving PN and/or EN presents unique clinical challenges for both diabetic and nondiabetic hospitalized patients with hyperglycemia. Coherent approaches to this problem are important to avoid potential complications. Obtaining a better match between the carbohydrate dose and the insulin supply is likely to improve glucose control. Granting more attention to the glycemic impact of nutrition regimes in conjunction with deploying novel technologies such as CGM and glucose-responsive automation of insulin delivery through closed-loop systems may address these needs without increasing staff workload. Supplemental or alternate use of noninsulin pharmacological approaches may further open up new lines of research. Well-designed and adequately powered randomized controlled trials are necessary to define the optimal management of hyperglycemia and consequent clinical benefits in patients receiving nutrition support.

Supplementary Materials: The following are available online at http://www.mdpi.com/2077-0383/8/7/935/s1; Figure S1: Quality assessment of clinical trials according to modified Cochrane Risk of Bias tool [30]. Table S1: PubMed Search Strategy 12.04.2019, Table S2: Embase Search Strategy 10.04.2019, Table S3: Cochrane Central Register of Controlled Trials Search Strategy 10.04.2019, Table S4: ClinicalTrials.gov Search Strategy 10.04.2019, Table S5: PRISMA 2009 checklist [28], Table S6: MOOSE checklist [29].

Author Contributions: Conceptualization and methodology, L.B.; design and conduction of the search: C.I.L. and L.B.; writing—original draft preparation; C.I.L. and L.B.; writing—reviewing and editing: C.I.L., P.C., E.R., Z.S., T.M. and L.B; supervision: L.B.

Acknowledgments: We would like to thank Heidrun Janka for her help in improving the search strategies and Kai Holtmann for his help in improving the design of the figures.

Conflicts of Interest: The authors declare no conflict of interest related to this work.

References

1. Pasquel, F.J.; Spiegelman, R.; McCauley, M.; Smiley, D.; Umpierrez, D.; Johnson, R.; Rhee, M.; Gatcliffe, C.; Lin, E.; Umpierrez, E.; et al. Hyperglycemia during total parenteral nutrition: An important marker of poor outcome and mortality in hospitalized patients. *Diabetes Care* **2010**, *33*, 739–741. [CrossRef] [PubMed]
2. Davidson, P.; Kwiatkowski, C.A.; Wien, M. Management of Hyperglycemia and Enteral Nutrition in the Hospitalized Patient. *Nutr. Clin. Pract.* **2015**, *30*, 652–659. [CrossRef] [PubMed]
3. Pleva, M.; Mirtallo, J.M.; Steinberg, S.M. Hyperglycemic events in non-intensive care unit patients receiving parenteral nutrition. *Nutr. Clin. Pract.* **2009**, *24*, 626–634. [CrossRef] [PubMed]
4. Pancorbo-Hidalgo, P.L.; Garcia-Fernandez, F.P.; Ramirez-Perez, C. Complications associated with enteral nutrition by nasogastric tube in an internal medicine unit. *J. Clin. Nurs.* **2001**, *10*, 482–490. [CrossRef] [PubMed]
5. McCowen, K.C.; Malhotra, A.; Bistrian, B.R. Stress-Induced Hyperglycemia. *J. Clin. Nurs.* **2001**, *17*, 107–124. [CrossRef]
6. Herrmann, C.; Göke, R.; Richter, G.; Fehmann, H.C.; Arnold, R.; Göke, B. Glucagon-Like Peptide-1 and Glucose-Dependent Insulin-Releasing Polypeptide Plasma Levels in Response to Nutrients. *Digestion* **1995**, *56*, 117–126. [CrossRef] [PubMed]
7. Andrews, R.C.; Walker, B.R. Glucocorticoids and insulin resistance: Old hormones, new targets. *Clin. Sci.* **1999**, *96*, 513–523. [CrossRef] [PubMed]

8. Marathe, C.S.; Rayner, C.K.; Bound, M.; Checklin, H.; Standfield, S.; Wishart, J.; Lange, K.; Jones, K.L.; Horowitz, M. Small intestinal glucose exposure determines the magnitude of the incretin effect in health and type 2 diabetes. *Diabetes* **2014**, *63*, 2668–2675. [CrossRef] [PubMed]
9. Olveira, G.; Tapia, M.J.; Ocón, J.; Cabrejas-Gómez, C.; Ballesteros-Pomar, M.D.; Vidal-Casariego, A.; Arraiza-Irigoyen, C.; Olivares, J.; Conde-García, M.e.C.; García-Manzanares, A.; et al. Parenteral nutrition-associated hyperglycemia in non-critically ill inpatients increases the risk of in-hospital mortality (multicenter study). *Diabetes Care* **2013**, *36*, 1061–1066. [CrossRef] [PubMed]
10. Lin, L.Y.; Lin, H.C.; Lee, P.C.; Ma, W.Y.; Lin, H.D. Hyperglycemia correlates with outcomes in patients receiving total parenteral nutrition. *Am. J. Med Sci.* **2007**, *333*, 261–265. [CrossRef] [PubMed]
11. Cheung, N.W.; Napier, B.; Zaccaria, C.; Fletcher, J.P. Hyperglycemia is associated with adverse outcomes in patients receiving total parenteral nutrition. *Diabetes Care* **2005**, *28*, 2367–2371. [CrossRef] [PubMed]
12. Yuan, J.; Liu, T.; Zhang, X.; Si, Y.; Ye, Y.; Zhao, C.; Wang, Q.; Shen, X. Intensive Versus Conventional Glycemic Control in Patients with Diabetes During Enteral Nutrition After Gastrectomy. *J. Gastrointest. Surg.* **2015**, *19*, 1553–1558. [CrossRef] [PubMed]
13. Murad, M.H.; Coburn, J.A.; Coto-Yglesias, F.; Dzyubak, S.; Hazem, A.; Lane, M.A.; Prokop, L.J.; Montori, V.M. Glycemic Control in Non-Critically Ill Hospitalized Patients: A Systematic Review and Meta-Analysis. *J. Clin. Endocrinol. Metab.* **2012**, *97*, 49–58. [CrossRef] [PubMed]
14. Kang, Z.-Q.; Huo, J.-L.; Zhai, X.-J. Effects of perioperative tight glycemic control on postoperative outcomes: A meta-analysis. *Endocr. Connect.* **2018**, *7*, R316–R327. [CrossRef] [PubMed]
15. Umpierrez, G.E.; Smiley, D.; Zisman, A.; Prieto, L.M.; Palacio, A.; Ceron, M.; Puig, A.; Mejia, R. Randomized Study of Basal-Bolus Insulin Therapy in the Inpatient Management of Patients with Type 2 Diabetes (RABBIT 2 Trial). *Diabetes Care* **2007**, *30*, 2181. [CrossRef] [PubMed]
16. Turchin, A.; Matheny, M.E.; Shubina, M.; Scanlon, J.V.; Greenwood, B.; Pendergrass, M.L. Hypoglycemia and clinical outcomes in patients with diabetes hospitalized in the general ward. *Diabetes Care* **2009**, *32*, 1153–1157. [CrossRef]
17. Finfer, S.; Chittock, D.R.; Su, S.Y.; Blair, D.; Foster, D.; Dhingra, V.; Bellomo, R.; Cook, D.; Dodek, P.; Henderson, W.R.; et al. Intensive versus Conventional Glucose Control in Critically Ill Patients. *N. Engl. J. Med.* **2009**, *360*, 1283–1297. [CrossRef] [PubMed]
18. Association, A.D. 15. Diabetes Care in the Hospital. *Diabetes Care* **2019**, *42*, S173–S181. [CrossRef] [PubMed]
19. Umpierrez, G.E.; Hellman, R.; Korytkowski, M.T.; Kosiborod, M.; Maynard, G.A.; Montori, V.M.; Seley, J.J.; Van den Berghe, G.; Society, E. Management of hyperglycemia in hospitalized patients in non-critical care setting: An endocrine society clinical practice guideline. *J. Clin. Endocrinol. Metab.* **2012**, *97*, 16–38. [CrossRef] [PubMed]
20. McCulloch, A.; Bansiya, V.; Woodward, J.M. Addition of Insulin to Parenteral Nutrition for Control of Hyperglycemia. *JPEN* **2018**, *42*, 846–854. [CrossRef] [PubMed]
21. Aragon, D. Evaluation of nursing work effort and perceptions about blood glucose testing in tight glycemic control. *Am. J. Crit. Care* **2006**, *15*, 370–377. [PubMed]
22. Elia, M.; Ceriello, A.; Laube, H.; Sinclair, A.J.; Engfer, M.; Stratton, R.J. Enteral nutritional support and use of diabetes-specific formulas for patients with diabetes: A systematic review and meta-analysis. *Diabetes Care* **2005**, *28*, 2267–2279. [CrossRef] [PubMed]
23. Ojo, O.; Brooke, J. Evaluation of the role of enteral nutrition in managing patients with diabetes: A systematic review. *Nutrients* **2014**, *6*, 5142–5152. [CrossRef] [PubMed]
24. Rodbard, D. Continuous Glucose Monitoring: A Review of Recent Studies Demonstrating Improved Glycemic Outcomes. *Diabetes Technol. Ther.* **2017**, *19*, S25–S37. [CrossRef] [PubMed]
25. Pickup, J.C. Insulin-pump therapy for type 1 diabetes mellitus. *N. Engl J. Med.* **2012**, *366*, 1616–1624. [CrossRef] [PubMed]
26. Bally, L.; Thabit, H.; Hovorka, R. Closed-loop for type 1 diabetes—an introduction and appraisal for the generalist. *BMC Med.* **2017**, *15*, 14. [CrossRef] [PubMed]
27. Bally, L.; Thabit, H.; Hovorka, R. Glucose-responsive insulin delivery for type 1 diabetes: The artificial pancreas story. *Int. J. Pharm.* **2017**. [CrossRef] [PubMed]
28. Moher, D.; Liberati, A.; Tetzlaff, J.; Altman, D.G.; Group, P. Preferred reporting items for systematic reviews and meta-analyses: The PRISMA statement. *Int. J. Surg.* **2010**, *8*, 336–341. [CrossRef] [PubMed]

29. Stroup, D.F.; Berlin, J.A.; Morton, S.C.; Olkin, I.; Williamson, G.D.; Rennie, D.; Moher, D.; Becker, B.J.; Sipe, T.A.; Thacker, S.B.; et al. Meta-analysis of Observational Studies in EpidemiologyA Proposal for Reporting. *JAMA* **2000**, *283*, 2008–2012. [CrossRef]
30. Higgins, J.P.T.; Altman, D.G.; Gøtzsche, P.C.; Jüni, P.; Moher, D.; Oxman, A.D.; Savović, J.; Schulz, K.F.; Weeks, L.; Sterne, J.A.C. The Cochrane Collaboration's tool for assessing risk of bias in randomized trials. *BMJ* **2011**, *343*, d5928. [CrossRef]
31. Boughton, C.K.; Bally, L.; Martignoni, F.; Hartnell, S.; Herzig, D.; Vogt, A.; Wertli, M.M.; Wilinska, M.E.; Evans, M.L.; Coll, A.P.; et al. Fully closed-loop insulin delivery in inpatients receiving nutritional support: A two-center, open-label, randomized controlled trial. *Lancet Diabetes Endocri.* **2019**, *7*, 368–377. [CrossRef]
32. Olveira, G.; Abuin, J.; Lopez, R.; Herranz, S.; Garcia-Almeida, J.M.; Garcia-Malpartida, K.; Ferrer, M.; Cancer, E.; Luengo-Perez, L.M.; Alvarez, J.; et al. Regular insulin added to total parenteral nutrition vs. subcutaneous glargine in non-critically ill diabetic inpatients, a multicenter randomized clinical trial: INSUPAR trial. *Clin. Nutr.* **2019**. [CrossRef] [PubMed]
33. Hakeam, H.A.; Mulia, H.A.; Azzam, A.; Amin, T. Glargine Insulin Use Versus Continuous Regular Insulin in Diabetic Surgical Noncritically Ill Patients Receiving Parenteral Nutrition: Randomized Controlled Study. *JPEN* **2017**, *41*, 1110–1118. [CrossRef] [PubMed]
34. Lidder, P.; Flanagan, D.; Fleming, S.; Russell, M.; Morgan, N.; Wheatley, T.; Rahamin, J.; Shaw, S.; Lewis, S. Combining enteral with parenteral nutrition to improve postoperative glucose control. *Br. J. Nutr.* **2010**, *103*, 1635–1641. [CrossRef] [PubMed]
35. Tiyapanjanit, T.; Boonyavarakul, A. Comparative study between the Phramongkutklao's diabetic blenderized diets and commercial diabetic diets on glycemic variability in continuous tube fed patients with type 2 diabetes. *J. Med. Assoc. Thai.* **2014**, *97*, 1151–1156. [PubMed]
36. Leon-Sanz, M.; Garcia-Luna, P.P.; Sanz-Paris, A.; Gomez-Candela, C.; Casimiro, C.; Chamorro, J.; Pereira-Cunill, J.L.; Martin-Palmero, A.; Trallero, R.; Martinez, J.; et al. Glycemic and lipid control in hospitalized type 2 diabetic patients: Evaluation of 2 enteral nutrition formulas (low carbohydrate-high monounsaturated fat vs. high carbohydrate). *JPEN* **2005**, *29*, 21–29. [CrossRef]
37. Hyperglycemia in Patients with Stroke and Indication of Enteral Nutrition. Available online: https://ClinicalTrials.gov/show/NCT03422900 (accessed on 20 May 2019).
38. Li, F.F.; Zhang, W.L.; Liu, B.L.; Zhang, D.F.; Chen, W.; Yuan, L.; Chen, M.Y.; Zhai, X.F.; Wu, J.D.; Su, X.F.; et al. Management of glycemic variation in diabetic patients receiving parenteral nutrition by continuous subcutaneous insulin infusion (CSII) therapy. *Sci. Rep.* **2018**, *8*, 5888. [CrossRef]
39. Kruyt, N.D.; Biessels, G.J.; Vriesendorp, T.M.; Devries, J.H.; Hoekstra, J.B.; Elbers, P.W.; Kappelle, L.J.; Portegies, P.; Vermeulen, M.; Roos, Y.B. Subjecting acute ischemic stroke patients to continuous tube feeding and an intensive computerized protocol establishes tight glycemic control. *Neurocrit. Care* **2010**, *12*, 62–68. [CrossRef]
40. Korytkowski, M.T.; Salata, R.J.; Koerbel, G.L.; Selzer, F.; Karslioglu, E.; Idriss, A.M.; Lee, K.K.; Moser, A.J.; Toledo, F.G. Insulin therapy and glycemic control in hospitalized patients with diabetes during enteral nutrition therapy: A randomized controlled clinical trial. *Diabetes Care* **2009**, *32*, 594–596. [CrossRef]
41. Valero, M.A.; Leon-Sanz, M.; Escobar, I.; Gomis, P.; de la Camara, A.; Moreno, J.M. Evaluation of nonglucose carbohydrates in parenteral nutrition for diabetic patients. *Eur. J. Clin. Nutr.* **2001**, *55*, 1111–1116. [CrossRef]
42. Truong, S.; Park, A.; Kamalay, S.; Hung, N.; Meyer, J.G.; Nguyen, N.; Momenzadeh, A. Glycemic Control in Adult Surgical Patients Receiving Regular Insulin Added to Parenteral Nutrition vs. Insulin Glargine: A Retrospective Chart Review. *Nutr. Clin. Pract.* **2019**. [CrossRef] [PubMed]
43. Hijaze, D.; Szalat, A. Retrospective Evaluation of Glycemic Control with Basal-Bolus or Neutral Protamine Hagedorn Insulin Regimens in Patients Receiving Continuous Enteral Nutrition Therapy in Medicine Wards. *Nutr. Clin. Pract.* **2017**, *32*, 557–562. [CrossRef] [PubMed]
44. Neff, K.; Donegan, D.; MacMahon, J.; O'Hanlon, C.; Keane, N.; Agha, A.; Thompson, C.; Smith, D. Management of parenteral nutrition associated hyperglycemia: A comparison of subcutaneous and intravenous insulin regimen. *Ir. Med. J.* **2014**, *107*, 141–143. [PubMed]
45. Hsia, E.; Seggelke, S.A.; Gibbs, J.; Rasouli, N.; Draznin, B. Comparison of 70/30 biphasic insulin with glargine/lispro regimen in non-critically ill diabetic patients on continuous enteral nutrition therapy. *Nutr. Clin. Pract.* **2011**, *26*, 714–717. [CrossRef] [PubMed]

46. Dardai, E. Basics in clinical nutrition: Nutritional support in the diabetic patient. *e-SPEN* **2009**, *4*, e304–e307. [CrossRef]
47. Woods, H.F.; Alberti, K.G. Dangers of intravenous fructose. *Lancet* **1972**, *2*, 1354–1357. [CrossRef]
48. Thomas, D.W.; Edwards, J.B.; Gilligan, J.E.; Lawrence, J.R.; Edwards, R.G. Complications following intravenous administration of solutions containing xylitol. *Med. J. Aust.* **1972**, *1*, 1238–1246.
49. Thomas, D.W.; Gilligan, J.E.; Edwards, J.B.; Edwards, R.G. Lactic acidosis and osmotic diuresis produced by xylitol infusion. *Med. J. Aust.* **1972**, *1*, 1246–1248.
50. Keller, U. The sugar substitutes fructose and sorbite: An unnecessary risk in parenteral nutrition. *Schweiz Med. Wochenschr.* **1989**, *119*, 101–106.
51. Tappy, L.; Schwarz, J.M.; Schneiter, P.; Cayeux, C.; Revelly, J.P.; Fagerquist, C.K.; Jequier, E.; Chiolero, R. Effects of isoenergetic glucose-based or lipid-based parenteral nutrition on glucose metabolism, de novo lipogenesis, and respiratory gas exchanges in critically ill patients. *Crit. Care Med.* **1998**, *26*, 860–867. [CrossRef]
52. Ahrens, C.L.; Barletta, J.F.; Kanji, S.; Tyburski, J.G.; Wilson, R.F.; Janisse, J.J.; Devlin, J.W. Effect of low-calorie parenteral nutrition on the incidence and severity of hyperglycemia in surgical patients: A randomized, controlled trial. *Crit. Care Med.* **2005**, *33*, 2507–2512. [CrossRef] [PubMed]
53. Lee, H.; Koh, S.O.; Park, M.S. Higher dextrose delivery via TPN related to the development of hyperglycemia in non-diabetic critically ill patients. *Nutr. Res. Pract.* **2011**, *5*, 450–454. [CrossRef] [PubMed]
54. Forchielli, M.L.; Bongiovanni, F.; Platé, L.; Piazza, G.; Puggioli, C.; D'Alise, A.; Bersani, G. Insulin Instability in Parenteral Nutrition Admixtures. *JPEN* **2018**, *42*, 907–912. [CrossRef] [PubMed]
55. Mühlebach, S.; Franken, C.; Stanga, Z.; Working group for developing the guidelines for parenteral nutrition of The German Association for Nutritional Medicine. Practical handling of AIO admixtures-Guidelines on Parenteral Nutrition, Chapter 10. *Ger. Med. Sci.* **2009**, *7*, Doc18. [CrossRef]
56. Pasquel, F.J.; Gianchandani, R.; Rubin, D.J.; Dungan, K.M.; Anzola, I.; Gomez, P.C.; Peng, L.; Hodish, I.; Bodnar, T.; Wesorick, D.; et al. Efficacy of sitagliptin for the hospital management of general medicine and surgery patients with type 2 diabetes (Sita-Hospital): A multicentre, prospective, open-label, non-inferiority randomized trial. *Lancet Diabetes Endocrinol* **2017**, *5*, 125–133. [CrossRef]

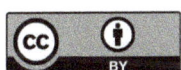

© 2019 by the authors. Licensee MDPI, Basel, Switzerland. This article is an open access article distributed under the terms and conditions of the Creative Commons Attribution (CC BY) license (http://creativecommons.org/licenses/by/4.0/).

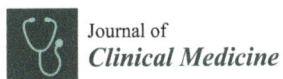

Review

Micronutrient Deficiencies in Medical and Surgical Inpatients

Mette M Berger *, Olivier Pantet, Antoine Schneider and Nawfel Ben-Hamouda

Service of Adult Intensive Care Medicine and Burns, Lausanne University Hospital (CHUV), BH 08.612, Rue du Bugnon 46, 1011 Lausanne, Switzerland
* Correspondence: Mette.Berger@chuv.ch; Tel.: +41-21-3142095

Received: 30 May 2019; Accepted: 21 June 2019; Published: 28 June 2019

Abstract: Inpatients are threatened by global malnutrition, but also by specific micronutrient (i.e., trace element and vitamins) deficiencies that frequently are overseen in the differential diagnosis of major organ dysfunctions. Some of them are related to specific geographic risks (iodine, iron, selenium, zinc, vitamin A), while others are pathology related, and finally many are associated with specific feeding patterns, including low dose enteral feeding. Among the pathologies in which laboratory blood investigations should include a micronutrient outwork, anemia is in the front line, followed by obesity with bariatric surgery, chronic liver disease, kidney disease, inflammatory bowel disease, cardiomyopathies and heart failure. The micronutrients at the highest risk are iron, zinc, thiamine, vitamin B12 and vitamin C. Admission to hospital has been linked with an additional risk of malnutrition—feeding below 1500 kcal/day was frequent and has been associated with a structural additional risk of insufficient micronutrient intake to cover basal needs. Although not evidence based, systematic administration of liberal thiamine doses upon admission, and daily complementation of inpatients' food and enteral feeding solutions with multi-micronutrient tablets might be considered.

Keywords: iron; copper; selenium; zinc; thiamine; vitamin B12; obesity; inflammation; enteral nutrition

1. Introduction

Malnutrition includes a wide spectrum of conditions [1] that may affect energy, substrates and micronutrients (i.e., trace elements and vitamins) to variable degrees. Deficiency is defined as a lack, or shortage of a specific micronutrient that is essential for the proper growth and metabolism of a human: 11 trace elements and 13 vitamins qualify as essential in humans [2,3].

Disease related malnutrition has shown to be frequent upon admission [4]. The proportion of patients that have been admitted to hospital in a poor nutritional status varies between nearly zero in trauma and up to 50% in oncologic pathologies [5,6], and has an important impact on costs [6]. Malnutrition affects all ages from pediatric [7] to geriatric admissions [8]. Elderly subjects constituted an important, increasing part of our population with specific physiopathologic characteristics [9]. In developing countries, socio-economic factors will generate specific deficiencies [10], which will also be present in migrant populations [11]. Further, some pathologies threaten more, particularly the micronutrient status. Finally, the geographic place of living in the world, including some western countries and the local soil characteristics, will have their own impact [12,13]. Iodine and iron deficiencies are the most well-known. The below text will review some of these undermining deficiencies.

The definition of deficiency requires knowing the specific needs of diseased patients—this information is generally not available. Micronutrient requirements have been determined for the healthy population with age specificities [3]. They are called dietary reference intakes (DRI), a concept that has replaced the recommended daily allowance (RDA). There is minimal data that exists about the needs during disease. Therefore, the present review, which is based on searches in PubMed and the

Cochrane library, is focused on conditions in adults that have been best documented, such as elderly patients, and some selected conditions. The issue of refeeding syndrome in hospitalized patients is be given particular attention.

2. Undermining Micronutrients Deficiencies

The causes of deficiency can globally be divided into three: Low availability, reduction of intakes, and malabsorption. Some geographic soil and nutrition specificities have threatened the entire populations' micronutrient status. This knowledge is not new [2], and the below text provides a brief summary of their impact on acute diseases.

Micronutrient deficiencies have been called the hidden hunger [14], as they are determining and aggravating factors for one's health status and quality of life. The close relation between fetal malnutrition and the development of chronic non-communicable diseases later in life has been repeatedly confirmed [10,15]. Vitamin A (in developing countries), iodine, and iron deficiencies (worldwide) are the most important in terms of global public health [16]. The below deficiencies have affected patients before their hospital admission and should be integrated in the differential diagnosis of the acute condition.

2.1. Iodine

Deficiencies early in life impairs cognition and growth. Iodine status is also a key determinant of thyroid disorders in adults. Iodine deficiency disorders have affected 740 million people. A severe deficiency causes goiter and hypothyroidism because, despite an increase in thyroid activity to maximize iodine uptake and recycling, iodine concentrations are insufficient to enable synthesis of thyroid hormones [17].

2.2. Iron

Deficiencies are a public health problem worldwide [18]. In the year 2000, it was estimated that iron deficiency anemia affected two billion people, mostly women and children. Anemia concerns roughly a third of the world's population [19], but anemia represents the end stage of an iron deficiency [20] which is largely prevalent in all categories of society [21]. The diagnosis of this deficiency is complex in acute and chronic diseases presenting an inflammatory response that modulates blood iron concentrations [20,22]. Its efficient treatment has often been prevented by beliefs such as the risk of iron administration causing additional oxidative stress or favoring infection. These concerns have not been confirmed [23]. The exploration of the iron status (deficiency < 7.1 µg/L or 12.5 mmol/L) included determining the presence of inflammation reflected by C-reactive protein (CRP) > 10 mg/L [24]. In addition to hemoglobin, and erythrocyte morphology (microcytosis, hypochromia), the following have been required: Serum ferritin (<30 ng/L), transferrin saturation (<15%), total iron-binding capacity (>13.1 µmol/L), soluble transferrin receptor (increased > 28.1 nmol/L) [20], and hepcidin (ranges men 0.6–23.3 nmol/L, women 0.4–19.7 nmol/L) [25].

With the availability of hepcidin as a marker of deficiency, the diagnosis should become easier [20,22,25]. Hepcidin is a hormone synthesized in the liver, secreted into the blood that systemically controls the rate of iron absorption as well as its mobilization from stores [26]. The synthesis of hepcidin is up-regulated by inflammatory cytokines (particularly interleukin-6), irrespective of the total level of iron in the body. This relationship most likely accounts for the development of anemia of chronic disease [27,28] (please see Section 3.7 for specificities in kidney diseases).

2.3. Selenium

Deficiencies have been an issue in Europe and in other parts of the world as the main source of human exposure is diet, which is related to the soil content [29]. Scientists have claimed that changes in climate and the organic carbon content of soil will lead to overall decreased soil Se concentrations, particularly in agricultural areas [30]. Europe and some parts of Australasia are particularly affected, while North America is spared by elevated soil content. Borderline Se status reduced endogenous antioxidant defenses via the reduction of the activity of the glutathione peroxidase (GPX) family of enzymes [31], which contributed to poor outcomes facing critical illness, and particularly sepsis [32]. In major trauma, the intravenous administration of selenium in combination with other micronutrients at 5 times DRI doses (see Table 1) resulted in normalization of plasma GPX3 activity and shortened hospital stays [33]. Nevertheless, the high dose single selenium trials (1000 µg/iv/day) in septic shock have been negative [34]. Therefore this strategy should not be considered, and has been advised against in the Surviving Sepsis Campaign 2017 recommendations [35].

Table 1. Micronutrient strategy in critically ill patients admitted to the Lausanne multidisciplinary ICU, according to disease and nutrition therapy.

Situation	Stress Profile in High Risk Patients in Organ Failure *	Parenteral Nutrition (and Combined Feeding)	Enteral Nutrition
Micro-Nutrients	1 vial multi-trace element (Addaven®, Fresenius Kabi, Oberdorf, Switzerland) + 5 mg Zinc + 1 vial multi-vitamin (Cernevit®, Baxter, Volketswil, Switzerland) + 500 mg vitamin C + 100 mg vitamin B1	Same as stress profile	Multi-micronutrient providing DRI needs (Supradyn®, Roche, Basel, Switzerland)
Duration Route	Diluted in 100 ml de NaCl 0.9% over 6 hours from admission for first 6 days during night shift	Daily with parenteral nutrition	Daily Mixed with enteral feeding

*: High risk conditions include shock (cardiogenic, septic, hypovolemic), pancreatitis, severe hepatopathy, major trauma, organ transplant, and malnutrition.

2.4. Zinc

Deficiencies were first identified in the 1960s [36], and have continued to plague multiple regions of the planet [37]. It has affected all ages, but particularly the elderly in western regions. Zinc deficiency affects cell-mediated immune dysfunction, susceptibility to infections, and increases oxidative stress. A randomized trial including 50 healthy elderly subjects tested the impact of a zinc-supplement (45 mg elemental Zn/day) orally for 12 months versus placebo [38]. First, the authors showed that compared to younger, healthy subjects, the elderly study subjects had lower plasma zinc, higher ex vivo generation of inflammatory cytokines and interleukin 10. The supplement resulted in a significant reduction of the incidence of infections and ex vivo generation of tumor necrosis factor alpha and plasma oxidative stress markers compared to the placebo group [38].

2.5. Copper

Deficiencies have also been shown to affect specific geographic areas—drinking water may or may not be rich in copper depending on the pipe composition. The deficiency is most frequently acquired [39], e.g., due to insufficient intakes in vulnerable populations, increased demands (pregnancy, lactation, wound healing), malabsorption (including high phytic content of vegetarian diets), increased losses (e.g., major burns, continuous renal replacement therapy), and from hereditary diseases [40,41].

2.6. Vitamin A

Deficiency is considered the world's most important cause of preventable blindness [42]. It affected 2.8 million children under five years of age. Tragically, the numbers have only grown over the last decades [20].

2.7. Vitamin D

Long known only for its role in calcium and bone homeostasis, and the development of osteoporosis, its deficiency seems to be a worldwide problem, and to particularly affect inpatients. The multiple effects of vitamin D are mediated by genomic and non-genomic effects, and include muscle function and metabolism, innate and adaptive immune system, lung epithelial function, cardiac function and numerous other functions as the specific nuclear vitamin D receptor are widely expressed throughout the body [43]. As shown in Table 1, low values can be found in nearly any severe condition. Many observational studies have consistently shown an association between low vitamin D levels and poor clinical outcomes. Nevertheless, high-quality evidence showing the benefits of vitamin D supplementation in inpatients is still lacking [44]. One of the largest studies (VITdAL-ICU) was analyzed retrospectively: 475 critically ill patients with 25(OH)D levels $\leq$ 20 ng/mL [45]. The deficiency was not associated with persistent critical illness, nor did supplementation with vitamin D3 mitigate the development of persistent critical illness. The actual evidence does not support general vitamin D screening and supplementation for the medical inpatient population in an acute care setting [44]. By contrast, screening of chronic kidney disease patients is probably rational (see Section 3.7).

3. Disease Specific Deficiency

The below Table 2 summarizes the most frequent deficits encountered in the different pathologies.

Table 2. Disease specific vitamins and in trace elements deficiencies.

Disease	Micronutrients at Risk
Alcoholism	Zn Vitamins A, D, E, K, B12, B9, B6, B1, B2, C
Anemia	Fe, Cu, Co Vitamins B12, B9
Cardiomyopathies/ Heart failure	Se, Fe Vitamin B1, D $^?$
Inflammatory bowel diseases	Se, Zn Vitamins B12, A, D, E, K
Liver diseases	Se, Zn Vitamins B12, A, D, E
Obesity and Bariatric surgery	Cu, Zn, Fe Vitamins A, D, E, K, B1, B9, B12, C
Kidney diseases (chronic & acute)	Chronic: Vitamins K, D Acute: B1, Fe, Se, Zn, Cu

$^?$: means uncertainty as to deficiency.

3.1. Alcoholism

Micronutrient deficiencies are commonly encountered in alcoholic patients, not only explained by a decrease of global dietary intake, but also because of maldigestion, malabsorption, impaired hepatic activation and an increased breakdown and excretion. The risk of developing micro and macronutrient deficiencies has been known to increase significantly when alcohol makes up more than 30 percent of total caloric intake [46].

All fat-soluble vitamins (A, D, E and K) are susceptible to be decreased [47], although vitamins A and K deficiencies are more common in the case of overt hepatic disease or chronic pancreatitis. Among water soluble vitamins, the vitamin B1 (thiamine) deficiency has been the most frequently described and feared [48], potentially leading to Wernicke's encephalopathy and its well-known triad (delirium, oculomotor abnormalities and ataxia). If left untreated, it can progress to the amnestic-confabulatory syndrome called Korsakoff. The therapeutic benefit of thiamin has been demonstrated in alcoholic patients even without severe Wernicke-Korsakoff encephalopathy [49]. In the emergency department, patients with acute alcohol intoxication have not all suffered thiamine deficiency [50,51]. A systematic review showed that thiamine and vitamin C were the most frequently identified deficiencies [51,52].

Nevertheless, considering the elevated prevalence of malnutrition in these patients, it is cautious and cheap, in case of hospital admission to provide 100–300 mg thiamine prior to any glucose IV infusion to prevent precipitating Wernicke's encephalopathy. Excessive alcohol consumption has also been linked to zinc and copper deficiency, which seems to be associated with a decreased quality of physical and mental life [53].

There has been one randomized trial testing the administration of 600 mg of benfotiamine in alcohol dependent patients—this thiamine analog was associated with a reduction of alcohol consumption, but no metabolic variables were tested [54]. In the absence of other randomized trials, most of the experts advocated the empiric administration to alcohol dependent patients of multivitamin cocktails, including in particular, thiamine (200–300 mg), folic acid, vitamin B6, and vitamin C upon admission.

3.2. Anemia

A third of the world's population is affected by anemia, and iron deficiency is involved in 50% of the cases [18]. The most common symptoms are paleness, fatigue, dyspnea and headache. Laboratory tests have shown low blood haemoglobin concentration (Hb < 130 g/L in men, <120 g/L in women and <110g/L in pregnancy) with microcytosis, hypochromia and serum ferritin below 30 µg/L. Iron deficiencies can be physiological (e.g., pregnancy), or pathological in case of blood loss (e.g., surgery, trauma, digestive tract bleeding), malabsorption (e.g., celiac disease, gastrectomy), chronic disease (cancer, chronic heart failure) or in some genetic disorders [19]. In the presence of iron-deficiency anemia, investigations to identify a cause of blood loss or malabsorption are required. Preventive iron supplementation should be prescribed in at-risk patients using the oral route, while treatment of in patients with a positive diagnosis [19], may require the intravenous route due to the frequent gastric intolerance and poor absorption of oral supplements.

Macrocytic anemia can be observed in vitamin B12 or/and vitamin B9 (folate) deficiencies. Vitamin B12 deficiencies occur in cases of severe malabsorption (bariatric surgery, gastrectomy, or autoimmune gastritis), in the abuse of nitrous oxide, and in cases of inherited metabolic disorders. Vitamin B12 supply is recommended after confirmed diagnosis. This treatment will be lifelong when the etiology of the deficiency is irreversible or unknown [55].

Copper deficiencies impair the activity of hephaestin, a copper-dependent ferroxidase responsible for transporting dietary iron from intestinal enterocytes into the circulatory system—its depression leads to iron deficiencies and low hemoglobin. Copper deficiency anemia has been treated with oral or intravenous copper supplementation [56]. Cobalt, a component of hydroxycobalamin, is considered one the most stimulator of erythrocyte production. In clinical practice, Cobalt administration is rare considering the high risk of toxicity of cobalt salts in humans [57].

3.3. Cardiomyopathies and Heart Failure

According to the European Society of Cardiology (ESC), cardiomyopathy (CM) is defined as a myocardial disorder in which the heart muscle is structurally and functionally abnormal, in the absence of coronary artery disease, hypertension, valvular disease and congenital heart disease [58]. CM can lead to heart failure (HF). Deficiencies in thiamine and selenium are nutritional factors that may be involved in the occurrence of such myocardial disorders [58,59] in malnutrition conditions, malabsorption, or exclusive parenteral nutrition (PN) [60–62]. Selenium deficiency cardiomyopathy is known as the Keshan disease in humans. It was initially described in China in 1935 in selenium-poor soils, with multiple case reports. In addition to the low plasma selenium levels, low glutathione peroxidase-1 activity has been reported in animals [63]. Some cases reported have been reversible by short-term oral or IV administration, and others have been fatal [60–63].

Thiamine plays a fundamental role in cellular metabolism, especially in the carbohydrate pathway. Severe and chronic thiamine deficiencies are known as Beriberi disease. The classic presentation includes neurologic features and encephalopathy. HF symptoms have been less frequent and have been associated to metabolic acidosis and hyperlactatemia (due to an inhibition of the pyruvate deshydrogenase) [64,65]. A fulminant form has also been described [64]. It has been shown that about 40% of the patients hospitalized for HF presented thiamine deficiencies [66]. Animal models have demonstrated that this deficiency causes cardiac disorders (cardiac hypertrophy, depressed cardiac contractility, and dysrhythmias) in the absence of beriberi. Finally, in human studies, the benefit of thiamine supplements in cases of chronic HF are unclear [66].

Iron deficiencies in HF are common (about 30–50%) in patients with chronic HF, independent of anemia, and have lead to skeletal muscle dysfunction. Recent ESC guidelines recommended screening for iron deficits in HF patients [28,59].

Recently, an association between vitamin D deficiency and HF has been suggested [67]. Vitamin D promoted cardioprotection in animals (anti-inflammatory, anti-apoptotic and anti-fibrotic mechanisms) [67].

3.4. Inflammatory Bowel Disease

Malnutrition is present in the vast majority of patients with inflammatory bowel disease (IBD), the deficiencies being more prevalent in Crohn's disease compared with ulcerative colitis and more important in active diseases [68]. Micronutrient deficiencies are essentially explained by the reduced dietary intake and the underlying malabsorption. They have been associated with prolonged hospitalization and higher mortality [69].

Fat-soluble vitamins are particularly prone to deficiency. A high prevalence of vitamin A and E deficiencies have been reported [70], but also of vitamin D, which has been suspected to play a role in the pathogenesis of IBD [71]. Vitamin K deficiencies are also frequent and correlated with disease activity [72].

Folate deficiencies are common in IBD and aggravated by treatment, such as sulfasalazine or methotrexate. Vitamin B12 has also been frequently observed, especially in Crohn's disease and after ileal resection of ≥30 cm [73]. Thiamin deficiency has also been reported, especially in IBD patients treated with parenteral nutrition [74].

Among trace elements, selenium deficiencies have been reported and may increase the severity of gut inflammation—the repletion data are conflicting [75]. Zinc deficiencies are also prevalent [76]. Iron deficiencies are very frequent and are the leading cause of anemia in patients with IBD. In the presence of inflammation, this diagnosis can be challenging and relies on the values of serum ferritin values.

3.5. Liver Disease

The liver plays a crucial role in maintaining systemic Zn homeostasis [77]. Chronic liver disease, such as chronic hepatitis, liver cirrhosis, or fatty liver, impairs Zn metabolism, and has resulted in Zn deficiency, which in turn has caused multiple metabolic abnormalities, including insulin resistance, hepatic steatosis and hepatic encephalopathy. Zn deficiency may also favor carcinogenesis of hepatocellular carcinoma (HCC). In chronic liver disease, low levels of selenium [78] have been generally observed. In comparison, copper levels have often been elevated [79]. It is argued that doses required to achieve an effect in chronic hepatitis are far beyond DRI with 150–200 mg/day [80].

In cases of liver disease secondary to alcoholism, please see 3.1 (same picture). Group B vitamin deficiencies, especially thiamine, are common in cirrhosis [81]. Unlike observations for alcoholic patients without liver disease, vitamin B12 levels have been frequently elevated in viral hepatitis, cirrhosis and hepatocellular carcinoma (HCC) [82]. This increase has been explained by the cytolysis of hepatocytes, and vitamin B12 being mainly stored in the liver.

Fat-soluble vitamin deficiencies have been observed in cases of alcoholism, but also in cholestasis with malabsorption and bile salt deficiency [83]. Levels of vitamins A, D and E should therefore be routinely checked as well as prothrombin time. However, prolonged prothrombin time does not purely reflect vitamin K deficiencies, but also reduced levels of coagulation factor V. Importantly, vitamin D has pleiotropic effects for liver disease, including anti-inflammatory, immune-modulatory and anti-fibrotic properties in addition to its classical skeletal effects. This may impact on disease progression [84], especially in HCC and non-alcoholic steatohepatitis, although any benefit from its repletion has not been formally proven by prospective studies [85].

3.6. Obesity & Bariatric Surgery

In patients with grade III obesity (body mass index ≥ 40 kg·m^{-2} or ≥ 35 kg·m^{-2} with comorbid conditions), bariatric surgery has become common. In 2013, over 450,000 bariatric surgeries were performed worldwide. Roux-en-Y gastric bypass, adjustable gastric band, and sleeve gastrectomy were the most frequent procedures [86,87]. Micronutrient deficiencies were observed before (in obese patients, vitamin C deficiency in about 40% and zinc deficiency is up to 50%) and after the surgery. Due to fat malabsorption and maldigestion, all fat-soluble vitamins are at risk. The bypass of the duodenum and proximal jejunum lead to thiamine deficiencies [86], leading to a risk of clinical Wernicke's encephalopathy [88]. Vitamin B9 is approximately 10%. Vitamin B12 deficiencies have been widely described in the literature because of their neurologic complications, especially an acquired myelopathy with paresthesias, ataxia and muscle weakness [89]. It is recalled that the intrinsic factor produced in the stomach is needed for ileal absorption of vitamin B12. The severity of a vitamin B6 deficiencies vary from peripheral neuropathy to seizures [89]. The common trace elements deficiencies after bariatric surgery include copper (absorbed in the stomach and the duodenum), iron (absorbed in the duodenum), and zinc (absorbed in the jejunum). The prevalence of copper deficiency has been reported to be as high as 90% post-surgery (70% for zinc). Further, systematic supplements of micronutrients are recommended after bariatric surgery by the American Society for Parenteral and Enteral Nutrition (ASPEN) [86] and the American Society for Metabolic and Bariatric Surgery clinical practice guidelines (ASMBS) [90].

3.7. Kidney Disease

Kidney disease, whether chronic (CKD) or acute, affects micronutrient homeostasis and might lead to either deficiency or toxic excess. Indeed, a decreased glomerular filtration rate might lead to accumulation of molecules normally excreted by the kidney such as selenium. On the other hand, renal replacement therapy when applied might lead to uncompensated losses of other micronutrients (copper). Finally, the loss of renal activation might lead to decreased biological activity (vitamin D). Unfortunately, the authors knowledge remains limited [91].

Anemia is commonly observed in CKD. Beyond the lack of erythropoietin, which is now clearly established and easily administered, it might also be associated with alterations in iron metabolism and inflammation. Oral corrections of iron deficiencies in pre-dialysis CKD patients have been shown to be an efficient option in a recent randomized trial [92]. The role of hepcidin, a key regulator of circulating iron level in CKD associated anemia is increasingly recognized. Indeed, the condition has been associated with elevated hepcidin serum levels as it is typically excreted by the kidney [93]. This leads to reduced iron availability and anemia. Its measurement and potential anti-hepcidin therapies could help managing anemia in CKD [27,94].

Subclinical vitamin K deficiencies have been shown to be clinically relevant as requirements have increased due to the vitamin K-dependent proteins required to inhibit calcification [95]. This vitamin governs the gamma-carboxylation of matrix Gla protein for inhibiting vascular calcification, and the vitamin D binding protein receptor is related to vitamin K gene expression [96]. Deficiency may favor vascular calcification.

Chronic dialysis is typically associated with elevated oxidative stress leading to low levels of zinc, selenium and GPX. A French team showed three decades ago that weekly administration of selenium with zinc was able to restore GPX activity and reduced thiobarbituric acid reactants (TBARs) plasma concentrations [97]. In a large cohort of 1278 patients on incident hemodialysis, it was observed that lower selenium and zinc concentrations were strongly and independently associated with death and all-cause hospitalization [98]. Trimestrial monitoring of selenium and zinc may thus be justified, with repletion in case of low values.

In acute kidney failure requiring continuous renal replacement therapy, other micronutrients such as thiamine and copper will be lost in the effluent fluid [39,40,99]. Copper losses causing low blood levels can be associated with severe arrhythmias and wound healing complications. Very low plasma levels (<8 mmol/L) might require active intravenous repletion with doses 6–10 mg/day, i.e., 5–10 times the usual DRI [40].

3.8. Migrant Populations

Being a migrant is not a disease, but a difficult social condition frequently associated with malnutrition for multiple reasons ranging from insufficient food intake, to exposure to unusual food or unbalanced diet due to incapacity to find the traditional foods. Migrants represent a growing category of inpatients. Micronutrients of concern have shown to be retinol, vitamin D, magnesium, potassium, copper, and selenium [11], in addition to iron.

3.9. Laboratory Investigations

Laboratory investigations of micronutrient deficiencies have often not been systematic except for 2 conditions: (1) Anemia outwork, which generally included determination of blood Vitamin B6, B12, iron, ferritin and transferrin; (2) screening before and the follow-up after bariatric surgery included thiamine, vitamin B12, folic acid, iron, zinc, copper, calcium and the liposoluble vitamins D, A, E and K were recommended [90]. In other conditions, the diagnosis lacked standardization. A pragmatic approach upon admission or during hospitalization could be to draw an additional blood sample for further diagnostic outwork, and to empirically administer multi-micronutrients without delay.

Inflammation causes a redistribution of micronutrients between the various compartments and generally reduces circulating levels. The intensity of inflammation has been reflected by CRP levels [24]. The example of vitamin D has been emblematic. While a CRP > 80 mg/L has been associated with a reduction of its blood concentration by 40% below reference ranges [24], CRP has never been mentioned in the vitamin D trials. CRP should belong to any micronutrients outwork as low levels do not necessarily indicate a deficiency.

4. Micronutrient Unavailability as Cause of Deficiency

4.1. Nutritional Sources

Hospital related malnutrition is a well know entity that is observed worldwide and is related to being bedridden [100]. A large proportion of patients only consume a third or half of the proposed meals [4]. In our hospital, a standard daily serving provides 1700–1800 kcal. If only half is consumed, the daily micronutrients cannot be covered.

The sickest patients are fed with enteral nutrition. Due to regulatory constraints, the industry must respect micronutrient recommendations intended for the general healthy population, the previously mentioned DRI. The concentrations of the products are calculated for feeding doses varying between 1500 and 2500 kcal/day. However, worldwide it has been shown that many patients receive no more than 1000 kcal/day by this route [101]. In addition, the most recent nutrition guidelines for critical care patients recommended ramping up the feeding over several days [102]. The consequences might be an even further reduction of nutrition delivery. By design, the enteral feeding solutions will not be able to cover needs as long as quantities below 1500 kcal per day are provided. Table 3 shows the detailed micronutrient provision for 1000 kcal/day provided by the 10 most frequently used enteral feeding solutions provided by 4 international companies on the Swiss market. While intakes below DRI of fluor and iodine may be less important during an acute phase, low intakes of iron and of the B vitamin group are a concern considering their essential role in energy (ATP synthesis) and carbohydrate metabolism. Moreover, as absorption is unreliable and as needs might be higher, several micronutrients such as vitamin C are just in the reference range, which may be insufficient.

Table 3. Energy, protein and micronutrient data for 1000 kcal for a selection of frequent products available on the Swiss market compared to the dietary reference intakes (DRI). The values which are below the DRI appear in red and bold characters; in violet-bold, those for which DRI is just covered.

Values for 1000 kcal	Abbott Promote Fibres Plus	Abbott Jevity Plus	Nestlé NovaSource GI Advance	Nestlé Isosource Energy	Nestlé Peptamen Intense	Fresenius K Fresubin 2 kcal HP	Fresenius K Fresubin HP Energy	Fresenius K Fresubin Intensive	Nutricia Nutrison Protein + Mulitf	Nutricia Nutrison	DRI Adults
Energy density kcal/ml	1.3	1.2	1.55	1.57	1.0	2.0	1.5	1.2	1.3	1.0	
Proteins g/1000 kcal	62.5	46.3	61.9	38.9	93.0	50.0	50.0	83.3	49.2	40.0	
Fer (Fe) mg	12.3	15.0	11.0	10.2	16.0	13.5	8.7	16.7	15.6	16.0	18
Zinc (Zn) mg	13.1	11.7	11.6	9.6	13	12	8.0	12.5	11.7	12	8
Cuivre (Cu) mg	1.5	1.7	1.5	1.5	1.8	1.5	0.7	1.7	1.8	1.8	0.9
Manganèse (Mn) mg	3.1	3.5	2.3	2.3	1.4	2.5	2.0	4.2	3.2	3.3	1.8
Fluor	0.0	0.0	1.0	1.3	1.6	1.5	0.7	1.7	1.0	1.0	3
Iode (I) µg	123	125	142	146	120	134	89	183	102	130	150
Molybdène (Mo) µg	92	108	116	115	170	100	67	117	102	100	45
Chrome (Cr) µg	54	67	97	96	60	67	45	92	65	67	20
Selenium (Se) µg	65	63	65	64	80	67	45	88	55	57	55
A (RE) µg	1154	700	1097	1083	650	925	613	1500	797	820	750
D µg	6.9	8.3	14.2	14	14	10	8.7	17	13.3	10	10
E (α-TE) mg	18.2	20	17.4	16.6	14	13.5	8.7	25	12.5	13	15
K µg	54	67	71	76	44	67	45	75	52	53	90
C mg	154	100	123	102	80	67	45	183	102	100	75
B1 mg	1.5	1.6	1.6	1.5	1.0	1.5	0.7	1.7	1.5	1.5	1.1
B2 Riboflavin mg	2.2	1.8	1.7	1.7	1.3	2.0	1.3	1.7	1.6	1.6	1.1
B3 Niacin mg	21.5	18.3	20.0	17.2	30	16	11	20	18	18	14
B5 Pantothenic acid mg	7.7	8.3	5.2	5.5	4.5	4.5	3.3	7.5	5.2	5.3	5
B6 Pyridoxin mg	2.2	2.2	1.8	1.8	1.7	1.5	0.8	2.5	1.6	1.7	1.5
B12 Cyancobalamin µg	4.6	2.9	3.8	3.7	2.9	2.5	2.0	4.2	2.0	2.1	2.4
B9 Folic acid µg	231	250	290	287	300	267	180	263	258	270	400
B8 Biotin µg	46	43	45	45	30	50	33	57	39	40	30
Choline mg	462	500	368	382	670	0	178	0	359	370	425

Regarding these low micronutrient doses, it might be justified to deliver standard multivitamin and trace element products daily providing DRI doses to the majority of inpatients. This strategy has been applied for many years in the Lausanne university hospital's ICU, as critically ill patients do have higher needs. In the sickest patients, multi-micronutrients cocktails have been delivered IV for the first 5 days [33], resulting in a shortening of the hospital stay, particularly in major trauma patients.

4.2. Geriatric Population

The qualification, elderly, encompasses patients aged 60 to over 100 years. While the younger seniors often are fit until the seventies, some physiological changes already occur that become exacerbated with growing age. The elderly often present with anorexia which is considered a complex geriatric syndrome and a risk factor for frailty [9]. These changes are associated with lower weight, and lower energy expenditure. The body undergoes specific changes—the gastric mucosa tends to atrophy, reducing vitamin B12 absorption. Indeed, the decline in vitamin B12 is independent of nutrition but caused by a decline of both the intestinal uptake and the renal reabsorption system for vitamin B12 [103]. The elderly also require higher doses of vitamin B6 and D to maintain health, which has been integrated into DRI recommendations for older subjects. Deficiencies can be overcome by supplementation, as shown by a large randomized controlled trial including 652 geriatric patients—daily oral nutrition supplements enriched with proteins, hydroxy-methyl-butyrate, vitamin D and other micronutrients reduced mortality [104].

4.3. Partial or Complete Starving upon Hospital Admission and Refeeding

The incidence and importance of the refeeding has often been underestimated [105]. The absence of a uniform definition participates in its underestimation [105]. Refeeding syndrome consists of metabolic changes that occur on the reintroduction of food or simply a glucose infusion. A few days of feeding grossly below needs will be sufficient to create the metabolic crisis which is characterized by sudden shifts in the electrolytes that are needed for energy and substrate (mainly glucose) metabolism. The NutritionDay survey, an initiative that analysed the relation between nutritional intakes and outcomes of a wide range of institutionalized and hospitalized patients worldwide, has shown that more than half of the patients admitted to hospital were eating less than half of their normal food intake before admission [106]. This places the majority of hospitalized patients at risk of a refeeding syndrome.

Some categories of patients, such as chronic, alcohol consumers, which are largely prevalent in western countries, being present in nearly 30% of hospital admissions, are at higher risk of thiamine deficiencies—these patients are at particularly high risk of refeeding syndrome and its worst neurologic complication, the Wernicke encephalopathy. A recent review of the literature confirmed the importance of administering intravenous thiamine to these patients in order to prevent severe sequelae [107]. The recommended doses ranged from 50–100 mg/day to 250–500 mg 3 times a day. The IV route was recommended due to the frequent presence of gastritis in these patients, which reduced absorption.

4.4. Economic Considerations

A Canadian prospective cohort study showed that approximately 40% of the 956 patients admitted to hospital were moderately to severely malnourished. These patients had longer hospital stays, and as a result, cost more than the well-nourished patients [108]. A European narrative review showed that malnutrition increased the length of hospital stays by 2.4 to 7.2 days [5]. Malnutrition led to an additional individual cost ranging between 1640 € and 5829 €.

Clinical evidences are lacking for empirical multi-micronutrient supplements. The cost of malnutrition attributable to micronutrient deficiencies have not been assessed in adult inpatients and several studies have failed to demonstrate significant beneficial effects of various micronutrient supplements in the general population [109]. Nevertheless, there are data suggesting a benefit, at least in the sickest patients [33,110].

However, data exists for children. A study focusing on estimates of disability-adjusted life years and their monetization showed that short-term economic costs of micronutrient malnutrition in India amounted to 0.8% to 2.5% of the gross domestic product [14]. The health and cost consequences of iodine, iron, vitamin A, and zinc deficiencies were assessed in Pakistani children: Societal costs amounted to 1.44% of gross domestic product and 4.45% of disability-adjusted life-years in Pakistan in 2013, which hindered the country's development [111].

When deciding about an empirical administration of micronutrients, the analytical costs of deficiency diagnosis must be considered. The European Society for Clinical Nutrition and Metabolism (ESPEN) monitoring recommendations indicate that some vitamin and trace element analysis (inductively coupled plasma mass spectrometry: ICP-MS) are expensive [112]. They are actually more expensive than the empirical administration. A semi-automatic weekly determination of blood selenium levels in our ICU resulted in major costs that could be contained by the decision to let blood sampling be prescribed only by the ICU nutritionists and dieticians in patients at risk [113].

A multi-micronutrient tablet costs 0.80 € (the IV dose in Table 1 costs 25 €), which is negligible compared to the cost of one day in hospital, or worse, in the ICU. This prescription is likely to be beneficial if the administration is standardized, and limited to the first week of hospitalization, and to patients on enteral feeding.

5. Conclusions

Micronutrient deficiencies and borderline status are more frequent than generally acknowledged. The most important potential acute deficiency that may compromise outcome is thiamine deficiency. Other deficiencies will impact on immune defenses and anabolic capacity. Therefore, an empirical and cheap complementation strategy, based on daily oral multi-micronutrient products providing DRI, may be justified for hospital inpatients for one week. It is important to state that the evidence from trials is still missing.

Author Contributions: Conceptualization M.M.B.; Search methodology M.M.B., N.B.-H., O.P.; validation, M.M.B., O.P., A.S. and N.B.-H.; writing—original draft preparation, M.M.B., O.P., N.B.-H.; writing—review and editing, N.B.-H., O.P., A.S., and M.M.B.

Conflicts of Interest: None of the authors have any conflicts of interest to declare.

Abbreviations

DRI	Dietary Reference Intakes
CKD	Chronic kidney disease
CM	cardiomyopathy
CRP	C-reactive protein
ESC	European Society of Cardiology
ESPEN	European Society for Clinical Nutrition and Metabolism
GPX	Glutathione peroxidase
HF	Heat failure
IBD	inflammatory bowel disease
IV	Intravenous
RDA	recommended daily allowance

References

1. Cederholm, T.; Jensen, G.L.; Correia, M.I.T.D.; Gonzalez, M.C.; Fukushima, R.; Higashiguchi, T.; Baptista, G.; Barazzoni, R.; Blaauw, R.; Coats, A.; et al. GLIM criteria for the diagnosis of malnutrition—A consensus report from the global clinical nutrition community. *Clin. Nutr.* **2019**, *38*, 1–9. [CrossRef] [PubMed]

2. Allen, L.; de Benoist, B.; Dary, O.; Hurrel, R. Guidelines on food fortification with micronutrients. In *World Health Organization (WHO) Food and Agricultural Organization (FAO) of the United Nations*; WHO: Geneva, Switzerland, 2006; pp. 1–376. Available online: http://www.who.int/nutrition/publications/guide_food_fortification_micronutrients.pdf (accessed on 25 June 2019).
3. Trumbo, P.; Yates, A.; Schlicker, S.; Poos, M. Dietary reference intakes: Vitamin A, vitamin K, arsenic, boron, chromium, copper, iodine, iron, manganese, molybdenum, nickel, silicon, vanadium, and zinc. *J. Am. Diet. Assoc.* **2001**, *101*, 294–301. [CrossRef]
4. Schuetz, P.; Fehr, R.; Baechli, V.; Geiser, M.; Deiss, M.; Gomes, F.; Kutz, A.; Tribolet, P.; Bregenzer, T.; Braun, N.; et al. Individualised nutritional support in medical inpatients at nutritional risk: A randomised clinical trial. *Lancet* **2019**, *393*, 2312–2321. [CrossRef]
5. Khalatbari-Soltani, S.; Marques-Vidal, P. The economic cost of hospital malnutrition in Europe; a narrative review. *Clin. Nutr. ESPEN* **2015**, *10*, e89–e94. [CrossRef] [PubMed]
6. Norman, K.; Pichard, C.; Lochs, H.; Pirlich, M. Prognostic impact of disease-related malnutrition. *Clin. Nutr.* **2008**, *27*, 5–15. [CrossRef] [PubMed]
7. Pawellek, I.; Dokoupil, K.; Koletzko, B. Prevalence of malnutrition in paediatric hospital patients. *Clin. Nutr.* **2008**, *27*, 72–76. [CrossRef] [PubMed]
8. Orlandoni, P.; Venturini, C.; Jukic Peladic, N.; Costantini, A.; Di Rosa, M.; Cola, C.; Giorgini, N.; Basile, R.; Fagnani, D.; Sparvoli, D.; et al. Malnutrition upon Hospital Admission in Geriatric Patients: Why Assess It? *Front. Nutr.* **2017**, *4*, 50. [CrossRef]
9. Sanford, A.M. Anorexia of aging and its role for frailty. *Curr. Opin. Clin. Nutr. Metab. Care* **2017**, *20*, 54–60. [CrossRef]
10. World Health Organisation. In *Nutrition for Health and Development: A Global Agenda for Combating Malnutrition*; Docemunt WHO/NHD/00.6; WHO: Geneva, Switzerland, 2000.
11. Castaneda-Gameros, D.; Redwood, S.; Thompson, J. Nutrient Intake and Factors Influencing Eating Behaviors in Older Migrant Women Living in the United Kingdom. *Ecol. Food Nutr.* **2018**, *57*, 50–68. [CrossRef]
12. Black, R. Global distribution and disease burden related to micronutrient deficiencies. *Nestle Nutr. Inst. Workshop Ser.* **2014**, *78*, 21–28. [CrossRef]
13. White, J.; Zasoski, R. Mapping soil micronutrients. *Field Crop. Res.* **1999**, *60*, 11–26. [CrossRef]
14. Stein, A.; Qaim, M. The human and economic cost of hidden hunger. *Food Nutr. Bull.* **2007**, *28*, 125–134. [CrossRef] [PubMed]
15. Diaz, J.; de las Cagigas, A.; Rodriguez, R. Micronutrient deficiencies in developing and affluent countries. *Eur. J. Clin. Nutr.* **2003**, *57* (Suppl. 1), S70–S72. [CrossRef]
16. World Health Orgniasation. Micronutrients. Available online: https://www.who.int/nutrition/topics/micronutrients/en/ (accessed on 25 April 2019).
17. Zimmermann, M.B.; Boelaert, K. Iodine deficiency and thyroid disorders. *Lancet Diabetes Endocrinol.* **2015**, *3*, 286–295. [CrossRef]
18. Stoltzfus, R. Defining iron-deficiency anemia in public health terms: A time for reflection. *J. Nutr.* **2001**, *131*, 565S–567S. [CrossRef] [PubMed]
19. Lopez, A.; Cacoub, P.; Macdougall, I.; Peyrin-Biroulet, L. Iron deficiency anaemia. *Lancet* **2016**, *367*, 907–917. [CrossRef]
20. Camaschella, C. Iron deficiency. *Blood* **2019**, *133*, 30–39. [CrossRef] [PubMed]
21. Schuepbach, R.; Bestmann, L.; Bechir, M.; Fehr, J.; Bachli, E. High prevalence of Iron deficiency among educated hospital employees in Switzerland. *Int. J. Biomed. Sci. IJBS* **2011**, *7*, 150–157.
22. Heming, N.; Montravers, P.; Lasocki, S. Iron deficiency in critically ill patients: Highlighting the role of hepcidin. *Crit. Care* **2011**, *15*, 210. [CrossRef]
23. Lasocki, S.; Piednoir, P.; Couffignal, C.; Rineau, E.; Dufour, G.; Lefebvre, T.; Puy, H.; Duval, X.; Driss, F.; Schilte, C. Does IV Iron Induce Plasma Oxidative Stress in Critically Ill Patients? A comparison with healthy volunteers. *Crit. Care Med.* **2016**, *44*, 521–530. [CrossRef]
24. Duncan, A.; Talwar, D.; McMillan, D.; Stefanowicz, F.; O'Reilly, D. Quantitative data on the magnitude of the systemic inflammatory response and its effect on micronutrient status based on plasma measurements. *Am. J. Clin. Nutr.* **2012**, *95*, 64–71. [CrossRef] [PubMed]

25. Galesloot, T.E.; Vermeulen, S.H.; Geurts-Moespot, A.J.; Klaver, S.M.; Kroot, J.; van Tienoven, D.; Wetzels, J.F.; Kiemeney, L.; Sweep, F.C.; den Heijer, M.; et al. Serum hepcidin: Reference ranges and biochemical correlates in the general population. *Blood* **2011**, *117*, e218–e225. [CrossRef] [PubMed]
26. Johnson-Wimbley, T.D.; Graham, D.Y. Diagnosis and management of iron deficiency anemia in the 21st century. *Ther. Adv. Gastroenterol.* **2011**, *4*, 177–184. [CrossRef] [PubMed]
27. Ueda, N.; Takasawa, K. Impact of Inflammation on Ferritin, Hepcidin and the Management of Iron Deficiency Anemia in Chronic Kidney Disease. *Nutrients* **2018**, *10*, 1173. [CrossRef] [PubMed]
28. Cohen-Solal, A.; Leclercq, C.; Deray, G.; Lasocki, S.; Zambrowski, J.; Mebazaa, A.; de Groote, P.; Damy, T.; Galinier, M. Iron deficiency: An emerging therapeutic target in heart failure. *Heart* **2014**, *100*, 1414–1420. [CrossRef]
29. Vinceti, M.; Filippini, T.; Wise, L.A. Environmental Selenium and human health: An update. *Curr. Environ. Health Rep.* **2018**, *5*, 464–485. [CrossRef] [PubMed]
30. Jones, G.D.; Droz, B.; Greve, P.; Gottschalk, P.; Poffet, D.; McGrath, S.P.; Seneviratne, S.I.; Smith, P.; Winkel, L.H. Selenium deficiency risk predicted to increase under future climate change. *Proc. Natl. Acad. Sci. USA* **2017**, *114*, 2848–2853. [CrossRef]
31. Rayman, M.P. Selenium and human health. *Lancet* **2012**, *379*, 1256–1268. [CrossRef]
32. Alhazzani, W.; Jacobi, J.; Sindi, A.; Hartog, C.; Reinhart, K.; Kokkoris, S.; Gerlach, H.; Andrews, P.; Drabek, T.; Manzanares, W.; et al. The effect of selenium therapy on mortality in patients with sepsis syndrome: A systematic review and meta-analysis of randomized controlled trials. *Crit. Care Med.* **2013**, *41*, 1555–1564. [CrossRef]
33. Berger, M.M.; Soguel, L.; Shenkin, A.; Revelly, J.P.; Pinget, C.; Baines, M.; Chiolero, R.L. Influence of early antioxidant supplements on clinical evolution and organ function in critically ill cardiac surgery, major trauma and subarachnoid hemorrhage patients. *Crit. Care* **2008**, *12*, R101. [CrossRef]
34. Bloos, F.; Trips, E.; Nierhaus, A.; Briegel, J.; Heyland, D.K.; Jaschinski, U.; Moerer, O.; Weyland, A.; Marx, G.; Grundling, M.; et al. Effect of sodium selenite administration and procalcitonin-guided therapy on mortality in patients with severe sepsis or septic shock: A randomized clinical trial. *JAMA Intern. Med.* **2016**, *176*, 1266–1276. [CrossRef] [PubMed]
35. Rhodes, A.; Evans, L.E.; Alhazzani, W.; Levy, M.M.; Antonelli, M.; Ferrer, R.; Kumar, A.; Sevransky, J.E.; Sprung, C.L.; Nunnally, M.E.; et al. Surviving Sepsis Campaign: International Guidelines for Management of Sepsis and Septic Shock: 2016. *Intensive Care Med.* **2017**, *43*, 304–377. [CrossRef] [PubMed]
36. Prasad, A.S. Zinc deficiency. *BMJ* **2003**, *326*, 409–410. [CrossRef] [PubMed]
37. Prasad, A.S. Impact of the discovery of human zinc deficiency on health. *J. Trace Elem. Med. Biol.* **2014**, *28*, 357–363. [CrossRef] [PubMed]
38. Prasad, A.S.; Beck, F.W.; Bao, B.; Fitzgerald, J.T.; Snell, D.C.; Steinberg, J.D.; Cardozo, L.I. Zinc supplementation decreases incidence of infections in the elderly: Effect of zinc on generation of cytokines and oxidative stress. *Am. J. Clin. Nutr.* **2007**, *85*, 837–844. [CrossRef] [PubMed]
39. Altarelli, M.; Ben-Hamouda, N.; Schneider, A.; Berger, M.M. Copper Deficiency—Causes, Manifestations, and Treatment. *Nutr. Clin. Prac.* **2019**. [CrossRef] [PubMed]
40. Ben-Hamouda, N.; Charrière, M.; Voirol, P.; Berger, M.M. Massive copper and selenium losses cause life-threatening deficiencies during prolonged continuous renal replacement. *Nutrition* **2017**, *34*, 71–75. [CrossRef] [PubMed]
41. Wapnir, R.A. Copper absorption and bioavailability. *Am. J. Clin. Nutr.* **1998**, *67*, 1054S–1060S. [CrossRef] [PubMed]
42. World Health Organization. The Global Burden of Disease: 2004 Update. 1. Cost of Illness. 2. World Health—Statistics. 3. Mortality—Trends. Available online: http://www.who.int/healthinfo/global_burden_disease/GBD_report_2004update_full.pdf (accessed on 30 August 2012).
43. Amrein, K.; Papinutti, A.; Mathew, E.; Vila, G.; Parekh, D. Vitamin D and critical illness: What endocrinology can learn from intensive care and vice versa. *Endocr. Connect.* **2018**, *7*, R304–R315. [CrossRef] [PubMed]
44. Gradel, L.; Merker, M.; Mueller, B.; Schuetz, P. Screening and Treatment of Vitamin D Deficiency on Hospital Admission: Is There a Benefit for Medical Inpatients? *Am. J. Med.* **2016**, *129*, 116.e111–116.e134. [CrossRef] [PubMed]

45. Viglianti, E.M.; Zajic, P.; Iwashyna, T.J.; Amrein, K. Neither vitamin D levels nor supplementation are associated with the development of persistent critical illness: A retrospective cohort analysis. *Crit. Care Resusc.* **2019**, *21*, 39–44. [PubMed]
46. Lieber, C.S. Alcohol: Its metabolism and interaction with nutrients. *Annu. Rev. Nutr.* **2000**, *20*, 395–430. [CrossRef] [PubMed]
47. Leo, M.A.; Lieber, C.S. Alcohol, vitamin A, and beta-carotene: Adverse interactions, including hepatotoxicity and carcinogenicity. *Am. J. Clin. Nutr.* **1999**, *69*, 1071–1085. [CrossRef] [PubMed]
48. Leevy, C.M. Thiamin deficiency and alcoholism. *Ann. N. Y. Acad. Sci.* **1982**, *378*, 316–326. [CrossRef] [PubMed]
49. Ambrose, M.L.; Bowden, S.C.; Whelan, G. Thiamin treatment and working memory function of alcohol-dependent people: Preliminary findings. *Alcohol. Clin. Exp. Res.* **2001**, *25*, 112–116. [CrossRef] [PubMed]
50. Li, S.F.; Jacob, J.; Feng, J.; Kulkarni, M. Vitamin deficiencies in acutely intoxicated patients in the ED. *Am. J. Emerg. Med.* **2008**, *26*, 792–795. [CrossRef]
51. Lee, H.J.; Shin, J.; Hong, K.; Jung, J.H. Vitamin C deficiency of Korean homeless vatients visiting to Emergency Department with acute alcohol intoxication. *J. Korean Med Sci.* **2015**, *30*, 1874–1880. [CrossRef]
52. Ijaz, S.; Jackson, J.; Thorley, H.; Porter, K.; Fleming, C.; Richards, A.; Bonner, A.; Savovic, J. Nutritional deficiencies in homeless persons with problematic drinking: A systematic review. *Int. J. Equity Health* **2017**, *16*, 71. [CrossRef]
53. Ordak, M.; Bulska, E.; Jablonka-Salach, K.; Luciuk, A.; Maj-Zurawska, M.; Matsumoto, H.; Nasierowski, T.; Wojnar, M.; Matras, J.; Muszynska, E.; et al. Effect of Disturbances of Zinc and Copper on the Physical and Mental Health Status of Patients with Alcohol Dependence. *Biol. Trace Elem. Res.* **2018**, *183*, 9–15. [CrossRef]
54. Manzardo, A.M.; He, J.; Poje, A.; Penick, E.C.; Campbell, J.; Butler, M.G. Double-blind, randomized placebo-controlled clinical trial of benfotiamine for severe alcohol dependence. *Drug Alcohol. Depend.* **2013**, *133*, 562–570. [CrossRef]
55. Green, R. Vitamin B12 deficiency from the perspective of a practicing hematologist. *Blood* **2017**, *129*, 2603–2611. [CrossRef] [PubMed]
56. Myint, Z.W.; Oo, T.H.; Thein, K.Z.; Tun, A.M.; Saeed, H. Copper deficiency anemia: Review article. *Ann. Hematol.* **2018**, *97*, 1527–1534. [CrossRef] [PubMed]
57. Oliveira, D.C.; Nogueira-Pedro, A.; Santos, E.W.; Hastreiter, A.; Silva, G.B.; Borelli, P.; Fock, R.A. A review of select minerals influencing the haematopoietic process. *Nutr. Res. Rev.* **2018**, *31*, 267–280. [CrossRef] [PubMed]
58. Elliott, P.; Andersson, B.; Arbustini, E.; Bilinska, Z.; Cecchi, F.; Charron, P.; Dubourg, O.; Kuhl, U.; Maisch, B.; McKenna, W.J.; et al. Classification of the cardiomyopathies: A position statement from the European Society Of Cardiology Working Group on Myocardial and Pericardial Diseases. *Eur. Heart J.* **2008**, *29*, 270–276. [CrossRef] [PubMed]
59. Ponikowski, P.; Voors, A.A.; Anker, S.D.; Bueno, H.; Cleland, J.G.F.; Coats, A.J.S.; Falk, V.; Gonzalez-Juanatey, J.R.; Harjola, V.P.; Jankowska, E.A.; et al. 2016 ESC Guidelines for the diagnosis and treatment of acute and chronic heart failure: The Task Force for the diagnosis and treatment of acute and chronic heart failure of the European Society of Cardiology (ESC)Developed with the special contribution of the Heart Failure Association (HFA) of the ESC. *Eur. Heart J.* **2016**, *37*, 2129–2200. [CrossRef] [PubMed]
60. Levy, J.B.; Jones, H.W.; Gordon, A.C. Selenium deficiency, reversible cardiomyopathy and short-term intravenous feeding. *Postgrad. Med. J.* **1994**, *70*, 235–236. [CrossRef] [PubMed]
61. Fleming, C.R.; Lie, J.T.; McCall, J.T.; O'Brien, J.F.; Baillie, E.E.; Thistle, J.L. Selenium deficiency and fatal cardiomyopathy in a patient on home parenteral nutrition. *Gastroenterology* **1982**, *83*, 689–693.
62. Burke, M.P.; Opeskin, K. Fulminant heart failure due to selenium deficiency cardiomyopathy (Keshan disease). *Med. Sci. Law* **2002**, *42*, 10–13. [CrossRef]
63. Oropeza-Moe, M.; Wisloff, H.; Bernhoft, A. Selenium deficiency associated porcine and human cardiomyopathies. *J. Trace Elem. Med. Biol.* **2015**, *31*, 148–156. [CrossRef]
64. Dabar, G.; Harmouche, C.; Habr, B.; Riachi, M.; Jaber, B. Shoshin Beriberi in Critically-Ill patients: Case series. *Nutr. J.* **2015**, *14*, 51. [CrossRef]
65. Ben-Hamouda, N.; Haesler, L.; Liaudet, L. Hyperlactatemia and lactic acidosis in the critically ill patient. *Rev. Med. Suisse* **2013**, *9*, 2335–2340. [PubMed]

66. Smithline, H.A. Thiamine for the treatment of acute decompensated heart failure. *Am. J. Emerg. Med.* **2007**, *25*, 124–126. [CrossRef] [PubMed]
67. Rai, V.; Agrawal, D.K. Role of Vitamin D in Cardiovascular Diseases. *Endocrinol. Metab. Clin. N. Am.* **2017**, *46*, 1039–1059. [CrossRef] [PubMed]
68. Kalantari, H.; Barekat, S.M.; Maracy, M.R.; Azadbakht, L.; Shahshahan, Z. Nutritional status in patients with ulcerative colitis in Isfahan, Iran. *Adv. Biomed. Res.* **2014**, *3*, 58. [CrossRef] [PubMed]
69. O'Sullivan, M. Symposium on The challenge of translating nutrition research into public health nutrition. Session 3: Joint Nutrition Society and Irish Nutrition and Dietetic Institute Symposium on 'Nutrition and autoimmune disease'. Nutrition in Crohn's disease. *Proc. Nutr. Soc.* **2009**, *68*, 127–134. [CrossRef] [PubMed]
70. Hashemi, J.; Asadi, J.; Amiriani, T.; Besharat, S.; Roshandel, G.R.; Joshaghani, H.R. Serum vitamins A and E deficiencies in patients with inflammatory bowel disease. *Saudi Med. J.* **2013**, *34*, 432–434. [PubMed]
71. Torki, M.; Gholamrezaei, A.; Mirbagher, L.; Danesh, M.; Kheiri, S.; Emami, M.H. Vitamin D Deficiency Associated with Disease Activity in Patients with Inflammatory Bowel Diseases. *Dig. Dis. Sci.* **2015**, *60*, 3085–3091. [CrossRef] [PubMed]
72. Nowak, J.K.; Grzybowska-Chlebowczyk, U.; Landowski, P.; Szaflarska-Poplawska, A.; Klincewicz, B.; Adamczak, D.; Banasiewicz, T.; Plawski, A.; Walkowiak, J. Prevalence and correlates of vitamin K deficiency in children with inflammatory bowel disease. *Sci. Rep.* **2014**, *4*, 4768. [CrossRef]
73. Bermejo, F.; Algaba, A.; Guerra, I.; Chaparro, M.; De-La-Poza, G.; Valer, P.; Piqueras, B.; Bermejo, A.; Garcia-Alonso, J.; Perez, M.J.; et al. Should we monitor vitamin B12 and folate levels in Crohn's disease patients? *Scand. J. Gastroenterol.* **2013**, *48*, 1272–1277. [CrossRef]
74. Larnaout, A.; El-Euch, G.; Kchir, N.; Filali, A.; Hamida, M.B.; Hentati, F. Wernicke's encephalopathy in a patient with Crohn's disease: A pathological study. *J. Neurol.* **2001**, *248*, 57–60. [CrossRef]
75. Hiller, F.; Oldorff, L.; Besselt, K.; Kipp, A.P. Differential acute effects of selenomethionine and sodium selenite on the severity of colitis. *Nutrients* **2015**, *7*, 2687–2706. [CrossRef] [PubMed]
76. Saod, W.M.; Darwish, N.T.; Zaidan, T.A.; Alfalujie, A.W.A. Trace Elements in Sera of Patients with Hepatitis B: Determination and Analysis. In Proceedings of the Advanced nanotechnology in engineering and medical sciences (ANEMS) – International conference 2017, Langkawi, Malaysia, 20–21 November 2017.
77. Vagianos, K.; Bector, S.; McConnell, J.; Bernstein, C.N. Nutrition assessment of patients with inflammatory bowel disease. *JPEN J. Parenter. Enter. Nutr.* **2007**, *31*, 311–319. [CrossRef] [PubMed]
78. Himoto, T.; Masaki, T. Associations between Zinc Deficiency and Metabolic Abnormalities in Patients with Chronic Liver Disease. *Nutrients* **2018**, *10*, 88. [CrossRef] [PubMed]
79. Agarwal, A.; Avarebeel, S.; Choudhary, N.S.; Goudar, M.; Tejaswini, C.J. Correlation of Trace Elements in Patients of Chronic Liver Disease with Respect to Child- Turcotte- Pugh Scoring System. *J. Clin. Diagn. Res.* **2017**, *11*, OC25–OC28. [CrossRef] [PubMed]
80. Murakami, Y.; Koyabu, T.; Kawashima, A.; Kakibuchi, N.; Kawakami, T.; Takaguchi, K.; Kita, K.; Okita, M. Zinc supplementation prevents the increase of transaminase in chronic hepatitis C patients during combination therapy with pegylated interferon alpha-2b and ribavirin. *J. Nutr. Sci. Vitaminol. (Tokyo)* **2007**, *53*, 213–218. [CrossRef] [PubMed]
81. Schenker, S.; Halff, G.A. Nutritional therapy in alcoholic liver disease. *Semin. Liver Dis.* **1993**, *13*, 196–209. [CrossRef] [PubMed]
82. Ermens, A.A.; Vlasveld, L.T.; Lindemans, J. Significance of elevated cobalamin (vitamin B12) levels in blood. *Clin. Biochem.* **2003**, *36*, 585–590. [CrossRef] [PubMed]
83. Lindor, K.D. Management of osteopenia of liver disease with special emphasis on primary biliary cirrhosis. *Semin. Liver Dis.* **1993**, *13*, 367–373. [CrossRef]
84. Konstantakis, C.; Tselekouni, P.; Kalafateli, M.; Triantos, C. Vitamin D deficiency in patients with liver cirrhosis. *Ann. Gastroenterol.* **2016**, *29*, 297–306. [CrossRef]
85. Kitson, M.T.; Roberts, S.K. D-livering the message: The importance of vitamin D status in chronic liver disease. *J. Hepatol.* **2012**, *57*, 897–909. [CrossRef]
86. Patel, J.J.; Mundi, M.S.; Hurt, R.T.; Wolfe, B.; Martindale, R.G. Micronutrient Deficiencies After Bariatric Surgery: An Emphasis on Vitamins and Trace Minerals [Formula: See text]. *Nutr. Clin. Pract.* **2017**, *32*, 471–480. [CrossRef] [PubMed]
87. Roust, L.R.; DiBaise, J.K. Nutrient deficiencies prior to bariatric surgery. *Curr. Opin. Clin. Nutr. Metab. Care* **2017**, *20*, 138–144. [CrossRef] [PubMed]

88. Singh, S.; Kumar, A. Wernicke encephalopathy after obesity surgery: A systematic review. *Neurology* **2007**, *68*, 807–811. [CrossRef] [PubMed]
89. Koffman, B.M.; Greenfield, L.J.; Ali, I.I.; Pirzada, N.A. Neurologic complications after surgery for obesity. *Muscle Nerve* **2006**, *33*, 166–176. [CrossRef] [PubMed]
90. Parrott, J.; Frank, L.; Rabena, R.; Craggs-Dino, L.; Isom, K.; Greiman, L. American Society for Metabolic and Bariatric Surgery Integrated Health Nutritional Guidelines for the Surgical Weight Loss Patient 2016 Update: Micronutrient. *Surg. Obes. Relat. Dis.* **2017**, *13*, 727–741. [CrossRef] [PubMed]
91. Jankowska, M.; Rutkowski, B.; Debska-Slizien, A. Vitamins and Microelement Bioavailability in Different Stages of Chronic Kidney Disease. *Nutrients* **2017**, *9*, 282. [CrossRef] [PubMed]
92. Jensen, G.; Goransson, L.; Fernstrom, A.; Furuland, H.; Christensen, J. Treatment of iron deficiency in patients with chronic kidney disease: A prospective observational study of iron isomaltoside (NIMO Scandinavia). *Clin. Nephrol.* **2019**, *91*, 246–253. [CrossRef]
93. Valenti, L.; Messa, P.; Pelusi, S.; Campostrini, N.; Girelli, D. Hepcidin levels in chronic hemodialysis patients: A critical evaluation. *Clin. Chem. Lab. Med.* **2014**, *52*, 613–619. [CrossRef]
94. Santos-Silva, A.; Ribeiro, S.; Reis, F.; Belo, L. Hepcidin in chronic kidney disease anemia. *Vitam. Horm.* **2019**, *110*, 243–264. [CrossRef]
95. Cozzolino, M.; Mangano, M.; Galassi, A.; Ciceri, P.; Messa, P.; Nigwekar, S. Vitamin K in Chronic Kidney Disease. *Nutrients* **2019**, *11*, 168. [CrossRef]
96. Hou, Y.C.; Lu, C.L.; Zheng, C.M.; Chen, R.M.; Lin, Y.F.; Liu, W.C.; Yen, T.H.; Chen, R.; Lu, K.C. Emerging Role of Vitamins D and K in Modulating Uremic Vascular Calcification: The aspect of passive calcification. *Nutrients* **2019**, *11*, 152. [CrossRef] [PubMed]
97. Richard, M.; Ducros, V.; Foret, M.; Arnaud, J.; Coudray, C.; Fusselier, M.; Favier, A. Reversal of selenium and zinc deficiencies in chronic hemodialysis patients by intravenous sodium selenite and zinc gluconate supplementation—Time-course of glutathione peroxidase repletion and lipid peroxidation decrease. *Biol. Trace Elem. Res.* **1993**, *39*, 149–159. [CrossRef] [PubMed]
98. Tonelli, M.; Wiebe, N.; Bello, A.; Field, C.J.; Gill, J.S.; Hemmelgarn, B.R.; Holmes, D.T.; Jindal, K.; Klarenbach, S.W.; Manns, B.J.; et al. Concentrations of Trace Elements and Clinical Outcomes in Hemodialysis Patients: A prospective cohort study. *Clin. J. Am. Soc. Nephrol.* **2018**, *13*, 907–915. [CrossRef] [PubMed]
99. Berger, M.M.; Shenkin, A.; Bollmann, M.D.; Revelly, J.P.; Cayeux, M.C.; Schaller, M.D.; Tappy, L.; Chioléro, R. Trace element balances during continuous venovenous hemodiafiltration (CVVHD). *Kardiovasc. Med.* **2003**, *6* (Suppl. 5), 81S.
100. Schindler, K.; Themessl-Huber, M.; Hiesmayr, M.J.; Kosak, S.; Lainscak, M.; Laviano, A.; Ljungqvist, O.; Mouhieddine, M.; Schneider, S.; de van der Schueren, M.; et al. To eat or not to eat? Indicators for reduced food intake in 91,245 patients hospitalized on nutritionDays 2006–2014 in 56 countries worldwide: A descriptive analysis. *Am. J. Clin. Nutr.* **2016**, *104*, 1393–1402. [CrossRef] [PubMed]
101. Alberda, C.; Gramlich, L.; Jones, N.; Jeejeebhoy, K.; Day, A.G.; Dhaliwal, R.; Heyland, D.K. The relationship between nutritional intake and clinical outcomes in critically ill patients: Results of an international multicenter observational study. *Intensive Care Med.* **2009**, *35*, 1728–1737. [CrossRef] [PubMed]
102. Singer, P.; Reintam-Blaser, A.; Berger, M.M.; Alhazzani, W.; Calder, P.C.; Casaer, M.; Hiesmayr, M.J.; Mayer, K.; Montejo, J.M.; Pichard, C.; et al. ESPEN Guidelines: Nutrition in the ICU. *Clin. Nutr.* **2019**, *38*, 48–79. [CrossRef] [PubMed]
103. Pannerec, A.; Migliavacca, E.; De Castro, A.; Michaud, J.; Karaz, S.; Goulet, L.; Rezzi, S.; Ng, T.; Bosco, N.; Larbi, A.; et al. Vitamin B12 deficiency and impaired expression of amnionless during aging. *J. Cachexia Sarcopenia Muscle* **2018**, *9*, 41–52. [CrossRef]
104. Deutz, N.E.; Matheson, E.M.; Matarese, L.E.; Luo, M.; Baggs, G.E.; Nelson, J.L.; Hegazi, R.A.; Tappenden, K.A.; Ziegler, T.R.; Group, Nourish Study. Readmission and mortality in malnourished, older, hospitalized adults treated with a specialized oral nutritional supplement: A randomized clinical trial. *Clin. Nutr.* **2016**, *35*, 18–26. [CrossRef]
105. Friedli, N.; Stanga, Z.; Sobotka, L.; Culkin, A.; Kondrup, J.; Laviano, A.; Mueller, B.; Schuetz, P. Revisiting the refeeding syndrome: Results of a systematic review. *Nutrition* **2017**, *35*, 151–160. [CrossRef]
106. Sauer, A.; Goates, S.; Malone, A.; Mogensen, K.; Gewirtz, G.; Sulz, I.; Moick, S.; Laviano, A.; Hiesmayr, M. Prevalence of Malnutrition Risk and the Impact of Nutrition Risk on Hospital Outcomes: Results From nutritionDay in the U.S. *JPEN. J. Parenter. Enter. Nutr.* **2019**, [CrossRef] [PubMed]

107. Pruckner, N.; Baumgartner, J.; Hinterbuchinger, B.; Glahn, A.; Vyssoki, S.; Vyssoki, B. Thiamine Substitution in Alcohol Use Disorder: A Narrative Review of Medical Guidelines. *Eur. Addict. Res.* **2019**, *25*, 103–110. [CrossRef] [PubMed]
108. Curtis, L.; Bernier, P.; Jeejeebhoy, K.; Allard, J.; Duerksen, D.; Gramlich, L.; Laporte, M.; Keller, H. Costs of hospital malnutrition. *Clin. Nutr.* **2017**, *36*, 1391–1396. [CrossRef] [PubMed]
109. Hercberg, S.; Galan, P.; Preziosi, P.; Bertrais, S.; Mennen, L.; Malvy, D.; Roussel, A.; Favier, A.; Briancon, S. The SU.VI.MAX Study: A randomized, placebo-controlled trial of the health effects of antioxidant vitamins and minerals. *Arch. Intern. Med.* **2004**, *164*, 2335–2342. [CrossRef]
110. Visser, J.; Labadarios, D.; Blaauw, R. Micronutrient supplementation for critically ill adults: A systematic review and meta-analysis. *Nutrition* **2011**, *27*, 745–758. [CrossRef]
111. Wieser, S.; Brunner, B.; Tzogiou, C.; Plessow, R.; Zimmermann, M.B.; Farebrother, J.; Soofi, S.; Bhatti, Z.; Ahmed, I.; Bhutta, Z.A. Societal costs of micronutrient deficiencies in 6- to 59-month-old children in Pakistan. *Food Nutr. Bull.* **2017**, *38*, 485–500. [CrossRef]
112. Berger, M.M.; Reintam-Blaser, A.; Calder, P.C.; Casaer, M.; Hiesmayr, M.; Mayer, K.; Montejo, J.C.; Pichard, P.; Preiser, J.; van Zanten, A.; et al. Monitoring nutrition in the ICU. *Clin. Nutr.* **2019**, *38*, 584–593. [CrossRef]
113. Gagnon, G.; Voirol, P.; Soguel, L.; Boulat, O.; Berger, M.M. Trace element monitoring in the ICU: Quality and economic impact of a change in sampling practice. *Clin. Nutr.* **2014**, *34*, 422–427. [CrossRef]

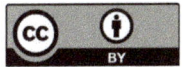

© 2019 by the authors. Licensee MDPI, Basel, Switzerland. This article is an open access article distributed under the terms and conditions of the Creative Commons Attribution (CC BY) license (http://creativecommons.org/licenses/by/4.0/).

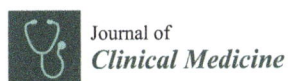

Review

Early Supplemental Parenteral Nutrition in Critically Ill Children: An Update

An Jacobs, Ines Verlinden, Ilse Vanhorebeek and Greet Van den Berghe *

Clinical Division and Laboratory of Intensive Care Medicine, Department of Cellular and Molecular Medicine, KU Leuven University Hospital, 3000 Leuven, Belgium; an.jacobs@kuleuven.be (A.J.); ines.verlinden@kuleuven.be (I.V.); ilse.vanhorebeek@kuleuven.be (I.V.)
* Correspondence: greet.vandenberghe@kuleuven.be; Tel.: +32-16-344021

Received: 13 May 2019; Accepted: 5 June 2019; Published: 11 June 2019

Abstract: In critically ill children admitted to pediatric intensive care units (PICUs), enteral nutrition (EN) is often delayed due to gastrointestinal dysfunction or interrupted. Since a macronutrient deficit in these patients has been associated with adverse outcomes in observational studies, supplemental parenteral nutrition (PN) in PICUs has long been widely advised to meeting nutritional requirements. However, uncertainty of timing of initiation, optimal dose and composition of PN has led to a wide variation in previous guidelines and current clinical practices. The PEPaNIC (Early versus Late Parenteral Nutrition in the Pediatric ICU) randomized controlled trial recently showed that withholding PN in the first week in PICUs reduced incidence of new infections and accelerated recovery as compared with providing supplemental PN early (within 24 h after PICU admission), irrespective of diagnosis, severity of illness, risk of malnutrition or age. The early withholding of amino acids in particular, which are powerful suppressors of intracellular quality control by autophagy, statistically explained this outcome benefit. Importantly, two years after PICU admission, not providing supplemental PN early in PICUs did not negatively affect mortality, growth or health status, and significantly improved neurocognitive development. These findings have an important impact on the recently issued guidelines for PN administration to critically ill children. In this review, we summarize the most recent literature that provides evidence on the implications for clinical practice with regard to the use of early supplemental PN in critically ill children.

Keywords: Pediatric Intensive Care Unit; enteral nutrition; early parenteral nutrition; critical illness

---

1. Introduction

Optimal nutritional support is considered of paramount importance for critically ill children admitted to the pediatric intensive care unit (PICU), since malnutrition and inadequate nutrient delivery have been associated with worse clinical outcome [1,2]. Moreover, critically ill children have limited macronutrient stores and relatively higher energy requirements than adults admitted to the intensive care unit (ICU), which can lead to substantial caloric and macronutrient deficits [2–4]. The feeding is thought to attenuate the metabolic stress response, prevent oxidative cellular injury and modulate immune responses, and has led to a shift from nutritional support as adjunctive care to actual therapy of the critically ill child [5]. The enteral route is preferred for providing nutrition [5]. However, critically ill children are often too ill to be fed normally by mouth, and nasogastric or nasoduodenal tube feeding is often not tolerated because of gastric dysmotility or ileus. Interruption of enteral feeding also occurs frequently for various reasons, like medical or surgical contraindications, or radiology, bedside or surgical procedures [6]. Therefore, parenteral nutrition (PN) is often initiated to supplement the insufficient enteral intake. Nonetheless, official guidelines on timing and thresholds of initiation, composition and doses of supplemental PN vary widely [5,7–9]. Moreover, concerns about overfeeding have led to even more uncertainty [9]. A recent survey showed significant differences in nutritional practices in PICUs worldwide, in terms of macronutrient goals, estimation of energy requirements, timing of nutrient delivery and thresholds for starting supplemental PN [10]. In this review, we summarize the most recent literature findings affecting evidence and clinical practices with regard to the use of early PN in critically ill children. We searched PubMed up to April 2019, without language restrictions, using different combinations of the search terms "parenteral nutrition", "PICU", "early" and "pediatric critical illness". We focused on publications of the last eight years, discussed in the context of earlier work.

2. Timing of PN Initiation

Several observational studies have shown that malnutrition is associated with worse clinical outcome [1,2,11]. A macronutrient deficit has been associated with infections, weakness, prolonged mechanical ventilation and delayed recovery. For that reason, guidelines used to recommend that when provision of enteral nutrition (EN) is insufficient, impossible or contraindicated, supplemental PN should be initiated [7,12,13]. However, observational studies cannot assign causality to an association. Hence, the association between inadequate nutrition and worse clinical outcome might merely exist because of a non-optimal nutritional support for the sickest children, which are at the highest risk of adverse outcome. Although it seems intuitive that providing early nutrition will be beneficial, it does not necessarily mean that nutritional support in the early phase of critical illness will improve clinical outcome [9]. In critically ill adults, the large multicenter EPaNIC (Early versus Late Parenteral Nutrition in ICU, n = 4640) randomized controlled trial (RCT) showed that withholding supplemental PN until day eight of an ICU stay (late PN), and thus accepting a substantial macronutrient deficit, was associated with fewer ICU infections, a shorter duration of mechanical ventilation and renal-replacement therapy and a shorter ICU and total hospital stay as compared with initiating supplemental PN early (within 48 h after ICU admission) [14]. Data generated by the broad international yearly survey of clinical nutrition practices "nutritionDay" revealed an important change in the pattern of PN prescription after publication of the EPaNIC results (Personal communication kindly shared by Prof. Dr. M. Hiesmayr, nutritionDay Project Leader). As compared with adults, critically ill children have limited stores of energy, fat and protein, as well as relatively higher energy requirements [2,3]. Since this makes them more vulnerable to a substantial caloric and macronutrient deficit, the effect of withholding supplemental PN in critically ill children could be different than in adults. Therefore, a multicenter PEPaNIC RCT (Early versus Late Parenteral Nutrition in the Pediatric ICU) was conducted [15] that investigated the same intervention in 1440 critically ill children aged 0–17 years in three PICUs in Belgium, the Netherlands and Canada. Withholding supplemental PN during the first week in critically ill children resulted in fewer new infections, a shorter dependency on mechanical ventilation and general intensive care and a shorter hospital stay as compared with providing PN early (within 24 h after PICU admission; see Figure 1). The clinical superiority of late PN was more pronounced in children than it was in adults, and was shown irrespective of diagnosis, severity of illness, risk of malnutrition or age of the child [15]. This last finding was surprising, since neonates are more susceptible to macronutrient deficits than older children [7], raising concerns by experts [16–18]. To address these concerns, a secondary analysis of the PEPaNIC trial was performed to investigate the effects of withholding PN for one week in 209 critically ill neonates who did not (or could hardly) tolerate EN [19]. Analyses were performed for term neonates aged up to four weeks, up to one week and younger than one day. Late PN resulted in fewer nosocomial infections in neonates aged up to one week and younger than one day, and in shorter dependency on intensive care and mechanical ventilation for all studied age groups of neonates. Hence, term neonates also benefited from withholding PN during the first week in the PICU, which is in agreement with findings for older children and adults [14,15]. Moreover, there was a more pronounced benefit of late PN in the youngest children, as shown in Figure 1. Since a macronutrient deficiency is presumed to be more detrimental during acute illness in undernourished children [5], a second subanalysis of the PEPaNIC RCT was performed, investigating the effects of withholding supplemental PN during the first PICU week in a subgroup of critically ill children who were undernourished upon admission to the PICU [20]. Undernourishment was defined as a weight-for-age z score lower than −2 in children younger than one year, and a body mass index-for-age z score lower than −2 in children one year or older. This identified 289 of 1440 PEPaNIC patients (20%) with undernourishment upon PICU admission. Among the undernourished patients, late PN reduced the absolute risk of new infections and shortened the duration of PICU stay. These effect sizes of late PN were even larger than in the main trial cohort of the PEPaNIC RCT. Late PN did not affect the safety outcomes of mortality, incidence of hypoglycemia or weight deterioration during PICU stay in the undernourished patients. A larger longitudinal study of all PEPaNIC patients with weight z scores available on admission and on the last day in the PICU showed that weight deterioration during PICU stay was associated with worse clinical outcomes, but that withholding supplemental PN during the first week did not alter weight z score deterioration during the PICU stay [21].

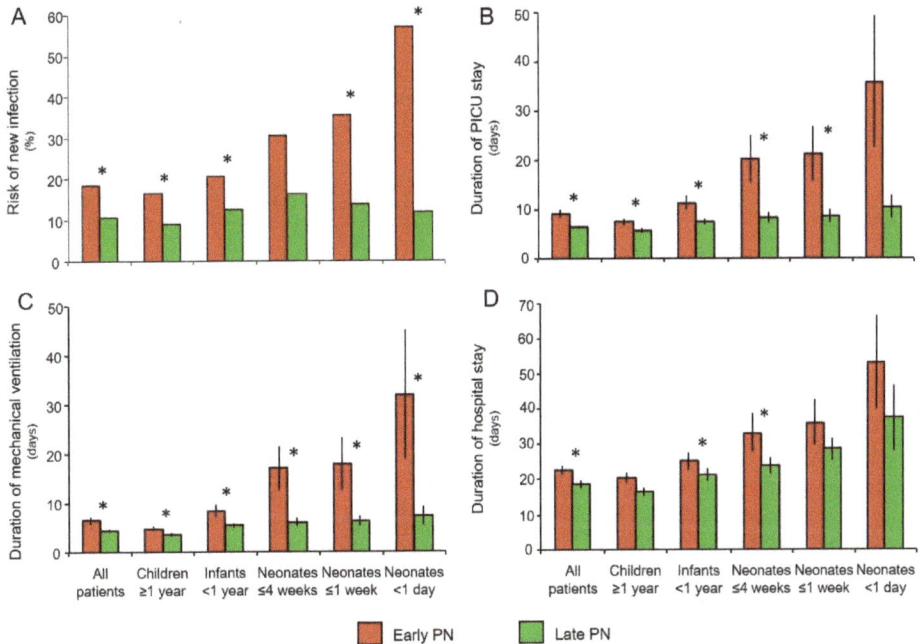

Figure 1. Bars represent incidence of (**A**) the risk of acquiring a new infection in PICUs (percentage), (**B**) duration (days) of PICU stay, (**C**) duration (days) of mechanical ventilation, and (**D**) duration (days) of total hospital stay. Whiskers indicate standard errors of the mean. Asterisks represent p values < 0.05 obtained with multivariable analysis adjusting for baseline risk factors (treatment center, age, risk of malnutrition (STRONGkids score), diagnosis upon admission and severity of illness (Pediatric Logistic Organ Dysfunction (PeLOD) score, and Pediatric Risk of Mortality 2 (PIM2) score) for all patients; treatment center, risk of malnutrition, diagnosis upon admission and severity of illness for children and infants; and treatment center, type of illness upon admission (medical, surgical cardiac, surgical other), severity of illness and weight for age z score for neonates).

The benefits of withholding supplemental PN during the first week in the PICU appeared not only present from a clinical point of view, but also from a health–economic perspective. A cost-effectiveness study indeed showed that the total direct medical costs were considerably lower with late PN as compared with early supplemental PN initiation [22]. This cost saving was beyond the expected lower costs for the use of PN itself, since avoidance of new infections by late PN yielded the largest cost reduction.

A possible limitation of the PEPaNIC RCT is the use of standard equations for the estimation of energy requirements instead of indirect calorimetry [23]. However, the use of indirect calorimetry for estimating energy expenditure does not seem to be accurate [24], or feasible [25], and is not frequently used in daily practice [10,26].

Apart from the PEPaNIC RCT, no other randomized controlled trial investigating the use or timing of supplemental PN in critically ill children has been published in the last eight years. A limited number of observational studies on the use of supplemental PN and over- and underfeeding in PICUs showed different results [2,24,27]. A retrospective single center study showed that late initiation of supplemental PN was associated with a higher nosocomial infection rate as compared with early initiation of supplemental PN [27]. In contrast, an observational study in 31 PICUs showed that the use of PN in general was associated with higher mortality [2]. Another retrospective study determining the incidence of over- and underfeeding in 139 children admitted to a tertiary PICU showed that underfeeding was associated with shorter durations of PICU and hospital stays, as well as with fewer ventilation days, as compared with appropriately fed and overfed patients [24]. However, the observational design of these studies holds a risk of bias by confounding variables, especially in nutritional research [28]. Therefore, comparison with the results of the PEPaNIC RCT is challenging. Further randomized controlled trials are warranted to determine the ideal time point for initiation of supplemental PN in PICUs.

3. Early PN Composition and the Role of Macronutrients

Although extensive guidelines on the composition of PN in critically ill children are available [5], a recent survey on nutritional practices in PICUs worldwide showed a wide variation in parenterally administered doses of protein, lipids and glucose [10]. Protein targets in particular seem to be a point of discussion. Several studies have assessed the association between protein delivery to and clinical outcome of critically ill children [2,29,30]. In an observational international cohort study that included 500 critically ill children, mortality at 60 days was higher in patients who received PN independently of the amount of energy or protein intake [2]. However, an important severity of illness bias has to be taken into account, since patients who are less sick are more likely to better tolerate EN. The study adjusted for severity of illness using admission scores, but data for calculating this severity of illness score were missing in 31% of the included patients, and the choice of severity of illness score differed between the participating centers [2]. Another large multicenter observational study of the same group showed an association between higher enteral protein intake and lower odds of mortality in more than 1200 mechanically ventilated critically ill children [29]. The effect was dose-dependent, and independent of energy intake. Again, the incomplete datasets and the lack of uniform usage for severity of illness scores, and the substantial number of patients who received EN, could potentially bias these observations. The authors reasoned that an increased demand in amino acids in catabolic disease, such as critical illness, could contribute to increased higher protein degradation from muscle to ensure bodily functions [29], which is associated with poor outcome [31]. By providing proteins, the synthesis of muscle proteins might be boosted, and thereby muscle loss could be prevented, possibly limiting the severity of intensive care unit-acquired weakness [32]. Nevertheless, a preplanned secondary analysis of the adult EPaNIC study did not support this concept, as increased macronutrient intake with early PN, including more amino acids, did not counteract muscle atrophy and actually increased the risk of developing clinically relevant muscle weakness in the ICU [33]. Interestingly, in a preplanned secondary analysis of the PEPaNIC RCT, the dose of amino acids was actually associated with more infections and a longer dependency on mechanical ventilation and other intensive medical care in children admitted to the PICU [30]. This risk of harm associated with early amino acid administration was elevated even at low doses of administered amino acids. A possible explanation for the difference between these results and the ones from the previously cited observational studies is the randomized design of the PEPaNIC trial, in which the doses of macronutrients differed from patient to patient and ranged widely [30]. In critically ill adults, three RCTs could not show benefits from early amino acid supplementation [34–37], but clinical trials on the effects of amino acid administration on clinical outcome in critically ill children in a randomized manner are lacking [38]. In contrast with the harm of amino acid administration, the secondary analysis of the PEPaNIC RCT suggested a benefit of glucose and lipid administration. Indeed, administering more glucose during the first three days of PICU stay was independently associated with fewer infections, and administering more lipids was independently associated with earlier PICU discharge [30]. Clearly, large-scale prospective RCTs in critically ill children are needed to identify the optimal composition of supplemental PN [9,38].

4. Impact of Early PN on Long-Term Outcome

Because of new insights in diagnostic and therapeutic measures in the field of pediatric critical care medicine [39], centralization of care [40] and specialized staff training and education [41,42], there has been an important decline in the mortality rate in PICUs over the last decades [43,44]. However, this improved survival has led towards a shift to considerable long-term morbidity, years after discharge [45,46]. This has been most thoroughly documented in regards to impairment of neurocognitive development, but it also includes growth retardation and may comprise poor physical functioning and reduced quality of life [47–50]. The fact that children are treated in the PICU during crucial developmental phases likely plays a role. Interestingly, it appears that, to a certain extent, neurocognitive outcome is modifiable, as shown by the attenuation of neurocognitive impairment with the prevention of hyperglycemia during intensive care [51]. Treatments in PICUs that have been shown to cause neurodevelopmental harm, such as anesthetic and analgesic agents [52,53] and toxicants such as phthalates that leach from indwelling medical devices [54], may also be targets for research into safer alternatives. Concerning nutrition in PICUs, in relation to long-term outcome, experts were concerned about the safety of withholding early supplemental PN in neonates in view of the more frequent episodes of hypoglycemia observed in the late PN arm of the PEPaNIC RCT [15,17]. However, in a previous large randomized controlled trial investigating the effect of tight glycemic control on morbidity and mortality in PICUs and on long-term neurocognitive development, a high incidence of brief hypoglycemia with tight glycemic control was not associated with harm to neurocognitive development, as documented four years later [51]. The proportion of neonates included in the PEPaNIC RCT was similar to that in the tight glycemic control trial [15,55]. In a preplanned two-year follow-up study, in which all patients included in the PEPaNIC RCT were approached for possible assessment of physical and neurocognitive development, exposure to hypoglycemia also did not associate with the investigated long-term outcomes [53]. Moreover, the main results of this follow-up study showed no adverse effects of withholding supplemental PN during the first week in PICUs on survival, anthropometrics, health status and neurocognitive development. In fact, omitting early supplemental PN in PICUs improved parent-reported executive functioning (inhibition, working memory, metacognition and overall executive functioning), externalizing behavioral problems and visual-motor integration two years later, as compared with early supplemental PN. In particular, a better inhibitory control was observed (Figure 2). Since poor inhibitory control in children contributes to impulsive and destructive behaviors that upset or harm others [56], delaying supplemental PN can have important consequences on daily life and social environments later in life. The long-term effects of late versus early supplemental PN were more pronounced in patients who were younger than one year of age at the time of PICU admission as compared with older children. This age-dependent vulnerability supports the hypothesis that the harm induced by early supplemental PN might be caused by a direct metabolic insult to the developing brain, since it was not statistically explained by the acute effects of the intervention itself, such as the increased incidence of new infections or delayed recovery. However, further research is warranted to unravel the underlying mechanisms that would provide support for this hypothesis. Although long-term outcomes and quality-of-life years after PICU discharge have gained great importance in research [45,46], investigating these outcomes is logistically challenging, expensive and time-consuming. To investigate whether these long-term effects persist or change over time, a four-year follow-up study of the PEPaNIC RCT is currently ongoing, of which the results are expected by 2020.

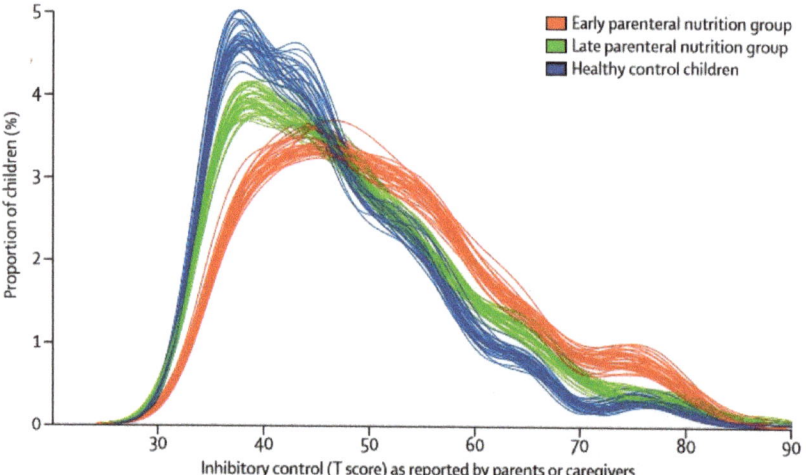

Figure 2. Density estimates for inhibitory function as reported by parents or caregivers. Densities, which correspond to the proportions of children with a certain score (equivalent to a smoothed histogram), are shown separately for healthy control children and for PEPaNIC participants who were randomly assigned to receive late PN or early PN. Higher scores indicate worse functioning. Each line corresponds to one of 31 imputed datasets. Figure reprinted from [53] with permission from Elsevier.

5. Potential Mechanisms Underlying Harm by Early PN

Several mechanisms may contribute to an adverse clinical impact of administering PN in the early phase of critical illness in children. As early PN has affected both short-term and long-term outcomes of patients, carryover effects persisting in the long term must play a role.

5.1. Potential Mechanisms Underlying the Adverse Impact of Early PN on Short-Term Outcome

As discussed, it was the administration of more amino acids that was associated with adverse short-term outcomes evoked by early PN in the PEPaNIC study [30]. The mechanisms underlying the potential harm of amino acids in this context remain to be unraveled, but it is possible to speculate. First, amino acids are powerful suppressors of autophagy [57], a pathway shown to be crucial in critically ill humans and animals for innate immunity and the removal of cellular damage [58,59]. Autophagy activation appeared suppressed in muscle from randomized adult patients exposed to early PN as compared with late PN in the EPaNIC trial, and amino acids in particular suppressed autophagy activation in a rabbit model of prolonged critical illness [33,58,59]. Second, macronutrients and amino acids in particular have long been assumed to counteract the hypercatabolic response to critical illness, which mobilizes amino acids by (mainly muscle) protein breakdown to guarantee substrate delivery to vital tissues [60]. More specifically, administration of exogenous amino acids was thought to circumvent the need for endogenous amino acid release and to stimulate muscle protein synthesis. However, once amino acid doses exceed anabolic capacity, they no longer stimulate muscle protein synthesis but are shuttled towards the liver for production of urea [61]. Such increased plasma urea concentrations were observed in early PN patients in the PEPaNIC RCT as compared with late PN patients [15]. In critically ill adults who received early PN, the administered amino acids did not counteract muscle wasting [33], but increased plasma urea and urinary nitrogen excretion (with a net waste of 63% of the extra nitrogen intake from early PN in the first two weeks) [62], which can cause harm to both liver and kidney. These results are in line with the EAT-ICU trial (Early goal-directed nutrition in ICU patients) results, in which increased urea production—but no beneficial effect on outcome—was seen with early goal-directed nutrition versus standard nutritional care in critically ill adults [63]. Altogether, these findings suggest that muscle wasting during the acute phase of critical illness may be considered an adaptive response designed to provide substrates for gluconeogenesis in order to meet the energy requirements of vital organs [32].

5.2. Potential Mechanisms Underlying the Adverse Impact of Early PN on Long-Term Outcome

Underlying mechanisms of the long-term harm caused by early PN in the context of critical illness remain largely unraveled. The clinical benefits of late PN observed far beyond the intervention window suggests that early PN induces carry-over "memory" effects with a negative impact on long-term outcome. Poor long-term outcomes in other conditions have been related to accelerated telomere shortening and the induction of aberrant so-called "epigenetic" changes. Importantly, inadequate nutrition may cause both adverse effects. Hence, these processes may also play a role in the developmental impairment of critically ill children and the adverse impact of early PN on neurocognitive development.

Telomeres are nucleoprotein complexes at the end of human chromosomes that shorten with each cell cycle. Telomere shortening can be accelerated by environmental and lifestyle factors [64,65], including excessive food consumption and/or unhealthy nutrition [66,67]. It has been demonstrated that critically ill children enter the PICU with significantly shorter leukocyte telomeres than matched healthy children [68]. More importantly, early PN had a telomere-shortening effect as compared with late PN in critically ill children between PICU admission and discharge, independent of baseline risk factors and post-randomization factors. Whether this accelerated telomere shortening contributes to long-term developmental impairment, and particularly the neurocognitive impairment caused by early PN, remains to be investigated.

The involvement of aberrant epigenetic changes in long-term consequences after acute events in life appears plausible. Epigenetics refers to the study of heritable changes in gene expression that do not involve changes in the underlying DNA sequence. Epigenetic changes play an important role in physical and neurocognitive development [69–72]. The most stable epigenetic change is the methylation or de-methylation of DNA. This is the attachment to or removal of a methyl group from a nucleotide, which occurs almost exclusively at the 5′ carbon in the cytosine residue of a CpG dinucleotide [69,70]. Alterations in DNA methylation have been implicated in the adverse effects of various environmental stressors, such as inadequate nutrition (both undernutrition and overfeeding), that have been shown to impact long-term health and disease [73]. Particularly during early life, DNA methylation changes may bring about long-term effects [71,72,74]. Data are needed on whether nutritional management in the early phase of critical illness induces aberrant changes in DNA methylation, which could explain the adverse impact of early PN on neurocognitive development.

6. Conclusions and Newest Guidelines

Nutritional support is considered to be an important aspect of patient care in PICUs [26], with large differences in PICUs worldwide regarding practices of supplemental PN for patients in whom EN as the preferred route is insufficient or impossible [5,10]. A large multicenter RCT showed that withholding supplemental PN throughout the first week in the PICU was clinically superior for short-term outcome as compared with initiating supplemental PN within 24 h after admission [19]. This was the case independent of age [19] or nutritional status [20]. The administered amino acids in particular appeared to explain the adverse impact of early provision of PN, possibly via suppression of required autophagy activation and the shuttling of amino acids to urea production with harmful effects to the liver and kidney. In the long-term, omitting PN during the first week of pediatric critical illness did not show harm, and actually improved executive functioning, behavioral problems and visual-motor integration, as compared with administering PN early. These findings had an important impact on recent ESPGHAN (European Society for Pediatric Gastroenterology Hepatology and Nutrition) pediatric PN guidelines [60], in which it is advised to consider withholding PN, including amino acids, for one week in critically ill infants, children and adolescents. However, the lack of other RCTs in this specific field makes it challenging to compare these findings with other available recent studies. Further research, in the form of multicenter RCTs, is warranted to determine the optimal composition and ideal timing of initiation of supplemental PN in critically ill children.

Author Contributions: A.J., I.V. (Ilse Vanhorebeek) and G.V.d.B. were responsible for the design of the review article. A.J. performed comprehensive literature search. A.J., I.V. (Ines Verlinden) and I.V. (Ilse Vanhorebeek) wrote the article. G.V.d.B. revised it carefully and gave a significant scientific contribution to its content.

Funding: This work was supported by ERC Advanced Grants from the Ideas programme of the European Union Seventh Framework Programme (AdvG-2012-321670) and Horizon 2020 Programme (AdvG-2017-785809) to G.V.d.B.; by the Methusalem programme of the Flemish Government (through the University of Leuven to G.V.d.B. and I.V. (Ilse Vanhorebeek), METH14/06); and by the Agency for Innovation through Science and Technology, Flanders, Belgium (through the University of Leuven to G.V.d.B., IWT/070695/TBM.

Conflicts of Interest: The authors declare no conflict of interest.

References

1. Pollack, M.M.; Ruttimann, U.E.; Wiley, J.S. Nutritional depletions in critically ill children: Associations with physiologic instability and increased quantity of care. *JPEN J. Parenter. Enter. Nutr.* **1985**, *9*, 309–313. [CrossRef] [PubMed]
2. Mehta, N.M.; Bechard, L.J.; Cahill, N.; Wang, M.; Day, A.; Duggan, C.P.; Heyland, D.K. Nutritional practices and their relationship to clinical outcomes in critically ill children–An international multicenter cohort study. *Crit. Care Med.* **2012**, *40*, 2204–2211. [CrossRef] [PubMed]
3. Oosterveld, M.J.; Van Der Kuip, M.; De Meer, K.; De Greef, H.J.; Gemke, R.J. Energy expenditure and balance following pediatric intensive care unit admission: A longitudinal study of critically ill children. *Pediatr. Crit. Care Med.* **2006**, *7*, 147–153. [CrossRef] [PubMed]
4. Joosten, K.F.; Kerklaan, D.; Verbruggen, S.C. Nutritional support and the role of the stress response in critically ill children. *Curr. Opin. Clin. Nutr. Metab. Care* **2016**, *19*, 226–233. [CrossRef] [PubMed]
5. Mehta, N.M.; Skillman, H.E.; Irving, S.Y.; Coss-Bu, J.A.; Vermilyea, S.; Farrington, E.A.; McKeever, L.; Hall, A.M.; Goday, P.S.; Braunschweig, C. Guidelines for the provision and assessment of nutrition support therapy in the pediatric critically Ill patient: Society of critical care medicine and american society for parenteral and enteral nutrition. *Pediatr. Crit. Care Med.* **2017**, *18*, 675–715. [CrossRef] [PubMed]
6. Mehta, N.M.; McAleer, D.; Hamilton, S.; Naples, E.; Leavitt, K.; Mitchell, P.; Duggan, C. Challenges to optimal enteral nutrition in a multidisciplinary pediatric intensive care unit. *JPEN J. Parenter. Enter. Nutr.* **2010**, *34*, 38–45. [CrossRef] [PubMed]
7. Koletzko, B.; Goulet, O.; Hunt, J.; Krohn, K.; Shamir, R.; Parenteral Nutrition Guidelines Working Group; European Society for Clinical Nutrition and Metabolism; European Society of Paediatric Gastroenterology, Hepatology and Nutrition. 1. guidelines on paediatric parenteral nutrition of the European Society of Paediatric Gastroenterology, Hepatology and Nutrition (ESPGHAN) and the European Society for Clinical Nutrition and Metabolism (ESPEN), supported by the European Society of Paediatric Research (ESPR). *J. Pediatr. Gastroenterol. Nutr.* **2005**, *41* (Suppl. 2), S1–S4. [PubMed]
8. Fivez, T.; Kerklaan, D.; Mesotten, D.; Verbruggen, S.; Joosten, K.; Van den Berghe, G. Evidence for the use of parenteral nutrition in the pediatric intensive care unit. *Clin. Nutr.* **2017**, *36*, 218–223. [CrossRef] [PubMed]
9. Joffe, A.; Anton, N.; Lequier, L.; Vandermeer, B.; Tjosvold, L.; Larsen, B.; Hartling, L. Nutritional support for critically Ill children. *Cochrane Database Syst. Rev.* **2016**. [CrossRef]
10. Kerklaan, D.; Fivez, T.; Mehta, N.M.; Mesotten, D.; van Rosmalen, J.; Hulst, J.M.; Van den Berghe, G.; Joosten, K.F.; Verbruggen, S.C. Worldwide survey of nutritional practices in PICUs. *Pediatr. Crit. Care Med.* **2016**, *17*, 10–18. [CrossRef]
11. Martinez, E.E.; Mehta, N.M. The science and art of pediatric critical care nutrition. *Curr. Opin. Crit. Care* **2016**, *22*, 316–324. [CrossRef]
12. Joffe, A.; Anton, N.; Lequier, L.; Vandermeer, B.; Tjosvold, L.; Larsen, B.; Hartling, L. Nutritional support for critically Ill children. *Cochrane Database Syst. Rev.* **2009**. [CrossRef]

13. Mehta, N.M.; Compher, C.; ASPEN Board of Directors. ASPEN clinical guidelines: Nutrition support of the critically ill child. *JPEN J. Parenter. Enter. Nutr.* **2009**, *33*, 260–276. [CrossRef]
14. Casaer, M.P.; Mesotten, D.; Hermans, G.; Wouters, P.J.; Schetz, M.; Meyfroidt, G.; Van Cromphaut, S.; Ingels, C.; Meersseman, P.; Muller, J.; et al. Early versus late parenteral nutrition in critically ill adults. *N. Engl. J. Med.* **2011**, *365*, 506–517. [CrossRef]
15. Fivez, T.; Kerklaan, D.; Mesotten, D.; Verbruggen, S.; Wouters, P.J.; Vanhorebeek, I.; Debaveye, Y.; Vlasselaers, D.; Desmet, L.; Casaer, M.P.; et al. Early versus late parenteral nutrition in critically Ill children. *N. Engl. J. Med.* **2016**, *374*, 1111–1122. [CrossRef]
16. Goulet, O.; Jochum, F.; Koletzko, B. Early or late parenteral nutrition in critically Ill children: Practical implications of the PEPaNIC trial. *Ann. Nutr. Metab.* **2017**, *70*, 34–38. [CrossRef]
17. Groenendaal, F. Early versus late parenteral nutrition in critically Ill children. *N. Engl. J. Med.* **2016**, *375*, 384. [CrossRef]
18. Vichayavilas, P.; Gist, K.; Kaufman, J. More and sooner, but not necessarily better. *J. Thorac. Dis.* **2016**, *8*, 1877–1879. [CrossRef]
19. Van Puffelen, E.; Vanhorebeek, I.; Joosten, K.F.M.; Wouters, P.J.; Van den Berghe, G.; Verbruggen, S. Early versus late parenteral nutrition in critically ill, term neonates: A preplanned secondary subgroup analysis of the PEPaNIC multicentre, randomised controlled trial. *Lancet Child Adolesc. Health* **2018**, *2*, 505–515. [CrossRef]
20. Van Puffelen, E.; Hulst, J.M.; Vanhorebeek, I.; Dulfer, K.; Van den Berghe, G.; Verbruggen, S.C.A.T.; Joosten, K.F.M. Outcomes of delaying parenteral nutrition for 1 week vs initiation within 24 h among undernourished children in pediatric intensive care: A subanalysis of the PEPaNIC randomized clinical trial. *JAMA Netw. Open* **2018**, *1*, e182668. [CrossRef]
21. Van Puffelen, E.; Hulst, J.M.; Vanhorebeek, I.; Dulfer, K.; Van den Berghe, G.; Joosten, K.F.M.; Verbruggen, S. Effect of late versus early initiation of parenteral nutrition on weight deterioration during PICU stay: Secondary analysis of the PEPaNIC randomised controlled trial. *Clin. Nutr.* **2019**. [CrossRef] [PubMed]
22. Van Puffelen, E.; Polinder, S.; Vanhorebeek, I.; Wouters, P.J.; Bossche, N.; Peers, G.; Verstraete, S.; Joosten, K.F.M.; Van den Berghe, G.; Verbruggen, S.; et al. Cost-effectiveness study of early versus late parenteral nutrition in critically ill children (PEPaNIC): Preplanned secondary analysis of a multicentre randomised controlled trial. *Crit. Care* **2018**, *22*, 4. [CrossRef] [PubMed]
23. Li, Y.; Huang, Y. Early versus late parenteral nutrition in critically Ill children. *N. Engl. J. Med.* **2016**, *375*, 384–385. [CrossRef] [PubMed]
24. Larsen, B.M.K.; Beggs, M.R.; Leong, A.Y.; Kang, S.H.; Persad, R.; Garcia Guerra, G. Can energy intake alter clinical and hospital outcomes in PICU? *Clin. Nutr. ESPEN* **2018**, *24*, 41–46. [CrossRef] [PubMed]
25. Beggs, M.R.; Garcia Guerra, G.; Larsen, B.M.K. Do PICU patients meet technical criteria for performing indirect calorimetry? *Clin. Nutr. ESPEN* **2016**, *15*, 80–84. [CrossRef] [PubMed]
26. Van der Kuip, M.; Oosterveld, M.J.; van Bokhorst-de van der Schueren, M.A.; de Meer, K.; Lafeber, H.N.; Gemke, R.J. Nutritional support in 111 pediatric intensive care units: A European survey. *Intensive Care Med.* **2004**, *30*, 1807–1813. [CrossRef]
27. Wang, D.; Lai, X.; Liu, C.; Xiong, Y.; Zhang, X. Influence of supplemental parenteral nutrition approach on nosocomial infection in pediatric intensive care unit of Emergency Department: A retrospective study. *Nutr. J.* **2015**, *14*, 103. [CrossRef]
28. Ioannidis, J.P.A. The challenge of reforming nutritional epidemiologic research. *J. Am. Med. Assoc.* **2018**, *320*, 969–970. [CrossRef]
29. Mehta, N.M.; Bechard, L.J.; Zurakowski, D.; Duggan, C.P.; Heyland, D.K. Adequate enteral protein intake is inversely associated with 60-d mortality in critically ill children: A multicenter, prospective, cohort study. *Am. J. Clin. Nutr.* **2015**, *102*, 199–206. [CrossRef]
30. Vanhorebeek, I.; Verbruggen, S.; Casaer, M.P.; Gunst, J.; Wouters, P.J.; Hanot, J.; Guerra, G.G.; Vlasselaers, D.; Joosten, K.; Van den Berghe, G. Effect of early supplemental parenteral nutrition in the paediatric ICU: A preplanned observational study of post-randomisation treatments in the PEPaNIC trial. *Lancet Respir. Med.* **2017**, *5*, 475–483. [CrossRef]
31. Fan, E.; Dowdy, D.W.; Colantuoni, E.; Mendez-Tellez, P.A.; Sevransky, J.E.; Shanholtz, C.; Himmelfarb, C.R.; Desai, S.V.; Ciesla, N.; Herridge, M.S.; et al. Physical complications in acute lung injury survivors: A two-year longitudinal prospective study. *Crit. Care Med.* **2014**, *42*, 849–859. [CrossRef]

32. Preiser, J.C. High protein intake during the early phase of critical illness: Yes or no? *Crit. Care* **2018**, *22*, 261. [CrossRef]
33. Hermans, G.; Casaer, M.P.; Clerckx, B.; Guiza, F.; Vanhullebusch, T.; Derde, S.; Meersseman, P.; Derese, I.; Mesotten, D.; Wouters, P.J.; et al. Effect of tolerating macronutrient deficit on the development of intensive-care unit acquired weakness: A subanalysis of the EPaNIC trial. *Lancet Respir Med.* **2013**, *1*, 621–629. [CrossRef]
34. Doig, G.S.; Simpson, F.; Bellomo, R.; Heighes, P.T.; Sweetman, E.A.; Chesher, D.; Pollock, C.; Davies, A.; Botha, J.; Harrigan, P.; et al. Intravenous amino acid therapy for kidney function in critically ill patients: A randomized controlled trial. *Intensive Care Med.* **2015**, *41*, 1197–1208. [CrossRef]
35. Ferrie, S.; Allman-Farinelli, M.; Daley, M.; Smith, K. Protein requirements in the critically Ill: A randomized controlled trial using parenteral nutrition. *JPEN J. Parenter. Enter. Nutr.* **2016**, *40*, 795–805. [CrossRef]
36. Rugeles, S.J.; Rueda, J.D.; Diaz, C.E.; Rosselli, D. Hyperproteic hypocaloric enteral nutrition in the critically ill patient: A randomized controlled clinical trial. *Indian J. Crit. Care Med.* **2013**, *17*, 343–349. [CrossRef]
37. Gunst, J.; Vanhorebeek, I.; Thiessen, S.E.; Van den Berghe, G. Amino acid supplements in critically ill patients. *Pharmacol. Res.* **2018**, *130*, 127–131. [CrossRef]
38. Coss-Bu, J.A.; Hamilton-Reeves, J.; Patel, J.J.; Morris, C.R.; Hurt, R.T. Protein requirements of the critically Ill pediatric patient. *Nutr. Clin. Pract.* **2017**, *32*, 128S–141S. [CrossRef]
39. Carcillo, J.A. What's new in pediatric intensive care. *Crit. Care Med.* **2006**, *34*, S183–S190. [CrossRef]
40. Pearson, G.; Shann, F.; Barry, P.; Vyas, J.; Thomas, D.; Powell, C.; Field, D. Should paediatric intensive care be centralised? Trent versus Victoria. *Lancet* **1997**, *349*, 1213–1217. [CrossRef]
41. Gupta, P.; Tang, X.; Rettiganti, M.; Lauer, C.; Kacmarek, R.M.; Rice, T.B.; Markovitz, B.P.; Wetzel, R.C. Association of house staff training with mortality in children with critical illness. *Acta Paediatr.* **2016**, *105*, e60–e66. [CrossRef] [PubMed]
42. Pollack, M.M.; Patel, K.M.; Ruttimann, E. Pediatric critical care training programs have a positive effect on pediatric intensive care mortality. *Crit. Care Med.* **1997**, *25*, 1637–1642. [CrossRef] [PubMed]
43. Burns, J.P.; Sellers, D.E.; Meyer, E.C.; Lewis-Newby, M.; Truog, R.D. Epidemiology of death in the PICU at five U.S. teaching hospitals. *Crit. Care Med.* **2014**, *42*, 2101–2108. [CrossRef] [PubMed]
44. Namachivayam, P.; Shann, F.; Shekerdemian, L.; Taylor, A.; van Sloten, I.; Delzoppo, C.; Daffey, C.; Butt, W. Three decades of pediatric intensive care: Who was admitted, what happened in intensive care, and what happened afterward. *Pediatr. Crit. Care Med.* **2010**, *11*, 549–555. [CrossRef] [PubMed]
45. Rennick, J.E.; Childerhose, J.E. Redefining success in the PICU: New patient populations shift targets of care. *Pediatrics* **2015**, *135*, e289–e291. [CrossRef] [PubMed]
46. Verstraete, S.; Van den Berghe, G.; Vanhorebeek, I. What's new in the long-term neurodevelopmental outcome of critically ill children. *Intensive Care Med.* **2018**, *44*, 649–651. [CrossRef]
47. Aspesberro, F.; Mangione-Smith, R.; Zimmerman, J.J. Health-related quality of life following pediatric critical illness. *Intensive Care Med.* **2015**, *41*, 1235–1246. [CrossRef]
48. Madderom, M.J.; Reuser, J.J.; Utens, E.M.; van Rosmalen, J.; Raets, M.; Govaert, P.; Steiner, K.; Gischler, S.J.; Tibboel, D.; van Heijst, A.F.; et al. Neurodevelopmental, educational and behavioral outcome at 8 years after neonatal ECMO: A nationwide multicenter study. *Intensive Care Med.* **2013**, *39*, 1584–1593. [CrossRef]
49. Sterken, C.; Lemiere, J.; Vanhorebeek, I.; Van den Berghe, G.; Mesotten, D. Neurocognition after paediatric heart surgery: A systematic review and meta-analysis. *Open Heart* **2015**, *2*, e000255. [CrossRef]
50. Buysse, C.M.; Vermunt, L.C.; Raat, H.; Hazelzet, J.A.; Hop, W.C.; Utens, E.M.; Joosten, K.F. Surviving meningococcal septic shock in childhood: Long-term overall outcome and the effect on health-related quality of life. *Crit. Care* **2010**, *14*, R124. [CrossRef]
51. Mesotten, D.; Gielen, M.; Sterken, C.; Claessens, K.; Hermans, G.; Vlasselaers, D.; Lemiere, J.; Lagae, L.; Gewillig, M.; Eyskens, B.; et al. Neurocognitive development of children 4 years after critical illness and treatment with tight glucose control: A randomized controlled trial. *J. Am. Med. Assoc.* **2012**, *308*, 1641–1650. [CrossRef] [PubMed]
52. Van Zellem, L.; Utens, E.M.; de Wildt, S.N.; Vet, N.J.; Tibboel, D.; Buysse, C. Analgesia-sedation in PICU and neurological outcome: A secondary analysis of long-term neuropsychological follow-up in meningococcal septic shock survivors. *Pediatr. Crit. Care Med.* **2014**, *15*, 189–196. [CrossRef] [PubMed]
53. Verstraete, S.; Verbruggen, S.C.; Hordijk, J.A.; Vanhorebeek, I.; Dulfer, K.; Guiza, F.; van Puffelen, E.; Jacobs, A.; Leys, S.; Durt, A.; et al. Long-term developmental effects of withholding parenteral nutrition for 1 week in

the paediatric intensive care unit: A 2-year follow-up of the PEPaNIC international, randomised, controlled trial. *Lancet Respir Med.* **2018**. [CrossRef]

54. Verstraete, S.; Vanhorebeek, I.; Covaci, A.; Guiza, F.; Malarvannan, G.; Jorens, P.G.; Van den Berghe, G. Circulating phthalates during critical illness in children are associated with long-term attention deficit: A study of a development and a validation cohort. *Intensive Care Med.* **2016**, *42*, 379–392. [CrossRef] [PubMed]

55. Vlasselaers, D.; Milants, I.; Desmet, L.; Wouters, P.J.; Vanhorebeek, I.; van den Heuvel, I.; Mesotten, D.; Casaer, M.P.; Meyfroidt, G.; Ingels, C.; et al. Intensive insulin therapy for patients in paediatric intensive care: A prospective, randomised controlled study. *Lancet* **2009**, *373*, 547–556. [CrossRef]

56. Utendale, W.T.; Hubert, M.; Saint-Pierre, A.B.; Hastings, P.D. Neurocognitive development and externalizing problems: The role of inhibitory control deficits from 4 to 6 years. *Aggress. Behav.* **2011**, *37*, 476–488. [CrossRef] [PubMed]

57. Meijer, A.J. Amino acid regulation of autophagosome formation. *Methods Mol. Biol.* **2008**, *445*, 89–109. [CrossRef]

58. Deretic, V.; Saitoh, T.; Akira, S. Autophagy in infection, inflammation and immunity. *Nat. Rev. Immunol.* **2013**, *13*, 722–737. [CrossRef]

59. Derde, S.; Vanhorebeek, I.; Guiza, F.; Derese, I.; Gunst, J.; Fahrenkrog, B.; Martinet, W.; Vervenne, H.; Ververs, E.J.; Larsson, L.; et al. Early parenteral nutrition evokes a phenotype of autophagy deficiency in liver and skeletal muscle of critically ill rabbits. *Endocrinology* **2012**, *153*, 2267–2276. [CrossRef]

60. Van Goudoever, J.B.; Carnielli, V.; Darmaun, D.; Sainz de Pipaon, M.; The ESPGHAN/ESPEN/ESPR/CSPEN Working Group on Pediatric Parenteral Nutrition. ESPGHAN/ESPEN/ESPR/CSPEN guidelines on pediatric parenteral nutrition: Amino acids. *Clin. Nutr.* **2018**, *37*, 2315–2323. [CrossRef]

61. Rennie, M.J.; Bohe, J.; Wolfe, R.R. Latency, duration and dose response relationships of amino acid effects on human muscle protein synthesis. *J. Nutr.* **2002**, *132*, 3225S–3227S. [CrossRef] [PubMed]

62. Gunst, J.; Vanhorebeek, I.; Casaer, M.P.; Hermans, G.; Wouters, P.J.; Dubois, J.; Claes, K.; Schetz, M.; Van den Berghe, G. Impact of early parenteral nutrition on metabolism and kidney injury. *J. Am. Soc. Nephrol.* **2013**, *24*, 995–1005. [CrossRef] [PubMed]

63. Allingstrup, M.J.; Kondrup, J.; Wiis, J.; Claudius, C.; Pedersen, U.G.; Hein-Rasmussen, R.; Bjerregaard, M.R.; Steensen, M.; Jensen, T.H.; Lange, T.; et al. Early goal-directed nutrition versus standard of care in adult intensive care patients: The single-centre, randomised, outcome assessor-blinded EAT-ICU trial. *Intensive Care Med.* **2017**, *43*, 1637–1647. [CrossRef] [PubMed]

64. Blackburn, E.H.; Epel, E.S.; Lin, J. Human telomere biology: A contributory and interactive factor in aging, disease risks, and protection. *Science* **2015**, *350*, 1193–1198. [CrossRef] [PubMed]

65. Epel, E.S.; Blackburn, E.H.; Lin, J.; Dhabhar, F.S.; Adler, N.E.; Morrow, J.D.; Cawthon, R.M. Accelerated telomere shortening in response to life stress. *Proc. Natl. Acad. Sci. USA* **2004**, *101*, 17312–17315. [CrossRef]

66. Pendergrass, W.R.; Penn, P.E.; Li, J.; Wolf, N.S. Age-related telomere shortening occurs in lens epithelium from old rats and is slowed by caloric restriction. *Exp. Eye Res.* **2001**, *73*, 221–228. [CrossRef]

67. Crous-Bou, M.; Fung, T.T.; Prescott, J.; Julin, B.; Du, M.; Sun, Q.; Rexrode, K.M.; Hu, F.B.; De Vivo, I. Mediterranean diet and telomere length in Nurses' Health Study: Population based cohort study. *Br. Med. J.* **2014**, *349*, g6674. [CrossRef]

68. Verstraete, S.; Vanhorebeek, I.; van Puffelen, E.; Derese, I.; Ingels, C.; Verbruggen, S.C.; Wouters, P.J.; Joosten, K.F.; Hanot, J.; Guerra, G.G.; et al. Leukocyte telomere length in paediatric critical illness: Effect of early parenteral nutrition. *Crit. Care* **2018**, *22*, 38. [CrossRef]

69. Qureshi, I.A.; Mehler, M.F. Understanding neurological disease mechanisms in the era of epigenetics. *JAMA Neurol.* **2013**, *70*, 703–710. [CrossRef]

70. Radford, E.J. Exploring the extent and scope of epigenetic inheritance. *Nat. Rev. Endocrinol.* **2018**, *14*, 345–355. [CrossRef]

71. Groom, A.; Elliott, H.R.; Embleton, N.D.; Relton, C.L. Epigenetics and child health: Basic principles. *Arch. Dis. Child.* **2011**, *96*, 863–869. [CrossRef] [PubMed]

72. Relton, C.L.; Groom, A.; St Pourcain, B.; Sayers, A.E.; Swan, D.C.; Embleton, N.D.; Pearce, M.S.; Ring, S.M.; Northstone, K.; Tobias, J.H.; et al. DNA methylation patterns in cord blood DNA and body size in childhood. *PLoS ONE* **2012**, *7*, e31821. [CrossRef] [PubMed]

73. Waterland, R.A.; Michels, K.B. Epigenetic epidemiology of the developmental origins hypothesis. *Ann. Rev. Nutr.* **2007**, *27*, 363–388. [CrossRef] [PubMed]
74. Abel, J.L.; Rissman, E.F. Running-induced epigenetic and gene expression changes in the adolescent brain. *Int. J. Dev. Neurosci.* **2013**, *31*, 382–390. [CrossRef] [PubMed]

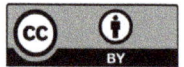

© 2019 by the authors. Licensee MDPI, Basel, Switzerland. This article is an open access article distributed under the terms and conditions of the Creative Commons Attribution (CC BY) license (http://creativecommons.org/licenses/by/4.0/).

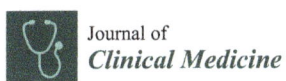

Review
Nutritional Laboratory Markers in Malnutrition

Ulrich Keller

FMH Endocrinology-Diabetology, Fichtlirain 33, CH-4105 Biel-Benken, Basel, Switzerland; ulrich.keller@unibas.ch

Received: 10 May 2019; Accepted: 29 May 2019; Published: 31 May 2019

Abstract: Serum visceral proteins such as albumin and prealbumin have traditionally been used as markers of the nutritional status of patients. Prealbumin is nowadays often preferred over albumin due to its shorter half live, reflecting more rapid changes of the nutritional state. However, recent focus has been on an appropriate nutrition-focused physical examination and on the patient's history for diagnosing malnutrition, and the role of inflammation as a risk factor for malnutrition has been more and more recognized. Inflammatory signals are potent inhibitors of visceral protein synthesis, and the use of these proteins as biomarkers of the nutritional status has been debated since they are strongly influenced by inflammation and less so by protein energy stores. The current consensus is that laboratory markers could be used as a complement to a thorough physical examination. Other markers of the nutritional status such as urinary creatinine or 3-methylhistidine as indicators of muscle protein breakdown have not found widespread use. Serum IGF-1 is less influenced by inflammation and falls during malnutrition. However, its concentration changes are not sufficiently specific to be useful clinically as a marker of malnutrition, and serum IGF-1 has less been used in clinical trials. Nevertheless, biomarkers of malnutrition such as prealbumin may be of interest as easily measurable predictors of the prognosis for surgical outcomes and of mortality in severe illnesses.

Keywords: malnutrition; inflammation; nutritional assessment; biomarkers; albumin; prealbumin; IGF-1; elderly; prognostic marker

---

1. Introduction

Malnutrition has a substantial clinical and socioeconomic significance; it increases rates of complications in hospitalized patients and healthcare-associated costs. Its prevalence has been estimated in hospitals of Western countries to be 30–50% and in long-term care facilities up to 85% depending on the definition and the type of population studied [1–3].

One of the problems of diagnosing malnutrition is the lack of a unified definition and of standard methods for screening and diagnosis.

Malnutrition results from a mismatch of nutritional requirements with intake. In many malnourished patients, there is an associated disease-related inflammation, resulting in a complex interplay between the two. Inflammation influences both, requirements and intake. It promotes malnutrition and adverse outcomes by provoking anorexia and by altering metabolism with elevation of resting energy expenditure and by increasing muscle catabolism [4].

The appreciation that inflammation plays a major role in the pathophysiology of malnutrition is often lacking, and many clinicians assume that weight loss is the single most important criterion for a malnourished state. This has led to frequent underrecognition of the condition [5].

The purpose of this review is to review the published literature on the role of laboratory biomarkers as a tool to diagnose malnutrition, to assess nutritional risk and to monitor nutritional intervention.

2. Role of Biomarkers in Published Screening Tools to Assess the Risk of Malnutrition

About half of all published risk scores of malnutrition use serum laboratory markers such as visceral proteins, and others do not (Table 1).

Table 1. Anthropometric parameters and biomarkers in various nutritional assessment and screening tools (adapted from [3] with an update, in chronological order of publication.

Nutritional Assessment and Screening Tool	Anthropometric Parameters and History	Biomarkers
Prognostic Nutritional Index [6]	Triceps skin fold	Albumin, transferrin, skin sensitivity
Prognostic Inflammatory and Nutritional Index [7]	None	Albumin, prealbumin, C-reactive protein, α1-acid glycoprotein
Subjective Global Assessment (SGA) [8]	Weight history, diet history, primary diagnosis, stress level, physical symptoms (s.c. fat, muscle wasting, edema), functional capacity, gastrointestinal symptoms	None
Birmingham Nutrition Risk Score [9]	Weight loss, BMI, appetite, ability to eat, stress factor, (severity of diagnosis)	None
Nutrition Risk Classification [10]	Weight loss, percentage ideal body weight, dietary intake, gastrointestinal function	None
Mini Nutritional Assessment (MNA; [11])	Weight data, height, mid-arm circumference, calf circumference, diet history, appetite, feeding mode	Albumin, prealbumin, cholesterol, lymphocyte count
Malnutrition Screening Tool [12]	Appetite, unintentional weight loss	None
Simple Screening Tool [13]	Body mass index (BMI), percentage weight loss	Albumin
Full nutritional assessment [14]	BMI, information on unintended weight loss, triceps skinfold thickness, mid-arm muscle circumference	Serum albumin, prealbumin, and total lymphocyte count
Malnutrition Universal Screening Tool (MUST) [15]	BMI, change in weight, presence of acute disease	None
Nutritional Risk Screening (NRS) 2002 [1]	Weight loss, BMI, food intake, diagnosis (severity)	None
Short Nutrition Assessment Questionnaire [16]	Recent weight history, appetite, use of oral supplement or tube feeding	None
Controlling nutritional status (CONUT) [17]	None	Serum albumin, total cholesterol and total lymphocyte count
Maastricht Index [18]	Percentage ideal body weight	Albumin, prealbumin, lymphocyte count
Nutritional Risk Index [19]	Present and usual body weight	Albumin
Elderly Nutritional Indicators for Geriatric Malnutrition Assessment (ENIGMA) [20]	Nutritional history	Albumin, hemoglobin, total cholesterol and lymphocyte count

Results of these screening tests vary considerably, as shown in a Greek study in elderly subjects [2]. These authors found the highest validity coefficient for MUST but a lower specificity for NRS 2000 which has frequently been used.

A consensus committee of the European and US nutritional societies (ESPEN and ASPEN) proposed three sub-definitions of malnutrition. "Starvation-related malnutrition" is present when there is chronic starvation without inflammation; "chronic disease-related malnutrition" is defined as a condition when inflammation is chronic and of mild to moderate degree, and "acute disease or injury-related malnutrition" occurs when inflammation is acute and of severe degree [21]. The criteria for diagnosis of these sub-definitions were energy intake, weight loss, body fat, muscle mass, fluid accumulation and grip strength but no biomarkers [22]. Among ancillary parameters, serum visceral proteins were mentioned, but since they would rather reflect the state of inflammation it was proposed to use them with caution to diagnose malnutrition.

A meta-regression published recently [23] assessed the role of biomarkers in describing the severity of malnutrition according to established and validated nutritional assessment tools. A total of 111 studies (observational and cohort studies; randomized controlled trials were not available) were included, representing 52,911 participants from various clinical settings. The BMI ($p < 0.001$) and concentrations of albumin ($p < 0.001$), hemoglobin ($p < 0.001$), total cholesterol ($p < 0.001$), prealbumin ($p < 0.001$) and total protein ($p < 0.05$) among subjects at high risk of malnutrition assessed by MNA were significantly lower than those with low risk. Similar results were observed for malnutrition identified by SGA and NRS 2002. When patients with acute illnesses were included, the predictive value of albumin and prealbumin was distinctly reduced, confirming the conclusion that they are more markers of inflammation than of malnutrition. The authors concluded that BMI, hemoglobin, and total cholesterol were useful markers of malnutrition in older adults.

3. Serum Visceral Proteins as Biomarkers of the Nutritional Status

Visceral proteins are mostly synthesized in the liver. Poor protein and energy intake, impaired liver synthetic function as well as inflammatory status result in low circulating levels of visceral proteins. During inflammatory states and increased production of acute-phase proteins the liver reprioritizes protein synthesis, and lowers as a mirror visceral protein synthesis to a degree which correlates with the severity of the injury.

3.1. Serum Albumin

Albumin is the most abundant protein in human serum. It has been used for decades as an indicator of malnutrition in patients in clinically stable conditions (review and meta-analysis [24]). Serum albumin concentrations decrease with increasing age by approx. by 0.1 g/L per year; however, age itself is not a cause of distinct hypoalbuminemia.

There is a clear relationship between serum albumin concentrations and all-cause mortality in elderly subjects [25]. In patients with a hip fracture, albumin levels below 35 g/L were associated with higher rates of post-operative complications such as sepsis and higher overall mortality. Significant loss of muscle mass has been observed in elderly people with low albumin levels. Inflammatory states and in particular, high concentrations of the cytokines IL-6 and TNF-alpha, were two of the main factors causing low levels of serum albumin [24]. Systemic inflammation not only reduces albumin synthesis but increases its degradation and promotes its transcapillary leakage.

Other studies also found this protein to be a good predictor of surgical outcome [26,27]. Compared to nine other risk variables, serum albumin was the strongest predictor. These findings were confirmed in a later study [26], but whether hypoalbuminemia was due to undernutrition or advanced disease was not clarified in these trials.

When serum albumin as a biomarker for the differential diagnosis of unexplained weight loss (involuntary weight loss of more than 5 kg in the previous 6 months) was included in a study from Spain in 306 referred patients, a little more than one-third were ultimately diagnosed with a malignancy. Multivariate analysis found the strongest predictors of a neoplasm were age >80 years, white blood cell count $> 12,000/mm^3$ and serum albumin < 3.5 g/dL [28].

Albumin has been criticized as a player in nutritional assessment due to its lack of specificity and long half-life (approximately 20 days) [29]. Serum albumin concentrations not only decrease during decreased synthesis due to inflammatory cytokines as mentioned above or to hepatic insufficiency, they may also decrease following renal losses in nephrotic syndrome and to losses via the GI tract in protein-losing enteropathies [30].

3.2. Serum Prealbumin

Prealbumin, also named transthyretin, is a transport protein for thyroid hormone and is synthesized by the liver and partly catabolized by the kidneys. Serum prealbumin concentrations less than 10 mg/dL are associated with malnutrition [31].

The use of prealbumin has been advocated as a nutritional marker, particularly during refeeding and in the elderly [32]. The main advantage of prealbumin compared to albumin is its shorter half-life (two to three days) (Table 2), making it a more favorable marker of acute changes of the nutritional state. In addition, prealbumin was not influenced by intestinal protein losses in patients with protein-losing enteropathy [30].

Table 2. Characteristics of serum visceral proteins used as nutritional markers.

Protein	Molecular Weight	Half-Life	Reference Range
Albumin	65,000	20 days	3.30 to 4.80 g per dL
Transferrin	76,000	10 days	0.16 to 0.36 g per dL
Prealbumin	54,980	2 days	16 to 35 mg per dL
Retinol-binding protein	21,000	1/2 day	3–6 mg/dL

Table adapted from Spiekerman AM [33].

Prealbumin levels may be increased in the setting of renal dysfunction, corticosteroid therapy or dehydration, whereas they can be decreased during physiological stress, infection, liver dysfunction, and over-hydration [34].

An algorithm that uses prealbumin has recently been proposed as a practical guide to help the clinician to stratify general medical and intensive care patients by risk of complications and outcome [34]. Prealbumin screening should only performed when an acute inflammatory state (CRP > 15 mg/L) was excluded. A prealbumin level of < 0.11 g/L was associated with increased mortality and length of stay, and an increase by less than 0.04 g/L per week indicated failure of nutritional therapy.

An increase in the C-reactive protein/prealbumin ratio in medical intensive care unit patients has been associated with mortality [35], and a low C-reactive protein/prealbumin ratio in surgical patients predicted the successful closure of gastrointestinal fistulas [36]. Routine measurement of prealbumin has been advocated to be a useful nutritional and prognostic indicator in non-ICU patients without inflammation [34].

Several publications reported a role for prealbumin in predicting prognosis (mostly survival) in various clinical conditions such as gastric cancer [37], lung cancer [38] and cardiovascular diseases [39].

3.3. Albumin and Prealbumin in Starved and Otherwise Healthy Malnourished Subjects

A systematic review assessed the role of albumin and prealbumin in otherwise healthy subjects who were severely nutrient- deprived due to poor access to food or unwillingness to eat, mostly due to anorexia nervosa [40]. The study showed that serum albumin and prealbumin levels were maintained even in the presence of distinct weight loss, and they were lowered only during extreme starvation (BMI < 11 kg/m^2). The authors concluded that serum visceral proteins are not predictive of nutritional deprivation and should not be used to guide nutritional therapy in this group of patients.

3.4. Transferrin

This acute-phase reactant is a transport protein for iron. It has a relatively long half-life (approx. 10 days), and has also been used as a marker of the nutritional status [41] It is influenced by other factors including iron status, liver disease and inflammatory state. Like prealbumin, transferrin levels increase with renal failure [42]. Some authors found transferrin measurements useful for nutritional assessment [43], other did not [44].

During iron-deficiency the levels of transferrin are elevated whereas they are decreased in iron-overload states. Serum transferrin increased in parallel to prealbumin during nutritional intervention in critically ill children [45]. Serum levels decrease in the setting of severe malnutrition, but this marker has been found to be unreliable in the assessment of mild malnutrition and of fat-free mass in a group of elderly Italian patients [46].

3.5. Retinol-Binding Protein (RBP)

This is a low molecular weight protein with the physiological role to transport retinol from the liver to target organs. It represents the visceral protein with the shortest half-life (approx. 12 h) [33]. According to a review [47] it provides similar responses to energy intake to prealbumin, but it is more difficult to measure than the latter and it is influenced by the vitamin A status. For these reasons there RBP measurements have not found widespread application.

4. Laboratory Markers of Malnutrition Other Than Visceral Proteins

4.1. Urinary Creatinine

Creatinine is the end product of creatine which consists of 3 amino acids and is mainly present in muscle. Provided that renal function is intact its excretion reflects creatinine production which in turn is a mirror of skeletal muscle turnover. Each mmol of creatinine in urine is derived from 1.9 kg skeletal muscle [47]. The disadvantages are that it is slowly responding to changes of the nutritional status and that it depends on renal function and requires 24 h urine collections.

4.2. Urinary 3-Methylhistidine

3-methylhistidine is a component of muscle fibers and is not reutilized by the body. Its urinary excretion reflects the amount of fat-free mass and it can be used as a measure of the rate of muscle protein breakdown. It is less dependent on renal function than creatinine; it is often expressed per mmol of urinary creatinine [47]. Both assay of urinary creatinine and 3-methylhistidine have not found widespread use mainly due to the fact that urinary collections are often cumbersome, their excretion may increase after meat intake and they show a relatively poor sensitivity to monitor changes of body protein stores.

4.3. Serum Cholesterol

As can be seen in Table 1, some nutritional screening tools used total serum cholesterol as parameter of malnutrition. Serum cholesterol concentrations show a U-shaped relationship with mortality, and low levels have been associated with increased mortality [48]. However, sensitivity and specificity to monitor malnutrition are low.

4.4. Delayed Hypersensitivity and Blood Lymphocyte Count

The local inflammatory response to a s.c. injection of an antigen is impaired during severe malnutrition. At the same time, maturation of lymphocytes may be reduced in malnourished patients so that total circulating lymphocyte concentration falls to less than 1500/mm^3 (reference range 2000–3500) [47].

These abnormalities can be taken as supporting evidence for protein-energy malnutrition, however, they are not specific and insensitive, and concomitant diseases and a severe stress reaction may also have an effect. Both markers respond slowly to correction of the nutritional status. These reasons limit their use as diagnostic tools for malnutrition.

4.5. Serum Insulin-Like Growth Factor 1 (IGF-1)

IGF-1 (formerly called Somatomedin C) is a ubiquitous growth factor, and the circulating form is mainly produced by the liver. Pituitary growth hormone stimulates its release. Its serum half-life is short (approx. 24 h), and it is largely bound in plasma to binding proteins (mainly IGF BP 3). Fasting lowers plasma IGF-1 levels more than 4 fold and IGF-1 concentrations increases during nutritional repletion. A correlation between energy intake (and less so of protein intake) and plasma IGF-1 concentrations has been reported [49]. IGF-1 levels were a reliable index of protein-energy undernutrition in elderly patients in the recovery period after surgery for hip fracture; however, according to this trial, this marker was also influenced by inflammation [50]. In contrast, IGF-1 levels were not clearly influenced by inflammation in other groups of surgical patients [51,52]. IGF-1 concentrations are altered by liver disease, renal impairment and severe trauma such as burns [47]. Nevertheless, IGF-1 performed better during nutritional rehabilitation to monitor protein and energy status than albumin or transferrin [53]. Drawback of IGF-1 measurements is the fact that their serum concentrations are influenced by other factors such as the acute-phase response. More recently, there has been interest in free IGF-I which holds promise as a nutritional marker (review in [54]. In spite of the earlier positive reports, IFG-1 measurements have not been advocated in more recent publications.

4.6. Serum Leptin

Decreased serum leptin concentrations combined with elevated prothrombin time has been reported in malnourished hospitalized patients with end-stage liver disease [55].

4.7. Serum Nesfatin-1

Nesfatin-1 is an anorexigenic molecule and seems to play a role in appetite regulation and energy homeostasis. Serum nesfatin-1 concentrations have been shown to be increased in chronically malnourished but otherwise healthy children [56].

4.8. Serum Zinc

Zinc is the most abundant trace element in man beside iron; it is present in all body tissues and fluids and is an essential component of many enzymes. Zinc deficiency has been associated with impaired taste and smell, reduced immunity and increased risk of pneumonia [57]. In cases of severe zinc deficiency, skin lesions, anemia, diarrhea, anorexia, decreased lymphocyte function, impaired visual function and mental retardation may be observed. Several psychological functions were impaired in elderly subjects with zinc deficiency [58].

Zinc deficiency is due to low intake of zinc-containing foods such as meat and to decreased absorption caused by intestinal malabsorption [57]. According to a large sample of the TromsØ study, the risk of zinc deficiency was increased 3 fold in subjects at high risk of malnutrition, particularly in men [59]. Assessment of the zinc status carries the problems that only a small fraction of body zinc is circulating, and most serum zinc is bound to albumin. Therefore, albumin deficiency makes interpretation of serum zinc levels difficult. In spite of the widespread functions of zinc in the body and the potential importance replacing zinc in subjects with zinc deficiency, there is little high-quality evidence of the therapeutic benefit of zinc replacement in adult subjects. A randomized controlled trial in children with protein-energy malnutrition and zinc deficiency showed benefits of zinc replacement [60]. It is likely that zinc deficiency in subjects at risk of malnutrition remains often unrecognized.

4.9. Other Essential Micronutrients (Trace Elements and Vitamins)

Laboratory assessment of other trace elements such as iron is not specifically mentioned as part of current nutritional screening tools. This does not mean that in cases with clinical suspicion of micronutrient deficiency this should not be performed. The same can be stated for laboratory screening for vitamin deficiencies, in particular, those of vitamins A, B1, B6, B12, D, and folate.

5. Biomarkers of Nutritional Risk in Some Specific Clinical Conditions

5.1. Geriatric Patients

Dementia: Eating and swallowing problems increase the risk of malnutrition. According to a study from a memory clinic in the Netherlands, about 14% of community-dwelling subjects with newly diagnosed dementia were at risk of malnutrition [61]. These authors pointed out that it is important to detect malnutrition in dementia as early as possible.

In patients with dementia, the nutritional history may only be obtainable by asking family caregivers about appetite and weight change of patients. However, it is unknown whether nutritional information provided by family caregivers are reliable, and therefore biomarkers of malnutrition would be of particular interest.

A recent study compared biochemical blood markers among patients with Alzheimer's disease (AD), dementia with Lewy bodies (DLB), and frontotemporal lobar degeneration (FTLD) [62]. A total of 339 dementia outpatients and their family caregivers participated. Low serum albumin was 7.2 times more prevalent among patients with DLB and 10.1 times more prevalent among those with FTLD than among those with AD, with adjustment for age. The levels of biochemical markers were not significantly correlated with cognitive function. These authors proposed that a multidimensional approach including serological biomarkers such as albumin are needed to assess malnutrition in patients with dementia.

Sarcopenia in the elderly: A clinical investigation performed in elderly persons supported the view that prealbumin levels are useful surrogate indicators of lean body mass (LBM). Compared to serum albumin and RBP, prealbumin showed the highest positive correlation with LBM [46]. In order to improve its predictive potency for sarcopenia the reference values for prealbumin should be adapted to the corresponding age and sex [32]. Ingenbleek proposed that routine screening for protein malnutrition using prealbumin should be performed in elderly subjects [63].

5.2. Chronic Kidney Disease

A position paper from the International Society of Renal Nutrition and Metabolism (ISRNM) stated that serum biomarkers played a particular role in diagnosing malnutrition in patients with kidney failure [64]. Protein-energy wasting can be observed in chronic and in acute kidney disease, and protein-energy wasting is diagnosed according to this publication when low serum biomarkers (albumin, prealbumin, or cholesterol), reduced body mass and reduced muscle mass are present.

Serum prealbumin levels were positively correlated with body cell mass in pre-dialytic kidney patients [65]. Serum biomarkers were part of a new nutritional risk index for predicting mortality in Japanese hemodialysis patients [66]. Cox proportional hazard models indicated that in addition to low BMI, low albumin, low creatinine, and low serum cholesterol predicted independently and significantly mortality within one year.

6. Conclusions

The role played by serum biomarkers in diagnosing or monitoring malnutrition is controversial, particularly in more recent reports. This is explained by their relatively low specificity and by the fact that underlying diseases such as inflammation exert a major influence, particularly on serum visceral proteins. In addition, the role of biomarkers to guide nutritional therapy has not been studied in large randomized controlled trials. A recent randomized controlled multicenter trial in hospitalized patients with malnutrition might fill this gap in the near future [67]. Nevertheless, biomarkers such as prealbumin are valid prognostic indicators of disease outcome and of mortality in patients at risk of malnutrition.

Acknowledgments: The page charges for this article were covered by the Swiss Society for Clinical Nutrition.

Conflicts of Interest: The author declares no conflict of interest.

References

1. Kondrup, J.; Rasmussen, H.H.; Hamberg, O.; Stanga, Z. Nutritional risk screening (NRS 2002): A new method based on an analysis of controlled clinical trials. *Clin. Nutr.* **2003**, *22*, 321–336. [CrossRef]

2. Poulia, K.-A.; Yannakoulia, M.; Karageorgou, D.; Gamaletsou, M.; Panagiotakos, D.B.; Sipsas, N.V.; Zampelas, A. Evaluation of the efficacy of six nutritional screening tools to predict malnutrition in the elderly. *Clin. Nutr.* **2012**, *31*, 378–385. [CrossRef] [PubMed]
3. Mueller, C.; Compher, C.; Ellen, D.M. ASPEN Clinical Guidelines. *J. Parenter. Enter. Nutr.* **2011**, *35*, 16–24. [CrossRef]
4. Jensen, G.L. Malnutrition and Inflammation—"Burning Down the House". *J. Parenter. Enter. Nutr.* **2015**, *39*, 56–62. [CrossRef] [PubMed]
5. Kirkland, L.L.; Kashiwagi, D.T.; Brantley, S.; Scheurer, D.; Varkey, P. Nutrition in the hospitalized patient. *J. Hosp. Med.* **2013**, *8*, 52–58. [CrossRef] [PubMed]
6. Buzby, G.P.; Mullen, J.L.; Matthews, D.C.; Hobbs, C.L.; Rosato, E.F. Prognostic nutritional index in gastrointestinal surgery. *Am. J. Surg.* **1980**, *139*, 160–167. [CrossRef]
7. Ingenbleek, Y.; Carpentier, Y.A. A prognostic inflammatory and nutritional index scoring critically ill patients. *Int. J. Vitam. Nutr. Res.* **1985**, *55*, 91–101.
8. Detsky, A.S.; Baker, J.P.; Johnston, N.; Whittaker, S.; Mendelson, R.A.; Jeejeebhoy, K.N. What is subjective global assessment of nutritional status? *J. Parenter. Enter. Nutr.* **1987**, *11*, 8–13. [CrossRef]
9. Reilly, H.M.; Martineau, J.K.; Moran, A.; Kennedy, H. Nutritional screening—Evaluation and implementation of a simple Nutrition Risk Score. *Clin. Nutr.* **1995**, *14*, 269–273. [CrossRef]
10. Kovacevich, D.S.; Boney, A.R.; Braunschweig, C.L.; Perez, A.; Stevens, M. Nutrition Risk Classification: A Reproducible and Valid Tool for Nurses. *Nutr. Clin. Pract.* **1997**, *12*, 20–25. [CrossRef]
11. Vellas, B.; Guigoz, Y.; Garry, P.J.; Nourhashemi, F.; Bennahum, D.; Lauque, S.; Albarede, J.L. The mini nutritional assessment (MNA) and its use in grading the nutritional state of elderly patients. *Nutrition* **1999**, *15*, 116–122. [CrossRef]
12. Ferguson, M.; Capra, S.; Bauer, J.; Banks, M. Development of a valid and reliable malnutrition screening tool for adult acute hospital patients. *Nutrition* **1999**, *15*, 458–464. [CrossRef]
13. Laporte, M.; Villalon, L.; Thibodeau, J.; Payette, H. Validity and reliability of simple nutrition screening tools adapted to the elderly population in healthcare facilities. *J. Nutr. Health Aging* **2001**, *5*, 292–294. [PubMed]
14. Thorsdottir, I.; Gunnarsdottir, I.; Eriksen, B. Screening Method Evaluated by Nutritional Status Measurements can be Used to Detect Malnourishment in Chronic Obstructive Pulmonary Disease. *J. Am. Diet. Assoc.* **2001**, *101*, 648–654. [CrossRef]
15. Elia, M. The 'MUST' Report. Nutritional Screening for Adults: A Multidisciplinary Responsibility. Development and Use of the 'Malnutrition Universal Screening Tool' (MUST) for Adults. 2003. Available online: https://eprints.soton.ac.uk/362499/ (accessed on 10 March 2019).
16. Kruizenga, H.M.; Van Tulder, M.W.; Seidell, J.C.; Thijs, A.; Ader, H.J.; Van Bokhorst-de van der Schueren, M.A. Effectiveness and cost-effectiveness of early screening and treatment of malnourished patients. *Am. J. Clin. Nutr.* **2005**, *82*, 1082–1089. [CrossRef]
17. De Ulíbarri, J.I.; González-Madroño, A.; De Villar, N.; González, P.; González, B.; Mancha, A.; Rodriguez, F.; Fernández, G. CONUT: A tool for controlling nutritional status. First validation in a hospital population. *Nutr. Hosp.* **2005**, *20*, 38–45.
18. Kuzu, M.A.; Terzioğlu, H.; Genç, V.; Erkek, A.B.; Özban, M.; Sonyürek, P.; Elhan, A.H.; Torun, N. Preoperative Nutritional Risk Assessment in Predicting Postoperative Outcome in Patients Undergoing Major Surgery. *World J. Surg.* **2006**, *30*, 378–390. [CrossRef]
19. The Veterans Affairs Total Parenteral Nutrition Cooperative Study Group. Perioperative Total Parenteral Nutrition in Surgical Patients. Available online: https://www.nejm.org/doi/10.1056/NEJM199108223250801?url_ver=Z39.88-2003&rfr_id=ori%3Arid%3Acrossref.org&rfr_dat=cr_pub%3Dwww.ncbi.nlm.nih.gov (accessed on 10 March 2019).
20. Ng, T.P.; Nyunt, M.S.Z.; Gao, Q.; Wee, S.L.; Yap, P.; Yap, K.B. Elderly Nutritional Indicators for Geriatric Malnutrition Assessment (ENIGMA): Development and validation of a nutritional prognostic index. *Clin. Nutr. ESPEN.* **2017**, *22*, 54–63. [CrossRef]
21. Jensen, G.L.; Mirtallo, J.; Compher, C.; Dhaliwal, R.; Forbes, A.; Grijalba, R.F.; Hardy, G.; Kondrup, J.; Labadarios, D.; Nyulasi, I.; et al. Adult Starvation and Disease-Related Malnutrition. *J. Parenter. Enter. Nutr.* **2010**, *34*, 156–159. [CrossRef]

22. White, J.V.; Guenter, P.; Jensen, G.; Malone, A.; Schofield, M. Consensus Statement: Academy of Nutrition and Dietetics and American Society for Parenteral and Enteral Nutrition. *J. Parenter. Enter. Nutr.* **2012**, *36*, 275–283. [CrossRef]
23. Zhang, Z.; Pereira, S.L.; Luo, M.; Matheson, E.M. Evaluation of Blood Biomarkers Associated with Risk of Malnutrition in Older Adults: A Systematic Review and Meta-Analysis. *Nutrients* **2017**, *9*, 829. [CrossRef]
24. Cabrerizo, S.; Cuadras, D.; Gomez-Busto, F.; Artaza-Artabe, I.; Marín-Ciancas, F.; Malafarina, V. Serum albumin and health in older people: Review and meta analysis. *Maturitas* **2015**, *81*, 17–27. [CrossRef]
25. Corti, M.-C.; Guralnik, J.M.; Salive, M.E.; Sorkin, J.D. Serum Albumin Level and Physical Disability as Predictors of Mortality in Older Persons. *JAMA* **1994**, *272*, 1036–1042. [CrossRef] [PubMed]
26. Kudsk, K.A.; Tolley, E.A.; DeWitt, R.C.; Janu, P.G.; Blackwell, A.P.; Yeary, S.; King, B.K. Preoperative albumin and surgical site identify surgical risk for major postoperative complications. *J. Parenter. Enter. Nutr.* **2003**, *27*, 1–9. [CrossRef]
27. Gibbs, J.; Cull, W.; Henderson, W.; Daley, J.; Hur, K.; Khuri, S.F. Preoperative Serum Albumin Level as a Predictor of Operative Mortality and Morbidity: Results from the National VA Surgical Risk Study. *Arch. Surg.* **1999**, *134*, 36–42. [CrossRef] [PubMed]
28. Hernández, J.L.; Riancho, J.A.; Matorras, P.; González-Macías, J. Clinical evaluation for cancer in patients with involuntary weight loss without specific symptoms. *Am. J. Med.* **2003**, *114*, 631–637. [CrossRef]
29. Levitt, D.G.; Levitt, M.D. Human serum albumin homeostasis: A new look at the roles of synthesis, catabolism, renal and gastrointestinal excretion, and the clinical value of serum albumin measurements. *Int. J. Gen. Med.* **2016**, *9*, 229–255. [CrossRef] [PubMed]
30. Takeda, H.; Ishihama, K.; Fukui, T.; Fujishima, S.; Orii, T.; Nakazawa, Y.; Shu, H.J.; Kawata, S. Significance of rapid turnover proteins in protein-losing gastroenteropathy. *Hepato-Gastroenterology* **2003**, *50*, 1963–1965.
31. Beck, F.K.; Rosenthal, T.C. Prealbumin: A Marker for Nutritional Evaluation. *Am. Fam. Physician* **2002**, *65*, 1575–1580. [PubMed]
32. Ingenbleek, Y. Plasma Transthyretin as a Biomarker of Sarcopenia in Elderly Subjects. *Nutrients* **2019**, *11*, 895. [CrossRef]
33. Spiekerman, A. Nutritional assessment (protein Nutriture). *Anal. Chem.* **1995**, *67*, 429–436. [CrossRef]
34. Dellière, S.; Cynober, L. Is transthyretin a good marker of nutritional status? *Clin. Nutr.* **2017**, *36*, 364–370. [CrossRef] [PubMed]
35. Li, L.; Dai, L.; Wang, X.; Wang, Y.; Zhou, L.; Chen, M.; Wang, H. Predictive value of the C-reactive protein-to-prealbumin ratio in medical ICU patients. *Biomark. Med.* **2017**, *11*, 329–337. [CrossRef]
36. Harriman, S.; Rodych, N.; Hayes, P.; Moser, M.A. The C-reactive protein-to-prealbumin ratio predicts fistula closure. *Am. J. Surg.* **2011**, *202*, 175–178. [CrossRef] [PubMed]
37. Shen, Q.; Liu, W.; Quan, H.; Pan, S.; Li, S.; Zhou, T.; Ouyang, Y.; Xiao, H. Prealbumin and lymphocyte-based prognostic score, a new tool for predicting long-term survival after curative resection of stage II/III gastric cancer. *Br. J. Nutr.* **2018**, *120*, 1359–1369. [CrossRef]
38. Shimura, T.; Shibata, M.; Inoue, T.; Owada-Ozaki, Y.; Yamaura, T.; Muto, S.; Hasegawa, T.; Shio, Y.; Suzuki, H. Prognostic impact of serum transthyretin in patients with non-small cell lung cancer. *Mol. Clin. Oncol.* **2019**, *10*, 597–604. [CrossRef]
39. Wang, W.; Wang, C.-S.; Ren, D.; Li, T.; Yao, H.-C.; Ma, S.-J. Low serum prealbumin levels on admission can independently predict in-hospital adverse cardiac events in patients with acute coronary syndrome. *Medicine* **2018**, *97*, e11740. [CrossRef] [PubMed]
40. Lee, J.L.; Oh, E.S.; Lee, R.W.; Finucane, T.E. Serum Albumin and Prealbumin in Calorically Restricted, Nondiseased Individuals: A Systematic Review. *Am. J. Med.* **2015**, *128*, 1203. [CrossRef]
41. Shetty, P.S.; Jung, R.T.; Watrasiewicz, K.E.; James, W.P. Rapid-turnover transport proteins: AN index of subclinical protein-energy malnutrition. *Lancet* **1979**, *314*, 230–232. [CrossRef]
42. Bharadwaj, S.; Ginoya, S.; Tandon, P.; Gohel, T.D.; Guirguis, J.; Vallabh, H.; Jevenn, A.; Hanouneh, I. Malnutrition: Laboratory markers vs nutritional assessment. *Gastroenterol. Rep.* **2016**, *4*, 272–280. [CrossRef] [PubMed]
43. Fletcher, J.P.; Little, J.M.; Guest, P.K. A Comparison of Serum Transferrin and Serum Prealbumin as Nutritional Parameters. *J. Parenter. Enter. Nutr.* **1987**, *11*, 144–147. [CrossRef]
44. Roza, A.M.; Tuitt, D.; Shizgal, H.M. Transferrin—A Poor Measure of Nutritional Status. *J. Parenter. Enter. Nutr.* **1984**, *8*, 523–528. [CrossRef]

45. Briassoulis, G.; Zavras, N.; Hatzis, T. Malnutrition, nutritional indices, and early enteral feeding in critically ill children. *Nutrition* **2001**, *17*, 548–557. [CrossRef]
46. Sergi, G.; Coin, A.; Enzi, G.; Volpato, S.; Inelmen, E.M.; Buttarello, M.; Peloso, M.; Mulone, S.; Marin, S.; Bonometto, P. Role of visceral proteins in detecting malnutrition in the elderly. *Eur. J. Clin. Nutr.* **2006**, *60*, 203–209. [CrossRef]
47. Shenkin, A.; Cederblad, G.; Elia, M.; Isaksson, B. Laboratory assessment of protein-energy status. *Clin. Chim. Acta.* **1996**, *253*, S5–S9. [CrossRef]
48. Neaton, J.D.; Blackburn, H.; Jacobs, D.; Kuller, L.; Lee, D.-J.; Sherwin, R.; Shih, J.; Stamler, J.; Wentworth, D. Serum Cholesterol Level and Mortality Findings for Men Screened in the Multiple Risk Factor Intervention Trial. *Arch. Intern. Med.* **1992**, *152*, 1490–1500. [CrossRef]
49. Isley, W.L.; Underwood, L.E.; Clemmons, D.R. Dietary components that regulate serum somatomedin-C concentrations in humans. *J. Clin. Investig.* **1983**, *71*, 175–182. [CrossRef]
50. Campillo, B.; Paillaud, E.; Bories, P.N.; Noel, M.; Porquet, D.; Le Parco, J.C. Serum levels of insulin-like growth factor-1 in the three months following surgery for a hip fracture in elderly: Relationship with nutritional status and inflammatory reaction. *Clin. Nutr.* **2000**, *19*, 349–354. [CrossRef]
51. López-Hellin, J.; Baena-Fustegueras, J.A.; Schwartz-Riera, S.; García-Arumí, E. Usefulness of short-lived proteins as nutritional indicators surgical patients. *Clin. Nutr.* **2002**, *21*, 119–125. [CrossRef]
52. Burgess, E.J. Insulin-Like Growth Factor 1: A Valid Nutritional Indicator during Parenteral Feeding of Patients Suffering an Acute Phase Response. *Ann. Clin. Biochem.* **1992**, *29*, 137–144. [CrossRef]
53. Unterman, T.G.; Vazquez, R.M.; Slas, A.J.; Martyn, P.A.; Phillips, L.S. Nutrition and somatomedin. XIII. Usefulness of somatomedin-C in nutritional assessment. *Am. J. Med.* **1985**, *78*, 228–234. [CrossRef]
54. Livingstone, C. Insulin-like growth factor-I (IGF-I) and clinical nutrition. *Clin. Sci.* **2013**, *125*, 265–280. [CrossRef]
55. Rachakonda, V.; Borhani, A.A.; Dunn, M.A.; Andrzejewski, M.; Martin, K.; Behari, J. Serum Leptin Is a Biomarker of Malnutrition in Decompensated Cirrhosis. *PLoS ONE* **2016**, *11*, e0159142. [CrossRef]
56. Acar, S.; Çatlı, G.; Küme, T.; Tuhan, H.; Gürsoy Çalan, Ö.; Demir, K.; Böber, E.; Abaci, A. Increased concentrations of serum nesfatin-1 levels in childhood with idiopathic chronic malnutrition. *Turk. J. Med. Sci.* **2018**, *48*, 378–385.
57. Tuerk, M.; Fazel, N. Zinc deficiency. *Curr. Opin. Gastroenterol.* **2009**, *25*, 136–143. [CrossRef]
58. Marcellini, F.; Giuli, C.; Papa, R.; Gagliardi, C.; Dedoussis, G.; Herbein, G.; Fulop, T.; Monti, D.; Rink, L.; Jajte, J.; et al. Zinc status, psychological and nutritional assessment in old people recruited in five European countries: Zincage study. *Biogerontology* **2006**, *7*, 339–345. [CrossRef]
59. Kvamme, J.-M.; Grønli, O.; Jacobsen, B.K.; Florholmen, J. Risk of malnutrition and zinc deficiency in community-living elderly men and women: The Tromsø Study. *Public Health Nutr.* **2015**, *18*, 1907–1913. [CrossRef]
60. Makonnen, B.; Venter, A.; Joubert, G. A Randomized Controlled Study of the Impact of Dietary Zinc Supplementation in the Management of Children with Protein–Energy Malnutrition in Lesotho. II: Special Investigations. *J. Trop. Pediatr.* **2003**, *49*, 353–360. [CrossRef]
61. Droogsma, E.; Van Asselt, D.Z.B.; Scholzel-Dorenbos, C.J.M.; Van Steijn, J.H.M.; Van Walderveen, P.E.; Van Der Hooft, C.S. Nutritional status of community-dwelling elderly with newly diagnosed Alzheimer's disease: Prevalence of malnutrition and the relation of various factors to nutritional status. *J. Nutr. Health Aging* **2013**, *17*, 606–610. [CrossRef]
62. Koyama, A.; Hashimoto, M.; Tanaka, H.; Fujise, N.; Matsushita, M.; Miyagawa, Y.; Hatada, Y.; Fukuhara, R.; Hasegawa, N.; Todani, S.; et al. Malnutrition in Alzheimer's Disease, Dementia with Lewy Bodies, and Frontotemporal Lobar Degeneration: Comparison Using Serum Albumin, Total Protein, and Hemoglobin Level. *PLoS ONE* **2016**, *11*, e0157053. [CrossRef]
63. Ingenbleek, Y. Why should plasma transthyretin become a routine screening tool in elderly persons? *J. Nutr. Health Aging* **2009**, *13*, 640–642. [CrossRef]
64. Fouque, D.; Kalantar-Zadeh, K.; Kopple, J.; Cano, N.; Chauveau, P.; Cuppari, L.; Franch, H.; Guarnieri, G.; Ikizler, T.A.; Kaysen, G.; et al. A proposed nomenclature and diagnostic criteria for protein–energy wasting in acute and chronic kidney disease. *Kidney Int.* **2008**, *73*, 391–398. [CrossRef]
65. Rymarz, A.; Bartoszewicz, Z.; Szamotulska, K.; Niemczyk, S. The Associations between Body Cell Mass and Nutritional and Inflammatory Markers in Patients with Chronic Kidney Disease and in Subjects Without Kidney Disease. *J. Ren. Nutr.* **2016**, *26*, 87–92. [CrossRef]

66. Kanda, E.; Kato, A.; Masakane, I.; Kanno, Y. A new nutritional risk index for predicting mortality in hemodialysis patients: Nationwide cohort study. *PLoS ONE* **2019**, *14*, e0214524. [CrossRef]
67. Schuetz, P.; Fehr, R.; Baechli, V.; Geiser, M.; Deiss, M.; Gomes, F.; Kutz, A.; Tribolet, P.; Bregenzer, T.; Braun, N.; et al. Individualised Nutritional Support in Medical Inpatients at Nutritional Risk: A Randomised Clinical Trial. *Lancet* **2019**. Available online: http://www.sciencedirect.com/science/article/pii/S0140673618327764 (accessed on 20 May 2019). [CrossRef]

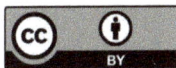

© 2019 by the author. Licensee MDPI, Basel, Switzerland. This article is an open access article distributed under the terms and conditions of the Creative Commons Attribution (CC BY) license (http://creativecommons.org/licenses/by/4.0/).

MDPI
St. Alban-Anlage 66
4052 Basel
Switzerland
Tel. +41 61 683 77 34
Fax +41 61 302 89 18
www.mdpi.com

Journal of Clinical Medicine Editorial Office
E-mail: jcm@mdpi.com
www.mdpi.com/journal/jcm

www.ingramcontent.com/pod-product-compliance
Lightning Source LLC
LaVergne TN
LVHW070123100526
838202LV00016B/2221